OCULAR SURFACE DISORDERS

OCULAR SURFACE DISORDERS

Jose M. Benitez-del-Castillo, MD, PhD
Professor and Chair of Ophthalmology
Department of Ophthalmology
Complutense University
Hospital Clinico San Carlos
Madrid
Spain

Michael A. Lemp, MD
Clinical Professor of Ophthalmology
Georgetown University
Washington, DC
George Washington University
Washington, DC
USA

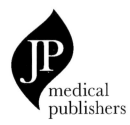

JP medical publishers

London • St Louis • Panama City • New Delhi

© 2013 JP Medical Ltd.
Published by JP Medical Ltd, 83 Victoria Street, London, SW1H 0HW, UK
Tel: +44 (0)20 3170 8910   Fax: +44 (0)20 3008 6180
Email: info@jpmedpub.com   Web: www.jpmedpub.com

The rights of Jose M. Benitez-del-Castillo and Michael A. Lemp to be identified
as editors of this work have been asserted by them in accordance with the
Copyright, Designs and Patents Act 1988.

Medical knowledge and practice change constantly. This book is designed
to provide accurate, authoritative information about the subject matter
in question. However readers are advised to check the most current
information available on procedures included and check information from the
manufacturer of each product to be administered, to verify the recommended
dose, formula, method and duration of administration, adverse effects
and contraindications. It is the responsibility of the practitioner to take all
appropriate safety precautions. Neither the publisher nor the editors assume
any liability for any injury and/or damage to persons or property arising from
or related to use of material in this book.

This book is sold on the understanding that the publisher is not engaged in
providing professional medical services. If such advice or services are required,
the services of a competent medical professional should be sought.

ISBN: 978-19-0781-631-4

British Library Cataloguing in Publication Data
A catalogue record for this book is available from the British Library

Library of Congress Cataloging in Publication Data
A catalog record for this book is available from the Library of Congress

JP Medical Ltd is a subsidiary of Jaypee Brothers Medical Publishers (P) Ltd,
New Delhi, India.

Publisher:	Geoff Greenwood
Development Editor:	Gavin Smith
Design:	Designers Collective Ltd

Typeset, indexed, printed and bound in India.

Preface

Ocular Surface Disorders is a comprehensive and definitive text on the diseases of the ocular surface. A few decades ago, the concept of the ocular surface, the tear film, the corneal and conjunctival epithelium, the lacrymal and Meibomian glands, and the naso-lacrimal ducts as a functional unit was not understood. The surface of the eye is an important and vital component of vision. The smooth, wet surface of the cornea serves as the major refractive surface of the visual system, which, along with corneal transparency, enables light to proceed to the macula. The ocular surface is exposed to the outside world where it is subject to desiccation, injury, and pathogens. A robust interaction between its different components is essential to protect the ocular surface and preserve vision.

This book has been written by a galaxy of eminent international contributors and draws together current knowledge of the epidemiology, clinical expression, pathophysiology and available medical and surgical therapy for ocular surface diseases. The aim of the book is to assist ocular surface specialists, general ophthalmologists, optometrists, and residents to understand the underlying facets of the physiology and pathophysiology of the ocular surface. This will provide a better context for identifying patients at risk of developing ocular surface diseases (mainly dry eye disease, including its two major subtypes, aqueous tear deficiency and evaporative dry eye), for accurately diagnosing patients, assessing disease severity, developing a treatment plan and monitoring the response to therapy.

In summary, this book provides the tools to improve care for patients with ocular surface disorders.

Jose M. Benitez-del-Castillo
Michael A. Lemp

Contents

Contributors

Jorge L. Alio, MD, PhD, FEBO
Professor and Chairman of Ophthalmology
Miguel Hernandez University
Alicante
Vissum Corporation
Spain

Monica Alves, MD, PhD
Professor of Ophthalmology
Department of Ophthalmology
Pontific Catholic University of Campinas
Campinas – SP
Brazil

Brianne Anthony, BS
Clinical Research Manager
Virginia Eye Consultants
Norfolk, Virginia
USA

Pasquale Aragona, MD, PhD
Professor of Ophthalmology
Department of Experimental Medical-Surgical Sciences
Ocular Surface Diseases Unit
University of Messina
Messina
Italy

Cheryl A. Arcinue, MD
Clinical Research Fellow
Massachusetts Eye Research and Surgery Institution (MERSI)
Ocular Immunology and Uveitis Foundation (OIUF)
Cambridge, Massachusetts
USA

Diego M. Aristizabal, MD
Professor of Cornea and Refractive Surgery
Associate Professor of Cornea
University of Antioquia
Clofán Clinic
Medellín, Antioquia
Colombia

Pedro Arriola-Villalobos, MD, PhD
Associate Adjunct Surgeon
Department of Cornea, External Diseases and Uveitis
Hospital Clinico San Carlos
Madrid
Spain

Penny A. Asbell, MD, FACS, MBA
Professor of Ophthalmology
Director of Cornea and Refractive Services
Cornea Fellowship Program Director
Department of Ophthalmology
Icahn School of Medicine at Mount Sinai
New York, New York
USA

Eva Avendaño, MD
Cornea and External Disease Service
Department of Ophthalmology
"La Mancha-Centro" General Hospital
Alcázar de San Juan
Spain

John D. Awad, BS Human Biology
Medical Student
The University of Texas Medical School at Houston
Houston, Texas
USA

Stefano Barabino, MD, PhD
Adjunct Professor of Ocular Surface and Contact Lenses
Ophthalmology Clinic
Department of Neuroscience, Rehabilitation, Ophthalmology, Genetics and Maternal-Child Health Services
University of Genoa
Genoa
Italy

Christophe Baudouin, MD, PhD
Professor of Ophthalmology
Quinze-Vingts National Ophthalmology Hospital
Vision institute, University of Paris 6
Paris
France

Oliver J. Baylis, BMedSci, BM BS, MRCOphth
Department of Ophthalmology
Royal Victoria Infirmary
Institute of Genetic Medicine
Newcastle University
Newcastle-upon-Tyne
UK

Jose Benitez-del-Castillo, MD, PhD
Professor and Chair
Department of Ophthalmology
Complutense University of Madrid
Hospital Clinico San Carlos
Madrid
Spain

Stefano Bonini, MD
Full Professor of Ophthalmology
Department of Ophthalmology
Campus Bio-Medico University of Rome
Rome
Italy

Javier Celis Sánchez, MD
Director of Cornea and External Disease Service
Department of Ophthalmology
"La Mancha-Centro" General Hospital
Alcázar de San Juan
Spain

Richard Chu, DO
Medical Director
Chu Eye Institute
Fort Worth, Texas
USA

J. Richard O. Collin, MA, FRCS, FRCOphth, DO
Professor of Ophthalmology
Moorfields Eye Hospital
London
UK

Ana P. Cotrim, DDS, PhD
Staff Clinician
Sjögren's Syndrome and Salivary Gland Dysfunction
Unit – MPTB
National Institutes of Dental and Craniofacial Research
National Institutes of Health
Bethesda, Maryland
USA

Reza Dana, MD, MSc, MPH
Claes H. Dohlman Professor of Ophthalmology
Vice Chairman and Associate Chief of Ophthalmology
Director of Cornea and Refractive Surgery, Senior
Scientist and W. Clement Stone Scholar
Massachusetts Eye and Ear Infirmary
Harvard Medical School
Department of Ophthalmology
Boston, Massachusetts
USA

David Diaz-Valle, MD, PhD
Associate Professor of Ophthalmology
Complutense University of Madrid
Head of Ocular Surface and Inflammation Department
Hospital Clinico San Carlos
Madrid
Spain

Elío Díez-Feijóo V, MD
Ophthalmologist
The Surgical Clinical Institute of Ophthalmology (ICQO)
Bilbao
Spain

Giovanni DiSandro, Jr., MD
Instructor
Eastern Virginia Medical School
Department of Ophthalmology
Norfolk, Virginia
USA

Serge Doan, MD
Hospital Practitioner Department of Ophthalmology
Bichat Hospital and Adolphe de Rothschild
Ophthalmological Foundation
Paris
France

Murat Dogru, MD, PhD
Visiting Associate Professor
Department of Ophthalmology
Keio University School of Medicine
Tokyo
Japan

Claes H. Dohlman, MD, PhD
Professor of Ophthalmology
Massachusetts Eye and Ear Infirmary
Harvard Medical School
Boston, Massachusetts
USA

Juan A. Durán, MD, PhD
Professor of Ophthalmology
The Surgical Clinical Institute of Ophthalmology (ICQO)
University of the Basque Country
Bilbao
Spain

Daniel Elies, MD
Institute of Ocular Microsurgery (IMO)
Barcelona
Spain

Francisco C. Figueiredo, MD, PhD, FRCOphth
Professor of Ophthalmology
Department of Ophthalmology and Institute of
Genetic Medicine
Newcastle University
Newcastle upon Tyne
UK

Eszter Fodor, MD
Assistant Professor of Ophthalmology
Department of Ophthalmology
Semmelweis University
Budapest
Hungary

C. Stephen Foster, MD, FACS, FACR
Founder and President, Massachusetts Eye Research
and Surgery Institution
Ocular Immunology and Uveitis Foundation
Cambridge, Massachusetts
Clinical Professor of Ophthalmology
Harvard Medical School
Boston, Massachusetts
USA

Eric E. Gabison, MD, PhD
Associate Professor of Ophthalmology
Bichat Hospital and Adolphe de Rothschild
Ophthalmological Foundation
Paris
France

Gerd Geerling, MD
Professor of Ophthalmology, Director and Chair
Department of Ophthalmology
University Hospital Düsseldorf
Heinrich-Heine-University
Düsseldorf
Germany

Georgi As. Georgiev, PhD
Professor in Chemistry of Biointerfaces and
Biomembranes
Model Membranes Laboratory
Department of Biochemistry
St Kliment Ohridski University of Sofia
Sofia
Bulgaria

Fernando Gonzalez del Valle, MD
Chief, Department of Ophthalmology
"La Mancha-Centro" General Hospital
Alcázar de San Juan
Spain

Arturo E. Grau, MD
Ophthalmologist
Cornea, External Disease and Refractive Surgery
Dr Sótero del Río Hospital
Pontifical Catholic University of Chile
Santiago
Chile

Oscar Gris, MD, PhD
Department of Cornea and Refractive Surgery
Institute of Ocular Microsurgery (IMO)
Autonomous University of Barcelona
Barcelona
Spain

Jose Güell, MD, PhD
Cornea, Cataract and Refractive Surgery Specialist
Associate Professor of Ophthalmology
Autonomous University of Barcelona
Director of Cornea and Refractive Surgery Unit
Institute of Ocular Microsurgery (IMO)
Barcelona
Spain

Rocío Herrero-Vanrell, PhD
Professor of Pharmaceutical Technology
Department of Pharmaceutical Technology
Faculty of Pharmacy
Complutense University (UCM)
Madrid
Spain

Thanh Hoang-Xuan, MD
Professor of Ophthalmology
American Hospital of Paris
Neuilly-sur-Seine
France

Maria T. Iradier, MD, PhD
Associate Professor of Ophthalmology
Complutense University of Madrid
Ocular Surface and Inflammation Unit
Hospital Clinico San Carlos
Iradier Eye Clinic
Madrid
Spain

Tetsuya Kawakita, MD
Assistant Professor
Department of Ophthalmology
Keio University School of Medicine
Tokyo
Japan

Nora Khatib, MD
Department of Ophthalmology
University of Maryland Medical Center
Baltimore, Maryland
USA

Takashi Kojima, MD, PhD
Visiting Assistant Professor
Department of Ophthalmology
Keio University School of Medicine
Tokyo
Japan

Friedrich E. Kruse, MD
Professor and Chairman
Department of Ophthalmology
University of Erlangen-Nuremberg
Erlangen
Germany

Alessandro Lambiase, MD, PhD
Associated Professor in Ophthalmology
Department of Ophthalmology
University of Rome Campus Bio-Medico
Rome
Italy

Michael A. Lemp, MD
Clinical Professor of Ophthalmology
Georgetown University
Washington, DC
George Washington University
Washington, DC
USA

Andrea Leonardi, MD
Assistant Professor in Ophthalmology
Department of Neuroscience
Ophthalmology Unit
University of Padua
Padua
Italy

Maria Lopez-Valladares, MD, PhD
Ophthalmology Attending Physician and Surgeon
Cornea and Ocular Surface Unit
Department of Ophthalmology
University Hospital Complex of Santiago de Compostela
University of Santiago de Compostela
Santiago de Compostela
Spain

Miguel J. Maldonado, MD, PhD, FEBO
Director of the Refractive Surgery Unit and Associate
Professor of Ophthalmology
University Institute of Applied Ophthalmology (IOBA)
University of Valladolid
Valladolid
Spain

Felicidad Manero, MD
Institute of Ocular Microsurgery
Barcelona
Spain

Flavio Mantelli, MD, PhD
Ophthalmologist
IRCCS G. B. Bietti Foundation for Study and Research in
Ophthalmology
Rome
Italy

Davi Lazarini Marques
Medical Student
Department of Ophthalmology
Faculty of Medicine of Ribeirao Preto
University of Sao Paulo
Sao Paulo
Brazil

Rosalia Mendez-Fernandez, MD
Ophthalmologist
Ocular Surface and Inflammation Unit
Hospital Clinico San Carlos
Madrid
Spain

Diana Mesa, MD
Cornea and External Disease Service
Department of Ophthalmology
"La Mancha-Centro" General Hospital
Alcázar de San Juan
Spain

Austin K. Mircheff, PhD
Professor of Physiology and Biophysics
Department of Physiology and Biophysics
University of Southern California
Keck School of Medicine
Senior Scientist
Doheny Eye Institute
Los Angeles, California
USA

Merce Morral, MD, PhD
Cornea, Cataract and Refractive Surgery Specialist
Clinical Institute of Ophthalmology
Hospital Clinic of Barcelona
Barcelona
Spain

M. Emilia Mulet, MD, PhD
Ophthalmologist
VISSUM Ophthalmological Institute of Alicante
Miguel Hernandez University
Alicante
Spain

Nambi Nallasamy, MD
Harvard Medical School
Harvard-MIT Division of Health Sciences and Technology
Boston, Massachusetts
USA

Jason J. Nichols, OD, MPH, PhD
University of Houston
College of Optometry
The Ocular Surface Institute
Houston, Texas
USA

Kelly K. Nichols, OD, MPH, PhD, FAAO
FERV Professor (Foundation for Education and Research in Vision)
The Ocular Surface Institute
University of Houston
College of Optometry
Houston, Texas
USA

Terrence P. O'Brien, MD
Professor of Ophthalmology
Charlotte Breyer Rodgers Distinguished Chair
Ocular Microbiology Laboratory
Bascom Palmer Eye Institute
University of Miami
Miller School of Medicine
Miami, Florida
USA

Diana Isabel Pachón Suárez, MD
Research Fellow
Massachusetts Eye Research and Surgery Institution (MERSI)
Cambridge, Massachusetts
USA

Friedrich P. Paulsen, MD
Professor of Anatomy
Department of Anatomy II
Friedrich Alexander University
Erlangen-Nuremberg
Germany

Jay S. Pepose, MD, PhD
Professor of Clinical Ophthalmology and Visual Sciences
Washington University School of Medicine
St. Louis, Missouri
Founder and Director
Pepose Vision Institute
Chesterfield, Missouri
USA

Roswell R. Pfister, MD, fARVO
Clinical Professor of Ophthalmology
University of Alabama
President and CEO
The Eye Research Foundation
Birmingham, Alabama
USA

Heiko Pult, PhD, MSc
Founder, Optometry and Vision Research
CEO Horst Riede GmbH
Weinheim, Germany
Honorary Research Fellow
Cardiff University, School of Optometry and Vision Sciences
Cardiff, UK

Domenico Puzzolo, MD
Professor of Histology Department of Biomedical Sciences and Morphofunctional Imaging,
University of Messina,
Messina
Italy

Mujtaba A. Qazi, MD
Director, Clinical Studies
Pepose Vision Institute
Chesterfield, Missouri
Associate Staff
Washington University School of Medicine
St. Louis, Missouri
USA

Laura Rania, MD, PhD
Assistant Professor of Ophthalmology
Department of Experimental Medical-Surgical Sciences,
Ocular Surface Diseases Unit,
University of Messina,
Messina
Italy

Saaeha Rauz, MBBS, PhD, FRCOphth
Senior Lecturer/Consultant Ophthalmologist
Academic Unit of Ophthalmology and Centre for Translational Inflammation Research
School of Immunity and Infection
College of Medical and Dental Sciences
University of Birmingham
Birmingham
UK

Peter S. Reinach, PhD
Visiting Professor of Ophthalmology
Department of Ophthalmology
Faculty of Medicine of Ribeirao Preto
University of Sao Paulo
Sao Paulo
Brazil

Eduardo M. Rocha, MD, PhD
Associate Professor
Department of Ophthalmology
Faculty of Medicine of Ribeirao Preto
University of Sao Paulo
Sao Paulo
Brazil

Teresa Rodríguez-Ares, MD, PhD
Professor of Ophthalmology
Cornea and Ocular Surface Unit
Department of Ophthalmology
University Hospital Complex of Santiago de Compostela
University of Santiago de Compostela
Santiago de Compostela
Spain

Maurizio Rolando, MD
Professor of Ophthalmology
ISPRE Ophthalmologic, Genoa
Eye Clinic, University of Genoa
Genoa
Italy

Perry Rosenthal, MD
Founder-President, Boston Eye Pain Foundation
Massachusetts Eye and Ear Infirmary
Boston, Massachusetts
USA

Marta Sacchetti, MD, PhD
Ophthalmologist
Cornea and Ocular Surface Unit
San Raffaele Hospital, IRCCS
Milan
Italy

Maite Sainz de la Maza, MD, PhD
Associate Professor of Ophthalmology Clinical Institute
of Ophthalmology
Hospital Clinic of Barcelona
Barcelona
Spain

Borja Salvador Culla, MD
Research Fellow in Ophthalmology
Massachusetts Eye and Ear Infirmary
Harvard Medical School
Boston, Massachusetts
USA

Valerie P. Saw, MBBS(Hons), FRANZCO, PhD
Consultant Ophthalmic Surgeon
Moorfields Eye Hospital NHS Foundation Trust
NIHR Biomedical Research Centre
Moorfields Eye Hospital NHS Foundation Trust and the
UCL Institute of Ophthalmology
London
UK

Stefan Schrader, MD, PhD
Consultant in Ophthalmology
Department of Ophthalmology
University Hospital Düsseldorf
Heinrich-Heine-University
Düsseldorf
Germany

Niraj S. Shah, MD
Ophthalmology Resident
Department of Ophthalmology
Eastern Virginia Medical School
Norfolk, Virginia
USA

Hosam Sheha, MD, PhD
Director of Clinical Research
Ocular Surface Center
Miami, Florida
USA

John D. Sheppard, MD, MMSc
President, Virginia Eye Consultants
Professor of Ophthalmology, Microbiology and
Molecular Biology
Ophthalmology Residency Research Program Director
Clinical Director, Thomas R. Lee Center for Ocular
Pharmacology
Eastern Virginia Medical School
Medical Director, Lion's Eye Bank of the Eastern Shore
Norfolk, Virginia
USA

Hasanain Shikari, MD, DNB
Massachusetts Eye and Ear Infirmary
Harvard Medical School
Department of Ophthalmology
Massachusetts
USA

Frank H.W. Tost, MD, PhD
Professor of Ophthalmology
University Eye Hospital
Ernst Moritz Arndt University
Greifswald
Germany

Rosario Touriño, MD, PhD
Attending Surgeon and Consultant, Cornea and External
Disease
Cornea and Ocular Surface Unit
Department of Ophthalmology
University Hospital Complex of Santiago de Compostela
University of Santiago de Compostela
Santiago de Compostela
Spain

Carlo Enrico Traverso, MD
Professor and Chairman, Ophthalmology Clinic
Department of Neuroscience, Rehabilitation,
Ophthalmology, Genetics and Maternal-Child Health
Services
University of Genoa
Genoa
Italy

Scheffer C. G. Tseng, MD, PhD
Director, Ocular Surface Center
Miami, Florida
USA

Kazuo Tsubota, MD
Professor of Ophthalmology
Department of Ophthalmology
Keio University School of Medicine
Tokyo
Japan

Christiana Valente, MD
Ophthalmologist
Department of Ophthalmology
Santa Croce and Carle Hospital
Cuneo
Italy

David H. Verity, MD, MA, FRCOphth
Consultant Ophthalmic Surgeon
Adnexal Department
Moorfields Eye Hospital
London
UK

David E. Wang
Research Associate
Johns Hopkins University
Maryland
USA

Katherine A. Weibel, OD
Optometrist
University of Houston
College of Optometry
The Ocular Surface Institute
Houston, Texas
USA

Geraint P. Williams, BSc, MBBCh, PhD, FRCOphth
Academic Clinical Lecturer in Ophthalmology
Academic Unit of Ophthalmology and Centre for
Translational Inflammation Research
School of Immunity and Infection
College of Medical and Dental Sciences
University of Birmingham
Birmingham
UK

Richard W. Yee, MD
Clinical Professor of Ophthalmology
The University of Texas Medical School at Houston
Houston, Texas
USA

Samuel C. Yiu, MD, PhD
Associate Professor of Ophthalmology
Department of Ophthalmology
Johns Hopkins University
Wilmer Eye Institute
Baltimore, Maryland
USA

Norihiko Yokoi, MD, PhD
Professor of Ophthalmology
Department of Ophthalmology
Kyoto Prefectural University of Medicine
Kyoto
Japan

Chapter 1

Functional anatomy of ocular surface and tear film and pathophysiological developments in the course of evaporative dry eye

Friedrich P. Paulsen

■ INTRODUCTION

The tear film is central to our visual system. It preserves a smooth surface for light refraction, lubricates the eyelids and the exposed ocular surface (cornea and conjunctiva), supplies nutrients to the cornea, removes foreign materials from the cornea and conjunctiva, and protects the ocular surface against pathogens employing both the innate and adaptive immune systems.

The tear film has traditionally been grasped as a triple-layered structure comprising an inner hydrophilic layer of membrane-bound mucins, which moistens the ocular surface via the main part, a middle aqueous layer, and a thin outer lipid layer, supported by the middle layer, that slows evaporation and functions as a stabilizing component. This model is still regarded as essentially correct, but it has now been realized that the structure is far more dynamic and complex, whereby the components interact in many different ways.

The tear film together with the glands and cells that produce it—lacrimal glands, ocular surface, eyelids, and the sensory and motor nerves connecting these—has been assigned the general term lacrimal functional unit (LFU) (Stern et al. 1998). Disease in or damage to any component of the LFU can destabilize the tear film and lead to dry eye disease (DED), a condition expressed by signs and/or symptoms of ocular irritation, redness, and foreign body sensations. DED afflicts millions of people around the world and is more common in women and the elderly (Gayton 2009).

Although DED may be caused by a deficiency in the aqueous component of tears, it is more commonly associated with hyperevaporation of tears—evaporative dry eye (DEWS 2007; Tong et al. 2010). Meibomian gland dysfunction (MGD), which refers to a diffuse abnormality of the meibomian glands, is considered to be the most common cause of evaporative dry eye (Schaumberg et al. 2011; Tong et al. 2010), but it may also be responsible for inflammatory conditions of the eyelids that do not necessarily manifest as classic DED (Blackie et al. 2010). A knowledge of the basic pathophysiology of the LFU, particularly of its individual structures, is essential in understanding the diagnosis and treatment of DED.

■ ANATOMY OF THE LACRIMAL APPARATUS AND OCULAR SURFACE

The ocular surface and its adnexa comprise the cornea; the conjunctiva with the bulbar, the fornical, and palpebral segments; the main lacrimal gland; the eyelid glands, that is, the meibomian gland; the glands of Moll and accessory lacrimal glands; the nasolacrimal system (also known as nasolacrimal ducts or efferent tear ducts) with the upper and lower puncta; paired lacrimal canaliculi; the lacrimal sac; and nasolacrimal duct. The nasolacrimal ducts collect the tear fluid from the ocular surface and convey it into the nasal cavity (Figure 1.1). All the other structures contribute to formation of the preocular tear film. The term 'lacrimal apparatus' includes the lacrimal gland and the accessory lacrimal glands, which secrete a complex fluid (tears). Its excretory ducts convey fluid to the surface of the eye where the fluid forms part of the tear film. Also the paired lacrimal canaliculi, the lacrimal sac, and the nasolacrimal duct belong to the 'lacrimal apparatus.'

■ Lacrimal gland

The main lacrimal gland is located in the anterior part of the superolateral region of the orbit (Figure 1.2). The levator palpebrae superioris muscle divides it into two parts. The orbital segment is located within the lacrimal fossa on the medial part of the zygomatic process of the frontal bone, just within the orbital margin. The smaller palpebral segment is located inferior to the levator palpebrae superioris in the superolateral segment of the eyelid. In terms of function, the lacrimal gland synthesizes, stores, and secretes a number of different proteins and peptides (>500), water, and electrolytes, which are released as tears onto the surface of the eye as part of the tear film via the excretory duct system. The lacrimal gland is a multilobed, tubuloalveolar, serous-type gland (Figure 1.3a). Discharge from the tubules does not use any characteristic excretory duct system (histological distinction from serous salivary glands) on its way into the interlobular excretory

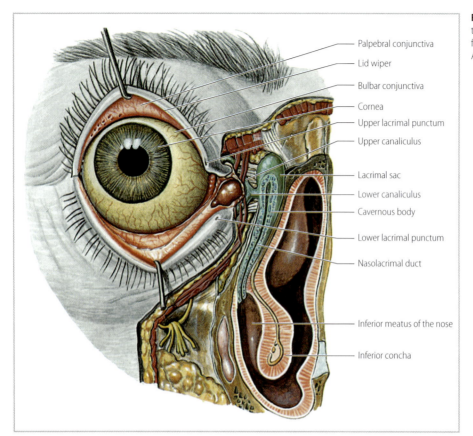

Palpebral conjunctiva
Lid wiper
Bulbar conjunctiva
Cornea
Upper lacrimal punctum
Upper canaliculus
Lacrimal sac
Lower canaliculus
Cavernous body
Lower lacrimal punctum
Nasolacrimal duct
Inferior meatus of the nose
Inferior concha

Figure 1.1 Structures of the ocular surface and the nasolacrimal ducts (redrawn with permission from Paulsen F, Waschke J. (eds). Sobotta – Atlas der Anatomie, 23rd edn. München: Elsevier, 2010).

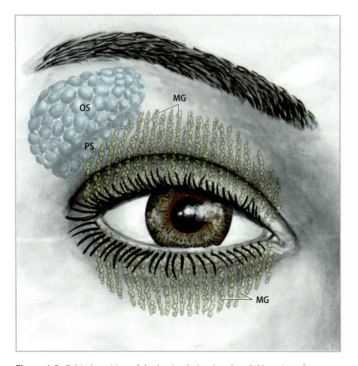

MG
OS
PS
MG

Figure 1.2 Orbital position of the lacrimal gland and eyelid location of meibomian glands. The lacrimal gland is located in the anterior part of the superolateral region of the orbit. The tendon of levator palpebrae superioris muscle divides it into two parts. The orbital segment (OS) is located within the lacrimal fossa on the medial part of the zygomatic process of the frontal bone, just within the orbital margin. The smaller palpebral segment (PS) is located inferior to the levator palpebrae superioris in the superolateral segment of the eyelid. Each tarsal plate contains a row of meibomian glands (MG).

ducts. The human lacrimal gland features 8–10 main excretory ducts (**Figure 1.3b**), which open onto the surface of the eye in front of the lateral portion of the superior conjunctival fornix. The secretory part of the gland is the ring-like acinus, composed of secretory cells—the acinar cells. Since several secretory units open into each secretory duct, the lacrimal gland is said to be 'branched.' Acinar cells comprise about 80% of the mass of the lacrimal gland. The ductal cells of the excretory duct system can modify the secretory product of the acinar cells.

The acinar cells of the lacrimal gland are polarized secretory cells with unidirectional secretion of their protein substances. Receptors for neurotransmitters and neuropeptides are located in the basolateral membrane of the acinar cells. The lacrimal gland is densely innervated (for a review, see Hodges & Dartt 2003) with release of the transmitters and peptides in close proximity to acinar cell membranes. These basolateral membranes also contain several of the transport proteins and ionic channels required for secretion of electrolytes and water (Hodges & Dartt 2003). It has been demonstrated that acinar cells are influenced by various hormones, including androgens and estrogens. Excretory lacrimal gland ducts are lined by one or two layers of cuboidal cells. The cells have been shown to secrete water and electrolytes for the most part, and also show a limited protein secretion potential. The main excretory ducts often contain single or grouped goblet cells forming intraepithelial glands near their transition into the conjunctival fornix. Acinar and ductal cells are basally surrounded by myoepithelial cells. Similar to the salivary glands, the myoepithelial cells are thought to contribute to secretion transport. They express receptors for several neurotransmitters that are known to stimulate acinar cell protein secretion (Hodges et al. 1997; Lemullois et al. 1996).

The lacrimal gland is considered to be an integral part of the ocular mucosal immune system. It contains populations of lymphocytes,

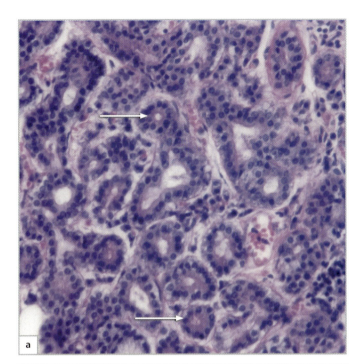

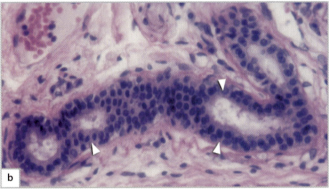

Figure 1.3 Histology of the lacrimal gland. (a) Section through the lacrimal gland showing lacrimal tubuli and acini. The secretory part of the gland is the ring-like acinus (arrows) that is composed of secretory cells, the acinar cells. (b) Section through a main excretory duct that is lined by two rows of excretory duct cells (arrowheads). These are able to modify the secretions. H&E staining.

plasma cells [expressing all immunoglobulins (IgA, IgG, IgE, IgM, IgD)], mast cells, macrophages, and dendritic cells. Of the mononuclear cells, over 50% are plasma cells, and most secrete IgA—a critical component of the ocular mucosal immune system (for a review, see Pflugfelder & Stern 2005; Stern & Pflugfelder 2004).

Ocular surface and eyelids

The ocular surface (**Figure 1.1**) consists of the epithelial cells of the cornea and the conjunctiva. It is nourished and protected by the tears. The corneal epithelium (**Figure 1.4a**) consists of a multicellular layer of non-keratinized, squamous epithelial cells, which is continuous with the epithelium of the bulbar conjunctiva. The bulbar conjunctiva curves in its anterior extension at the fornix to reflect onto the posterior surface of the eyelids as the palpebral conjunctiva. The conjunctiva covering the lid margin and bulbar conjunctiva is a modified non-keratinized, stratified squamous epithelium (**Figure 1.4b**), whereas the palpebral conjunctiva comprises stratified, non-keratinized squamous

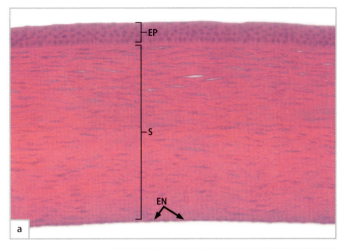

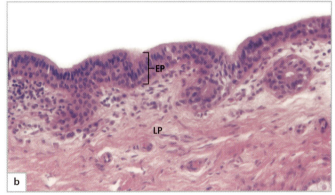

Figure 1.4 Histology of the cornea and conjunctiva. (a) Section through the cornea demonstrating a superficial lining with a multicellular layer of non-keratinized, squamous epithelial cells (EP), stromal layer(S), and one row of endothelial cells (EN). (b) Section through the conjunctiva revealing a modified non-keratinized, stratified squamous epithelium (EP) with an underlying lamina propria (LP) of connective tissue. H&E staining.

epithelium that converts toward the fornix into columnar epithelium. All areas of the conjunctival epithelium contain mucin-secreting goblet cells often arranged in groups to form small intraepithelial mucin-producing glands.

The outer surface of the corneal and conjunctival epithelia is characterized by a specialized interface between the tear fluid and epithelial cells that stabilizes the fluid layer. This interface includes undulating membrane ridges on the apical membrane of the cells, termed microplicae, as well as a polysaccharide matrix known as the glycocalyx. This matrix covers the cell surface including the microplicae and is apparently loosely bound to the mucin layer of the tear film.

The blinking action of the eyelids spreads the tears across the ocular surface (**Figures 1.5a** and **1.5b**), afterward draining the fluid from the eye through two small (about 0.3 mm) openings, the superior and inferior nasal puncta, located on the medial aspect of the upper and lower eyelid margins (**Figure 1.5c**). These open into narrow drainage tubes, the superior and inferior canaliculi, which then join to form the common canaliculus and drain the fluid into the lacrimal sac comprising the widened top portion of the nasolacrimal duct. The upper and lower eyelid margins converge medially at the rounded medial canthus and laterally at the angular lateral canthus to form the boundaries of an adjustable opening in front of the eye, the palpebral opening. The outer (anterior) skin surface of the lid is covered by thin, stratified, keratinized squamous epithelium—the thinnest epidermis

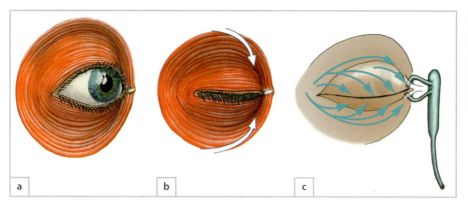

Figure 1.5 Blinking action of the orbicularis eye muscle. (a) Muscle in open eye condition. (b) For the blink the palpebral part of the muscle contracts from temporally to nasally in a time shift. (c) The blinking action of the eyelids spreads the tears across the ocular surface and drains the fluid from the eye through the superior and inferior lacrimal puncta into the efferent tear duct system.

in the body. The posterior surface is lined by the palpebral conjunctiva as mentioned above (**Figure 1.6**).

The mucocutaneous junction (**Figure 1.7**) is the designation of the eyelid margin separating the tear-wettable conjunctival mucous membrane from the oil-wettable marginal skin. It is a transition zone just behind the meibomian gland orifices where keratinized stratified squamous epithelial cells of the eyelid skin abruptly change to non-keratinized epithelial cells of the palpebral conjunctiva toward the fornix (**Figure 1.7**) (for a review, see Knop et al. 2011). This inner border is critically important for ocular surface integrity as it spreads the meibomian gland secretions over the preocular tear film. It is also known as the Marx's line and can be stained with Rose Bengal and other dyes. In younger persons it forms a smooth, continuous line parallel to the posterior lid margin, becoming more irregular in older persons (Norn 1985).

Each eyelid (**Figure 1.6**) is rigidified by an internal plate of dense connective tissue, the tarsus (containing the large aggrecan molecules responsible for the stiffness of the tarsus), as well as muscles and muscular insertions. The orbicularis oculi muscle, responsible for eyelid closure, is located in the middle of the lid, whereas the tendon of the levator palpebral muscle, one of the muscles that raise the upper eyelid, inserts into the tarsus. A superficial projection of Riolan's muscle (part of the orbicularis oculi muscle), known as the gray line, is visible

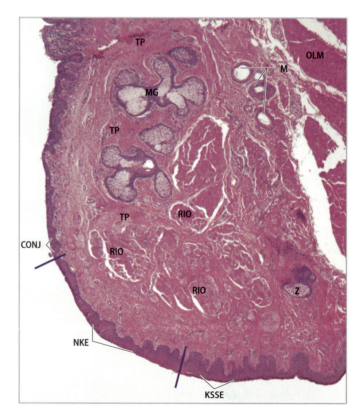

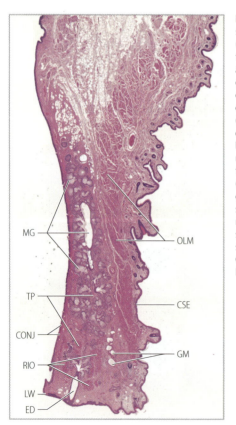

Figure 1.6 Sagittal section through an upper eyelid showing the tarsal plate (TP), acini of a meibomian gland (MG), orbicularis eye muscle (OLM), conjunctival epithelium (CONJ), and epithelium of the outer side of the lid (CSE). Near the lid rim the lower part of the main excretory duct (ED) of a meibomian gland is visible. It is surrounded by Riolan's muscle (RIO). CSE, stratified, keratinized squamous epithelium; GM, glands of Moll; LW, lid wiper. H&E staining.

Figure 1.7 Sagittal section through the so-called area of the lid wiper of an eyelid where a mucocutaneous junction is observed. Two lines demonstrate the areas of epithelial changes at the mucocutaneous junction. It is a transition zone where keratinized stratified squamous epithelial cells of the eyelid skin (KSSE) change abruptly to non-keratinized epithelial cells (NKE) and the mucocutaneous junction between the eyelid margin and the conjunctival mucous membrane (Marx's line). OLM, orbicularis eye muscle; M, glands of Moll; Z, gland of Zeis; RIO, Riolan's muscle; TP, tarsal plate; MG, parts of a meibomian gland. H&E staining.

on the lid margin, dividing it into anterior and posterior portions. Two or three rows of eyelashes are located near the anterior margin of the eyelids. The apocrine or ciliary glands (glands of Moll) (**Figure 1.8a**) open near the eyelashes, whereas sebaceous glands (the glands of Zeiss) are associated with the eyelashes. The lipid component of the tear film is secreted by the meibomian glands opening onto the lid margin (see below). The eyelids also contain small accessory lacrimal glands in the conjunctival fornix (Krause's and Wolfring's glands) that contribute to the aqueous component of the tear film and show a histology (although they are much smaller) that corresponds to that of the main lacrimal glands.

MEIBOMIAN GLANDS

Each tarsal plate contains a row of branched alveolar sebaceous glands (**Figure 1.2**), unrelated to the eyelashes, known as the meibomian glands. The glands are named after Heinrich Meibom (1638–1700), the German physician who first described them in detail. There are approximately 30–40 glands in the upper eyelid and about 25 in the lower lid.

The meibomian glands (a special type of sebaceous glands) are of the holocrine type (secretion involves extrusion of their entire content). Most sebaceous glands are associated with hairs (such as

the glands of Zeiss), but the meibomian glands belong to the small category of free sebaceous glands, which otherwise occur only in the outer auditory meatus, lips, external genitals, and nipples. In a healthy state, these glands secrete a clear, oily fluid known as meibum.

Each gland is composed of clusters of secretory acini (10–15 per gland) arranged in circular form around a long central duct and connected to it by short ductules (**Figure 1.6**). There is typically one ductule for two acini. The final part of the central duct, the excretory duct, opens onto the lid margin just anterior to the mucocutaneous junction. This location, between the hydrophilic mucosa and the lipophilic dermis, ensures that the meibomian lipid is readily transferred to the surface of the tear film during blinking. The luminal diameter of each acinus is about 30–50 mm. The ductules are around 150 mm long, lined by four-layered, non-keratinized basal epithelium (**Figure 1.8b**). They typically enter the long central duct obliquely. The central duct normally has a diameter of 100–150 mm and is also lined with four layers of squamous, non-keratinized epithelium (**Figure 1.8c**). It extends throughout the total length of the gland and the terminal part is encircled by Riolan's muscle fibers. The four-layered, non-keratinized epithelium continues into the excretory duct, gradually increasing from four layers to eight about 0.5 mm internal to the orifice. In a normal, youthful eye, meibomian gland orifices are open and visible as small gray rings on the posterior lid margin when viewed with the

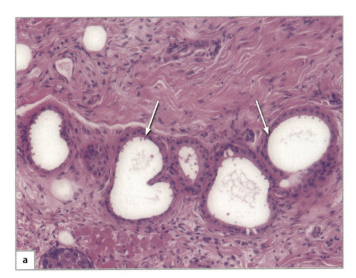

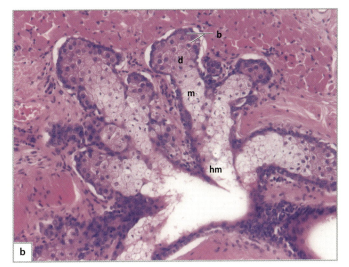

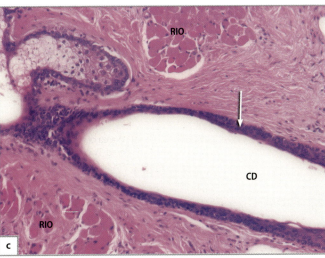

Figure 1.8 Histological sections through a gland of Moll (a) and a meibomian gland (b, c). (a) The figure reveals several sections through one glandular tube (arrows) of a gland of Moll. (b) Section through several acini of a meibomian gland. The acini are completely filled with secretory meibocytes. The meibocytes undergo a maturation process starting as basal (b) cells, then differentiate (d), mature (m), and become finally hypermature (hm). They lead into a ductule that is around 150 μm long and lined by four layers of squamous, non-keratinized epithelium. (c) The ductules typically enter the long central duct (CD) obliquely. Central duct of a meibomian gland normally has a diameter of 100–150 μm and is also lined with four layers of squamous, non-keratinized epithelium (arrow). RIO, Riolan's muscle.

slit lamp (Foulks & Bron 2003; Kozak et al. 2007). The structure of the orifices becomes less apparent in advanced age, while in patients with MGD the gland orifices are often compromised due to stenosis or closure. This loss of architecture is an important clinical sign of MGD.

Little information is available on physiological regulation of the meibomian glands, although parasympathetic, sympathetic, and sensory nerve fibers are all located in the region (Knop et al. 2011; Seifert & Spitznas 1996). Androgen receptors are present, which, if activated, promote lipogenesis and suppress keratinization (Sullivan et al. 2009). It is known that androgen deficiency can result in MGD and evaporative dry eye (Sullivan et al. 2002), and that application of testosterone can improve symptoms in MGD sufferers (Schiffman et al. 2006). Conversely, estrogens have been shown to reduce lipid synthesis (Sullivan et al. 2002) and promote DED (Schaumberg et al. 2001). In addition, use of the antiacne drug isotretinoin, which inhibits androgen-induced stimulation of the sebaceous glands, also leads to deterioration of meibomian gland architecture and promotes MGD (Lambert & Smith 1988; Mathers et al. 1991).

The acini are completely filled with secretory cells known as meibocytes (**Figure 1.8b**). These cells undergo a maturation process, and at the end of this process, they form the meibum through apoptosis. Four stages of meibocyte maturation are recognized: basal, differentiating, maturing, and hypermature. Basal meibocytes are considered to be a type of stem cell; they contain an abundance of smooth endoplasmic reticulum surrounding lipid vesicles. During the maturation process they move along the acinus, the nucleus disappears, and the size of the lipid-containing vesicles increases along with the lipid content, giving the cells a foamy, pale aspect. Finally, the cells undergo apoptosis, leaving behind a lipid mass (the meibum), which is secreted via the ducts.

Transport within the ductule system occurs due to the pressure exerted by the differentiation of new meibocytes and by contraction of the orbicularis eye muscle during eye closure, which causes mechanical tension on the tarsal plate, and is also influenced by the action of Riolan's muscle. The specific function of Riolan's muscle is not yet known but it may prevent secretion of meibum when the eyelids are closed (Lipham et al. 2002). The meibum is supplied to the skin of the lid margin, where it forms shallow reservoirs on the upper and lower lid margins from which the tear film lipid layer is formed and replenished. Studies have shown that, in the blink upstroke, aliquots of lipid may be directly squirted from some glands into the tear film lipid layer (Linton et al. 1961; Yokoi et al. 1999). This indicates that, while the meibomian glands secrete their lipids continuously into the lid reservoirs, delivery also occurs directly into the tear film lipid layer by the force of lid action during blinking. It has been determined that only 45% of adult glands are active at any given time (Norn 1987), suggesting that each gland goes through a cycle of activity followed by a period of quiescence. Forced expression of meibomian glands has shown that the glands on the nasal side are considerably more active than those on the temporal side (Korb & Blackie 2008).

During blink upstroke, lipid spreads from the lower marginal lid reservoir onto the tear film to form the tear film lipid layer, whereby polar lipids and other surfactant components of the tear film lipid layer, such as mucins and surfactant proteins, interact with the aqueous phase of the tear film to reduce surface tension (**Figure 1.9**). Once formed, the tear film lipid layer maintains relative stability from blink to blink until it is abruptly reconstituted by mixing of lipid from both reservoirs with that of the tear film lipid layer—the beginning of a new cycle (Bron et al. 2004).

The composition of meibomian lipids is different from those produced by sebaceous hair follicles. The main types of lipids involved

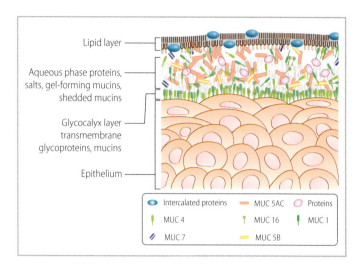

Figure 1.9 Depiction of present understanding of the structure of the tear film showing secreted and membrane-anchored mucins (MUC) together with proteins and lipids.

are non-polar wax esters and sterol esters (60–70%), both of which are highly hydrophobic, although small amounts of other lipids, such as free fatty acids and alcohols, derived from the ester fractions, are also found along with some monoglycerides, diglycerides, and neutral fats (Butovitch et al. 2008; Green-Church et al. 2011; McCulley & Shine 1997; Nicolaides et al. 1981). The wax esters comprise a complex mixture, with oleic acid being the most prominent. Recent studies have reported negligible levels of phospholipids in meibomian secretions (Butovich 2009). Phospholipids have previously been cited as the basis for the interaction between the tear film lipid layer and the aqueous subphase of the tear film required for tear film spread (McCulley & Shine 1997). However, as mentioned above, it is now thought that surfactant proteins and mucins are more important factors in the process. The nature and mixture of the lipids present in meibum give them a melting range of 19–33°C, which means that they are fluid on the tear film. The lipid composition of meibum changes with age and in MGD, while the secretion may also be modified after delivery due to the lipases produced by ocular bacteria (McCulley & Shine 2003). A number of proteins also appear to be produced by the meibomian glands. One of these, psoriasin, is in the S100 calcium-binding protein group (S100A7) and functions mainly as an element of the innate immune defense system. It is produced by the epithelial lining of the excretory ducts. The highest ocular concentration of this protein is found in the meibomian glands, although it is also produced by the cornea and conjunctiva (Garreis et al. 2011). The concentration of psoriasin in the tear fluid is higher than anywhere else in the body. Interestingly, a very recent publication analyzed changes in gene expression in human MGD, revealing multiple changes. The nature of these alterations, including the upregulation of genes encoding small proline-rich proteins and S100 calcium-binding proteins of which group psoriasin is a member, suggests that keratinization plays an important role in the pathogenesis of MGD (Liu et al. 2011).

PREOCULAR TEAR FILM

Aqueous component

The aqueous component of the tear film, comprising primarily water, electrolytes, and tear proteins, is secreted by the main lacrimal gland located in the anterior portion of the superolateral region of the orbit, and by the accessory lacrimal glands (Krause's and Wolfring's glands) located in the eyelids (**Figure 1.9**). Acinar cells (polarized secretory cells) comprise about 80% of the mass of the lacrimal gland.

Mucin component

The mucin component of tears comes from the conjunctival goblet and epithelial cells, corneal epithelial cells, acinar cells, and excretory duct cells of the lacrimal gland and probably also from acinar cells of the accessory lacrimal glands (Jumblatt et al. 2003; Paulsen et al. 2004).

Mucins are high-molecular-weight, heavily glycosylated proteins produced by epithelial tissues. As to their molecular structure, mucins are classed as secreted or cell-surface-associated (also known as membrane-associated) (Hattrup & Gendler 2008; Thornton et al. 2008). Two types of secreted mucins have been identified: large gel-forming mucins and smaller non-polymeric mucins. The corneal and conjunctival epithelia express three cell-surface-associated mucins: MUC1, MUC4, and MUC16 (Gipson et al. 2004; Paulsen & Berry 2006). The main gel-forming mucin found at the ocular surface is MUC5AC. It is expressed by the goblet cells of the conjunctiva, whereas a small non-polymeric mucin, MUC7, as well as a further gel-forming mucin, MUC5B, is expressed by acinar cells of the lacrimal gland (Gipson et al. 2004; Paulsen & Berry 2006). MUC1, MUC4, MUC16, and MUC5AC are the main mucins that have been detected in human tear fluid (Spurr-Michaud et al. 2007).

Trefoil factor family (TFF) peptides, the molecules involved in mucosal maintenance and repair throughout the body, are also intimately associated with the mucin component of tears and have been demonstrated to be synthesized by conjunctival goblet cells (Langer et al. 1999) as well as by corneal epithelial cells under pathological and inflammatory conditions (Paulsen et al. 2008; Steven et al. 2004).

Mucins and TFF peptides perform a number of essential functions that collectively provide protection to the ocular surface. Mucins are present both in the epithelial glycocalyx and in tear fluid. Membrane-anchored mucins are part of the glycocalyx, together with a variety of other polysaccharide-based components, and provide a continuous barrier across the surface of the eye that prevents pathogen penetration. The high-molecular-weight secreted mucins and TFF peptides are responsible for the rheological properties of the tear film, but TFF peptides also have a variety of other physiological functions such as promotion of epithelial cell migration and healing (Hoffmann et al. 2001; Paulsen and Berry 2006). Reduced production of ocular mucins and TFF peptides, resulting in altered tear rheology, is an important factor in the pathogenesis of DED (Paulsen & Berry 2006).

In evaporative dry eye, excessive evaporation of water from the ocular surface leads to tear hyperosmolarity, regarded as the central causal mechanism in ocular surface inflammation and symptoms in all forms of DED (DEWS 2007). In animal models, hyperosmolarity has been shown to stimulate a cascade of inflammatory events in the epithelial surface cells involving the generation of inflammatory cytokines such as IL-1β and TNF-α, and matrix metalloproteinases (Li et al. 2004; Luo et al. 2004). This inflammatory response is interpreted as leading to apoptotic death of surface epithelial cells, including goblet cells (Nelson & Wright 1984; Rivas et al. 1998; Yeh et al. 2003). In fact, goblet cell loss is a feature of every form of DED, and it is, therefore, not surprising that the levels of the gel-forming mucin MUC5AC are reduced in DED (Argüeso et al. 2002; Zhao et al. 2001).

Lipid layer

As stated previously, the lipid layer derives primarily from the meibomian glands situated in the eyelids. It performs many vital functions such as providing a clear optical surface for the cornea, interfering with bacterial colonization, retarding tear overflow, and inhibiting tear evaporation (Bron et al. 2004).

The tear film lipid layer can be observed using interferometry, a technique involving the study of the interference patterns produced when split light beams are reflected back from the surface of the eye. The lipid layer is observed to spread upward during the upstroke of the blink and becomes comparatively stable after ≤1 second (Goto & Tseng 2003; Owens & Phillips 2001). Through interferometry, thinning of the tear film lipid layer has been observed in cases of lipid tear deficiency (Goto & Tseng 2003). In order to explain the ability of the hydrophobic tear film lipid layer to spread over the aqueous component of the tear film, it has been suggested that the tear film lipid layer may contain two phases: a thin polar phase adjacent to the aqueous-mucin phase and a thick non-polar phase associated with both the polar phase and the air interface (McCulley & Shine 1997).

Studies have shown that polar lipids alone cannot lower surface tension to the level found in tears, for which reason it is now thought that proteins and mucins also contribute to the thin inner portion of the tear film lipid layer (Bron et al. 2004; Miano et al. 2005). It has therefore been suggested that the outer layer of the tear film comprises a complex mixture of islands of proteins, islands of lipids, islands of mucins, and various mixtures of these components (Millar et al. 2010) (**Figure 1.9**). In this model, the outer layer is considered to be a non-collapsible, viscoelastic gel, an arrangement permitting the lowest free energy states of the proteins in contact with the lipids. The surfactant-associated proteins SP-B and SP-C, with low molecular weights, are hydrophobic proteins known to lower surface tension in the lung (Whitsett & Weaver 2002). These proteins have also been identified at the ocular surface and in tears (Bräuer & Paulsen 2008) and it has been suggested that they might be embedded into the lipid component of the tear film, orientated according to their amphiphilic character (Bräuer & Paulsen 2008; Millar et al. 2011, Palaniappan et al. 2013).

Nasolacrimal ducts

The upper and lower canaliculus, lacrimal sac, and nasolacrimal duct are subsumed under the terms 'nasolacrimal ducts,' 'efferent tear ducts,' or 'lacrimal passages' (**Figures 1.1** and **1.5**). After birth, the function of the nasolacrimal ducts is to drain tear fluid into the inferior nasal meatus. The nasolacrimal ducts comprise a bony passage and a membranous lacrimal passage (Duke-Elder 1961). The bony passage is formed at the anterior end by the frontal maxillary process and at the posterior end by the lacrimal bone. The membranous lacrimal passages include the lacrimal canaliculi, the lacrimal sac, and the nasolacrimal duct (for reviews, see Paulsen 2003; Paulsen et al. 2003).

The upper and lower canaliculi feature a lining of pseudostratified/stratified columnar epithelium and are surrounded by a dense ring of connective tissue as well as by fibers of Horner's muscle (the lacrimal portion of the orbicularis oculi muscle) (Halben 1904). The lacrimal sac and nasolacrimal duct are lined with a double-layered epithelium comprising a superficial columnar layer and a deep, flattened layer of basal cells (Duke-Elder 1961; Tsuda 1952). The two layers sometimes appear to be a pseudostratified epithelium. The cytoplasm of superficial epithelial cells contains numerous secretory vesicles (Paulsen et al. 1998) and they have been shown to secrete many different antimicrobial proteins and peptides (Paulsen et al. 2001, 2002a). Besides the epithelial cells, goblet cells are integrated in the epithelium as single cells or, more frequently, in a characteristic arrangement forming intraepithelial mucous glands (Paulsen et al. 1998; Werncke 1905). Moreover, kinociliae (motile ciliae) have been described as occurring commonly in some epithelial cells (Radnot 1977; Radnot & Bölcs 1971). However, most epithelial cells are lined with microvilli (for a review, see Paulsen 2003). Rivas et al. (1991) described small serous glands in the lamina propria, particularly in the fundus of the lacrimal sac.

The walls of the lacrimal sac and nasolacrimal duct comprise a helical system of different connective tissue fibers. Wide luminal plexi with specialized blood vessels are embedded in this helical system, which functions as a cavernous body (Ayub et al. 2003; Paulsen et al. 2000a). The vascular system is connected caudally to the cavernous body of the inferior turbinate. Upon lid closure, the system distends and may be 'wrung out' due to its medial attachment and helically arranged fibrillar structures, resulting in distal drainages of tear fluid (Thale et al. 1998). The embedded blood vessels and epithelial layer are under vegetative control. This was evidenced by a high density of nerve fibers and the presence of various neuropeptides (Paulsen et al. 2000b). Regulated via this innervation, the specialized blood vessels control blood flow by the opening and subsidence of the cavernous body, while regulating tear outflow at the same time. Relevant related functions include a role in epiphora in response to emotional stimuli.

The nasolacrimal ducts are integral to the ocular mucosal immune system. There is usually a diffuse infiltrate of variable intensity within the lamina propria consisting mainly of T lymphocytes with scattered CD20- and CD45RA-positive B cells as well as many plasma cells, most of them IgA positive. Aggregated follicles are present in nearly one third of nasolacrimal ducts, fulfilling the criteria for mucosa-associated lymphoid tissue or tear-duct-associated lymphoid tissue (for a review, see Paulsen 2003; Paulsen et al. 2000c, 2002b, 2003).

As a draining and secretory system, the nasolacrimal ducts play a role in tear transport and non-specific immune defenses. Components of tear fluid are also absorbed in the nasolacrimal passage and transported into the surrounding vascular system (Paulsen et al. 2002d).

It has been suggested that tear fluid components are constantly being absorbed into the blood vessels of the surrounding cavernous body under normal conditions. These vessels are connected to the blood vessels of the outer eye and may be involved in a feedback signal for tear fluid production, which is thus stopped in the absence of absorption of these tear components (Paulsen et al. 2003).

MEIBOMIAN GLAND DYSFUNCTION AND EVAPORATIVE DRY EYE

MGD is known to destabilize the tear film and increase tear evaporation. It is also considered to be the key trigger for development of evaporative DED. Risk factors for development of MGD are aging (Den et al. 2006), androgen deficiency, isotretinoin use and possibly postmenopausal estrogen therapy, and wearing contact lenses

(Arita et al. 2009), where loss of lipids and proteins to the contact lens surface may be important.

Evaporative dry eye can also result from a reduced blink rate or an increase in the exposed evaporative surface of the eye such as in proptosis, exophthalmos, high myopia, poor lid apposition or lid deformity, and increased width of the palpebral fissure (Gilbard & Farris 1983, Rolando et al. 1985). Increased ocular surface exposure also occurs in certain gaze positions such as upgaze (Tsubota & Nakamori 1995), and in activities that induce upgaze, such as playing pool.

A reduced blink rate, which extends the period during which the ocular surface is exposed to water loss before the next blink (Tsubota & Nakamori 1995), may occur during the performance of certain tasks involving concentration, for example working at computers, video terminals (Nakamori et al. 1997), watching television, or it may be a feature of an extrapyramidal disorder such as Parkinson's disease (Biousse et al. 2004).

The main cause of MGD appears to be excretory duct obstruction due to hyperkeratinization and an increase in the viscosity of the meibum produced (Knop et al. 2011). This is followed by cystic dilatation of glandular ducts, acinal cell atrophy, and loss of secretory meibocytes. MGD also facilitates bacterial growth on the lid margins—probably because some of the protective proteins secreted by the glands are now absent—and promotes inflammation in the adjacent conjunctiva. Colonizing bacteria have lipases that break down the non-polar wax and sterol esters into triglycerides and free fatty acids (polar lipids), thus changing the normal composition of the meibum (Knop et al. 2011, McCulley & Shine 2003). Studies indicate that in MGD, secretions contain more protein, significantly higher levels of branched-chain fatty acids, and lower levels of saturated fatty acids (Borchman et al. 2010). These changes result in meibum that is less fluid and more viscous, which results in less flow out of the gland orifice and less casual lipid on the lid margin.

Ocular surface damage in the early stages of evaporative dry eye is thought to result in reflex stimulation of the lacrimal gland. There is also a reflex increase in blink rate. These responses, combined with the fact that the lacrimal gland is still functioning normally, initially compensate for tear film hyperosmolarity. Increased tear secretion has been reported in patients with MGD compared to normal persons, although a shorter tear film break-up time, and enhanced fluorescein and Rose Bengal staining was still demonstrated (Shimazaki et al. 1995).

A number of reports indicate impairment of corneal sensitivity in chronic DED (Bourcier et al. 2005, Xu et al. 1995), suggesting that the initial period of increased reflex sensory activity as described above is followed by a chronic period of reduced sensory input. This is thought to result from the effects of inflammatory mediators on sensory nerve terminals supplying the ocular surface (Benitez-del-Castillo et al. 2007). Over the longer term, the initial compensatory response would therefore be expected to diminish and a reduction in aqueous flow has been reported in MGD sufferers in some studies (Goto and Tseng 2003, Tomlinson & Khanal 2005).

ACKNOWLEDGMENTS

Many thanks to Michael Beall for his help with the text and Jörg Pekarsky for drawing Figures 1.2, 1.5 and 1.9.

■ REFERENCES

Argüeso P, Balaram M, Spurr-Michaud S, et al. Decreased levels of the goblet cell mucin MUC 5AC in tears of Sjögren's syndrome patients. *Invest Ophthalmol Vis Sci* 2002; **43**:1004–1011.

Arita R, Itoh K, Inoue K, et al. Contact lens wear is associated with decrease of meibomian glands. *Ophthalmology* 2009; **116**:379–384.

Ayub M, Thale A, Hedderich J, Tillmann B, Paulsen F. The cavernous body of the human efferent tear ducts functions in regulation of tear outflow. *Invest Ophthalmol Vis Sci* 2003; **44**:4900–4907.

Benitez-Del-Castillo JM, Acosta MC, Wassfi MA, et al. Relation between corneal innervation with confocal microscopy and corneal sensitivity with noncontact esthesiometry in patients with dry eye. *Invest Ophthalmol Vis Sci* 2007; **48**:173–181.

Biousse V, Skibell BC, Watts RL, et al. Ophthalmological features of Parkinson's disease. *Neurology* 2004; **27**:177–180.

Blackie CA, Korb DR, Knop E, et al. Nonobvious obstructive meibomian gland dysfunction. *Cornea* 2010; **29**:1333–1345.

Borchman D, Yappert MC, Foulks GN. Changes in human meibum lipid with meibomian gland dysfunction using principal component analysis. *Exp Eye Res* 2010; **91**:246–256.

Bourcier T, Acosta MC, Borderie V, et al. Decreased corneal sensitivity in patients with dry eye. *Invest Ophthalmol Vis Sci* 2005; **46**:2341–2345.

Bräuer L, Paulsen F. Tear film and ocular surfactants. *J Epithel Biol Pharmacol* 2008; **1**:62–67.

Bron AJ, Tiffany JM, Gouveia SM, Yokoi N, Voon LW. Functional aspects of the tear film lipid layer. *Exp Eye Res* 2004; **78**:347–360.

Butovich IA. The meibomian puzzle: combining pieces together. *Prog Retin Eye Res* 2009; **28**:483–498.

Butovitch IA, Millar TJ, Ham BM. Understanding and analysing meibomian lipids: a review. *Curr Eye Res* 2008; **33**:405–420.

Den S, Shimizu K, Ikeda T, et al. Association between meibomian gland changes and aging, sex, or tear function. *Cornea* 2006; **25**:651–656.

DEWS. The definition and classification of dry eye disease: report of the definition and classification subcommittee of the International dry eye workshop. *Ocul Surf* 2007; **5**:75–92.

Duke-Elder S. Trachoma and allied infections. *Trans Ophthalmol Soc UK* 1961; **81**:343–349.

Foulks GN, Bron AJ. Meibomian gland dysfunction: a clinical scheme for description, diagnosis, classification, and grading. *Ocul Surf* 2003; **1**:107–126.

Garreis F, Gottschalt M, Paulsen F. Antimicrobial peptides as a major part of the innate immune defense at the ocular surface. *Dev Ophthalmol* 2010; **45**:16–22.

Garries F, Gottschalt M, Schlorf T, Gläser R, Harder J, Worlitzsch D, Paulsen FP. Expression and regulation of antimicrobial peptide psoriasin (S100A7) at the ocular surface and in the lacrimal apparatus. *Invest Ophthalmol Vis Sci* 2011; **52**:4914–4922.

Gayton JL. Etiology, prevalence, and treatment of dry eye disease. *Clin Ophthalmol* 2009; **3**:405–412.

Gilbard JP, Farris RL. Ocular surface drying and tear film osmolarity in thyroid eye disease. *Acta Ophthalmol* 1983; **61**:108–116.

Gipson IK, Hori, Y, Argüeso P. Character of ocular surface mucins and their alteration in dry eye disease. *Ocul Surf* 2004; **2**:131–148.

Goto E, Tseng SC. Differentiation of lipid tear deficiency dry eye by kinetic analysis of tear interference images. *Arch Ophthalmol* 2003; **121**:173–180.

Green-Church K, Butovich I, Willcox M, et al. Report of the tear film lipids and lipid-protein interactions in health and disease subcommittee of the International Workshop on Meibomian Gland Dysfunction. *Invest Ophthalmol Vis Sci* 2011; **52**:1979–1993.

Halben R. Beiträge zur Anatomie der Tränenwege. Albrecht von Graefe's Arch. *Klin Exp Ophthalmol* 1904; **57**:61–92.

Hattrup CL, Gendler SJ. Structure and function of the cell surface (tethered) mucins. Ann Rev Physiol 2008; 70:431–437.

Hodges RR, Dartt DA. Regulatory pathways in lacrimal gland epithelium. *Int Rev Cytol* 2003; **231**:129–200.

Hodges RR, Zoukhri D, Sergheraert C, Zieske JD, Dartt DA. Identification of vasoactive intestinal peptide receptor subtypes in the lacrimal gland and their signal-transducing components. *Invest Ophthalmol Vis Sci* 1997; **38**:610–619.

Hoffmann W, Jagla W, Wiede A. Molecular medicine of TFF-peptides: from gut to brain. *Histol Histopathol* 2001; **16**:319–334.

Jumblatt MM, McKenzie RW, Steele PS, Emberts CG, Jumblatt JE. MUC7 expression in the human lacrimal gland and conjunctiva. *Cornea* 2003; **22**:41–45.

Knop E, Knop N, Millar T, Obata H, Sullivan DA. The international Workshop on Meibomian gland dysfunction: report of the subcommittee on anatomy, physiology, and pathophysiology of the meibomian gland. *Invest Ophthalmol Vis Sci* 2011; **52**:1938–1978.

Korb DR, Blackie CA. Meibomian gland diagnostic expressibility: correlation with dry eye symptoms and gland location. *Cornea* 2008; **27**:1142–1147.

Kozak I, Bron AJ, Kucharova K, et al. Morphologic and volumetric studies of the meibomian glands in elderly human eyelids. *Cornea* 2007; **26**:610–614.

Lambert RW, Smith RE. Pathogenesis of blepharoconjunctivitis complicating 13-cis-retinoic acid (isotretinoin) therapy in a laboratory model. *Invest Ophthalmol Vis Sci* 1988; **29**:1559–1564.

Langer G, Jagla W, Bebrens-Baumann W, Walter S, Hoffmann W. Secretory peptides TFF1 and TFF3 synthesised in human conjunctival goblet cells. *Invest Ophthalmol Vis Sci* 1999; **40**:2220–2224.

Lemullois M, Rossignol B, Maudit P. Immunolocalization of myoepithelial cells in isolated acini of rat exorbital lacrimal gland: cellular distribution of muscarinic receptors. *Biol Cell* 1996; **86**:175–181.

Li DQ, Chen Z, Song XJ, Luo L, Pflugfelder SC. Stimulation of matrix metalloproteinases by hyperosmolarity via a JNK pathway in human corneal epithelial cells. *Invest Ophthalmol Vis Sci* 2004; **45**:4302–4311.

Linton RG, Curnow DH, Riley WJ. The meibomian glands: an investigation into the secretion and some aspects of the physiology. *Br J Ophthalmol* 1961; **45**:718–723.

Lipham WJ, Tawfik HA, Dutton JJ. A histologic analysis and three-dimensional reconstruction of the muscle of Riolan. *Ophthal Plast Reconstr Surg* 2002; **18**:93–98.

Liu S, Richards SM, Lo K, et al. Changes in gene expression in human meibomian gland dysfunction. *Invest Ophthalmol Vis Sci* 2011; **52**:2727–2740.

Luo L, Doshi A, Farley W, et al. Experimental dry eye stimulates production of inflammatory cytokines and MMP-9 and activates MAPK signalling pathways on the ocular surface. *Invest Ophthalmol Vis Sci* 2004; **45**:4293–4301.

Mathers WD, Shields WJ, Sachdev MS, Petroll WM, Jester JV. Meibomian gland morphology and tear osmolarity: changes with Accutane therapy. *Cornea* 1991; **10**:286–290.

Mcculley JP, Shine W. A compositional based model for the tearfilm lipid layer. *Trans Am Ophthalmol Soc* 1997; **95**:79–88.

Mcculley JP, Shine WE. Meibomian gland function and the tear lipid layer. *Ocul Surf* 2003; **1**:97–106.

Miano F, Calcara M, Millar TJ, Enea V. Insertion of tear proteins into a meibomian lipids film. *Colloids Surf B Biointerfaces* 2005; **44**:49–55.

Millar TJ, Mudgil P, Khanal S. Meibomian glands and lipid layer. In: *Encyclopedia of the Eye, vol. 3. Amsterdam: Elsevier,* 2010:**13**–20.

Nakamori K, Odawara M, Nakajima T, Mizutani T, Tsubota K. Blinking is controlled primarily by ocular surface conditions. *Am J Ophthalmol* 1997; **124**:24–30.

Nelson JD, Wright JC. Conjunctival goblet cell densities in ocular surface disease. *Arch Ophthalmol* 1984; **102**:1049–1051.

Nicolaides N, Kaitaranta JK, Rawdah TN, et al. Meibomian gland studies: comparison of steer and human lipids. *Invest Ophthalmol Vis Sci* 1981; **20**:522–536.

Norn M. Meibomian orifices and Marx's line. Studied by triple vital staining. *Acta Ophthalmol (Copenh)* 1985; **63**:698–700.

Norn M. Expressibility of meibomian secretion. Relation to age, lipid precorneal film, scales, foam, hair and pigmentation. *Acta Ophthalmol (Copenh)* 1987; **65**:137–142.

Owens H, Phillips J. Spreading of tears after a blink: velocity and stabilization time in healthy eyes. *Cornea* 2001; **20**:484–487.

Palaniappan CK, Schütt BS, Bräuer L, Schicht M, Millar TJ. Effects of keratin and lung surfactant proteins on the surface activity of meibomian lipids. *Invest Ophthalmol Vis Sci* 2013; **54**:2571–2581.

Paulsen F. The human nasolacrimal ducts. *Adv Anat Embryol Cell Biol* 2003; **170**:1–106.

Paulsen F, Berry MS. Mucins and TFF peptides of the tear film and lacrimal apparatus. *Prog Histochem Cytochem* 2006; **41**:1–53.

Paulsen F, Hallmann U, Paulsen J, Thale A. Innervation of the cavernous body of the human efferent tear ducts and function in tear outflow mechanism. *J Anat* 2000b; **197**:373–381.

Paulsen F, Hinz M, Schaudig U, et al. TFF peptides in the human efferent tear ducts. *Invest Ophthalmol Vis Sci* 2002c; **43**:3359–3364.

Paulsen F, Langer G, Hoffmann W, Berry M. Human lacrimal gland mucins. *Cell Tissue Res* 2004; **316**:167–177.

Paulsen F, Paulsen J, Thale A, Schaudig U, Tillmann B. Organized mucosa associated lymphoid tissue in human nasolacrimal ducts. *Adv Exp Med Biol* 2002b; **506**:873–876.

Paulsen F, Paulsen J, Thale A, Tillmann B. Mucosa-associated lymphoid tissue (MALT) in the human efferent tear ducts. *Virchows Arch* 2000c; **437**:185–189.

Paulsen F, Pufe T, Schaudig U, et al. Protection of human efferent tear ducts by antimicrobial peptides. *Adv Exp Med Biol* 2002a; **506**:547–553.

Paulsen F, Pufe T, Schaudig U, et al. Detection of natural peptide antibiotics in human nasolacrimal ducts. *Invest Ophthalmol Vis Sci* 2001; **42**:2157–2163.

Paulsen F, Schaudig U, Thale A. Drainage of tears—impact on the ocular surface and lacrimal system. *Ocular Surf* 2003; **1**:180–191.

Paulsen F, Thale A, Hallmann U, Schaudig U, Tillmann B. The cavernous body of the human efferent tear ducts–function in tear outflow mechanism. *Invest Ophthalmol Vis Sci* 2000a; **41**:965–970.

Paulsen F, Thale A, Kohla G, et al. Functional anatomy of human lacrimal duct epithelium. *Anat Embryol (Berl)* 1998; **198**:1–12.

Paulsen F, Thale A, Schaudig U. Ableitende Tränenwege und Trockenes Auge. *Ophthalmologe* 2002d; **99**:566–574.

Paulsen F, Woon CW, Varoga D, et al. Intestinal trefoil factor/TFF3 promotes re-epithelialization of corneal wounds. *J Biol Chem* 2008; **283**:13418–13427.

Pflugfelder SC, Stern ME. Dry eye: inflammation of the lacrimal functional unit. In: Kriegelstein GK, Weinreb RN (eds), Uvetitis and immunological disorders. *Berlin, Heidelberg: Springer,* 2005:11–22.

Radnot M, Bölcs S. Fine structure of the epithelial cell surfaces in the lacrimal sac. *Klin Monatsbl Augenheilkd* 1971; **159**:158–164.

Radnot M. Die Flimmerhaare des Tränensackepithels. *Klin Monatsbl Augenheilkd* 1977; **170**:428–432.

Rivas L, Rodriguez JJ, Murube J. Glandulas seosas en el saco lagrimal. *Arch Soc Esp Oftal* 1991; **60**:173–176.

Rivas L, Toledano A, Alvarez MI, et al. Ultrastructural study of the conjunctiva in patients with keratoconjunctivitis sicca not associated with systemic disorders. *Eur J Ophthalmol* 1998; **8**:131–136.

Rolando M, Refojo MF, Kenyon KR. Tear water evaporation and eye surface diseases. *Ophthalmologica* 1985; **190**:147–149.

Schaumberg DA, Buring JE, Sullivan DA, Dana MR. Hormone replacement therapy and dry eye syndrome. *JAMA* 2001; **286**:2114–2119.

Schaumberg DA, Nichols JJ, Papas EB, et al. The international workshop on meibomian gland dysfunction: report of the subcommittee on the epidemiology of, and associated risk factors for, MGD. *Invest Ophthalmol Vis Sci* 2011; **52**:1994–2005.

Schiffman RM, Bradford R, Bunnell B. A multi-center, double-masked, randomized, vehicle-controlled, parallel group study to evaluate the safety and efficacy of testosterone ophthalmic solution in patients with meibomian gland dysfunction. *Invest Ophthalmol Vis Sci* 2006; **47**:E-abstract 5608.

Seifert P, Spitznas M. Immunocytochemical and ultrastructural evaluation of the distribution of nervous tissue and neuropeptides in the meibomian gland. *Graefes Arch Clin Exp Ophthalmol* 1996; **234**:648–656.

Shimazaki J, Sakata M, Tsubota K. Ocular surface changes and discomfort in patients with meibomian gland dysfunction. *Arch Ophthalmol* 1995; **113**:1266–1270.

Spurr-Michaud S, Argüeso P, Gipson I. Assay of mucins in human tear fluid. *Exp Eye Res* 2007; **84**:939–950.

Stern ME, Beuerman RW, Fox RI, et al. The pathology of dry eye: the interaction between the ocular surface and lacrimal glands. *Cornea* 1998; **17**:584–589.

Stern ME, Pflugfelder SC. Inflammation in dry eye. *Ocular Surf* 2004; **2**:124–130.

Steven P, Schafer G, Nolle B, et al. Distribution of TFF peptides in corneal disease and pterygium. *Peptides* 2004; **25**:819–825.

Sullivan DA, Jensen RV, Suzuki T, Richards SM. Do sex steroids exert sex-specific and/or opposite effects on gene expression in lacrimal and meibomian glands. *Mol Vis* 2009; **15**:1553–1572.

Sullivan DA, Sullivan BD, Evans JE, et al. Androgen deficiency, Meibomian gland dysfunction, and evaporative dry eye. *Ann N Y Acad Sci* 2002; **966**:211–222.

Thale A, Paulsen F, Rochels R, Tillmann B. Functional anatomy of human efferent tear ducts—a new theory of tear outflow. *Graefe´s Arch Clin Exp Ophthalmol* 1998; **236**:674–678.

Thornton DJ, Rousseau K, McGuckin MA. Structure and function of the polymeric mucins in airways mucus. *Ann Rev Physiol* 2008; **70**:459–86.

Tomlinson A, Khanal, S. Assessment of tear film dynamics: quantification approach. *Ocul Surf* 2005; **3**:81–95.

Tong L, Chaurasia SS, Mehta JS, Beuerman RW. Screening for meibomian gland disease: its relation to dry eye subtypes and symptoms in a tertiary referral clinic in Singapore. *Invest Ophthalmol Vis Sci* 2010; **5**:3449–3454.

Tsubota K, Nakamori K. Effects of ocular surface area and blink rate on tear dynamics. *Arch Ophthalmol* 1995; **113**:155–158.

Tsuda K. On the histology of ductulus lacrimalis in adult, especially on its innervation. Tohoku. *J Exp Med* 1952; **56**:233–243.

Werncke T. Ein Beitrag zur Anatomie des Tränensackes, speziell zur Frage der Tränensackdrüsen. *Klin Monatsbl Augenheilkd* 1905; **43**:191–205.

Whitsett JA, Weaver TE. Hydrophobic surfactant proteins in lung function and disease. *N Engl J Med* 2002; **347**:2141–2418.

Xu KP, Yagi Y, Tsubota K. Decrease in corneal sensitivity and change in tear function in dry eye. *Cornea* 1995; **15**:235–239.

Yeh S, Song XJ, Farley W, et al. Apoptosis of ocular surface cells in experimentally induced dry eye. *Invest Ophthalmol Vis Sci* 2003; **44**:124–129.

Yokoi N, Mossa F, Tiffany JM, Bron AJ. Assessment of meibomian gland function in dry eye using meibometry. *Arch Ophthalmol* 1999; **117**:723–729.

Zhao H, Jumblatt JE, Wood TO, Jumblatt MM. Quantification of MUC5AC protein in human tears. *Cornea* 2001; **20**:873–877.

Chapter 2 Classification of ocular surface disease

Friedrich E. Kruse

◼ INTRODUCTION

The integrity of the ocular surface depends on interaction of the cellular components with the tear film. It has been established that the components of the ocular surface (lid margin and meibomian glands, conjunctiva and mucin secreting cells, as well as cornea) act as a functional unit, together with the lacrimal gland and the interconnecting innervation (DEWS 2007, Nichols et al. 2011, Stern et al. 1998, 2004, Tseng & Tsubota 1977). Furthermore, integrity of the ocular surface requires the three major components of the tear film: the lipid phase, the aqueous phase, and the mucin phase. A poorly lubricated ocular surface is vulnerable to environmental challenges and can undergo various pathological changes. Alterations in any of the components of the ocular surface cause disturbances of the entire tear film system, which can lead to pathological changes of the surface.

Although disorders of the tear film are by far the most common reasons for ocular surface disease, both the cells of the cornea and the conjunctiva can become dysfunctional. Thus, ocular surface disease can be due to:

- Disorders of the corneal epithelium
- Disorders of the conjunctival epithelium
  - Conjunctival inflammation
  - Goblet cell dysfunction
- Disorders of the tear film

Since disorders of the tear film will be described in detail in Chapters 3 to 5, we will limit the classification of ocular surface disease to disorders of the corneal and conjunctival epithelium.

◼ DISORDERS OF THE CORNEAL EPITHELIUM

◼ Limbal stem cell deficiency

The corneal epithelium is characterized by a continuous process of cell renewal, which is necessary for the maintenance of a constant mass of corneal epithelial cells. Impairment of the self-renewing capacity of the corneal epithelium results in a specific clinical entity, which is called limbal stem cell deficiency.

◼ Definition of limbal stem cell deficiency

Limbal stem cell deficiency is a disease caused by a decrease in the population and/or function of corneal epithelial progenitor cells that leads to the inability to sustain normal homeostasis of the corneal epithelium. It is primarily characterized by conjunctivalization, which means replacement of normal corneal epithelium by conjunctival epithelium. Other features that may be present are neovascularization,

recurrent or persistent epithelial defects, ocular surface inflammation, and scarring. The usual consequences are decreased vision and an impaired quality of life.

Functional limbal stem cells as a prerequisite for regeneration and repair

Under normal conditions, corneal wounds heal by centripetal movement of neighboring corneal epithelium and closure of epithelial wounds is initially independent of cell division. Subsequent adjustment of the depleted cell mass depends on cell proliferation and differentiation. Proliferation of corneal epithelial cells originates in stem cells with unlimited capacity for cell division. Corneal epithelial stem cells are exclusively located in the basal limbal epithelium and cannot be detected in the peripheral or central epithelium. The hypothesis of limbal stem cells' progenitor role is of importance for both the understanding of corneal surface pathology and the development of therapies aimed for the reconstruction of the abnormal corneal surface. Numerous experimental studies have established that corneal regeneration is only possible in the presence of functional limbal stem cells, and that malfunction of these cells results in typical alterations of the corneal surface.

◼ Pathological features of limbal stem cell deficiency

The most important feature of limbal stem cell deficiency is the presence of goblet cells on the corneal surface. Histology shows an irregular epithelium of variable thickness containing numerous cells that can be stained with Alcian blue or periodic acid-Schiff (PAS). These goblet cells may be present in all parts of the cornea, including the center. The presence of goblet cells is the only certain diagnostic criterion for limbal stem cell deficiency; we think it is mandatory to prove their existence before making a diagnosis. This is particularly important when patients are subjected to any form of stem cell transplantation that requires immunosuppression with the inherent risk of significant side effects. Proof of goblet cells can be obtained either by biopsy or, more elegantly, by non-invasive impression cytology (Puangsricharern & Tseng 1995). Immunohistochemically, both the absence of a cornea-type differentiation (such as the absence of keratin K-3) and the presence of mucin in goblet cells have been shown by monoclonal antibodies (Huang & Tseng 1987, Kenyon 1990). In addition, goblet cells can be seen by confocal microscopy of the corneal surface.

The pathophysiological characteristics of conjunctival epithelium on the corneal surface can explain several of the biomicroscopic features of limbal stem cell deficiency that are visible on slit-lamp investigation. Although the lateral connection of corneal epithelial cells is established by firm tight junctions, the interconnection of conjunctival epithelial cells is relatively loose. This could explain the dull, irregular aspect of the corneal surface. The observation that conjunctival epithelium is more permeable than corneal epithelium explains increased staining with fluorescein in limbal stem cell deficiency, which can be appreciated as delayed fluorescence staining (Dua & Forrester 1990, Dua et al. 1994). Increased permeability may also contribute to the generation of band keratopathy in corneas with limbal deficiency. Loose intercellular contact might favor the influx of leukocytes from the tear film, thus explaining chronic inflammatory changes that are prevalent in many patients with limbal stem cell deficiency. Normal corneal epithelium is attached to the basement membrane by hemidesmosomal structures that are not formed by conjunctival basal cells. This lack of hemidesmosomes might explain the tendency of the patients with limbal stem cell deficiency to develop recurrent epithelial defects. Furthermore, numerous reports have shown that the integrity and function of the corneal stroma depends on a healthy corneal epithelium. On a cellular level, cross-talk between these two cell types is mediated by polypeptide growth factors that are known to govern cellular differentiation (Li & Tseng 1995, You et al. 1999). Each cell type seems to express a unique set of cytokines. Therefore, when the corneal epithelium is replaced by conjunctival cells, the cytokine repertoire in the epithelial compartment is most likely changed. This could, in part, explain stromal pathology such as opacification and haze that might be due to prolonged activation of myofibroblasts. Subepithelial and stromal vascularization is another important histopathological feature of limbal deficiency. As mentioned, the presence of blood vessels seems to be important for the maintenance of the conjunctival phenotype, possibly for supplying retinoids that are crucial for the differentiation of goblet cells. Although it is not known how corneal neovascularization develops, several angiogenic and antiangiogenic growth factors have been identified, and there seems to be some evidence to suggest that the corneal epithelium might contain antiangiogenic factors, whereas the conjunctiva expresses angiogenic factors (Chang et al. 2000). Furthermore, inflammatory cytokines play a major role in corneal angiogenesis. In an experimental setting, limbal deficiency with vascularization of the corneal surface recurred much more frequently in severely inflamed eyes than in eyes with full immunosuppression (Tsai & Tseng 1995).

Diseases associated with limbal stem cell deficiency

Clinical manifestations of limbal stem cell deficiency can be classified according to the extent of severity, as well as origin (Table 2.1).

Partial limbal deficiency is characterized by various degrees of peripheral conjunctivalization while the visual axis is still covered by corneal epithelium. Sequential observation of patients with limbal injuries has established that limbal epithelial wounds heal by circumferential movement of small buds of remaining limbal epithelium (Dua & Forrester 1990). In large defects, these migrating limbal sheets cannot meet; instead, conjunctival epithelium crosses the compromised limbal barrier, resulting in partial limbal stem cell deficiency. Partial limbal deficiency can be found in most patients with large limbal and corneal defects. It has been established that conjunctival epithelium can cross the limbal barrier in such patients and that such areas tend to increase with time (Dua 1998, Dua & Forrester 1990, Dua et al. 1994). Consequently, mechanical scraping of the invading conjunctival epithelium to allow the neighboring limbal epithelium to cover the defect has been suggested (Dua et al. 1994).

Total limbal deficiency is characterized by conjunctivalization of the entire corneal surface. In some patients, the corneal surface can still contain islands of functional corneal epithelium, and the borders between these two cell types may not be clearly demarcated from each other. This mixed phenotype represents a mosaic pattern (Dua 1998). Depending on the cause of the disease, primary limbal deficiency can be differentiated from secondary limbal deficiency. Primary limbal deficiency is characterized by the absence of external factors such as injuries, mechanical damage, or medication. Although rare, three disease entities can be attributed to the loss or functional impairment of stem cells: aniridia, multiple endocrine deficiency, and congenital erythrokeratodermia. The extent of corneal changes in aniridia is highly variable. A subset of patients with aniridia express irregular and hazy epithelium with neovascularization. In such eyes, observation of goblet cells in the corneal epithelium by impression cytology suggests an ingrowth of conjunctival epithelium due to loss of the limbal barrier (Nishida et al. 1995). Two patients with multiple endocrine deficiencies also showed goblet cells on the corneal surface. In congenital erythrokeratodermia, which was initially described by Burns (1915), a clear but irregular corneal epithelium that contains goblet cells is traversed by blood vessels (Kruse et al. 1993). A majority of ocular surface disorders that are caused by the absence or dysfunction of corneal stem cells are of secondary origin. Most importantly, chemical and thermal burns cause damage to limbal epithelium and vasculature. The extent of this damage is the cornerstone of various classifications for prognosis after the acute injury (Hughes 1946a, 1946b, Roper-Hall 1965, Thoft 1979). Increased permeability of the limbal vasculature leads to an influx of leukocytes that can alter cellular proliferation and differentiation (Brown et al. 1969, Hughes 1946a, Matsua & Smelser 1973). In contrast to minor injuries, in which a loss of corneal epithelium is combined with minor limbal damage, larger defects of the limbal circumference cannot heal by sliding of the adjacent healthy limbal epithelium (Dua & Forrester 1990). In partial limbal damage and in severe inflammation, a localized loss of the limbal barrier occurs with invasion of conjunctival epithelium (Dua & Forrester 1990, Faulkner et al. 1981, Mann & Pullinger 1942). Exposure to irradiation can also induce limbal stem cell dysfunction. Depending on the dose and the recovery of limbal stem cells, damage can be either permanent or transient (Fujishima et al. 1996).

Table 2.1 Ocular surface diseases associated with limbal stem cell deficiency

Primary limbal stem cell deficiency
Aniridia
Multiple endocrine deficiency
Erythrokeratodermia
Secondary limbal stem cell deficiency
Chemical burns
Thermal burns
Irradiation
Contact lens
Iatrogenic limbal deficiency
Multiple limbal surgeries
Inflammation
Stevens–Johnson syndrome
Ocular mucous membrane pemphigoid
Postinfection

DISORDERS OF THE CONJUNCTIVAL EPITHELIUM

Inflammation of the conjunctival epithelium

The conjunctiva has a simple histological structure that limits the response to inflammatory stimuli. This explains why different causes for conjunctival inflammation can induce seemingly similar clinical pictures.

Acute conjunctival inflammation (hyperemia, chemosis, and cellular exudate)

Hyperemia due to dilation of blood vessels in response to inflammatory mediators is the most frequent acute response to inflammation. Increased permeability leads to chemosis, secondary to accumulation of fluid in the perivascular space. Increased adhesion of leukocytes to the wall of blood vessels allows for diapedesis and formation of a cellular exudate consisting of leukocytes, plasma cells, lymphocytes, and immunoglobulins. Hyperemia, chemosis, and cellular exudate are non-specific reactions that are found in various forms of conjunctival inflammation.

Membranous and pseudomembranous conjunctivitis

Severe conjunctivitis can lead to the formation of membranes as well as pseudomembranes. True membranes are caused by coagulation of an exudate with a high concentration of fibrin within the epithelium and stroma. Due to the location within the conjunctiva, removal of the membranes with forceps causes bleeding. In contrast, pseudomembranes are caused by coagulation of an exudate that contains fibrin and necrotic conjunctival cells. Pseudomembranes are deposited on the intact surface of an intact conjunctival epithelium and can be removed without bleeding. The most common causes for membranous and pseudomembranous conjunctivitis are listed in **Table 2.2**.

Ulcerative, necrotizing, and hemorrhagic conjunctivitis

During very severe inflammation of the conjunctival epithelium, necrosis can lead to ulcerative changes and exposure of the stroma. Damage of stromal blood vessels may cause significant leukocytic infiltration as well as induces bleeding. The most common forms of ulcerative conjunctivitis are shown in **Table 2.3**.

Follicular conjunctivitis

The formation of follicles by the conjunctiva is an important clinical sign that significantly facilitates the differential diagnosis of conjunctival inflammation. The morphology of conjunctival follicles is characterized by small, oval, or round elevations, that are pale, grayish in color. The outline and direction of blood vessels on the surface of the follicle are important for the diagnosis. Vessels originate in the periphery of the follicle and point toward the center without reaching it. Histology shows lymphoid hyperplasia with secondary vascularization from the periphery of the follicle. In contrast to papillary hypertrophy, in which vessels originate in the center, the epithelium above the follicles is not thinned. Causes of follicular hypertrophy are listed in **Table 2.4**.

Table 2.2 Ocular surface diseases associated with membranes or pseudomembranes

Membranes
Virus
Adenovirus measles
Herpes simplex
Variola
Bacteria
Corynebacterium diphtheriae
Neisseria gonorrhoeae
Pneumococcus
Streptococcus
Pseudomonas aeruginosa
Immunologic disease
Stevens–Johnson syndrome
Toxic epidermal necrolysis (Lyell's syndrome)
Conjunctivitis lignosa
Pseudomembranes
Virus
Adenovirus
Herpes simplex virus
Herpes zoster
Vaccinia
Bacteria
Staphylococcus
Pneumococcus
Meningococcus
Pseudomonas aeruginosa
Escherichia coli
Mycobacterium tuberculosis
Fungi
Candida albicans
Chemical and thermal burn
Immunologic disease
Ocular mucous membrane pemphigoid
Linear IgA disease
Bullous pemphigoid
Epidermolysis bullosa acquisita
Stevens–Johnson syndrome
Toxic epidermal necrolysis

Chronic conjunctival inflammation

Although acute conjunctivitis is generally self-limiting, it may enter a chronic stage. Chronic conjunctivitis is characterized by persistent hyperemia. Increased production of mucus is due to an increase of goblet cells during the early phase of chronic conjunctivitis. The following histopathological changes develop in chronic conjunctivitis.

Table 2.3 Ocular surface disease associated with ulcerative, necrotizing, and hemorrhagic conjunctivitis

Virus
Herpes zoster
Adenovirus
Enterovirus 70
Immunologic disease
Stevens–Johnson syndrome
Toxic epidermal necrolysis (Lyell's syndrome)
Chemicals, physical injury
Chemical or thermal injury
Bacterial toxins
Staphylococcus
Neisseria

Table 2.4 Ocular surface diseases associated with formation of follicles

Infectious
Acute
Virus
Adenovirus
Herpes simplex virus
Newcastle disease
Enterovirus 70
Chlamydia oculogenitalis
Chronic
Chlamydia
C. trachomatis
C. psittacosis
Bacteria
Moraxella
Borrelia burgdorferi
Virus
Epstein–Barr
Measles
Non-infectious
Drug-induced
Iodine-desoxyuridine
Eserine
Atropine
Cosmetics
Immunological reactions
Molluscum contagiosum
Antigens of exogenous origin (plants, animals, chemicals)
Antigens of endogenous origin (measles, rubella)
Uncorrected refractive errors

■ Papillary hypertrophy

Papillary hypertrophy is a result of chronic epithelial and stromal hyperplasia that causes round, hyperemic elevations of the conjunctiva. Vessels originate in the center of the papillae, a sign that serves to differentiate papillary hypertrophy from follicles. Initial changes are characterized by hyperemia and an inflammatory infiltrate in the stroma consisting of lymphocytes, plasma cells, mast cells, and granulocytes. In the chronic state, the conjunctival epithelium is pushed upward by the formation of stromal granulation tissue and fibrosis. The existence of fibrillary bands that reach from subepithelial tissue to the tarsal plate is responsible for the formation of indentations between papillae. The size of papillae is variable and reaches from small hyperemic changes to larger cobblestones and giant papillary changes. The formation of papillary changes is a rather unspecific sign.

■ Subepithelial scarring and formation of symblepharon

Persistent chronic inflammation leads to subepithelial fibrosis and deposition of collagen fibers that appear as faint whitish lines. Chronic inflammation with destruction of the basement membrane and proliferation of the subepithelial tissue can cause significant fibrosis. It results in foreshortening of the fornix and formation of symblepharon. Although symblepharon formation is a non-specific sign of chronic inflammation, its presence is frequently induced by the disease entities listed in **Table 2.5**.

Table 2.5 Ocular surface diseases associated with formation of symblepharon

Immunologic disorders
Ocular mucous membrane pemphigoid
Stevens–Johnson syndrome
Lyell's syndrome (toxic epidermal necrolysis)
Herpetiform dermatitis (Duhring)
Linear IgA disease
Acquired epidermolysis bullosa
Atopic keratoconjunctivitis
Bacteria
Corynebacterium diphtheriae
Borrelia burgdorferi
Chlamydia
Chlamydia trachomatis
Virus
Adenovirus
Herpes zoster
Chemicals, drugs, physical injury
Chemical burn
Thermal burn
Drug-induced pseudopemphigoid

Granulomatous conjunctivitis

Depending on the type of inflammation, the size of conjunctival granulomas can vary from very small lesions, which may be missed upon slit-lamp investigation (e.g. sarcoidosis), to large elevated nodules of yellow-whitish color surrounded by an area of hyperemic conjunctiva. Depending on the underlying pathology, a diffuse type can be differentiated from a zonular type. Diffuse granulomas result from an undirected infiltration of lymphocytes with proliferation of endothelial cells. In contrast, zonular granulomas are characterized by a specific architecture. The causing pathogen (e.g. a foreign body) is located in the center, surrounded by a ring of epitheloid cells and giant cells. The outermost zone of the granuloma is made up of lymphocytes, plasma cells, and eosinophilic granulocytes. The most common forms of conjunctivitis associated with the formation of either diffuse or zonular granuloma are summarized in **Table 2.6**.

Conjunctival inflammation in the context of ocular allergy

Based on the underlying pathomechanism, several forms of chronic conjunctivitis can be classified as related to allergy, as shown in **Table 2.7**.

Perennial and seasonal conjunctivitis are the most frequent forms of ocular allergy. They are characterized by benign pathological changes with mild epithelial hyperplasia and an increase in the number of goblet cells. A scant inflammatory infiltrate is found in the substantia propria consisting of mast cells and esosinophils. The tarsal conjunctiva shows papillary hypertrophy. Upon contact with antigens, a type I hypersensitivity reaction causes the production of antibodies by B-lymphocytes. The increase of IgE and antibodies can be measured in serum and tears (Ballow et al. 1984, Dart et al. 1986). When the conjunctiva encounters new contact, antigens bind to IgE on the surface of mast cells, which leads to degranulation and the release of inflammatory mediators such as histamine, leukotriene, and prostaglandins. These mediators cause both dilation of vessels and secondary tissue damage due to recruitment of additional inflammatory cells. The identification of the role of mast cells and the release of inflammatory mediators has enabled the development of medications for the treatment of seasonal or perennial conjunctivitis, such as mast cell stabilizers and antihistamines.

Atopic conjunctivitis is a chronic disease that is based on several abnormalities of the immune system, such as delayed hypersensitivity responses to pathogens (McGready & Buckley 1975) and defective T-cell function (Foster et al. 1991). Inflammatory mediators induce the expression of class II antigens and cause a pseudoglandular hyperplasia (Roat et al. 1993). The conjunctival changes are characterized by giant papillary conjunctivitis of the lower tarsus, which can lead to linear tarsal scars, fornix foreshortening, and symblepharon. Trantas dots at the limbus are caused by focal accumulations of eosinophils. Corneal changes associated with atopic dermatitis can be severe, and may lead to scarring and vascularization.

Vernal keratoconjunctivitis mimics several clinical features of atopic disease. The immunological changes are caused by type I and IV hypersensitivity reactions. Similar to atopic disease, one of the most important pathophysiological mechanisms is the release of inflammatory mediators such as histamine by degranulating mast cells and eosinophils (Trocme et al. 1989). Plasma cells synthesize IgA, IgG, and IgE in the conjunctiva (Allensmith et al. 1977). A basophilic hypersensitivity reaction is characterized by changes of the vascular endothelium such as hyperplasia, hypertrophy, and necrosis, together with the existence of basophilic granulocytes (Collin & Allensmith 1977). Increased vascular permeability, fibrovascular hypertrophy of subepithelial tissue, and deposition of fibrin lead to the formation of giant papillary changes that are mostly located in the tarsal conjunctiva. In the limbal variant of vernal conjunctivitis, papillae are smaller and inflammatory degenerations of the epithelium cause formation of pseudocysts containing degenerated epithelial cells. The reason might be a possible failure to terminate the production of IgE in response to specific antigens (Rachelefsky et al. 1976). In addition, the conjunctival epithelium and stroma contain focal accumulations of mast cells and eosinophilic granulocytes (Trantas dots). Corneal

Table 2.6 Ocular surface diseases associated with formation of granuloma

Bacteria
Mycobacterium leprae
Mycobacterium tuberculosis
Treponema pallidum
Hemophylus ducreii
Yersinia
Cat scratch disease (Afipia felis, Bartonella henselae)
Listeria
Franciscella tularensis
Rickettsia
Chlamydia
Virus
Epstein–Barr virus
Other infectious organisms
Actinomycosis
Blastomycosis
Sporotrichosis
Leptospirosis
Systemic disease
Sarcoidosis
Wegener's granulomatosis
Allergic granulomas
Parasites
Toxocara canis
Shistosoma
Onchocerca
Caterpillar hairs
Allergic granulomas without detectable antigen
Foreign body granulomas
Organic material
Plants
Insects
Non-organic material
Sutures
Plastics (e.g. stuffed toys)

Table 2.7 Ocular surface diseases associated with allergy

Seasonal conjunctivitis
Perennial conjunctivitis
Atopic keratoconjunctivitis
Vernal keratoconjunctivitis
Giant papillary conjunctivitis
Contact dermatitis

changes include superficial keratitis, formation of (shield) ulcers, and stromal opacities frequently located at the limbus.

Giant papillary conjunctivitis is caused by a multitude of immunological changes that partly resemble those found in vernal or atopic keratoconjunctivitis (Allensmith et al. 1979, 1981, Trocme et al. 1989). Conjunctival changes are often associated with the use of contact lenses, suggesting that components of the plastic material or contents of storage or cleaning solutions might function as immunologic stimuli. Conjunctivitis due to allergic contact dermatitis is based on a type of delayed hypersensitivity reaction.

■ Conjunctival inflammation in the context of collagen vascular disease

The term collagen vascular disease is used to represent a group of systemic disorders characterized by vasculitis and inflammation of connective tissue. Ocular surface disease related to collagen vascular disorder not only involves the conjunctiva, but also causes peripheral ulcerative disease of the cornea with damage to epithelium and stroma. The onset of ocular symptoms is, in most cases, a sign of increased activity of the systemic disease. Since ocular symptoms may precede systemic manifestation, the ophthalmologist is responsible for initiating a systemic workup and should teach the rheumatologist about the association between ocular manifestations and a potentially life-threatening increase in disease activity. The clinical manifestations of ocular surface disease due to different forms of collagen vascular disease are very similar. The differential diagnosis includes the following disorders: rheumatoid arthritis, Wegener's granulomatosis, panarteritis nodosa, systemic lupus erythematosus, and relapsing polychondritis.

Rheumatoid arthritis seems to be based on the presence of a special subset of histocompatibility antigens with possible cross-reactivity to bacterial or viral antigens (Harris 1990, McMichael et al. 1977). Bacterial heat shock proteins can mimic human leukocyte antigens (HLA) antigens and are incriminated in triggering inflammation (Ford & Schulzer 1994). Keratoconjunctivitis sicca or dry eye disease (DED) is the most common manifestation of rheumatoid arthritis and is part of secondary Sjögren's syndrome. Lymphocyte infiltration of the lacrimal gland is associated with acinar atrophy and proliferation of fibroblasts leading to secretory dysfunction (Williamson et al. 1973). The conjunctival epithelium undergoes stratification with subsequent loss of goblet cells and infiltration of T-cells and neutrophilic granulocytes in the ok (Raphael et al. 1988).

Wegener's granulomatosis is characterized by necrotizing granulomas of the respiratory tract, generalized focal necrotizing vasculitis, and glomerulonephritis. Similar to other connective tissue disease, a special HLA configuration is present. Bacterial and viral infections are thought to trigger the disease (Pinching et al. 1980). The detection of antineutrophil cytoplasmic antibodies greatly facilitates the diagnosis of Wegener's granulomatosis (Van der Woude et al. 1985). Ocular manifestations involve eyelids and the orbit, as well as episclera and sclera. Conjunctival inflammation is often associated with scleritis, episcleritis, or peripheral ulcerative disease of the cornea. Yellowish elevated areas of inflammation share similarities with granulomas or giant papillae. The conjunctiva contains inflammatory infiltrates consisting of lymphocytes, plasma cells, giant cells, and neutrophilic, as well as eosinophilic, granulocytes. Histology does not resemble the necrotizing vasculitis, which is characteristic of Wegener's granulomatosis, but shows similarities to pyogenic granulomas or chalazia (Jordan & Addison 1994).

Periarteritis nodosa is a necrotizing vasculitis that affects various organs. Conjunctival involvement is characterized by chemosis, subconjunctival hemorrhage, and yellowish, avascular zones (Purcell et al. 1984). Histology shows signs of vasculitis with fibrinoid necrosis of conjunctival vessels. Characteristically, necrotizing vasculitis can be found adjacent to normal segments of vessels with only moderate hyperplasia of endothelial cells and slight lymphocytic infiltration. Immune complex deposition of IgG and IgM, as well as complement, is found in conjunctival vessels (Purcell et al. 1984).

■ Other forms of conjunctival inflammation

Ligneous conjunctivitis is a rare membranous conjunctivitis primarily affecting infants and adolescents. Most likely based on a familial predisposition, the immune response that is mediated by lymphocytes is characterized by the formation of thick, yellowish membranes on the tarsal conjunctiva consisting of eosinophilic material, mucopolysaccharides, fibrin, and IgG (Eagle et al. 1986, Holland et al. 1989). The conjunctival epithelium is thickened with papillomatous changes and dyskeratosis. The inflammatory infiltrate is composed of lymphocytes (more T-helper cells than suppresser cells), plasma cells, macrophages, and polymorphonuclear granulocytes (Holland et al. 1989). Vessels show thickened walls suggestive of vasculitis (Kosik et al. 1980).

Also of unknown origin, superior limbic keratoconjunctivitis is often bilateral in adults with characteristic Rose Bengal staining of the superior limbus. The pathogenesis might be due to environmental factors, or mechanical irritation. Keratinization, acanthosis, and dyskeratosis of the conjunctival epithelium occur together with alterations of cell nuclei (Theodore & Ferry 1970, Wander & Mukusawa 1981).

Conjunctivitis in floppy eyelid syndrome is characterized by papillary hypertrophy with thickening and partial keratinization of the epithelium. The subepithelial inflammatory infiltrate consists of lymphocytes and plasma cells (Arocker-Mettinger et al. 1986, Culbertson & Ostler 1981).

■ Goblet cell dysfunction

One of the most important functional properties of the conjunctival epithelium is the secretion of glycoproteins, especially mucins. Mucins are secreted by either goblet cells or secretory epithelial cells (Greiner et al. 1985). They are of great importance for the interaction between the ocular surface epithelium and the tear film. Hyposecretion of mucins results from goblet cell deficiency. It is the common denominator of conjunctival scarring in the context of chronic conjunctival inflammation. On the basis of the underlying pathophysiology, goblet cell deficiency can be classified as shown in **Table 2.8**.

Table 2.8 Ocular surface diseases associated with goblet cell deficiency

Malnutrition
Vitamin A deficiency
Oculocutaneous disease
Ocular mucous membrane pemphigoid
Bullous pemphigoid
Linear IgA disease
Dermatitis herpetiformis (Duhring)
Epidermolysis bullosa acquisita
Stevens–Johnson syndrome (Erythema multiforme majus)
Toxic epidermal necrolysis (Lyell syndrome)
Porphyria cutanea tarda
Erythroderma ichthyosiform congenita
Hydroa vacciniforme
Atopic keratoconjunctivitis
Acne rosacea
Drugs
Pseudopemphigoid
Miscellaneous conjunctival inflammation
Sjögren's syndrome
Systemic sclerosis (scleroderma)
Graft-versus-host disease
Inflammatory bowel disease
Reiter's syndrome
Infectious conjunctivitis
Viral conjunctivitis
Adenovirus
Herpes simplex
Varicella zoster
Bacterial conjunctivitis
Borrelia burgdorferi
Corynebacterium diphtheriae
Beta-hemolytic streptococcus Staphylococcus
Treponema pallidum
Chlamydia
Chemical or physical factors
Acid burn
Alkali burn
Thermal burn
Irradiation
Trauma

Goblet cell deficiency due to vitamin A deficiency

Experimental evidence suggests that retinoids are essential for the normal differentiation of goblet cells. Furthermore, in vitro data

suggest that retinoic acid may also be important for the differentiation of limbal progenitor cells of the corneal epithelium (Kruse & Tseng 1994). Systemic vitamin A deficiency due to malnutrition is common in the developing world. In contrast, malabsorption secondary to gastrointestinal and hepatic diseases as well as surgical interventions is the leading cause of vitamin A deficiency in industrialized countries. An early sign of vitamin A deficiency is the reduction of goblet cells that are associated with dull, irregular surface of the conjunctiva due to squamous metaplasia (Pfister & Renner 1978). Histology of whitish, elevated Bitot spots shows loss of epithelial and goblet cells, basophilic intracellular granuloma, as well as keratinization of superficial cell layers (Sommer et al. 1981).

Goblet cell deficiency associated with mucocutaneous disease

Conjunctivitis associated with mucocutaneous disorders is one of the leading causes of goblet cell dysfunction, which develops secondary to cicatricial changes due to cytotoxic (type II and IV) immune reactions.

Cicatricial pemphigoid is a chronic dermatosis characterized by vesiculobullous eruptions of the mucosa (Mondino et al. 1979). The disease process is mediated by various autoantibodies that bind to antigens in the basement membrane zone (Foster 1986, Smith et al. 1993). Immunofluorescence shows a linear pattern of deposition (Leonard et al. 1988). The release of cytokines leads to activation of fibroblasts and scar formation (Bernauer et al. 1993, Foster 1986). The early phase is characterized by subtle subconjunctival fibrosis that leads to a disappearance of the caruncle. The late phase is characterized by fibrosis and keratinization with loss of goblet cells, as well as symblepharon formation in bullous pemphigoid; linear deposition of IgG and complement occurs together with inflammatory infiltrates (Frith et al. 1989).

Pemphigus vulgaris is characterized by subepithelial deposition of autoantibodies. Involvement of the conjunctiva is rare and characterized by hyperemia with mucoid discharge rather than conjunctival scarring (Hodak et al. 1990, Schwab et al. 1992).

Linear IgA disease shows a linear arrangement of antibodies in the basement membrane zone. The histopathology of another chronic bullous, cutaneous disease, dermatitis herpetiformis (Duhring) is characterized by granular deposition of IgA along the basement membrane zone (Chorzelski et al. 1971), Epidermolysis bullosa acquisita is a rare autoimmune mechanobullous disease that is also characterized by linear deposition of IgG and fibrin along basement membranes, as well as by the accumulation of electron-dense amorphous material (Lin et al. 1994, Zierhut et al. 1989).

Erythema multiforme, Stevens–Johnson syndrome, and toxic epidermal necrolysis (Lyell) form another group of diseases with common clinical and pathophysiological characteristics. In contrast to mucocutaneous diseases described above, they are characterized by acute onset of inflammation. The major form of Stevens–Johnson syndrome involves two or more mucosal surfaces together with vesiculobullous skin lesions. Toxic epidermal necrolysis (Lyell) is the most severe form of Stevens–Johnson syndrome, and clinical manifestations may resemble a thermal injury. In both forms, the acute inflammation can change into a chronic conjunctivitis (Foster et al. 1988). Probably based on a specific genetic background, most cases of Stevens–Johnson syndrome seem to be triggered by systemic, and sometimes even topical, medication (Bianchine et al. 1968, Chan et al. 1990, Mondino et al. 1982, Rubin 1977).

Histopathological changes due to a type III hypersensitivity reaction represent an IgA-mediated necrotizing vasculitis with deposition of immune complexes (Wuepper et al. 1980). During the acute phase, a diffuse, non-specific inflammatory response has been described, and pseudomembranous or membranous conjunctivitis occurs. In chronic conjunctivitis, the proliferation of basal conjunctival epithelial cells is increased while the number of goblet cells is continuously decreased, suggesting that goblet cell differentiation might be impaired (Nelson & Wright 1984, Weisman et al. 1992).

Porphyria cutanea tarda is based on an abnormality of the porphyrin-heme metabolism that renders ocular tissues sensitive to photochemical damage causing conjunctival inflammation with the formation of blisters and scarring. Other rare causes of goblet cell deficiency in the context of cicatrizing oculocutaneous disease are erythroderma ichthyosiformis and hydroa vacciniforme.

Drug-induced pseudopemphigoid causes depletion of goblet cells associated with ophthalmic medications, most commonly, preservatives contained in glaucoma medications. Although based on a different mechanism, clinical and histopathological changes are almost indistinguishable from those in cicatricial pemphigoid (Fiore et al. 1987, Hirst et al. 1982, Pouliquen et al. 1986).

Goblet cell deficiency in systemic inflammatory disease

In Sjögren's syndrome, chronic conjunctival inflammation in the context of keratoconjunctivitis sicca results in progressive loss of goblet cells and epithelial stratification (Abdel-Khalek et al. 1978). Scleroderma causes chronic conjunctivitis, which is associated with microangiopathy including teleangiectasia and varicosis. Histopathology is characterized by loss of goblet cells, epithelial thinning, and keratinization together with mild lymphocytic infiltrates (Hogan 1969, West & Barnett 1979). Graft-versus-host disease is a T-cell-mediated reaction of hematopoetic stem cells against host antigens. Conjunctival inflammation can be severe with subconjunctival hemorrhage, ulcerations, and formation of pseudomembranes (Jack et al. 1983). Aqueous tear deficiency is often present leading to severe keratoconjunctivitis sicca (DED) (Jabs et al. 1989, Jack et al. 1983).

DISORDERS OF THE TEAR FILM

Disorders of the tear film are a very common cause of ocular surface disease. The entities that can cause ocular pathology will be described in Chapters 3 to 5.

REFERENCES

Abdel-Khalek LMR, Williamson J, Lee WR. Morphological changes in the human conjunctival epithelium. II. In keratoconjunctivitis sicca. Br J Ophthalmol 1978; 62:800–806.

Allensmith MR, Baird RS, Greiner JV. Vernal conjunctivitis and contact lens-associated giant papillary conjunctivitis compared and contrasted. Am J Ophthalmol 1979; 87:544–555.

Allensmith MR, Baird RS, Greiner JV. Density of goblet cells in vernal conjunctivitis and contact lens-associated giant papillary conjunctivitis. Arch Ophthalmol 1981; 99:884–885.

Allensmith MR, Hahn GS, Simon MA. Tissue, tear and serum IgE concentrations in vernal conjunctivitis. Am J Ophthalmol 1977; 81:506–511.

Arocker-Mettinger E, Haddad R, Konrad K, Steinkogler FJ. Floppy eyelid syndrome. Light and electron microscopic observations. Klin Mbl Augenkeilk 1986; 188:596–598.

Ballow M, Mendelson L, Donshik P, Rooklin A, Rapacz P. Pollen-specific IgG antibodies in the tears of patients with allergic-like conjunctivitis. J Allergy Clin Immunol 1984; 73:376–380.

Bernauer W, Wright P, Dart JK, Leonard JN, Lightman S. The conjunctiva in acute and chronic mucous membrane pemphigoid. An immunohistochemical analysis. Ophthalmology 1993; 100:339–346.

Bianchine JR, Macaraeg PVJ Jr, Lasagna L, et al. Drugs as etiologic factors in the Stevens–Johnson syndrome. Am J Med 1968; 44:390–405.

Brown SI, Wassermann HE, Dunn MW. Alkali burns of the cornea. Arch Ophthalmol 1969; 82:91–94.

Burns FS. A case of generalized congenital keratodermia. J Cutan Dis 1915; 33:255–261.

Chan HL, Stern RS, Arndt KA, et al. The incidence of erythema multiforme, Stevens–Johnson syndrome, and toxic epidermal necrolysis. A population-based study with particular reference to reactions caused by drugs among outpatients. Arch Dermatol 1990; 126:43–47.

Chang JH, Azar DT, Hernandez-Quintela HC, et al. Characterization of angiostatin in the mouse cornea. Invest Ophthalmol Vis Sci 2000; 41:S832.

Chorzelski TP, Beutner EH, Jablonska S, Blaszcyk M, Tviftshauser C. Immunofluorescence studies in the diagnosis of dermatitis herpetiformis and its differentiation from bullous pemphigoid. J Invest Dermatol 1971; 65:373–380.

Collin HB, Allensmith MA. Basophils in vernal conjunctivitis in humans: an electron microscopic study. Invest Ophthalmol Vis Sci 1977; 16:858–864.

Culbertson W, Ostler JB. The floppy eyelid syndrome. Am J Ophthalmol 1981; 92:568–575.

Dart JKG, Buckley RJ, Monnickendan P, Prasad J. Perennial allergic conjunctivitis: definition, clinical characteristics and prevalence. A comparison with seasonal allergic conjunctivitis. Trans Ophthalmol Sco UK 1986; 105:513–520.

DEWS. The definition and classification of dry eye disease: report of the Definition and Classification Subcommittee of the International Dry Eye WorkShop (2007). Ocul Surf 2007; 5:75–92.

Dua HS. The conjunctiva in corneal epithelial wound healing. Br J Ophthalmol 1998; 82:1407–1411.

Dua HS, Forrester JV. The corneoscleral limbus in human corneal wound healing. Am J Ophthalmol 1990; 110:646–656.

Dua HS, Gomes JA, Singh A. Corneal epithelial wound healing. Br J Ophthalmol 1994; 78:401–408.

Eagle RC, Brooks JSJ, Katowitz JA, Weinberg JC, Perry HC. Fibrin is a major constituent of ligneous conjunctivitis. Am J Ophthalmol 1986; 101:493–504.

Faulkner WJ, Kenyon KR, Rowsey JJ, et al. Chemical burns of the human ocular surface: clinicopathological studies in 14 cases. Invest Ophthalmol Vis Sci 1981; 20:S8.

Fiore PM, Jacobs IH, Goldberg DH. Drug induced ocular pemphigoid. A spectrum of diseases. Arch Ophthalmol 1987; 105:1660–1663.

Ford DK, Schulzer M. Synovial lymphocytes indicate "bacterial" antigens may cause some cases of rheumatoid arthritis. J Rheum 1994; 21:1447–1449.

Foster CS. Cicatricial pemphigoid. Trans Am Ophthalmol Soc 1986; 84:527–663.

Foster CS, Fong LP, Azar D, Kenyon KR. Episodic conjunctival inflammation after Stevens–Johnson syndrome. Ophthalmology 1988; 95:453–462.

Foster CS, Rice BA, Dutt JE. Immunopathology of atopic keratoconjunctivitis. Ophthalmology 1991; 98:1190–1196.

Frith PA, Venning VA, Wojnarowska F, Millard PR, Bron AJ. Conjunctival involvement in cicatricial and bullous pemphigoid: a clinical and immunopathological study. Br J Ophthalmol 1989; 73:52–56.

Fujishima H, Shimazaki J, Tsubota K. Temporary corneal stem cell dysfunction after radiation therapy. Br J Ophthalmol 1996; 80:911–914.

Greiner JV, Weidman TA, Korb DR, Allansmith MR. Histochemical analysis of secretory vesicles in nongoblet conjunctival epithelial cells. Acta Ophthalmol (Copenh) 1985; 63:89–92.

Harris ED Jr. Mechanism of disease: rheumatoid arthritis—pathophysiology and implications for therapy. N Engl J Med 1990; 322:1277–1289.

Hirst LW, Werblin T, Nowak M. Drug induced cicatrizing conjunctivitis simulating ocular pemphigoid. *Cornea* 1982; **1**:121–128.

Hodak E, Kremer I, David M, et al. Conjunctival involvement in pemphigus vulgaris: a clinical, histopathologic and immunofluorescence study. *Br J Dermatol* 1990; **123**:615–620.

Hogan EC. Ophthalmic manifestations of progressive systemic sclerosis. *Br J Ophthalmol* 1969; **53**:388–392.

Holland EJ, Chan CC, Kuwabara T, et al. Immunohistologic findings and results of treatment with cyclosporine in ligneous conjunctivitis. *Am J Ophthalmol* 1989; **107**:160–166.

Huang AJW, Tseng SCG. Development of monoclonal antibodies to rabbit ocular mucin. *Invest Ophthalmol Vis Sci* 1987; **28**:1483–1491.

Hughes WR Jr. Alkali burns of the eye. I. Review of the literature and summary of the present knowledge. *Arch Ophthalmol* 1946a; **35**:423.

Hughes WR Jr. Alkali burns of the eye. II. Clinical and pathologic course. *Arch Ophthalmol* 1946b; **36**:189–214.

Jabs DA, Wingard J, Green WR, et al. The eye in bone marrow transplantation. III. Conjunctival graft-vs-host disease. *Arch Ophthalmol* 1989; **107**:1343–1348.

Jack MK, Jack GM, Sale GE, Shulman HM, Sullivan KM. Ocular manifestation of graft versus host disease. *Arch Ophthalmol* 1983; **103**:1080–1084.

Jordan DR, Addison DJ. Wegener's granulomatosis. Eyelid and conjunctival manifestations as the presenting features in two individuals. *Ophthalmology* 1994; **101**:602–607.

Kenyon KR, Bulusoglu G, Zieske JD. Clinical pathologic correlations of limbal autograft of limbal autograft transplantation. *Invest Ophthalmol Vis Sci* 1990; **31**:S1.

Kosik D, Landolt E, Speiser P. Conjunctivitis lignosa. *Klin Mbl Augenheilk* 1980; **176**:640–643.

Kruse FE, Rohrschneider K, Blum M, et al. Ocular findings in progressive erythrokeratodermia. *Ger J Ophthalmol* 1993; **2**:368.

Kruse FE, Tseng SCG. Retinoic acid regulates clonal growth and differentiation of cultured limbal and peripheral corneal epithelium. *Invest Ophthalmol Vis Sci* 1994; **35**:2405–2420.

Leonard JN, Hobday CM, Haffenden GP, et al. Immunofluorescence studies in ocular cicatricial pemphigoid. *Br J Dermatol* 1988; **118**:209–217.

Li D-Q, Tseng SCG. Three patterns of cytokine expression involved in epithelial-fibroblast interaction of human ocular surface. *J Cell Phys* 1995; **163**:61–79.

Lin AN, Murphy F, Brodie SE, Carter DM. Review of ophthalmic findings in 204 patients with epidermolysis bullosa. *Am J Ophthalmol* 1994; **118**:384–390.

Mann I, Pullinger BD. A study of mustard gas lesions of the eyes of rabbits and man. *Proc R Soc Med* 1942; **35**:229–244.

Matsua H, Smelser GK. Epithelium and stroma in alkali burned corneas. *Arch Ophthalmol* 1973; **89**:396–401.

McGready SJ, Buckley RH. Depression of cell-mediated immunity in atopic eczema. *J Allergy Clin Immunol* 1975; **56**:393–406.

McMichael AJ, Sazuki T, McDevitt HO, Payne RO. Increased frequency of HLACw3 and HLADw4 in rheumatoid arthritis. *Arthritis Rheum* 1977; **20**:1037–1042.

Mondino BJ, Brown SI, Biglan AW. HLA antigens in Stevens–Johnson syndrome with ocular involvement. *Arch Ophthalmol* 1982; **100**:1453–1554.

Mondino BJ, Brown SI, Rabin BS. HLA antigens in ocular cicatricial pemphigoid. *Arch Ophthalmol* 1979; **97**:479.

Nelson JD, Wright JC. Conjunctival goblet cell densities in ocular surface disease. *Arch Ophthalmol* 1984; **102**:1049–1051.

Nichols KK, Foulks GN, Bron AJ, et al. The international workshop on meibomian gland dysfunction: executive summary. *Invest Ophthalmol Vis Sci* 2011; **52**:1922–1929.

Nishida K, Kinoshita S, Ohashi Y, Kuwayama Y. Ocular surface abnormalities in aniridia. *Am J Ophthalmol* 1995; **120**:368–375.

Pfister RR, Renner ME. The corneal and conjunctival surface in vitamin A deficiency: a scanning electron microscopic study. *Invest Ophthalmol Vis Sci* 1978; **17**:874–883.

Pinching AJ, Rees AJ, Pussell BA, et al. Relapses in Wegener's granulomatosis: the role of infection. *Br Med J* 1980; **281**:836–838.

Pouliquen Y, Patey A, Foster CS, Goichot L, Savoldelli M. Drug-induced cicatricial pemphigoid affecting the conjunctiva: light and electron microscopic features. *Ophthalmology* 1986; **93**:775–781.

Puangsricharern V, Tseng SCG. Cytologic evidence of corneal diseases with limbal stem cell deficiency. *Ophthalmology* 1995; **102**:1476–1485.

Purcell JJ, Bikenkamp R, Tsai CC. Conjunctival lesions in panarteritis nodosa. A clinical and immunopathologic study. *Arch Ophthalmol* 1984; **102**:736–738.

Rachelefsky GS, Opelz G, Mickey MR, et al. Defective T cell function in atopic dermatitis. *J Allergy Clin Immunol* 1976; **57**:569–576.

Raphael M, Bellefqih S, Piette JC, et al. Conjunctival biopsy in Sjögren's syndrome: correlations between histological and immunohisto chemical features. *Histopathology* 1988; **13**:191–202.

Roat MI, Ohij M, Hunt LVE, Thoft RA. Conjunctival epithelial hypermitosis and goblet cell hyperplasia in atopic keratoconjunctivitis. *Am J Ophthalmol* 1993; **116**:456–463.

Roper-Hall MJ. Thermal and chemical burns. *Trans Ophthalmol Soc UK* 1965; **85**:631–646.

Rubin Z. Ophthalmic sulfonamide-induced Stevens–Johnson syndrome. *Arch Dermatol* 1977; **113**:235–236.

Schwab IR, Plotnik RD, Mannis MJ. Pemphigus and pemphigoid. *Arch Ophthalmol* 1992; **110**:171.

Smith EP, Taylor TB, Meyer LJ, Zone JJ. Identification of a basement membrane zone antigen reactive with circulating IgA antibody in ocular cicatricial pemphigoid. *J Invest Dermatol* 1993; **101**:619–623.

Sommer A, Green WR, Kenyon KR. Bitot's spots responsive and nonresponsive to vitamin A. Clinicopathologic correlations. *Arch Ophthalmol* 1981; **99**:2014–2027.

Stern ME, Beurman RW, Fox RI, et al. The pathology of dry eye: the interaction between the ocular surface and lacrimal glands. *Cornea* 1998; **17**:584–598.

Stern ME, Gao J, Siemasko KF, Beuerman RW, Pflugfelder SC. The role of the lacrimal functional unit in the pathophysiology of dry eye. *Exp Eye Res* 2004; **78**:409–416.

Theodore FH, Ferry AP. Superior limbic keratoconjunctivitis. Clinical and pathological correlations. *Arch Ophthalmol* 1970; **84**:481–484.

Thoft RA. Chemical and thermal injury. *Int Ophthalmol Clin* 1979; **19**:243–256.

Trocme SD, Kephart GM, Allensmith MR, Bourne WM, Gleich GS. Conjunctival deposition of eosinophil granule major basic protein in vernal conjunctivitis and contact lens-associated giant papillary conjunctivitis. *Am J Ophthalmol* 1989; **108**:57–63.

Tsai RJ, Tseng SCG. Effect of stromal inflammation on the outcome of limbal transplantation for corneal surface reconstruction. *Cornea* 1995; **14**:439–449.

Tseng SC, Tsubota K. Important concepts for treating ocular surface and tear disorders. *Am J Opthalmol* 1997; **124**: 825–835.

Van der Woude FJ, Rasmussen N, Lebatto S, et al. Autoantibodies against neutrophils and monocytes: tool for diagnosis and marker for disease activity in Wegener's granulomatosis. *Lancet* 1985; **1**:425–429.

Wander AH, Mukusawa T. Unusual appearance of condensed chromatin in conjunctival cells in superior limbic keratitis. *Lancet* 1981; **2**:42.

Weisman SS, Char DH, Herbort CP, Ostler HB, Kaleta-Michaels S. Alteration of human conjunctival proliferation. *Arch Ophthalmol* 1992; **110**:357–359.

West RH, Barnett AJ. Ocular involvement in scleroderma. *Br J Ophthalmol* 1979; **63**:845–847.

Williamson J, Gibson AAM, Wilson T, et al. Histology of the lacrimal gland in keratoconjunctivitis sicca. *Br J Ophthalmol* 1973; **57**:852–855.

Wuepper KD, Watson PA, Kazmierowski JA. Immune complexes in erythema multiforme and the Stevens–Johnson syndrome. *J Invest Dermatol* 1980; **74**:368–371.

You L, Kruse FE, Pohl J, Völcker H. Bone morphogenetic proteins and growth and differentiation factors in the human cornea. *Invest Ophthalmol Vis Sci* 1999; **40**:296–311.

Zierhut M, Thiel HJ, Weidle EG, et al. Ocular involvement in epidermolysis bullosa acquisita. *Arch Ophthalmol* 1989; **107**:398–401.

Chapter 3 — Definition and classification of dry eye disease

Michael A. Lemp, Jose M. Benitez-del-Castillo

INTRODUCTION

While there are a variety of diseases that involve the ocular surface, dry eye disease (DED) is by far the most common, affecting up to 20% of the general populations in Europe, North America, and Asia. The manifestations of DED are multiple and change in different stages of development of disease (Schaumberg et al. 2003). Recognition of the widespread effects of DED has grown in recent decades along with its differentiating characteristics.

NOMENCLATURE

DED has a number of names associated with it. In the older literature, the term 'keratoconjunctivitis sicca' has been prominently used. This implies an inflammatory character to the disease, a finding that has been widely acknowledged in the last two decades. More common is the use of the term 'dry eye syndrome,' which implies an association of a symptom complex unlinked to a well-defined pathogenesis. With recent advances in our understanding of the pathological processes active in the disease, the term 'DED' is in common use to denote that a discrete set of pathological events are operative in this disease. An alternative term, 'dysfunctional tear syndrome,' has been proposed to acknowledge changes in tear composition and the fact that not all cases of DED demonstrate a lack of tear production (Behrens 2006). Both terms are in use but there is general recognition of the term 'dry eye' in the general medical and lay communities and even in foreign languages. This argues for the term DED, which will be used here.

DEFINITION

There have been several attempts to define DED over the past 20 years. Two of these have been the result of international consensus conferences in which recognized experts have agreed on the elements contained in the definition. The first of these was the National Eye Institute/Industry Dry Eye Workshop (Lemp 1995), which defined DED as 'a disorder of the tear film due to tear deficiency or excessive evaporation, which causes damage to the interpalpebral ocular surface and is associated with symptoms of ocular discomfort.'

In a follow-up consensus meeting of the International Dry Eye Workshop (DEWS 2007), a more expansive definition reflecting recent research was promulgated: 'Dry eye is a multifactorial disease of the tears and ocular surface that results in symptoms of discomfort, visual disturbance, and tear film instability with potential damage to the ocular surface. It is accompanied by increased osmolarity of the tear film and inflammation of the ocular surface.'

Integral to an understanding of this definition is the recognition that DED results from a dysfunction of the lacrimal functional unit, which consists of the ocular surface (cornea, conjunctiva, and meibomian glands), the lacrimal glands, lids (Stern et al. 1998), and (more recently recognized) the nasolacrimal ducts, all integrated via sensory afferent fibers, which elicit afferent impulses via the pterygopalatine ganglion terminating in the lacrimal gland, nasopharynx, and orbit, and via the somatic efferent fibers of the 7th cranial nerve, which controls the blink reflex. In addition, there is a rich sympathetic supply to the epithelium and vasculature of the ocular surface and glands. These connections are responsible for the homeostatic control of the ocular surface in response to environmental stress. In healthy eyes, these responses support a robust and stable tear film; this control breaks down with the development of DED.

Damage to any part of this finely tuned system, including the nerves subserving the responses, compromises the homeostasis of the lacrimal functional unit, which is important in maintaining a stable tear film for clear vision, and leads to sensory changes. Most commonly, this is manifested as ocular irritation, although in many cases alterations in perception of pain lead to hyperalgesia in early disease and paradoxically decreased sensory perception in more severe DED. The role of ocular irritation in DED has undergone a reassessment recently. Although considered an essential feature of DED (DEWS 2007) and advanced in a proposal to rename the disease as chronic ocular pain syndrome (Rosenthal & Borsook 2012), recent research has demonstrated that up to 40% of patients with clear objective evidence of DED are asymptomatic for pain (Sullivan et al. 2012a). The pathways in which cold sensory receptors become noci(pain)ceptors in the presence of ocular simulation have further increased our appreciation of the complex mechanisms involved in this disease process (Belmonte & Gallar 2011). Another recently appreciated aspect of DED is the commonly evident effect of the unstable tear film on vision. Degradation of image between blinks, also described as ocular fatigue, is a common feature of the disease that is not often reported by patients until brought to their attention.

Typical compensatory responses particularly in mild-moderate DED include increased reflex tearing, increased blinking, squinting, increased meibomian gland secretion, and inflammatory changes in the ocular surface and glandular secretory cells.

RISK FACTORS

DED is typically described as a multifactorial disease. Although practically all diseases are multifactorial, what is meant is that initiation of the disease process is associated with a number of other disease conditions. Generally accepted risk factors for the development of DED include female gender, aging, androgen deficiency, contact lens wear, systemic drug effects, and refractive surgery. These conditions are represented in Figure 3.1 from the International Dry Eye Workshop as the outer ring entities in brown. Dysfunction in these conditions gives rise to a vicious cycle of events that magnify each other. Their interactions are detailed in the caption (DEWS 2007). The final common pathway, however, of expression of DED is that of an unstable and hyperosmolar tear film, which leads to inflammation and tissue damage, decreased vision, and, in most cases, ocular surface pain.

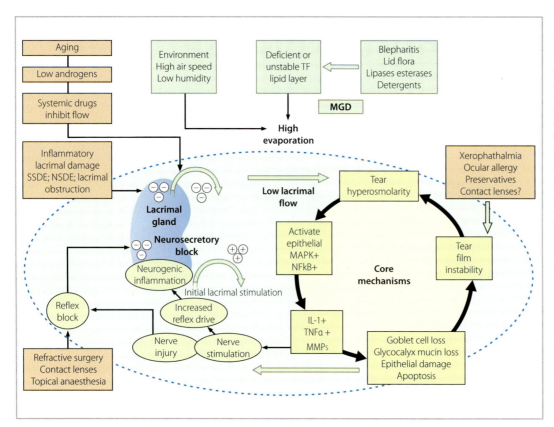

Figure 3.1 Mechanisms of dry eye disease (DED). The core mechanisms of DED are driven by tear hyperosmolarity and tear film instability. The cycle of events is shown on the right of the figure. Tear hyperosmolarity causes damage to the surface epithelium by activating a cascade of inflammatory events at the ocular surface and a release of inflammatory mediators into the tears. Epithelial damage involves cell death by apoptosis, a loss of goblet cells, and disturbance of mucin expression, leading to tear film instability. This instability exacerbates ocular surface hyperosmolarity and completes the vicious circle. Tear film instability can be initiated without the prior occurrence of tear hyperosmolarity, by several etiologies, including xerophthalmia, ocular allergy, topical preservative use, and contact lens wear. Reproduced with permission from DEWS (2007). MGD (Meibomian gland dysfunction); NSDE = non-Sjögren´s syndrome dry eye; SSDE = Sjögren´s syndrome dry eye.

As each of these elements comes into play, inflammation increases, with further tissue damage and, ultimately, dysfunction of both major secretory processes, that is, lacrimal and meibomian gland secretion. Table 3.1 contains a list of conditions associated with non-Sjögren's DED (DEWS 2007). Prominent among the risk factors for development of DED is systemic autoimmune disease, most notably Sjögren's syndrome, in which the lacrimal glands are attacked and suffer autoimmune-induced inflammatory damage. Meibomian gland dysfunction (MGD) (see below) is also a major feature of Sjögren's-associated DED probably due to the mechanisms discussed above.

CLASSIFICATION

One of the most useful classification systems for DED is that of the DEWS report (DEWS 2007). Another classification system, the Madrid Triple Classification, is a comprehensive schema detailing the many subtypes of DED and is useful for understanding the complex character of the disease (Murrube et al. 2005). The more clinically useful classification of the DEWS report is an etiopathogenic system reflecting the major secretory elements involved. Figure 3.2, with its explanatory caption, reflects current opinion on the different pathogenetic pathways of disease. The major divisions are those of aqueous tear-deficient dry eye (ADDE) (lacrimal gland) and evaporative dry eye. The most common form of DED is MGD. Many textbooks and articles refer to blepharitis (a term implying inflammation of the eyelids) as a comorbid condition associated with DED. This diagram emphasizes that posterior blepharitis, otherwise known as MGD, is a major component of DED and indeed the most common form (see below).

Less common but, nonetheless, important conditions leading to evaporative dry eye are also listed in the figure.

DISTRIBUTION OF DRY EYE SUBTYPES

As mentioned, DED has been treated as synonymous with ADDE for many years. Recent publications have noted that MGD is a highly prevalent form of DED. In patients with Sjögren's-associated DED, MGD is reported to be present in approximately two thirds of cases in Japan (Uchino et al. 2006) and Singapore (Siak et al. 2012, Tong et al. 2010), giving rise to the perception that the prevalence of MGD is higher in Asian populations than others. But recent papers have reported similar prevalence in European and American populations as well (Lemp et al. 2012, Viso et al. 2011). In this most recent study, a significantly higher percentage of patients exhibited signs of MGD than ADDE; 86% of patients had evidence of MGD. This study did not have a large number of subjects with Sjögren's-associated DED and they may have exhibited more evidence of ADDE. The results, however, suggest that ADDE may occur secondary to MGD.

Recently, it has been suggested that patients presenting symptoms and signs consistent with DED but no definitive evidence of obstructive MGD may represent a condition termed as 'non-obvious obstructive MGD' (Blackie et al. 2010). This assumes that changes in the composition of the tear lipid can give rise to these results without overt evidence of gland obstruction or malfunction, and emphasizes the importance of examining the character of the expressed meibum, as these changes may precede sign of gland obstruction.

Table 3.1 Conditions associated with non-Sjögren's DED

Primary lacrimal gland deficiencies
Age-related DED
Congenital alacrima
Familial dysautonomia
Secondary lacrimal gland deficiencies
Lacrimal gland infiltration
Sarcoidosis
Lymphoma
AIDS
Graft-versus-host disease
Lacrimal gland ablation
Lacrimal gland denervation
Obstruction of the lacrimal gland ducts
Trachoma
Cicatricial pemphigoid and ocular mucous membrane pemphigoid
Erythema multiforme
Chemical and thermal burns
Reflex hyposecretion
Reflex sensory block
Contact lens wear
Diabetes
Neurotrophic keratitis
Reflex motor block
VII cranial nerve damage
Multiple neuromatosis
Exposure to systemic drugs

Reproduced with permission from DEWS (2007).

Analysis of data in a paper studying almost 300 subjects in Europe and the United States, and using a composite scale consisting of the most commonly used objective tests for DED (Korb 2000) plus a symptom score (Sullivan et al. 2010), demonstrates that as severity increases, both subtypes are present in individuals. This supports the contention that initiation of the pathogenic pathway of evaporative tear loss can lead to the development of ADDE via neurogenic inflammation outlined in **Figure 3.1**.

◼ TEAR FILM INSTABILITY AND HYPEROSMOLARITY: HALLMARKS OF DRY EYE DISEASE

The DEWS report includes tear instability and hyperosmolarity of the tears in the definition of DED. These are thought to be the hallmarks of DED, with tear hyperosmolarity being the principal pathogenic mechanism causing damage to the ocular surface (DEWS 2007). In healthy eyes, the lacrimal functional unit provides a stable tear film between blinks, providing for clear vision. The tear osmolarity is maintained at about 290 mOsmol/L, the same as that for blood serum from which it is derived. This fluid provides nourishment for the ocular surface cells and is continually replenished as an equal amount exits via the nasolacrimal ducts as is being secreted. In the development of DED, there is a breakdown in the homeostatic functional unit in response to environmental stress, leading to a rapid break-up of the tear film and a hyperconcentrated tear film, which is measured as osmolarity. Numerous studies have demonstrated the deleterious effects of a hyperosmolar solution on the ocular surface, resulting in the initiation of inflammatory cascades and recruitment of inflammatory cells with tissue destruction. Likewise, tear instability not only results in the degradation of vision between blinks, but also gives rise to the variability in clinical signs seen in DED (Sullivan et al. 2012b).

Both of these processes are inextricably linked and increase with increasing severity of the disease. Both can be measured by (1) an assay of tear osmolarity collected in a very small sample (50 nL) from

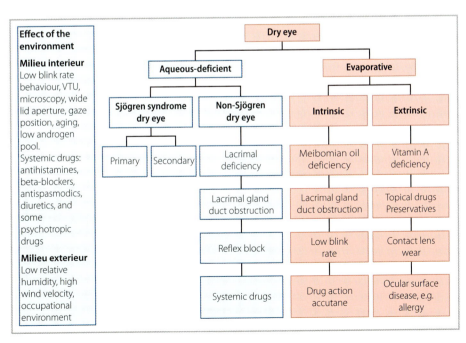

Figure 3.2 Major etiological causes of dry eye disease (DED). The left-hand box illustrates the influence of environment on an individual's risk to develop DED. The term 'environment' is used broadly, to include bodily states habitually experienced by an individual, the 'milieu interieur,' or the exposure to external conditions, the 'milieu exterieur.' This background may influence the onset and type of DED in an individual, which may be aqueous tear-deficient or evaporative in nature. Reproduced with permission from DEWS (2007).

the inferior marginal tear strip and (2) an assessment of tear break-up time viewed both with and without fluorescein dye. These latter measurements are somewhat subjective, but more objective measuring devices are under development. The use of these tests in the diagnosis and management of DED is detailed in subsequent chapters.

Increased tear osmolarity has been linked to activation of inflammatory cascades in the cornea and conjunctiva, elevated expression of HLA-DR markers in surface cells, initiation of pain, increased apoptotic ocular surface cell death, changes in behavior of ocular surface and tear mucins, and degradation of vision. In a study of subjects with DED, tear osmolarity, one of the commonly used objective tests for diagnosis, displayed a linear relationship to increasing severity of disease along a composite severity scale. Tear osmolarity is not only the best diagnostic metric (Lemp et al. 2011) but also thought to be the principal mechanism for tissue damage in DED (DEWS 2007).

RELATIONSHIP TO SYSTEMIC DISEASE

The majority of cases of DED are not associated with discernable systemic autoimmune disease. Those that are associated, however, are characteristically more severe, may have different inflammatory pathways operative early in disease, and may respond to different treatment strategies. DED is most commonly associated with Sjögren's syndrome, both primary and secondary. Among the secondary group of these conditions is rheumatoid arthritis, but most of the other conditions are also common. A great gender difference in prevalence, 4–9× greater prevalence in females, has been observed. This is discussed in greater detail in Chapter 12.

MGD, which is the most common subtype of DED, is associated with the skin condition, rosacea. In this genetically based dysfunction of the oil glands of the skin, the eyelids are frequently involved. An examination of the facial skin, particularly in the malar area of the face and nose for telangiectasia, can be an important clue to the presence of MGD. This is discussed elsewhere in the book.

Another systemic disease associated with DED is graft-versus-host disease in which a potentially vision-threatening disease can occur. Typically, there can be an acute onset affecting the lacrimal glands and the ocular surface. This condition is discussed in Chapter 13.

ROLE OF INFLAMMATION IN DRY EYE DISEASE

Inflammation is a key aspect of DED and is responsible for the destructive effects on the ocular surface and within the lacrimal glands. Although in mild-moderate disease there are few, if any, clinical signs of surface inflammation, histopathological investigations and analysis of tear cytokines reveal distinct evidence of inflammatory cells and elevated proinflammatory cytokines and associated proteins such as matrix metalloproteinases (MMPs) that break down intercellular adhesions (Chotikavanich et al. 2009). The exact entry points for these processes are, as yet, unclear. Animal models of DED demonstrate elevated proinflammatory tear cytokines and MMPs in addition to histopathological evidence of inflammation. Exactly where in the pathogenic processes inflammation enters might differ with different forms of the disease, for example, systemic-disease-associated forms such as Sjögren's DED or graft-versus-host (primary inflammation). In the more common age-associated or androgen-deficiency-associated disease, inflammation may be secondary to tear hyperosmolarity and instability. Nonetheless, inflammation is an important link in the chain of events leading to tissue destruction. It will be described in greater detail in the following chapters.

CLASSIFYING DRY EYE DISEASE BY SEVERITY

It is important to classify DED by severity, since different treatment regimens are appropriate for differing levels of disease severity. The most commonly used severity scale is an outgrowth of that first

Table 3.2 DED severity grading scheme

DED severity level	1	2	3	4*
Discomfort, severity, and frequency	Mild and/or episodic; occurs under environmental stress	Moderate episodic or chronic; stress or no stress	Severe frequent or constant without stress	Severe and/or disabling and constant
Visual symptoms	None or episodic mild fatigue	Annoying and/or activity-limiting episodic	Annoying, chronic, and/or constant limiting activity	Constant and/or possibly disabling
Conjunctival injection	None to mild	None to mild	±	+/++
Conjunctival staining	None to mild	Variable	Moderate to marked	Marked
Corneal staining (severity/location)	None to mild	Variable	Marked central	
Corneal/tear signs	None to mild	Mild debris, decreased meniscus	Filamentary keratitis, mucus clumping, increased tear debris	Filamentary keratitis, mucus clumping, increased tear debris
Lid/meibomian glands	MGD variably present	MGD variably present	Frequent	Trichiasis, keratinization, symblepharon
TFBUT (seconds)	Variable	≤10	≤5	Immediate
Schirmer's score (mm per 5 minutes)	Variable	≤10	≤5	≤2

Reproduced with permission from DEWS (2007).
Reprinted with permission from Behrens et al. (2006).
MGD, meibomian gland dysfunction; TFBUT, [fluorescein] tear film break-up time.
*Must have signs and symptoms.

presented in the Delphi panel report (Behrens et al. 2006) and then refined in the DEWS report (DEWS 2007) (**Table 3.2**). This categorical scale divides the disease into four levels based on a series of commonly performed objective tests and symptoms. While it provides a useful template for differentiating severity, it has several drawbacks. Categorical schemes such as this depend on a summation of results of clinical tests without incorporating individual test severity. Mild-moderate DED is characterized by conflicts in tests; for example, some are positive and some negative. In clinical trial use, investigators must supply numbers in the boxes for grades 1 and 2 and this is subject to wide variability depending on what formulation is being tested. For example, should corneal staining be positive in grade 1? A recent study has shown that <50% of subjects with mild-moderate disease have any corneal staining (Sullivan et al. 2010). Similarly, between 30% and 40% of subjects with mild-moderate disease are asymptomatic. Based on purely clinical presentation, a consensus report from Canada concluded that it is impossible to differentiate between grades 1 and 2 and has suggested a compressed 3-point scale (Jackson 2000). Attempts to demonstrate tear cytokine levels in DED have demonstrated little difference between levels 1 and 2.

An alternative objective approach to disease severity (Sullivan et al. 2010) proposes using a continuous composite severity score, which takes into account individual severity and frequency, adjusted to bring the differing scales into mathematical alignment. In this way, individual tests can be plotted against this composite severity. This is demonstrated in **Figure 3.3** (Sullivan et al. 2010), which plots tear osmolarity against the composite scale. Tear osmolarity, of all the commonly employed tests, demonstrates a linear relationship. All of the tests demonstrate increasing agreement with the composite severity in moderate to severe levels.

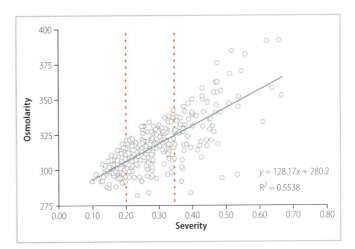

Figure 3.3 Composite severity index composed of six objective markers and one of symptoms, ocular surface disease index (OSDI), on the x-axis and osmolarity plotted on the y-axis. A linear relationship is seen. With permission from Sullivan et al. (2010).

SUMMARY

In this chapter, we have outlined current thinking on the best ways to classify DED. Advances in this area are being made at a rapid pace and further refinements are anticipated. The reader will, however, be well placed in understanding many of the aspects of this sometimes vexing disease, which should lead to better diagnosis and management of patients with more timely improvement of patient discomfort and restoration of a more normal ocular surface.

◼ REFERENCES

Behrens A, Doyle JJ, Stern L, et al; Dysfunctional tear syndrome study group. Dysfunctional tear syndrome: a Delphi approach to treatment recommendations. *Cornea* 2006; **25**:900–907.

Belmonte C, Gallar J. Cold thermoreceptors. Unexpected players in tear production and ocular dryness sensations. *Invest Ophthalmol Vis Sci* 2011; **52**:3888–3892.

Blackie CA, Korb DR, Knop E, et al. Nonobvious meibomian gland dysfunction *Cornea* 2010; **29**:1333–1345.

Chotikavanich S, de Paiva CS, Li de Q, et al. Production and activity of matrix metalloproteinase-9 on the ocular surface increase in dysfunctional tear syndrome. *Invest Ophthalmol Vis Sci* 2009; **50**:3203–3209.

DEWS. The definition and classification of dry eye disease: report of the Definition and Classification Subcommittee of the International Dry Eye Workshop. *Ocul Surf* 2007; **5**:75–92.

Jackson WB. Management of dysfunctional tear syndrome: a Canadian consensus. *Can J Ophthalmol* 2009; **44**:385–394.

Korb DR. Survey of preferred tests for diagnosis of the tear film and dry eye. *Cornea* 2000; **19**:483–486.

Lemp MA. Report of the National Eye Institute/Industry Workshop on Clinical Trials in Dry Eyes. *CLAO J* 1995; **21**:221–132.

Lemp MA, Bron AJ, Baudouin C, et al. Tear osmolarity in the diagnosis and management of dry eye disease. *Am J Ophthalmol* 2011; **151**:792–798.

Lemp MA, Crews LA, Bron AJ, Foulks GN, Sullivan BD. Distribution of aqueous-deficient and evaporative dry eye in a clinic-based patient cohort: a retrospective study. *Cornea* 2012; **31**:472–478.

Murrube J, Németh J, Höh H, et al. The Madrid triple classification of dry eye for practical clinical use. *Eur J Ophthalmol* 2005; **15**:660–667.

Rosenthal P, Borsook D. The corneal pain syndrome. Part 1. The missing piece of the dry eye puzzle. *Ocul Surf* 2012; **10**:2–14.

Schaumberg DA, Sullivan DA, Buring JE, Dana MR. Prevalence of dry eye syndrome among US women. *Am J Ophthalmol* 2003; **136**:318–326.

Siak JJ, Tong L, Wong WL, et al. Prevalence and risk factors of meibomian gland dysfunction. *Cornea* 2012; **31**:1223–1228.

Stern ME, Beuerman RW, Fox RI, et al. The pathology of dry eye: the interaction between the ocular surface and lacrimal glands. *Cornea* 1998; **17**:584–589.

Sullivan BD, Crews LA, Messmer EM, et al. Correlation between commonly used clinical tests in the management of dry eye disease. IOVS 2012a; 53:ARVO E-Abstract 550/A18.

Sullivan BD, Crews LA, Sönmez B, et al. Clinical utility of objective tests for dry eye disease: variability over time and implications for clinical trials and disease management. *Cornea* 2012b; **31**:1000–1008.

Sullivan BD, Whitmer D, Nichols KK, et al. An objective approach to dry eye severity. *Invest Ophthalmol Vis Sci* 2010; **51**:6125–6130.

Tong L, Chaurasia SS, Mehta JS, Beuerman RW. Screening for meibomian gland disease: its relation to dry eye subtypes and symptoms in a tertiary clinic in Singapore. *Invest Ophthalmol Vis Sci* 2010; **51**:3449–3454.

Uchino M, Dogru M, Yagi Y, et al. The features of dry eye disease in a Japanese elderly population. *Optom Vis Sci* 2006; **83**:797–802.

Viso E, Gude F, Rodriguez-Ares MT. The association of meibomian gland dysfunction and other common ocular disease with dry eye: a population-based study in Spain. *Cornea* 2011; **30**:1–6.

Chapter 4
The epidemiology of dry eye disease

Kelly K. Nichols, Katherine A. Weibel

INTRODUCTION

In order to fully understand the signs, symptoms, and treatment of any disease, it is imperative to first understand the relationship of the various factors that determine the distribution and frequency of the disease in a population. The study of this interconnected and complicated relationship is the study of epidemiology of dry eye disease (DED). This chapter will describe, in particular, the factors that help to explain the distribution of DED across the world, the similarities and differences, and what we know about the overlap and relationship between the various ocular surface disorders.

DEFINITION AND CHALLENGES IN OCULAR SURFACE EPIDEMIOLOGY

In the process of identifying the prevalence of a disease, a working definition is needed to guide the process. Thus, the definition of DED resulting from the 1995 National Eye Institute/Industry Workshop included ocular symptoms in addition to one or more ocular signs: 'Dry eye is a disorder of the tear film due to tear deficiency or excessive tear evaporation which causes damage to the interpalpebral ocular surface associated with symptoms of ocular surface associated with symptoms of ocular discomfort' (Lemp 1995). This original definition was updated in 2007 in the DEWS report and maintained many of the key features, and added components that further explored the etiology and underlying factors, while focusing on the multifaceted aspects of the disease: 'Dry eye is a multifactorial disease of the tears and ocular surface that results in symptoms of discomfort, visual disturbance, and tear film instability with potential damage to the ocular surface. It is accompanied by increased osmolarity of the tear film and inflammation of the ocular surface' (DEWS 2007a).

Although the definition has become fairly well-recognized and accepted, it is still challenging to distinguish who has DED and who does not and even, perhaps more pertinent, to decide how DED can (or should) be subcategorized (DEWS 2007a). Currently, there is no singular, definitive test to diagnose DED (DEWS 2007b). Additionally, there is not even an accepted, standardized combination of clinical tests to diagnose DED, although several are utilized clinically as well as in patient-based research. One reason for this lack of accepted tests may be the absence of correlation between subjective feelings of irritation and discomfort and the results of clinical DED tests (DEWS 2007b; Nichols et al. 2004b). Yet another reason might be the lack of repeatability for DED clinical tests (Nichols et al. 2004a); however, newer objective osmolarity testing (Eperjesi et al. 2012) as well as modifications to existing testing such as tear film break-up time (TFBUT) (Pult & Riede-Pult 2012) demonstrates improved reliability and repeatability. Furthermore, much of DED diagnosis is based upon 'subjective' symptoms that may be influenced by varied levels of pain tolerance and cognitive responses to physical sensations found among different individuals (DEWS 2007b).

PREVALENCE

An accurate snapshot into the prevalence of DED is difficult to capture since various studies have employed different definitions of 'DED' as well as different study methods, that is, surveys, examinations, or a combination of both (DEWS 2007b). Current estimation of DED prevalence in the United States among women younger than 50 years is about 5.7%, which increases to 9.9% at older than 75 years and more. Age-adjusted prevalence is about 7.8% for women older than 50 years and more (Schaumberg et al. 2003). Meanwhile, the prevalence of DED among men of age 50–54 years is estimated at 3.9% and increases to 7.7% for men older than 80 years and more. The age-standardized prevalence was 4.3% for men older than 50 years and more (Schaumberg et al. 2009). In both studies, cross-sectional surveys were filled out by thousands of women and men. The definition of DED for both included either a clinical diagnosis of DED or severe symptoms of constant or frequent dryness and irritation (Schaumberg et al. 2003, 2009). In addition, a study in Taiwan including Chinese individuals older than 65 years found that 33.7% of the 1361 participants were symptomatic of DED (one or more symptoms often or all of the time) and 96% displayed at least one positive clinical sign such as TFBUT $\leq$10 sec. positive corneal staining, or a Schirmer's score $\leq$5 mm/5 min (Lin et al. 2003). However, in overview of eight large epidemiological studies of DED, a prevalence range of approximately 5–35% was revealed (DEWS 2007b). Once again, there was a difference in DED definitions, populations, and age groups. In general, trends in the prevalence of DED have emerged; namely, the disease seems to affect women more than men (Lin et al. 2003, Moss et al. 2000, Schaumberg et al. 2003, 2009) and its frequency increases with age (Moss et al. 2000, Schaumberg et al. 2003, 2009).

Since 2007, new prevalence data on DED have been published routinely. Several recent examples include a cross-sectional survey conducted in July 2010 of 1902 senior high school students in Shouguang, a county of Shandong Province, China, where the prevalence of DED was found to be 23.7%, which is significant because DED is clinically considered to be a disease of the elderly. In contrast, a recent study of US military veterans at the Miami and Broward Veterans Affairs eye clinics (Galor et al. 2011) showed an overall DED prevalence of 12% in male and 22% in female patients, with female gender imparting a 2.40 × increased risk [95% confidence interval (CI) 2.04–2.81] over male gender. This demonstrates the importance of using consistent definitions of DED in the assessment of prevalence when comparing across studies. **Table 4.1** highlights the most commonly reported prevalence studies, including updates from the 2007 DEWS epidemiology report (DEWS 2007b).

Table 4.1 A summary of the most commonly reported prevalence studies on dry eye disease (DED)

Study	Sample size	Year	Age group (years)	Prevalence (%)
Salisbury Eye Study (Schein et al. 1997, 1999)	2,420	1999	≥65	14.6
Beaver Dam (Munoz et al. 2000)	3,722	2000	≥48	14.4
Sumatra (Lee et al. 2002)	1,058	2002	≥21	27.5
Women's Health Study (Schaumberg et al. 2003)	36,995	2003	≥49	7.8
Blue Mountains (Chia et al. 2003)	1,075	2003	≥50	16.6
Melbourne Visual Impairment Project (Chia et al. 2003)	926	2003	≥40	5.5
Shihpa (Lin et al. 2003)	2,038	2003	≥65	33.7
Japanese High School (Uchino et al. 2008)	3,433	2008	15–18	4.3, males; 8.0, females
Physician's Health Studies I and II (Schaumberg et al. 2009)	25,655	2009	≥50, ≥80	3.9, 7.7
Beijing Eye study (Jie et al. 2009)	4,439	2009	≥40	21
Henan Eye Study (Guo et al. 2010)	657	2010	≥65	30.3
Miami Veterans (Galor et al. 2011)	16,862	2011	≥65	12, males; 22, females
Koumi, Japan (Uchino et al. 2011)	2,791	2011	≥40	12.5, males 21.6, females
Korea (Han et al. 2011)	657	2011	≥65	30.3
Shouguang, China High School (Zhang et al. 2012)	1,902	2012	15–18	23.7

INCIDENCE

The incidence of a disease may be thought of as the rate at which new cases of that specific condition arise over a specific time period. The incidence of DED was discovered to be 13.3% over a 5-year time interval (Moss et al. 2004), and was followed by a 10-year report demonstrating an incidence of 21.6% (95% CI 19.9–23.3%) (Moss et al. 2008). The incidence of DED was significantly associated with increasing age. In addition, after adjusting for age, the incidence was greater for individuals who had a history of allergy or diabetes, who used antihistamines or diuretics, and who reported poorer self-rated health. Moreover, the incidence was less for individuals who used angiotensin-converting enzyme inhibitors or who consumed alcohol (Moss et al. 2004). Follow-up data from the same research team demonstrated similar findings, with the additional new findings of higher incidence after adjusting for age, thyroid disease not treated with hormones, and use of antianxiety medications, antidepressants, oral steroids, or vitamins (Moss et al. 2008). In addition to previously reported variables, incidence was lower for those with a sedentary lifestyle (Moss et al. 2008).

Several medical conditions have been found to increase DED risk, including post-traumatic stress disorder [odds ratio (OR) 1.97, 95% CI 1.75–2.23], depression (OR 1.91, 95% CI 1.73–2.10), thyroid disease (OR 1.81, 95% CI 1.46–2.26), and sleep apnea (OR 2.20, 95% CI 1.97–2.46) (all analyses adjusted for gender and age). The use of several systemic medications, including antidepressant medications (OR 1.97, 95% CI 1.79–2.17), antianxiety medications (OR 1.74, 95% CI 1.58–1.91), and antibenign prostatic hyperplasia medications (OR 1.68, 95% CI 1.51–1.86), was likewise associated with an increased risk of DED (Moss et al. 2004, 2008). Recent findings validate the association of post-traumatic stress disorder, depression, and medications taken for these conditions with DED; whether causal or a downstream effect, depression is commonly reported by patients with DED and may have clinical significance in managing the condition.

FINANCIAL BURDEN OF DED

The financial burden of DED may be significant especially when one considers the high prevalence of this condition (Mizuno et al. 2012). The financial burden results from costs such as office visits, surgical interventions, prescription and over-the-counter medications, specialized eyewear, and humidifiers (DEWS 2007b). Indirect costs such as lost work time, decreased productivity, and alterations in the work environment also contribute to the economic burden (DEWS 2007b). The financial burdens are recognized in many countries around the world. A recent Japanese study included 118 patients, 47 of whom had Sjögren's syndrome (SS) and an average age of 64.1 ± 11.2 years, consistent with the typical age of a DED patient. The direct cost per person was determined to be US$530 per year (Mizuno et al. 2012). Furthermore, a study involving six European countries found that the average cost to manage DED patients per year was about US$622 (Clegg et al. 2006). These costs included office visits, medications, and surgical procedures such as tarsorrhaphy and punctual plug occlusion (Clegg et al. 2006). Furthermore, another study estimated that office visits for SS patients were estimated at US$211 in 2003 (Reddy et al. 2004). Finally, a 2009 study estimated that in the United States alone, 7–10 million individuals spent $320 million per year on artificial tear preparations (Gayton 2009). Indirect costs of DED are a cause for concern for the patient as they often involve loss of work time. One study estimated the opportunity cost of multiple office visits per year for DED to be about US$500 (Mizuno et al. 2012). Furthermore, it has been estimated that because of ocular discomfort, DED patients and SS patients do not attend 2–5 days of work per year, respectively, yet the loss of productive work hours can far exceed that time estimate (Nelson et al. 2000). Of the severe DED patients in the study, 11% were forced to cut back on working hours and experienced DED symptoms 191–208 working days per year (Nelson et al. 2000). The economic burden of DED, therefore, appears significant and detrimental.

■ QUALITY OF LIFE

DED has a displayed a significant correlation with a decline in quality of life in a number of studies (Mertzanis et al. 2005, Miljanovic et al. 2007, Pflugfelder 2008, Schiffman et al. 2003). Persons who suffer from DED are likely to report very frequent symptoms of both dryness and irritation (DEWS 2007b), and these symptoms are commonly included in many definitions of DED in epidemiological studies. Individuals diagnosed with DED or severe symptoms were found to have measurably more difficulty than those without DED in carrying out common and important tasks. These tasks included reading, completing professional work, using a computer, driving at night or during the day, and watching television (Miljanovic et al. 2007). Furthermore, a utility assessment was conducted among individuals diagnosed with DED (Schiffman et al. 2003) to quantify patient preferences for health outcomes. A typical utility assessment scale ranges from 0 to 1.0, and the closer the score is to 1.0, the better the quality of life (Schiffman et al. 2003). In this study, individuals rated their own DED at a mean value of (0.81) with a range of 0.16–0.97. Furthermore, they rated moderate DED at (0.78), severe DED at (0.72), and severe DED requiring tarsorrhaphy at (0.62). These results display the perceived decrease in quality of life in proportion to increasing severity of DED. In comparison, moderate to severe angina historically was reported at (0.71) and a disabling hip fracture at (0.65). The reported score for severe DED resulting in loss of utility was similar to the score reported for moderate to severe angina. This exposes the severity at which DED sufferers view their own condition (Schiffman et al. 2003), which is often underestimated by practitioners (Chalmers et al. 2005).

■ SPECIFIC OCULAR SURFACE CONDITIONS

■ Sjögren's syndrome

Sjögren's syndrome is considered an autoimmune disease characterized by chronic inflammation involving the exocrine glands, which may result in a severe form of DED and/or dry mouth (DEWS 2007a; Nikolov & Illei 2009). The syndrome has a strong female predominance; estrogens are believed to be contributory whereas androgens (e.g. testosterone) are believed to be protective (Nikolov & Illei 2009). It is estimated that SS affects women nine times more frequently than men (Segal et al. 2009). The peak of onset is around menopause, and the change in androgen–estrogen ratio is viewed as a risk factor, rather than the absolute level of estrogen; it is hypothesized that there exist contributing genetic, environmental, and random factors that may cause SS (Nikolov & Illei 2009). Ocular complaints may include burning, grittiness, fatigue, blurred vision, and watery eyes from reflex tearing, which can be significant to patients. Over time, there may be deterioration in ocular surface, ulceration, tear film debris, and mucus strands adhering to the cornea (Nguyen et al. 2007). In addition, the impact of SS on quality of life is substantial; patients have been reported more likely to be disabled and suffer pain, fatigue, depression, and cognitive symptoms than the controls (Segal et al. 2009). Depression was reported in 37% of SS patients versus 12% of controls (same age and gender) in a recent study (Segal et al. 2009). Moreover, SS patients were more likely to experience hospitalization and more frequent infections, and use multiple medications; patients' out-of-pocket dental expenses for the past year were reported three times greater than those for the peer group (Segal et al. 2009).

■ Meibomian gland dysfunction

Meibomian gland dysfunction (MGD) is defined as a 'chronic diffuse abnormality of the meibomian glands, commonly characterized by terminal duct obstruction and/or qualitative or quantitative changes in glandular secretion. This may result in alteration of the tear film, symptoms of eye irritation, clinically apparent inflammation and ocular surface disease' (Nelson et al. 2011). Currently, there exist a number of studies that evaluate symptoms as well as clinical correlates, such as lid telangiectasia, gland orifice capping, gland drop-out, and TFBUT, to help determine a more accurate prevalence of MGD in the context of DED (Schaumberg et al. 2011). The prevalence of MGD reported in the literature varies greatly from 3.5% to almost 70% and depends on the methods used to define MGD (Schaumberg et al. 2011). Even given these differences across studies, the prevalence in Asian populations appears higher than that reported in populations consisting mostly of Caucasians. For example, the reported prevalence was 60.8, 61.9, and 69.3% in the Shihpai Eye Study (Lin et al. 2003), the Japanese study (Uchino et al. 2006), and the Beijing Eye Study (Jie et al. 2009), respectively (Schaumberg et al. 2011). In contrast, the reported prevalence was 3.5% in the Salisbury Eye Evaluation Study (Schein et al. 1999) and 19.9% for the Melbourne Visual Impairment Project (Chia et al. 2003). However, each of these studies utilized different definitions of MGD, different clinical signs, and different age groups, so a direct comparison is cautioned (Schaumberg et al. 2011). Knop et al. (2011) provide an excellent and thorough explanation of MGD. They report possible causes of MGD including hyperkeratinization as a reason for obstructive MGD, which causes degenerative gland dilation and atrophy without inflammation. Factors enhancing epithelial keratinization include aging, hormonal alterations, medication toxicities, and even contact lens wear (Knop et al. 2011). Furthermore, it was reported that androgens promoted the production of lipids and decreased keratinization, and that androgen deficiency may lead to MGD (Schirra et al. 2006). Furthermore, abnormalities of the lid margin and also meibomian gland dropout increase significantly with age, notably for age >50 years (Den et al. 2006). Additionally, aging has been associated with significant changes in lipid profiles of human meibomian gland secretions. The secretions of polar and neutral lipids were greater for younger men and women (mean age 37.3 and 36.4 years) than for older men and women (mean age 70.1 and 70.6 years) (Sullivan et al. 2006). Moreover, increasing age was correlated with increasing opacification of meibomian gland secretions as well as eyelid and eyelid margin changes (Sullivan et al. 2006). It was hypothesized in this same study that an androgen deficiency, at least in part, may explain the effects of aging on meibomian glands.

■ Contact lens dry eye

Contact lens wear has been associated with DED. It is estimated that the frequency of contact lens contact lens dry eye is becoming the accepted terminology is about 50% with approximately 17 million wearers affected in the United States alone (Ramamoorthy & Sinnott 2008). In a study including 360 subjects, several factors were reported to be significantly associated with DED status, including recent lens refitting, artificial tear or rewetting drop usage, and high-water-content lenses (Ramamoorthy & Sinnott 2008). Patient-related factors associated with DED status included DED diagnosis or symptoms in the absence of contact lenses, decreased satisfaction with current contact lenses, reduced daily wear time, and reduced ability to wear lenses for as long as desired. Another large study ($n = 730$) to determine frequency and factors associated with contact lens dissatisfaction and discontinuation found that 26.3% expressed contact lens dissatisfaction and another 24.1% had permanently discontinued contact lens wear. The primary reason for both dissatisfaction and discontinuation was dryness and discomfort (Richdale et al. 2007). There are factors to consider regarding dry and contact lens wear. One may consider if these individuals have predisposing factors even before contact lens wear is attempted or if contact lenses, in fact, induce DED.

SUMMARY

In summary, the field of DED epidemiology has been steadily progressing over the past 5–10 years. New prevalence and incidence data, as well as data assessing associated factors, have increased significantly, and our understanding of fundamental epidemiological concepts related to DED is becoming widely accepted. The next 10 years seem equally promising.

REFERENCES

Chalmers RL, Begley CG, Edrington T, et al. The agreement between self-assessment and clinician assessment of dry eye severity. *Cornea* 2005; **24**:804–810.

Chia EM, Mitchell P, Rochtchina E, et al. Prevalence and associations of dry eye syndrome in an older population: the Blue Mountains Eye Study. *Clin Experiment Ophthalmol* 2003; **31**:229–232.

Clegg JP, Guest JF, Lehman A, Smith AF. The annual cost of dry eye syndrome in France, Germany, Italy, Spain, Sweden and the United Kingdom among patients managed by ophthalmologists. *Ophthalmic Epidemiol* 2006; **13**:263–274.

Den S, Shimizu K, Ikeda T, et al. Association between meibomian gland changes and aging, sex, or tear function. *Cornea* 2006; **25**:651–655.

DEWS. The definition and classification of dry eye disease: report of the Definition and Classification Subcommittee of the International Dry Eye WorkShop. *Ocul Surf* 2007a; **5**:75–92.

DEWS. The epidemiology of dry eye disease: report of the Epidemiology Subcommittee of the International Dry Eye WorkShop. *Ocul Surf* 2007a; **5**:93–107.

Eperjesi F, Aujla M, Bartlett H. Reproducibility and repeatability of the OcuSense TearLab osmometer. *Graefes Arch Clin Exp Ophthalmol* 2012; **250**:1201–1205.

Galor A, Feuer W, Lee DJ, et al. Prevalence and risk factors of dry eye syndrome in a United States veterans affairs population. *Am J Ophthalmol* 2011; **152**:377–384.e372.

Gayton JL. Etiology, prevalence, and treatment of dry eye disease. *Clin Ophthalmol* 2009; **3**:405–412.

Guo B, Lu P, Chen X, et al. Prevalence of dry eye disease in Mongolians at high altitude in China: the Henan eye study. *Ophthalmic Epidemiol* 2010; **17**:234–241.

Han SB, Hyon JY, Woo SJ, et al. Prevalence of dry eye disease in an elderly Korean population. *Arch Ophthalmol* 2011; **129**:633–638.

Jie Y, Xu L, Wu YY, et al. Prevalence of dry eye among adult Chinese in the Beijing Eye Study. *Eye (Lond)* 2009; **23**:688–693.

Knop E, Knop N, Miller T, et al. The international workshop on meibomian gland dysfunction: report of the subcommittee on anatomy, physiology, and pathophysiology of the meibomian gland. *Invest Ophthalmol Vis Sci* 2011; **52**:1938–1978.

Lee AJ, Lee J, Saw S-M, et al. Prevalence and risk factors associated with dry eye symptoms: a population based study in Indonesia. *Br J Ophthalmol* 2002; **86**:1347–1351.

Lemp MA. Report of the National Eye Institute/Industry workshop on Clinical Trials in Dry Eyes. *CLAO J* 1995; **21**:221–232.

Lin PY, Tsai SY, Cheng CY, et al. Prevalence of dry eye among an elderly Chinese population in Taiwan: The Shihpai Eye Study. *Ophthalmology* 2003; **110**:1096–1101.

Mertzanis P, Abetz L, Rajagopalan K, et al. The relative burden of dry eye in patients' lives: comparisons to a U.S. normative sample. *Invest Ophthalmol Vis Sci* 2005; **46**:46–50.

Miljanovic B, Dana R, Sullivan DA, et al. Impact of dry eye syndrome on vision-related quality of life. *Am J Ophthalmol* 2007; **143**:409–415.

Mizuno Y, Yamada M, Shigeyasu C. Annual direct cost of dry eye in Japan. *Clin Ophthalmol* 2012; **6**:755–760.

Moss SE, Klein R, Klein BE. Incidence of dry eye in an older population. *Arch Ophthalmol* 2004; **122**:369–373.

Moss SE, Klein R, Klein BE. Long-term incidence of dry eye in an older population. *Optom Vis Sci* 2008; **85**:668–674.

Moss SE, Klein R, Polz-Dacewicz M. Prevalence of and risk factors for dry eye syndrome. *Arch Ophthalmol* 2000; **118**:1264–1268.

Munoz B, West SK, Rubin GS, et al. Causes of blindness and visual impairment in a population of older Americans: The Salisbury Eye Evaluation Study. *Arch Ophthalmol* 2000; **118**:819–825.

Nelson JD, Helms H, Fiscella R, Southwell Y, Hirsch JD. A new look at dry eye disease and its treatment. *Adv Ther* 2000; **17**:84–93.

Nelson JD, Shimazaki J, Benitez-del-Castillo JM, et al. The international workshop on meibomian gland dysfunction: report of the definition and classification subcommittee. *Invest Ophthalmol Vis Sci* 2011; **52**:1930–1937.

Nguyen CQ, Cha SR, Peck AB. Sjögren's syndrome (SjS)-like disease of mice: the importance of B lymphocytes and autoantibodies. *Front Biosci* 2007; **12**:1767–1789.

Nichols KK, Mitchell GL, Zadnik K. The repeatability of clinical measurements of dry eye. *Cornea* 2004a; **23**:272–285.

Nichols KK, Nichols JJ, Mitchell GL. The lack of association between signs and symptoms in patients with dry eye disease. *Cornea* 2004b; **23**:762–770.

Nikolov NP, Illei GG. Pathogenesis of Sjögren's syndrome. *Curr Opin Rheumatol* 2009; **21**:465–470.

Pflugfelder SC. Prevalence, burden, and pharmacoeconomics of dry eye disease. *Am J Manag Care* 2008; **14**:S102–S106.

Pult H, Riede-Pult BH. A new modified fluorescein strip: its repeatability and usefulness in tear film break-up time analysis. *Cont Lens Anterior Eye* 2012; **35**:35–38.

Ramamoorthy P, Sinnott LT. Treatment, material, care, and patient-related factors in contact lens-related dry eye. *Optom Vis Sci* 2008; **85**:764–772.

Reddy P, Grad O, Rajagopalan K. The economic burden of dry eye: a conceptual framework and preliminary assessment. *Cornea* 2004; **23**:751–761.

Richdale K, Sinnott LT, Skadahl E, Nichols JJ. Frequency of and factors associated with contact lens dissatisfaction and discontinuation. *Cornea* 2007; **26**:168–174.

Schaumberg DA, Dana R, Buring JE, et al. Prevalence of dry eye disease among US men: estimates from the Physicians' Health Studies. *Arch Ophthalmol* 2009; **127**:763–768.

Schaumberg DA, Nichols JJ, Papas EB, et al. The international workshop on meibomian gland dysfunction: report of the subcommittee on the epidemiology of, and associated risk factors for, MGD. *Invest Ophthalmol Vis Sci* 2011; **52**:1994–2005.

Schaumberg DA, Sullivan DA, Buring JE, et al. Prevalence of dry eye syndrome among US women. *Am J Ophthalmol* 2003; **136**:318–326.

Schein OD, Hochberg MC, Munoz B, et al. Dry eye and dry mouth in the elderly: a population-based assessment. *Arch Intern Med* 1999; **159**:1359–1363.

Schein OD, Munoz B, Tielsch JM, et al. Prevalence of dry eye among the elderly. *Am J Ophthalmol* 1997; **124**:723–728.

Schiffman RM, Walt JG, Jacobsen G, et al. Utility assessment among patients with dry eye disease. *Ophthalmology* 2003; **110**:1412–1419.

Schirra F, Richards SM, Liu M, et al. Androgen regulation of lipogenic pathways in the mouse meibomian gland. *Exp Eye Res* 2006; **83**:291–296.

Segal B, Bowman SJ, Fox SJ, et al. Primary Sjögren's syndrome: health experiences and predictors of health quality among patients in the United States. *Health Qual Life Outcomes* 2009; **7**:46.

Sullivan BD, Evans JE, Dana MR, Sullivan DA. Influence of aging on the polar and neutral lipid profiles in human meibomian gland secretions. *Arch Ophthalmol* 2006; **124**:1286–1292.

Uchino M, Dogru M, Uchino Y, et al. Japan Ministry of Health study on prevalence of dry eye disease among Japanese high school students. *Am J Ophthalmol* 2008; **146**:925–929.e922.

Uchino M, Dogru M, Yagi Y, et al. The features of dry eye disease in a Japanese elderly population. *Optom Vis Sci* 2006; **83**:797–802.

Uchino M, Nishiwaki Y, Michikawa T, et al. Prevalence and risk factors of dry eye disease in Japan: Koumi study. *Ophthalmology* 2011; **118**:2361–2367.

Zhang Y, Chen H, Wu X. Prevalence and risk factors associated with dry eye syndrome among senior high school students in a county of Shandong Province, China. *Ophthalmic Epidemiol* 2012; **19**:226–230.

Chapter 5 — Discrimination of subtypes of dry eye disease: aqueous tear-deficient dry eye and evaporative dry eye

Maurizio Rolando

■ INTRODUCTION

Dry eye disease (DED) has been defined as a multifactorial disease of the tears and ocular surface that results in discomfort, visual disturbance, and tear film instability, with potential damage to the ocular surface. It is accompanied by increased osmolarity of the tear film and inflammation. The presence of symptoms is usually at the origin of the clinical diagnosis (DEWS 2007).

DED can be divided into conditions in which the production of the aqueous component of tears is inadequate [aqueous deficient dry eye (ADDE)] and conditions in which aqueous production is relatively normal but tear evaporation rate is increased [evaporative dry eye (EDE)]. It is now considered that evaporative causes of DED are more common, being responsible for almost two thirds of cases (Rolando et al. 2010).

At present, the most frequently reported noxious agent for the ocular surface structures in course of tear film dysfunction is tear osmolarity, which depends on evaporation rate divided by tear secretion rate and is an increasing function of this ratio (Ciprandi et al. 1994, Luo et al. 2005, Rolando et al. 1983b). From a theoretical point of view, in EDE, such a ratio is increased because the evaporation rate is increased, whereas in ADDE, the ratio is increased because the tear secretion rate is reduced.

Unfortunately, in the clinical practice the difference is not so sharp because a significant number of ADDEs show increased tear water evaporation (**Figure 5.1**).

Evaporation is controlled by both extrinsic and ocular factors. Extrinsic factors include the relative humidity, temperature, and flow velocity of the ambient air. Ocular factors include the surface temperature of the tear film. But the main controller of evaporation of water from the ocular surface is the lipid layer of the tear film, which acts as a barrier to evaporation from the aqueous part of the tear film (Tsubota & Yamada 1992). The resistance of the lipid layer to evaporation may be expected to depend not only on its thickness but also on its structure, composition, and dynamic behavior (**Table 5.1**).

It is common knowledge that at each blink, the lipid layer of the tear film is squeezed between the two lid margins and its architecture is very quickly rebuilt after the lids are opened and the lipids are spread over the aqueous layer of the film in a reproducible manner. For this to be optimal it is important to have not only an adequate amount of lipids but also good lipid molecules mixture with proper elasticity and ability to spread on water.

The ability to spread quickly is not only a function of the quality of the available lipids but also, according to Marangoni law of thin lipid

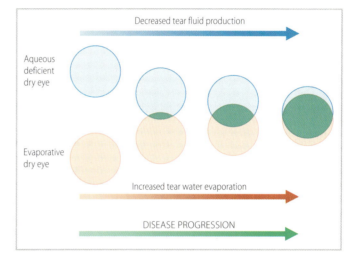

Figure 5.1 Hypothesis of the dynamic changes in the importance of the different pathogenetic factors during the evolution of dry eye disease. In aqueous deficient dry eyes the water volume changes and the qualitative changes of available glycoproteins can progressively impair the ability of the lipid layer to spread evenly and to be efficient in preventing water evaporation. On the other end, tear water evaporation building up an inflammatory status on the ocular surface seems to be able to reduce tear production from the lacrimal gland (Barabino et al. 2007).

films, a function of the volume and the compositional characteristics of the available aqueous fluid. A quality-wise altered composition of tensioactive proteins of the aqueous phase as well as an insufficient volume of fluid could hinder the ability of the lipids of the film to spread into an even, regular, effective lipid layer.

In severe ADDE, spreading may be undetectable, suggesting a major defect in the tear film lipid layer (TFLL) function. Delayed or absent spreading of the tear film could lead to an increase in water loss from the eye.

This could explain why the correlation between lipid thickness and evaporative tear film thinning can be sometimes poor (King-Smith et al. 2009) and why a higher than normal evaporation rate is frequent in ADDE as well (Rolando et al. 1983a).

The use of dynamic lipid interference pattern (DLIP) testing (Rolando et al. 2008) shows that the ability to reproduce the lipid interference patterns at each blink, for several times, which is a feature characteristic of normal eyes, is lost or highly diminished in DED patients, suggesting a difficulty in maintaining the proper dynamic performances of

Table 5.1 Factors affecting tear water evaporation

Intrinsic
Lipid layer composition and architecture
Lipid layer thickness
Lipid layer dynamics (ability to spread evenly and quickly)
Lipid-layer–aqueous-layer proteins interactions
Tear film water volume
Interpalpebral fissure size
Blink rate
Blink completeness
Ocular surface regularity

Extrinsic
Temperature
Relative humidity
Airflow
Air composition (lipid diluent in the environment, such as in sick building syndrome)
Use of contact lens

the lipid layer in these patients regardless of the original pathogenetic factor of the condition (**Figure 5.2**).

The evaluation of the possible causative risk factors could be important and their presence has to be balanced to help the assessment of the primary source of the tear dysfunction and the planning of an effective therapeutic strategy.

Due to the fact that aqueous deficiency is a cause of increased evaporation, that prolonged evaporation can slow down tear fluid production (Barabino et al. 2007), and that most symptoms and signs of DED are non-specific and relate to the resulting ocular surface damage rather than the cause of DED, differential diagnosis between ADDE and EDE can be difficult in many cases.

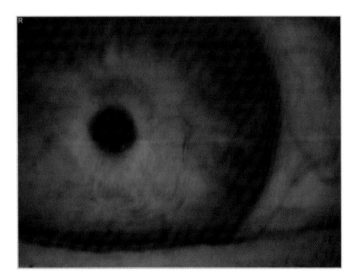

Figure 5.2 The lipid layer on the tear film surface has a memory. Interference patterns of lipids can be recognized quite easily on the tear film surface, and they, under normal conditions, tend to maintain and repeat their shape over several blinks (12–20), probably indicating good elasticity and ability of spreading as a result of the proper combination of several intrinsic characteristics such as lipid composition and quantity and availability of water and tensioactive proteins.

GENERAL PHYSICAL AND OCULAR EXAMINATION

Tear dysfunction is characterized by the presence of typical symptoms. Even if the description of its symptoms can vary from patient to patient due to specific personal physical characteristics or ethnic and cultural environment, burning, foreign body sensation, scratchy eyelids at movement, as well as pain, blurred vision, or photophobia are the most frequently reported complaints.

Some considerations about these common symptoms could be made in order to grasp some hint about the pathophysiological events occurring in our patient.

In normal subjects, forcedly keeping the eyelids wide open results in a growing sensation of burning after a while. This suggests that burning is somehow associated with evaporation of water from the ocular surface and can be arbitrarily interpreted as an indicator of the osmotic changes occurring on the tear film. On the other hand, foreign body sensation during blink could be interpreted as a lack of lubrication, suggesting a reduced volume of tear fluid available at the interface between the bulb and the lids indicating aqueous tear deficiency.

Unfortunately, because the two conditions are often concomitant in the clinically apparent DED, the presence or the predominance of one symptom over the other can only be suggestive but not highly significant for separation of an evaporative from an aqueous deficient tear dysfunction.

QUESTIONNAIRES

Current standard DED symptom questionnaires are not designed to differentiate between ADDE and EDE.

However, if the symptoms described are more associated with the lids, rather than the eye in general, then this could be indicative that some form of blepharitis or meibomian gland dysfunction (MGD) is involved and it suggests that further investigation of the meibomian glands is worthwhile. The recollection of personal habits, such as lid rubbing to relieve itching, is also of interest and a history of chalazion or hordeolum is also suggestive. In addition, since MGD is often associated with common skin diseases such as acne rosacea, atopic dermatitis, and seborrhoea sicca, as previously stated, a positive response to questions related to the presence or history of such conditions may be particularly important in the early asymptomatic form of the condition. In addition, MGD may be secondary to exposure to certain drugs, such as isotretinoin, or related to other environmental factors such as contact lens wear or smoking (Tomlinson et al. 2011).

While autoimmune diseases, bone marrow transplantation, cancer, menopausal hormone therapy, and sex hormone changes are significant risk factors for aqueous deficiency, the lack of essential fatty acids in the diet, low-humidity environments, computer use, contact lens wear, and less sharply keratorefractive surgery suggest hyperevaporation as the first agent in the DED cascade.

The evaluation of the presence of what we call an adverse environment will include physiological variation between individuals as well as the ambient conditions in which they live. A normal subject may have a low natural blink rate, or the blink rate may be slowed for behavioral or psychological reasons. The area of the palpebral aperture in the primary position varies between individuals and between ethnic groups, and the size of the exposed interpalpebral area affects the amount of water lost by evaporation from the ocular surface in a predictable way (Rolando 1983b).

FACE, LIDS, AND OCULAR EXAMINATION

Lid dysfunction and meibomian gland dysfunction

The face should be examined for signs of dermatitis, since this is often associated with lid disease (**Figure 5.3**).

It is true that, even if lipid changes associated with MGD are not the only cause of lipid layer malfunction and EDE, taking into consideration its frequency and the fact that most of the lipid layer constituents derive from the meibomian gland, a dysfunction or a disease of meibomian glands is accepted as the most common risk factor for EDE.

MGD is the main risk factor for EDE. It represents a progressive disorder of the meibomian glands of the eyelids that involves hyperkeratinization of the ductal epithelium of the glands and an increase in the viscosity of the secreted meibum, which can eventually lead to functional obstruction. The resulting reduction in the quantity, as well as a change in the quality of meibum on the lid margin and in the tear film, generally leads to tear film instability and EDE condition.

A number of morphological changes to the eyelids, particularly the eyelid margin and mucocutaneous junction, are typical of MGD and can be readily observed by everting and examining the lids. Thickening of the lid is a common feature of long-term MGD and is often associated with rounding of the posterior lid margin, giving it a convex appearance. Vascularization may also be pronounced (telangiectasis), while hyperkeratinization may impart an eczematous appearance to the cutaneous margin. The lid margin may appear to be irregular.

In MGD, the mucocutaneous junction, which represents the dividing line between the lipid-wettable skin of the lid margin and the water-wettable mucosa, becomes irregular and may appear to move anterior or more posterior to the gland orifices (**Figure 5.4**).

An early sign of MGD is elevation or pouting of the orifice, which is no longer flush with the surface. The orifice may also appear dilated. Finally, the orifice may become narrow and the punctum of the orifice may not be visible or may lose definition (meibomian gland drop out) (Tomlinson et al. 2011).

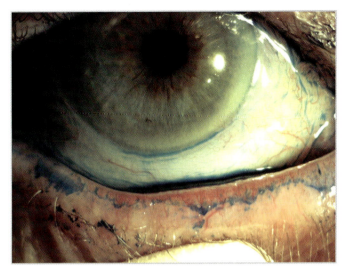

Figure 5.4 The convex appearance of the lid margin and the irregular scalloped profile of the mucocutaneous junction, evidentiated by lissamine green staining, reveal the presence of a long-lasting obstructive meibomian gland dysfunction with an inflammatory component in this eye.

APPLICATION OF GENERAL TESTS FOR DRY EYE

Measurement of the tear film break-up time and Schirmer's test

In theory, tear film break-up time (TFBUT) will be decreased in pure EDE, since changes in the lipid layer will make the tear film unstable. As a consequence, a low TFBUT together with a relatively normal Schirmer's value may be indicative of an EDE rather than ADDE. Unfortunately, because of the impact of pre-epithelial mucous layer on tear stability and the possible negative effect of chronic ocular surface stress on tear fluid production (Barabino et al. 2007), this is not always the case.

The Schirmer's test is used to assess the amount of tears secreted and is therefore primarily of benefit in diagnosing ADDE (DEWS 2007). Many studies have indicated that no significant differences exist in Schirmer's test values between patients with simple MGD and healthy control subjects. However, Schirmer's test scores have been shown to decrease with age, while signs of MGD, such as plugging of orifices, gland expressibility, and meibomian gland drop out, have been shown to increase.

By definition, a low Schirmer's test is the indicator of ADDE, while in early EDE, usually the Schirmer's test is in the normal range. Unfortunately, this is no longer the case in patients with a long-standing disorder in which the vicious cycle of ocular surface disease complicates the clinical patterns.

Vital staining

Lee and Tseng (1997) studied the patterns of vital staining in patients affected by lipid deficiency with unstable tear film and non-inflamed MGD. Vital staining was negative in 95 eyes (67%), positive on non-exposure zones in 30 eyes (21%), and positive on exposure zones in 17 eyes (12%).

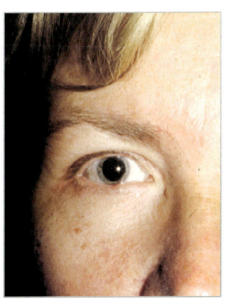

Figure 5.3 The observation of facial characteristics. It can give hints about the presence of dermatitis such as rosacea, which is a significant risk factor for meibomian gland dysfunction.

They suggested that preferential distribution of vital staining in the non-exposure zone characterizes lipid tear deficiency and helps to differentiate it from aqueous tear deficiency in patients with unstable tear film caused primarily by a lipid tear abnormality resulting from MGD (**Figure 5.5**).

One per cent lissamine staining as well as fluorescein staining observed through a yellow filter allows the observation of the mucocutaneous junction, which, in normals, is represented by a thin linear staining that thickens and appears irregular and scalloped in presence of MGD-related changes and can be a significant tool for an easy diagnosis.

OTHER MEASURES

Osmolarity

Measurement of tear osmolarity in presence of a theoretically adequate Schirmer's test is possibly the most reliable technique currently available for the diagnosis of EDE, with a value of 316 mOsmol/L producing an overall predictive accuracy of 89% for the diagnosis of DED (**Figure 5.6**).

Tear osmolarity used to be very difficult to measure in the clinic, but simple-to-use instruments are now becoming commercially available (Versura et al. 2010), and make measurement of tear osmolarity a more reasonable proposition in general clinical practice.

Evaporimetry

An increased evaporation rate of the tear film was first demonstrated in patients with ocular surface disease and posterior blepharitis (meibomitis) by Rolando and co-workers (1985) and measurement of tear film evaporation rate has subsequently been used in the study of DED. It has been confirmed (Mathers 1993) that the evaporation rate is increased in MGD, and has been suggested as a useful tool in differential diagnosis. However, at the present time, it remains a research tool.

Meibomian gland expression

In addition to the observation of morphological changes in the inner eyelids, meibomian gland expression is a mandatory technique to confirm the presence of changes in the quantity and quality of the lipids available for the ocular surface and it will suggest the amount of risk of tear water evaporation from the exposed ocular surface.

Meibum can be expressed from the glands by applying digital pressure on the lids. The quantity and quality of the fluid expressed and the amount of pressure required can be used to assess the presence and severity of MGD (Tomlinson et al. 2011).

Meiboscopy

Meiboscopy is a technique in which white light from a transilluminator is applied onto the cutaneous side of the everted eyelid, which allows observation and documentation of morphological changes in meibomian glands from the conjunctival side. A non-contact method of meibography, to get images of the meibomian glands eyelids from the mucosal side using infrared photography, has been developed (DEWS 2007).

Meibometry

Meibometry is a technique in which the meibomian lipids are blotted onto a loop of plastic tape from the central third of the lower lid margin and the amount of lipids taken up is measured optically or with a densitometer. The band becomes more or less translucent depending on the amount of oil associated with the lid margin. This method has shown that the lipid level of MGD sufferers is significantly lower than that of patients with tear-deficient dry eyes and normal subjects (Yokoi et al. 1999). Its clinical relevance has to be proved.

Tear meniscus radius, height, and cross-sectional area measurements

Tear meniscus measurement at the slit lamp with a McIntire lens is usually 0.23 ± 0.09 mm in normal eyes and 0.1 ± 0.04 mm in dry eyes.

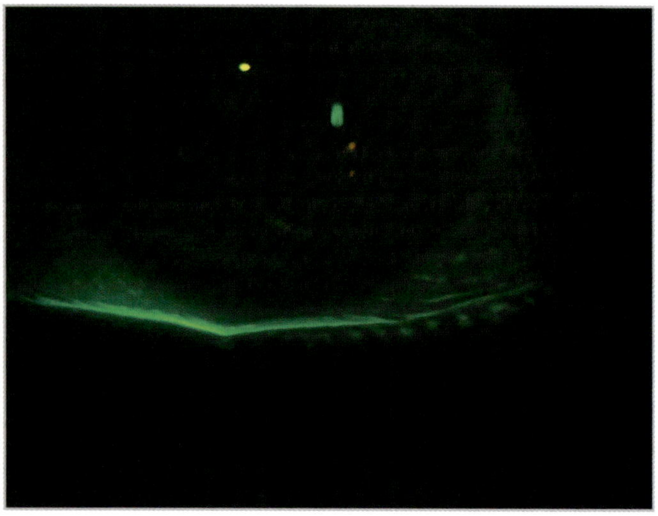

Figure 5.5 Fluorescein staining of the ocular surface reveals the irregular profile of the lid margin, irregular mucocutaneous junction, and a low-riding staining of the cornea, suggesting changes in lipid layer composition and function.

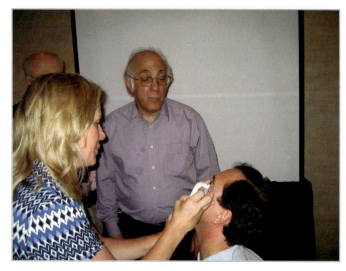

Figure 5.6 Measurement of tear meniscus osmolarity by means of the TearLab. The instrument provides quick, 'practically non-invasive' measurement of instant tear osmolarity.

If fluorescein instillation is used to improve accuracy, the resulting values are reliable and corresponding to the measurements performed before fluorescein instillation, if taken 4–7 minutes after the instillation of the dye (Lim & Lee 1991) (**Figure 5.7**).

Meniscometry

With this method, the subject is seated at a slit lamp, and is introduced coaxially; images of the tear meniscus (of either or both eyes), on which a target comprising a series of black and white stripes is projected, are recorded and transferred to a computer to calculate the radius of curvature of the meniscus (Dogru et al. 2006).

It has been shown that the meniscus radius is directly related to the total tear volume over the ocular surface (Yokoi et al. 2004). Furthermore, other data (Creech et al. 1998) suggest that the precorneal aqueous layer thickness is proportional to the meniscus radius, indicating that this technique is useful to diagnose aqueous deficiency conditions in a non-invasive way.

A study has shown a positive relationship between meniscus radius and initial velocity of the TFLL spread measured by dynamic interferometry, a significant indicator of tear film function, which strongly supports the concept that this parameter is influenced by tear volume, particularly tear film thickness. Thus, it is likely that the decrease in initial velocity of the TFLL spread in patients with ADDE is related to reduction in tear film thickness.

More recently, anterior segment optical coherence tomography (OCT) has been proposed as a good non-invasive method to measure tear meniscus parameters (Savini et al. 2006). Its major advantage compared to meniscometry is that room light is sufficient for monitoring the eye position and no visible light is required for the OCT system, which could cause some reflex tearing and result in an increase in tear meniscus size.

Interferometry

One requirement for maintaining a stable tear film is that a sufficient amount of superficial lipids must spread very rapidly onto a thin film with appropriate thickness and uniformity in order to give proper refractive qualities to the eye surface and control water evaporation.

Interferometry is a non-invasive technique that uses the interference patterns produced when split light beams are reflected back from the surface of the eye to assess tear film stability and spreading. Analysis of the interference patterns produced is done to differentiate between healthy and dry eyes and grade DED severity. It is also useful in differential diagnosis and can provide an indication of lipid layer thickness (Craig & Tomlinson 1997).

Tear lipid layer interference images can be observed using devices such as Tearscope (Keeler, Windsor, UK) or other more sophisticated techniques. Lipid layer thickness can be estimated using color comparison method. Kinetic analysis of interference images helps to measure lipid spread time.

It has been suggested that the thickness of the lipid layer, evaluated by interferometry by color comparison, is a good marker of protection from evaporation, but there are evidences that this is not the case as we can observe high evaporation rates in very thin but also in thick lipid layers.

Craig and Tomlinson (1997) studied the relation between evaporation rate and lipid layer patterns (and, hence, estimated lipid thickness) observed using a Tearscope. They found no significant differences in evaporation rates between different lipid patterns corresponding to medium lipid thickness, but evaporation rates were significantly increased, by about four times, in patients with no detectable lipid layer.

Unexpectedly, subjects with thick but abnormal lipid layers also experienced significantly increased evaporation.

More significant in identifying the functional ability of the lipid layer can be the observation and recording of its dynamic behavior. Goto and Tseng (2003), using kinetic analysis of tear interference images, found that although the tear lipid film spread time in normal eyes is short (0.3 ± 0.2 seconds), it is much longer in dry eyes with lipid and aqueous tear deficiency (3.5 ± 1.8 and 2.2 ± 1.1 seconds, respectively).

While ADDE tend to form vertical striped interference patterns, normal eyes have more horizontally shaped patterns on the surface of the lipid layer.

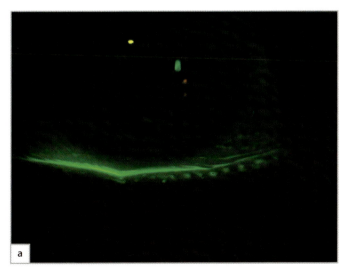 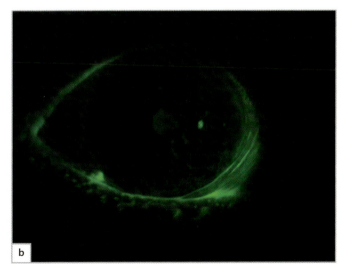

Figure 5.7 (a) A thick meniscus characterizes this eye with typical punctate staining of the lower cornea, suggesting an evaporative pathogenesis. (b) A very thin meniscus is present on the surface of this eye with extensive cornea damage and suggests a decreased tear production as the initial main pathogenic culprit for the disease.

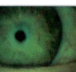

Figure 5.8 The dynamic lipid interference patterns (DLIP) test allows a numeric quantification of the ability of the lipid layer to maintain its interference pattern memory. The results of the test are expressed as the number of blinks preceding the inability to further recognize the previously identified interference pattern. (a) DLIP test results in a normal eye; at each blink the interference bands repeat the same pattern several times. (b) However, in a dry eye disease patient, after each blink the interference patterns change significantly.

Studies using interferometry have indicated that the TFLL remains stable over several blink cycles, before abruptly becoming restructured. The cycle of stability has been shown to be shortened in the presence of MGD, and this has been proposed as a measure of MGD-related disease in the DLIP test (Rolando et al. 2008).

The DLIP test has been introduced that allows a numeric quantification of the ability of the lipid layer in maintaining its interference pattern memory, which is a consistent typical feature of normal eyes.

In fact, remarkable morphological constancy of the interference patterns in normal subjects over successive blinks was reported by Mishima in the normal rabbit tear film (Mishima & Maurice 1961) and by Bron and Tiffany (2004) (EVER meeting, Alicante, October 2003). These studies suggest that substantial regions of the TFLL have a stable structure over a series of blinks. The DLIP test is based on the stability of the shape of the colored interference patterns in normal subjects, and on its irregular change of shape in patients with DED after a series of blinks. If this is the result of quantitative or qualitative primary lipid deficiencies, it is the consequence of the lack of an appropriate amount of water or of the lack of an appropriate substance allowing lipid spreading and stability (**Figures 5.8a and b**).

The test allows for a simple quantification of this specific behavior of the lipid layer and its results are expressed as the number of blinks preceding the inability to further recognize the identified interference pattern. The value of 6.5 consecutive blinks, providing the same consistent lipid layer interference pattern of the tear film, seems to be the best (sensitivity of 0.98 and a specificity of 0.95) in separating normal from dry eyes.

A positive DLIP test indicates that the inability to maintain a constant lipid pattern for more than six blinks is suggestive of dry eyes.

If this is associated with a normal secretion of tears (Schirmer's test >5.5 mm per 5 minutes), the suspicion of a relevant impact of evaporation caused by a malfunctioning lipid layer on the pathogenesis of the disease should be raised.

CONCLUSION

In conclusion, the separation of the two main classes of DED (ADDE and EDE) is not always easy in a clinical setting where often many of the tests are borderline and tend to change from one visit to the other.

In clear-cut cases, a normal tear secretion with thick meniscus but low break-up time (BUT) and/or bad dynamic behavior of the lipid layer should suggest an increased evaporation as the main source of dysfunction, while a thin, scanty meniscus or a Schirmer's test <5 mm per 5 minutes associated with a low BUT or a bad dynamic lipid behavior makes us think of aqueous deficiency.

When it is more diffuse, the clinical measurement of osmolarity will give a precious hint in evaluating how the ability to produce new tears can compensate the level of evaporation of the eye that we observe.

Due to the dynamic aspects and the changes in relevance of the pathogenetic factors during the evolution of DED with time, in a clinical setting, a clear-cut separation of the two main sources of tear film disease may be difficult. Nevertheless, the combination of the results of the different tests will allow us to address the therapy toward the particular dysfunction active on the ocular surface, correcting, if possible, the failures that maintain or aggravate the vicious cycles that are the basis of the disease.

REFERENCES

Barabino S, Rolando M, Chen L, Dana MR. Exposure to a dry environment induces strain-specific responses in mice. *Exp Eye Res* 2007; **84**:973–977.

Bron AJ, Tiffany JM. The contribution of meibomian disease to dry eye. *Ocul Surf* 2004; **2**:149–165.

Ciprandi G, Buscaglia S, Pesce G, et al. Effects of conjunctival hyperosmolar challenge in allergic subjects and normal controls. *Int Arch Allergy Immunol* 1994; **104**:92–96.

Craig JP, Tomlinson A. Importance of the lipid layer in human tear film stability and evaporation. *Optom Vis Sci* 1997; **74**:8–13.

Creech JL, Do LT, Fatt I, Radke CJ. In vivo tear-film thickness determination and implications for tear-film stability. *Curr Eye Res* 1998; **17**:1058–1066.

DEWS. The definition and classification of dry eye disease: report of the Definition and Classification Sub committee of the International Dry Eye WorkShop (2007). *Ocul Surf* 2007; **5**:75–92.

Dogru M, Ishida K, Matsumoto Y, et al. Strip meniscometry: a new and simple method of tear meniscus evaluation invest. *Ophthalmol Vis Sci* 2006; **47**:1895–1901.

Goto E, Tseng SCG. Kinetic analysis of tear interference images differentiates lipid tear deficient patients from normal subjects. *Arch Ophthalmol* 2003; **121**:173–180.

King-Smith P, Fink B, Nichols J, et al. The contribution of lipid layer movement to tear film thinning and breakup. *Invest Ophthalmol Vis Sci* 2009; **50**:2747–2756.

Lim KJ, Lee JH. Measurement of tear meniscus height using 0.25 fluorescein sodium. *Korean J Ophthalmol* 1991; **5**:34–36.

Lee SH, Tseng SC. Rose bengal staining and cytologic characteristics associated with lipid tear deficiency. *Am J Ophthalmol* 1997; **124**:736–750.

Luo L, Li DQ, Corrales RM, Pflugfelder SC. Hyperosmolar saline is a proinflammatory stress on the mouse ocular surface. *Eye Contact Lens* 2005; **31**:186–193.

Mathers WD. Ocular evaporation in meibomian gland dysfunction and dry eye. *Ophthalmology* 1993; **100**:347–351.

Mishima S, Maurice DM. The oily layer of the tear film and evaporation from the corneal surface. *Exp Eye Res* 1961; **1**:39–45.

Rolando M, Geerling G, Dua HS, Benítez-del-Castillo JM, Creuzot-Garcher C. Emerging treatment paradigms of ocular surface disease: proceedings of the Ocular Surface Workshop. *Br J Ophthalmol* 2010; **94**:1–9.

Rolando M, Refojo MF. Tear evaporimeter for measuring water evaporation rate from the tear film under controlled conditions in humans. *Exp Eye Res* 1983a; **36**:25–33.

Rolando M, Refojo MF, Kenyon KR. Increased tear evaporation in eyes with keratoconjunctivitis sicca. *Arch Ophthalmol* 1983b; **101**:557–558.

Rolando M, Refojo MF, Kenyon KR. Tear water evaporation and eye surface diseases. *Ophthalmological* 1985; **190**:147–149.

Rolando M, Valente C, Barabino S. New test to quantify lipid layer behavior in healthy subjects and patients with keratoconjunctivitis sicca. *Cornea* 2008; **27**:866–870.

Savini G, Barboni P, Zanini M. Tear meniscus evaluation by optical coherence tomography. *Ophthalmic Surg Lasers Imaging* 2006; **37**:112–118.

Tomlinson A, Bron AJ, Korb DR, et al. The international workshop on meibomian gland dysfunction: report of the diagnosis subcommittee. *Invest Ophthalmol Vis Sci* 2011; **52**:2006–2049.

Tsubota K, Yamada M. Tear evaporation from the ocular surface. *Invest Ophthalmol Vis Sci* 1992; **33**:2942–2950.

Versura P, Profazio V, Campos EC. Performance of tear osmolarity compared to previous diagnostic tests for dry eye diseases. *Curr Eye Res* 2010; **35**:553–564.

Yokoi N, Bron AJ, Tiffany JM, et al. Relationship between tear volume and tear meniscus curvature. *Arch Ophthalmol* 2004; **122**:1265–1269.

Yokoi N, Mossa F, Tiffany J, Bron AJ. Assessment of meibomian gland function in dry eye using meibometry. *Arch Ophthalmol* 1999; **117**:723–729.

Chapter 6 The clinical utility of objective tests (biomarkers)

Michael A. Lemp

INTRODUCTION

As described in Chapter 3, dry eye disease (DED) is a progressive and chronic disease involving the lacrimal glands, meibomian glands, the ocular surface, the afferent and efferent tracts distributing tears to the preocular surface tear film, the fornices, and the marginal tear strips. In normal subjects, the lacrimal function unit is well connected via a neural network, allowing this integrated unit to respond to changes in environmental stress and systemic effects on these components. This functional unit, which controls secretion from the lacrimal glands, mucin-producing elements of the ocular surface, and the meibomian glands of the eyelids, maintains a homeostatic tear film–ocular surface interaction, which provides remarkable stability. This, in turn, subserves visual function by providing a semistable tear film between blinks, which acts as the anterior refracting surface of the visual system (Stern et al. 1998).

In contrast, patients with DED demonstrate a loss of this homeostatic control resulting in an unstable, hyperconcentrated tear film, which demonstrates rapid break-up of the tear film between blinks, resulting in a decrease in visual acuity, contrast sensitivity, and, in most patients, symptoms of irritation. Studies have demonstrated a substantial loss of quality-of-life measures in these subjects. As the disease progresses, damage to the ocular surface is apparent and revealed by ocular staining. In aqueous tear-deficient dry eye (ADDE), tests of aqueous tear production, such as Schirmer's test, phenol red, and tear turnover, show a decrease. In evaporative dry eye (EDE), which is most commonly seen in meibomian gland dysfunction, changes in the appearance of the lid margin and the quantity of secretion of the meibomian glands are seen (DEWS 2007). As disease progresses, more of these different aspects of disease become apparent. The challenge in recognizing DED is primarily in early mild cases, which gives rise to symptoms of irritation in most but not all patients. This challenge is further complicated by the well-known lack of correlation between signs and symptoms in DED (Nichols et al. 2004). There is anecdotal evidence that many of the commonly recommended tests are not employed in clinical practice because they do not correlate well with a physician's overall assessment. This fact complicates not only diagnosis but also assessment of severity and establishment of useful endpoints for clinical trials in the development of new therapeutic intervention. Recent studies have revealed new information that allows us to place these tests in a better focus and establish their roles in the diagnosis and management of DED.

COMMONLY USED TESTS IN THE DIAGNOSIS OF DRY EYE DISEASE

A survey of practicing clinicians revealed the most commonly employed (or at least recommended) tests; these include the Schirmer's test (with and without anesthesia), corneal and conjunctival staining, tear film break-up time (TBUT), and assessment of lid margin for changes in appearance and in the quantity and quality of meibomian gland excretion (Korb 2000). There has been increased interest in biomarkers that reflect an overall measure of severity of disease, particularly because of the view of most clinicians that there is a lack of correlation between signs and symptoms. In general, the terms (bio) markers, surrogates, endpoints, outcomes, and others, have been used to describe a metric that is either objective or subjective, which accurately reflects the characteristics of disease, and has been defined as a 'laboratory measurement or a physical sign used as a substitute for a clinically meaningful endpoint that measures directly how a patient feels, functions or survives' (Ellenberg & Hamilton 1989). The value of such a metric lies in how accurately it can capture important aspects of the disease. Such measures are typically used clinically in diagnosis, assessment of disease severity, and response to therapy. In addition, physicians place value in symptoms reported by patients, which can be captured in questionnaires and quantitated. Let us consider the information about the most commonly used tests and assess the clinical utility of each of these tests.

Schirmer's test

Originally described in 1903, and used throughout the world, this is a test that aims to measure aqueous tear production, wherein a strip of filter paper is inserted over the inferior lid margin and the length of filter paper that is wetted is measured in millimeters after 5 minutes. Usually, a topical anesthetic is instilled prior to measurement to reduce the irritating effects of the strip on the conjunctiva, which can trigger reflex tearing. It has been thought that this might represent 'basal' tearing; however, it has been shown that while tearing is lessened by decreasing some of the sensory input, stimuli from the lid margin and lashes are unaffected. Therefore, most clinicians perform this test without anesthetic. There are several variations of this methodology such as the phenol red test, in which a color-impregnated thread is substituted for the strip. One limitation of this test is that it is a measure only of aqueous tear production and does not capture metrics pertaining to EDE. Additionally, it is susceptible to wide intrasubject, day-to-day, and visit-to-visit variation. More consistent readings are attainable with increasing severity of disease, as the test scoring has a lower boundary limit of 0 mm measurement. A recent study has demonstrated that in mild-to-moderate DED, Schirmer's test results lack sensitivity and are essentially a 'random number generator' (Sullivan et al. 2010). This test tends to improve in accuracy in moderate-to-severe disease in which most subjects have a mixed or hybrid form of the disease.

Tear film break-up time

Tear instability is a hallmark of the DED state. It affects vision and contributes to the loss of homeostatic control of the lacrimal functional unit, giving rise to the variability of many clinical tests used to assess this disease. Tear instability is, therefore, of particular interest, and accurate measurement of this factor could provide information that reflects a principal axis of the disease. The tear break-up test has been used as a measure of tear instability for decades. Most commonly, it is measured after the instillation of a defined volume of fluorescein, followed by assessment of the rapidity with which the tear film begins to break up after a blink. Values of <10 seconds have been recommended as diagnostic thresholds; however, more recently, the use of smaller volumes (5 mL) of instilled 2% fluorescein with a referent value of 5 seconds has been recommended. Unfortunately, this test suffers from limitations such as poor reproducibility and low performance accuracy, and the fact that other events such as the presence of surface irregularities will influence results.

Attempts to standardize the assessment of tear instability have centered on the development of automated visual capture of serial images using videokeratography to eliminate the subjective aspects of tear instability measurement. Several different algorithm-driven programs have been described. While more rapid interblink TBUTs have clearly been demonstrated in patients with DED, the range of normative values and relationships over the spectrum of DED severity are yet to be elucidated. Recently, there has been an interest in a group of patients in Japan complaining of symptoms of irritation, with little or no corneal staining and a short TBUT (Kaido et al. 2012). Whether these patients represent a new disease entity or an example of early mild DED, as described elsewhere, remains to be determined.

Ocular surface staining

The definition of DED expressed in the DEWS report emphasizes on damage to the ocular surface. For many years, damage has been assessed using vital dyes that increase visibility of areas of discontinuity on the corneal and conjunctival surfaces. Fluorescein solutions are common in current clinical practice to assess corneal disruptions; rose Bengal staining, and more recently lissamine green, has been implemented to visualize these areas of the conjunctiva. Ocular surface staining is used to diagnose DED, to assess its severity, and as a clinical endpoint in clinical trials for pharmaceutical effect.

It should be noted, however, that the precise nature of damage revealed by staining methods, and whether distinct clinical patterns of staining reflect different changes to the ocular surface, remain undefined. Traditionally, positive rose Bengal staining was thought to be due to a breakdown in the structure of the cell wall of conjunctival surface cells; however, experimental studies revealed that discontinuities in the mucin coating of the cells corresponded to the patterns of staining observed. Fluorescein staining of the corneal surface is thought to reflect a breakdown in the cell barrier to aqueous solutions, but the import of differences in staining patterns (punctate vs. confluent) is unclear (Foulks 2010). Recent reports have described changes in mucin expression in patients with DED, which may account for some of the patterns of corneal staining that have been seen. Although there are other grading systems that have been described, for example, the Baylor and the Ora systems, we will consider only those in general use.

Several grading systems for assessing severity of ocular surface staining have been developed. These include an older van Bijsterveld system, the National Eye Institute/Industry Report system, and the Oxford system. The latter two are the most commonly used systems in clinical trials. They differ in the subdivisions of the corneal and conjunctival surfaces, and the progression of severity (e.g. the Oxford progression is geometric).

Recent evaluation of corneal and conjunctival staining in DED, as measured using a composite index of severity over the entire range of

disease, demonstrated that in mild-to-moderate disease, <50% of subjects demonstrated any corneal staining (Sullivan et al. 2010). A slightly higher fraction of subjects displayed evidence of conjunctival staining; however, much higher percentages would be expected if staining were a precise indicator of the presence of disease. This exemplifies the problems that can arise if the presence of ocular surface staining is used for the diagnosis of disease. This demonstrates the danger in using just one of the currently widely used metrics for diagnosis. While staining provides an important piece of information, it is not necessarily informative for overall disease assessment. In summary, ocular surface staining remains a useful data point for assessing DED, but it can be misleading if considered alone. As with most of the tests, staining measurements become more informative in more advanced stages of disease but lack specificity in mild-to-moderate disease.

Tear osmolarity

For over half a century, it has been known that the osmolarity of the tears in DED is elevated. While several devices have been developed to measure the osmolarity of bodily fluids, the scanty volume of tears available for sampling in both normal subjects and DED patients has limited this measurement as a practical clinical tool. The introduction of a new technology employing collection of a 50-nL sample from the inferior marginal tear strip and rapid analysis via tear impedance has provided clinicians and researchers with a highly accurate tool (Lemp et al. 2011). Hyperosmolar tears are regarded as the central pathogenetic mechanism in DED. Hyperosmolarity, regardless of symptomatic status, has been shown to induce inflammation, including an upregulation of interleukin (IL)-1b, tumor necrosis factor-a, and matrix metalloprotein-9, and activation of c-Jun N-terminal kinase, extracellular signal-regulated kinase, and mitogen-activated protein kinase pathways. Additionally, hyperosmolarity has been shown to activate caspase-3 and cytochrome c pathways that cause spontaneous epithelial cell death. Hyperosmolarity causes decreased intracellular connections, loss of microplicae, cell membrane disruption, and increased desquamation. An increase in the concentration of tears also has functional consequences, wherein a hyperosmolar tear film has been directly associated with fluctuating vision. Most importantly, data suggest that an increase in osmolarity directly reduces the ability of the cornea and lid to maintain proper boundary lubrication, thereby increasing friction during each blink and likely manifesting long-term wear and lid epitheliopathies evident in DED.

In the recently published 2011 American Academy of Ophthalmology Preferred Practice Patterns on Dry Eye Syndrome, it is noted that 'tear osmolarity has been shown to be a more sensitive method of diagnosing and grading the severity of DED compared to corneal and conjunctival staining, tear break-up. Tear osmolarity was also found to be a superior correlate to a composite disease severity index as compared to the other most common tests for DED.' In addition, tear osmolarity has been shown to exhibit the lowest variability over time and the highest sensitivity to therapeutic intervention as compared to corneal staining, TBUT, Schirmer's tests, and meibomian gland grading (Sullivan et al. 2012). In effect, tear osmolarity gives a direct insight into the health of the ocular surface while predicting response to therapy before symptoms or the other signs have been resolved.

Despite the extensive literature detailing the effects of hyperosmolarity on the ocular surface, many clinicians have not had first-hand experience interpreting results, which can lead to confusion and incorrect conclusions surrounding its clinical utility. For diagnosis, the most important difference between osmolarity and other tests is that the unstable tear film and its effects on compensatory mechanisms require that both eyes be tested to make a proper determination. Once that is completed, a positive determination is made if either of the eyes is >308 mOsm/L or the difference between the eyes is ≥8 mOsm/L. Since a normal homeostatic tear film is isotonic with plasma osmolarity (290 mOsm/L), either the elevation of osmolarity or significant differences between eyes are indicators of tear film instability and an unhealthy ocular surface. For instance, a mildly symptomatic subject may exhibit a two-eye reading of 304/295 mOsm/L (right eye/left eye). While the two-eye maximum is clearly elevated from 290 mOsm/L, it is below the 308 mOsm/L threshold. However, given that the low analytical variance {±4mOsm/L [TearLabFDA510(k); www.accessdata.fda.gov/cdrh_docs/pdf8/K083184.pdf (Last accessed 02 April 2013)]} makes the number statistically equivalent to 308 mOsm/L, coupled with presence of symptoms and a ≥8-mOsm/L difference between the eyes, these findings are indicative of a loss of homeostatic control of the ocular surface, a hallmark of DED.

GRADING OF MEIBOMIAN GLAND DYSFUNCTION

The meibomian glands of the lid margins form an integral part of the lacrimal function unit providing for the outer lipid layer of the tear film, which decreases evaporative tear loss and facilitates lubricity for lid movement over the ocular surface. There are various schemes that have been described to capture the features of this disease, which is the most common subtype of DED. The one in most common use (Foulks & Bron 2003) has been optimized for clinical research, in which the vasculature and the excretion of the oil glands of the lids are noted and graded.

OTHER OBJECTIVE MARKERS OF DRY EYE DISEASE

Other tests that are in various stages of development include tear film interferometry and tear protein analysis. The former has been of interest with the development of more automated capture and measurement of tear film and lipid layer thickness. In general, there is a moderate correlation between thin lipid layers and symptoms of ocular irritation, but as yet, there is a paucity of normative and repeatability data necessary to determine its role in clinical practice and research.

Much more is known concerning the presence of proinflammatory protein markers in the tears of DED patients. Both cytokines and chemokines have been reported to increase in DED, particularly in moderate-to-severe forms of the disease as seen in patients with Sjögren's syndrome. Minimal distinction between normal subjects and patients with mild DED has been noted using measurements of cytokines and chemokines. Several of these molecular markers have been shown to increase in DED and to respond to treatment with topically applied cyclosporine A (Pflugfelder 2011). The advent of microarray technology, particularly, multiplex bead arrays and highly sensitive enzyme-linked immunosorbent assay tests for proteins, has spurred investigation aimed at identifying patterns of protein elevation; although, some obstacles remain in interpreting results of microwell arrays that produce interfering effects that can greatly reduce signal-to-noise ratio and limit the ability to obtain meaningful results. In spite of these potential concerns, a number of panels of these proteins have shown promise as diagnostic biomarkers and have been advanced as suitable markers for DED. Other promising

techniques have also recently been described for collecting and measuring cytokines present in tear fluid, including extraction of cytokines and MMPs from Schirmer's strips followed by Luminex analysis. Numerous cytokines and MMPs were detected in the tear samples of healthy volunteers using this methodology; however, future studies will be required to determine whether tear quantity and quality can be similarly measured in DED subjects. Other recent studies have presented normative values for the presence of cytokines and chemokines in tears. As further investigations refine the relations between these patterns, their association with severity of disease and response to treatment, and the emergence of simplified assays for clinical use, their utility may become clearer.

One particular proinflammatory marker that has received much recent attention is MMP-9. This protein is widespread in the body and is associated with tissue repair and remodeling. MMP-9 is present in very small amounts in normal tears and rises considerably in DED. While not specific for DED, MMP-9 activation is associated with tissue damage from inflammation, which is a prominent feature of DED in moderate-to-severe cases. Several studies have demonstrated the rise of MMP-9 in DED. In one study measuring tear levels of MMP-9, the protein was elevated across four levels of increasing disease severity (Chotikavanich et al. 2009). However, the actual expression levels were significantly lower for grades 1 and 2 than for grades 3 and 4. It is of interest to note that the categorization of subjects in the study was primarily based on corneal staining. Since other studies have shown that <50% of patients with mild-to-moderate disease have corneal staining (see below), it may be that MMP-9 correlates very well with staining, but not necessarily DED. MMP-9 levels in the tears have been shown to be elevated in ocular surface diseases other than DED. The recent commercialization of an office test for MMP-9 (RPS InflammaDry Detector), which is qualitative, may prove useful in identifying patients with a significant inflammatory component and, therefore, likely to respond to anti-inflammatory therapy; however, it should also be noted that RPS excludes the difficult-to-diagnose mild-to-moderate subjects [with ocular surface disease index (OSDI) between 1 and 13] in order to achieve the performance reported in its labeling. Given that MMP-9 correlates so well with staining, it is not clear whether the marker gives any additional information than ocular surface staining alone. Recently, Na et al. (2012) have determined cytokine and chemokine concentrations in the tears of DED patients and analyzed the possible relations with the clinical severity of DED. Patients were divided into four groups according to the Dry Eye Workshop severity classification. Tears were collected from 133 DED patients and 70 healthy controls. Concentrations of cytokines, chemokines, and soluble receptors in collected tear samples were analyzed. The levels of cytokines IL-1β, IL-6, IL-16, IL-33, granulocyte colony-stimulating factor, and transforming growth factor α were significantly higher in DED patients, while those of cytokines IL-4, IL-12, IL-17A, and interferon-γ were significantly lower. The levels of fractalkine [chemokine (C-X3-C motif) ligand 1; CX3CL1], monocyte chemotactic protein-1 [chemokine (C-C motif) ligand 2; CCL2], MIP-1δ [chemokine (C-C motif) ligand 15; CCL15], and ENA-78 [chemokine (C-X-C motif) ligand 5; CXCL5], respectively, and soluble receptors, soluble IL-1 receptor type 1 (sIL-1RI), soluble glycoprotein (sgp)130, sIL-6R, soluble epidermal growth factor receptor, and soluble tumor necrosis factor receptor 2 were higher in the DED patients. There were significant correlations between these molecules and the clinical severity of DED. The authors concluded that there is an increase in inflammatory cytokines IL-6 and IL-1β, during the earliest changes in DED patients, in addition to potential indicators of homeostatic process sIL-6R, sIL-6R, and sgp130. How exactly these 'earliest' DED cases were identified is unclear and the limitations of a categorical severity scale such as that of the DEWS report are discussed later in this chapter. The development of pathogenic inflammatory biomarkers will likely be clinically useful in diagnosing DED and its subtypes, and in directing treatment modalities.

In this era of advancing technology, broad studies at the proteomics level are becoming more affordable and feasible to carry out in patient populations. Thus, further research in these directions may identify other protein candidates and/or panels of proteins that represent clinically useful data to identify DED and its subtypes.

RELATIONSHIP BETWEEN INDIVIDUAL TESTS OF DRY EYE DISEASE

In recently published papers, it has been demonstrated that the commonly employed tests for DED diagnosis and management are variable over time (Sullivan et al. 2012). This is thought to be due primarily to the instability of the tear film seen in DED patients but not in normal healthy subjects. In this study, a cohort of 52 patients with DED was followed over a 3-month period, typical of a DED clinical trial. All objective tests and symptomatology, as measured by the OSDI, displayed significant variability, with tear osmolarity being the least variable (**Table 6.1**). In another recent study designed to test the correlation between subjective and objective tests, no correlations above $r^2 = 0.17$ were found between any signs or symptoms, except for corneal or conjunctival staining, which reported an $r^2 = 0.36$ (and measure similar events). In the multisite study, the average r^2 for osmolarity (0.07), TBUT (0.12), Schirmer's test (0.09), corneal (0.16) and conjunctival staining (0.17), meibomian grading (0.11), and OSDI (0.11) were consistently low. Similar results were observed in another study dataset. No consistent relation was found between common signs and symptoms of DED. Therefore, each type of measurement reveals different information about the condition of the ocular surface. Moreover, among patients who showed evidence of DED by consensus of clinical signs, only 57% reported symptoms (OSDI) consistent with a diagnosis of DED. These results demonstrate that symptoms alone are insufficient for the diagnosis and management of DED and argue for the clinical utility of a composite index of severity, which better reflects all aspects of the disease. Tear osmolarity results parallel this severity index.

Table 6.1 Tear film instability in DED

	Mild/Moderate (n = 16)	Severe (n = 36)	Overall (n = 52)
Osmolarity	5.9%	10.0%	8.7%
TBUT	16.0%	9.8%	11.7%
Schirmer's test	13.2%	9.5%	10.7%
Corneal	10.9%	12.3%	12.2%
Conjunctival	14.4%	14.8%	14.8%
MGD	14.5%	14.3%	14.3%
OSDI	3.8%	11.8%	9.3%

Standard Deviation/Dynamic Range of commonly used dry eye tests. Standard deviations were calculated using the more severe measurement on each day of observation. Values are expressed as percentages of the dynamic range for each test.

Composite index of disease severity

Given the statistical complexity inherent to the signs and symptoms of DED, there has been little guidance as to how to synthesize multiple data points into a single coherent index of overall disease severity. The traditional Delphi approach reprinted in the DEWS report outlines a 1–4 grading scheme, with 1 being mild or episodic DED and 4 being severe, constant, and disabling disease. Unfortunately, the Delphi schema does not supply a quantitative method for dealing with conflicts within individual patients, such as when a patient exhibits low break-up time but no apparent staining or symptoms. Conflicting data from a battery of clinical signs are more the norm than the exception. When coupled with a lack of consensus on any single gold standard test for DED, there is a need to quantitatively and objectively determine disease severity for clinical trials.

In creating a composite scale (Sullivan et al. 2010), clinical signs are combined by converting each data point into a common severity basis such as a scale of 0–4, or a 0–1 scheme, adding them together to generate a final severity score, then parsing the total into normal, mild-to-moderate, and severe categories. A similar but attenuated method was used in a seminal OSDI paper, as a means to check the performance of the symptom questionnaire. To create their index, the authors mixed Schirmer's test, lissamine green staining, and a subjective facial expression scale, with cutoffs for scoring determined by a literature review (e.g. Schirmer's normal values were >10 mm, mild-to-moderate values between 6–10 mm, and severe values <5 mm in length). For each sign, normal results were given 1 point, mild-to-moderate 2 points, and severe 3 points. The summed index was graded as ≤3 as normal, 4–7 as mild-to-moderate, and then 8–9 as severe. Although straightforward, there is a series of problems with this approach. Most importantly, when comparing signs against the total score, there is an inherent risk of ordinate bias against the composite abscissa. Few data are available about the facial expression scale used in the paper, but unsurprisingly, two measures of symptoms (OSDI and facial expressions) were shown to be very well correlated ($r = 0.669$). Especially when a composite is formed from a small number of variables, these biases can be significant. As a result, the OSDI showed a sensitivity of 60% against the physician rating, but jumped up to 80% sensitivity against the composite score with the facial expression as part of the abscissa. A second limitation of this approach is that in order to facilitate simplicity, the categories are discrete. A person with a 6/9 in lissamine green staining is given the same input to the total severity as someone with a with a 2/9 grading in staining or a 10 mm Schirmer's result. This resulting lack of resolution typically creates spurious false negatives or false positives in sensitivity and specificity analysis, which is unacceptable in regulatory environments.

A more recent attempt to create an objective, unbiased composite index outlined a continuous method for determining DED severity. In this approach, the standard procedure of relying upon clinical expertise to assign thresholds to each of seven quantitative measures was followed by fitting either a linear or an exponential function to the clinical breakpoints, depending on strength of fit. These functions were inverted, and allowed raw clinical data to be mapped on a common 0–1 scale without discretization (converting continuous differential equations into discrete ones). The next step, adding the individual dimensions together to form a final severity score, was accomplished by first rotating each dimension (equivalent to weighting each data point) by the amount of independent information the measure contributed to the composite. This independent components' analysis, unlike the direct linear addition approach used in previous studies, attempted to equalize correlation risk against the composite abscissa (point on the *x*-axis). Control data sets (random data with no clinical meaning) showed that the expected correlation was on the order $r^2 = 0.1$, which indicated the successful removal of bias for each clinical measure, that is, a sign that may provide the same, and thus redundant, information as another sign. This was in part due to the fact that there were many more inputs to the composite scale than in earlier attempts, so that any one measurement could not dominate the *x*-axis. Finally, the bases were geometrically combined to form a single normalized composite index from 0 to 1, with 0 having no evidence of disease and 1 the greatest. The resulting continuous index revealed the gross failure of threshold-based classification schemes for clinical trials (e.g. a patient must have *N* out of *M* tests above a threshold to qualify as a DED patient in the study), wherein basic thresholds failed to properly classify 63% of the mild-to-moderate subjects recruited for analysis.

The results of measuring the relation between the individual tests and the composite severity scale revealed that only one test—tear osmolarity—demonstrated a linear relation to the composite severity score (see Figure 3.3). This should not be too surprising since tear osmolarity is viewed as the central pathogenic mechanism resulting in damage to the ocular surface in DED. Thus, although it has been shown that osmolarity may be the ideal global biomarker correlating to disease severity—whether the DED is EDE, ADDE, or a hybrid—it does not define the etiology of the disease and the other biomarkers that remain useful in that role.

CONCLUSION

We have reviewed the major candidates for biomarker that will accurately reflect disease effects over the entire range of DED severity. There are a number of candidates that demonstrate good utility for subtypes of DED (i.e. ADDE or EDE), whereas others are still in early stages of testing and might prove to be of value with further development. Currently, however, only tear osmolarity has been found to serve as a clinically useful biomarker over a wide range of disease severity. It should be emphasized that the most commonly used objective tests (signs) do not correlate well, particularly in early DED. This means that they provide important but independent information about the disease; some of these become more reliable in more severe disease and/or are useful in differentiating subtypes of DED, that is, ADDE, EDE, or a mixed form of the disease. The increasing use of biomarkers may enable clinicians to more effectively recognize disease in patients, particularly at mild-to-moderate or early stages, and facilitate the evaluation of new treatment modalities for improved disease management.

REFERENCES

Chotikavanich S, de Paiva CS, Li de Q, et al. Production and activity of matrix metalloproteinase-9 on the ocular surface increase in dysfunctional tear syndrome. *Invest Ophthalmol Vis Sci* 2009; **50**:3203–3209.

DEWS. The definition and classification of dry eye disease: Report of the Definition and Classification Subcommittee of the International Dry Eye Workshop (2007). *Ocul Surf* 2007; **5**:75–92.

Ellenberg S, Hamilton JM. Surrogate endpoints in clinical trials: cancer. *Stat Med* 1989; **8**:405–413.

Foulks GN. Ocular surface cells: disease and repair. *Ocul Surf* 2010; **8**:47–48.

Foulks GN, Bron AJ. Meibomian gland dysfunction: a clinical scheme for description, diagnosis, classification, and grading. *Ocul Surf* 2003; **1**:107–126.

Kaido M, Ishida R, Dogru M, Tsubota K. Visual function changes after punctal occlusion with the treatment of short BUT type of dry eye. *Cornea* 2012; **31**:1009–1013.

Korb DR. Survey of preferred tests for diagnosis of the tear film and dry eye. *Cornea* 2000; **19**:483–486.

Lemp MA, Bron AJ, Baudouin C, et al. Tear osmolarity in the diagnosis and management of dry eye disease. *Am J Ophthalmol* 2011; **151**:792–798.

Na KS, Mok JW, Kim JY, Rho CR, Joo CK. Correlations between tear cytokines, chemokines, and soluble receptors and clinical severity of dry eye disease. *Invest Ophthalmol Vis Sci* 2012; **53**:5443–5450.

Nichols KK, Nichols JJ, GL Mitchell. The lack of association between signs and symptoms in patients with dry eye disease. *Cornea* 2004; **23**:762–770.

Pflugfelder SC. Tear dysfunction and the cornea: LXVIII Edward Jackson Memorial Lecture. *Am J Ophthalmol* 2011; **152**:900–909.e1.

Stern ME, Beuerman RW, Fox RI, et al. The pathology of dry eye; the interaction between the ocular surface and lacrimal glands. *Cornea* 1998; **17**:584–589.

Sullivan BD, Crews LA, Sönmez B, et al. Clinical utility of objective tests for dry eye disease: variability over time and implications for clinical trials and disease management. *Cornea* 2012; **31**:1008.

Sullivan BD, Whitmer D, Nichols KK, et al. An objective approach to dry eye severity. *Invest Ophthalmol Vis Sci* 2010; **51**:6125–6130.

Chapter 7

Tear dynamics and dry eye disease

Norihiko Yokoi, Georgi As. Georgiev

INTRODUCTION

Dry eye disease (DED) was defined by the International Dry Eye Workshop (DEWS) in 2007 as a multifactorial disease of the tears and ocular surface that results in discomfort, visual disturbance, and tear film (TF) instability, with potential damage to the ocular surface. It is accompanied by increased hyperosmolarity of the TF and inflammation of the ocular surface. This definition suggests the stratified structure of DED (**Figure 7.1**), which comprises a core mechanism, risk factors, and their connecting mechanisms. The core mechanism of DED comprises a vicious cycle between the TF and ocular surface epithelium. However, reflex tear secretion plays a role in the repair of the vicious cycle, which results in the attenuation of the core mechanism through the increase of aqueous tears (AT), leading to increased TF stability, and secretion of vitalizing factors such as epidermal growth factor, hepatocyte growth factor, tumor growth factor β, and vitamin A for the epithelium (Stern et al. 2004). This means that in the above-mentioned connecting mechanisms, aqueous tears deficiency (ATD) has the strongest impact because there is a positive relationship

between tear volume at the ocular surface and reflex tear secretion (Yokoi & Komuro 2004). Therefore, decreased reflex tear secretion in ATD may provide incomplete repair of the core mechanism, which is induced by ATD alone. As to the inflammation, it is possible that the vicious cycle results in that inflammation. However, according to the DEWS report, inflammation is not the result of, but instead is a part of the core mechanism, whereby hyperosmolarity and TF instability also constitute the common mechanism of DED.

There are at least four important connecting mechanisms between the risk factors and the core mechanism, through which the risk factors can enter into the vicious cycle. Those connecting mechanisms include (1) ATD, which is related to aging or drug usage (anticholinergic oral medicine, beta-blocker eye drops, etc.), diseases (Sjögren's syndrome, graft-versus-host disease, diabetes, etc.), and surgeries (brain surgery, etc.); (2) increased AT evaporation due to meibomian gland dysfunction, lifestyle-related factors including heavy visual display terminal work, air-conditioning, contact lens wear, and eye-closure difficulties such as lagophthalmos; (3) decreased wettability of ocular surface epithelium due to unknown causes or keratinization (Nishida et al. 1999) seen in severe inflammatory ocular surface diseases such as Stevens–Johnson syndrome, graft-versus-host disease, and ocular mucous membrane pemphigoid; and (4) increased friction between the bulbar conjunctiva or cornea and the palpebral conjunctiva during a blink, which is seen in superior limbic keratoconjunctivitis (Yokoi et al. 2003), conjunctivochalasis (CCh), entropion, and blepharoptosis. The fourth mechanism is not directly related to TF instability, but may worsen the epithelial damage and symptoms of DED. Even in DED cases, those risk factors and connecting mechanisms are often related duplicately.

RECENT MODEL FOR TEAR FILM AND TEAR FILM DYNAMICS

According to a recent model, the TF comprises the TF lipid layer (TFLL), aqueous-mucin (primarily MUC5AC) gel, and membrane-associated mucins located within the glycocalyx of surface epithelium. TF formation at eye opening comprises two major steps (**Figure 7.2**):

- AT deposition by the upper eyelid meniscus. The balance of surface tension and viscosity determines the thickness of tear fluid deposited onto the eye surface in the narrow region at the meniscus edge
- Subsequent TFLL spread that drags aqueous upward and ensures redistribution of AT

These two steps provide an explanation for the observations (Benedetto et al. 1984) that the superior TF thickens for about 1 second after a blink, whereas the inferior TF thins over a comparable time.

Decreased surface wettability of corneal epithelium may contribute to the instantaneous (prior to TFLL spread) TF break-up, immediately at eye opening (**Figure 7.3**, upper). The event typically occurs in the upper cornea, where the AT thickness at deposition is thinner and the

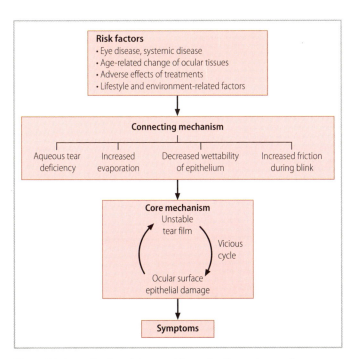

Figure 7.1 A stratification of the causal factors leading to dry eye disease (DED). DED is the outcome of risk factors, 'connecting' mechanisms, and a core mechanism that result in the symptoms. Risk factors are responsible for the core mechanism via the connecting mechanisms. Among the latter, increased friction is not directly related to tear film (TF) instability; however, it may worsen the epithelial damage and symptoms. Risk factors and the connecting mechanisms often have multiple interrelationships.

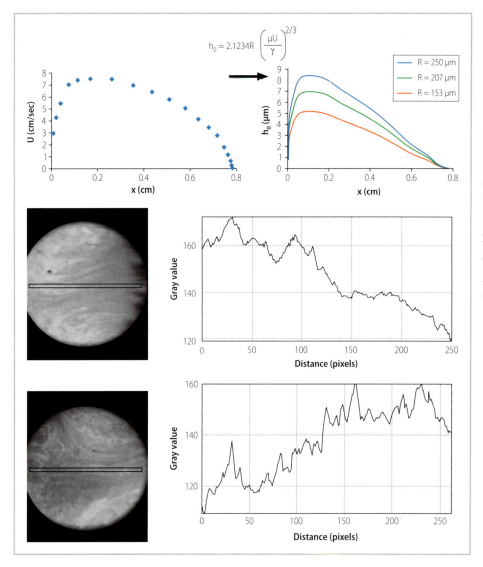

Figure 7.2 Step of precorneal tear film (TF) formation at eye opening (simplified scheme). Upper row, left panel: Upper eyelid velocity as a function of lid position; the origin of x is located at the lower lid margin. The dependence is calculated as explained by Jones et al. (2005). The data of upper eyelid velocity are converted in thickness by the denoted equation (Wong et al. 1996) where h0 = aqueous tear (AT) thickness at deposition; 2.1234 = numerical constant; R = upper menisci radius; μ = AT viscosity, 1.3x10-3 Pa s; γ = tear surface tension, 45 mN/m. Upper row, right panel: TF thickness profile calculated for various upper meniscus radii (Shen et al. 2009). Middle row: Intensity profile of the selected region in DR-1 video interferometer (Yokoi et al. 1996) images that illustrates the asymmetric deposition of AT by the eyelid prior to TF lipid layer (TFLL) spread; the thinner upper part of the TF is susceptible to dewetting. Bottom row: Intensity profile of selected region in DR-1 images that illustrates the upward drag of AT by the TFLL spread.

TF is most susceptible to dewetting if a micrometrically sized spot (a cluster of a few cells of decreased wettability) is present (Sharma & Ruckenstein 1989). The decreased wettability might be associated with the dysfunction and/or decreased expression of the membrane-associated mucins (Shanker et al. 1995, Sumiyoshi et al. 2008). The instantaneous break-up differs from the type of break-up that appears when an eye is kept open after the establishment of TF (**Figure 7.3**, lower). In the first type of break-up, a circular-like break-up ('spot break') can be seen, and in the second type, a linear-like break-up ('line break') is most typical. Considering that the 'spot break' can be attributed to the decreased wettability of the corneal surface epithelium, while the 'line break' can be attributed to the different mechanism of TF instability (e.g. evaporation; Kimball et al. 2010); these differences are considered quite important for deciding the correct treatment for DED. For the former, treatment for increasing wettability is necessary, but for the latter, treatment aimed at increasing TF stability is necessary. This might raise a question (Bron et al. 2009) regarding the classification of DED (DEWS 2007), where DED is divided into aqueous tear-deficient dry eye (ATDDE) and evaporative DED (dewettable DED, where the spot break is the main manifestation).

In Japan, currently, new eye drops (3% diquafosol sodium eye drops and 2% rebamipide eye drops) are commercially available that are reported to increase the expression of membrane-associated mucin together with goblet-cell-derived mucin (Takaoka-Shichijo & Nakamura 2011, Takaoka-Shichijo et al. 2011, Urashima et al. 2004). It is expected that these two, new eye drop medications will become candidates for treating the decreased wettability of the corneal surface, which can be confirmed by the spot break at the time of eye opening.

■ FUNCTION OF THE TEAR MENISCUS

The tear meniscus has a suction effect on AT at the meniscus due to negative capillary pressure (Δp) inside the meniscus, and this effect is greatly related to the tear dynamics and the dynamics of the precorneal TF. Δp can be described as

$$\Delta p = \gamma/R \qquad (1)$$

where g = surface tension of tears at the meniscus; and R = radius of the tear meniscus. On the other hand, due to the suction effect

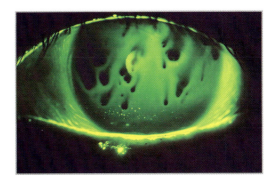

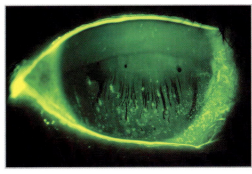

Figure 7.3 Two different types of tear film (TF) break-up. One is circular-like break-up ['spot break' (upper image)], which appears instantaneously at the time of eye opening. This can be attributed to the decreased wettability of the corneal surface epithelium. The other is linear-like break-up ['line break' (lower image)], which appears when the eye is kept open. This can be attributed to TF instability due to a different mechanism (e.g. facilitated evaporation); it should be noted that in the lower picture, three small spot breaks can also be observed at the center of the cornea just after eye opening.

inside the canaliculus produced by the action of the Horner's muscle (Kakizaki et al. 2005) at the time of eye opening, which results in the production of Δp inside the canaliculus, Δp counteracts with the $2\Delta p$ (the total of upper and lower meniscus). Accordingly, $K(\Delta p - 2\Delta p) = K(\Delta p - 2\gamma/R)$ (where K is a constant) should determine the tear volume that is sucked into the canaliculus (Mishima 1970). Based on this principle, a much lesser amount of tears must be sucked into the canaliculus in eyes with a smaller meniscus radius. The clinical implication of this theory is that tear clearance (or tear turnover) is delayed in ATDDE. Based on the inflammation theory for the core mechanism of DED, delayed tear clearance (de Paiva & Pflugfelder 2004) can result in the enhancement of inflammation, and from this point of view, ocular surface inflammation is more important for ATDDE.

TEAR FILM DYNAMICS IN AQUEOUS TEARS DEFICIENCY

It is clinically known that in cases of ATDDE, mucus also accumulates due to the delayed clearance, and this may sometimes be one of the symptoms of ATDDE. This mechanism is also responsible for the epithelial damage modified by mucin such as corneal filaments (Tanioka et al. 2009), mucus plaque, and patchy superficial punctate keratopathy (**Figure 7.4**). Considering the mucin-gel structure in TF, decreased aqueous tear content is thought to result in the disruption of secretory mucin, and due to delayed tear clearance, this mucin accumulates over the ocular surface, resulting in superficial corneal damage. However, the mechanism described below might also be associated with this damage.

RATE OF TEAR FILM LIPID LAYER SPREADING

A simple expression for the relationship between tear physical properties and TFLL spread rate is given by the Gibbs–Marangoni equation (Marangoni 1871), implemented for TF by Berger and Corrsin (1974)

$$U = \frac{h \times \Delta\gamma}{\mu \times L} \qquad (2)$$

where U = spread velocity of the TFLL; h = AT thickness; $\Delta\gamma$ = surface tension gradient (inverse relation between surface tension and TFLL thickness is assumed); μ = tear viscosity; and L = extent of TFLL spread.

Therefore, the rate of the surface-tension-driven spread of the TFLL is proportionally related to AT thickness. Thus, the attenuated TFLL spread measured in ATDDE (Yokoi et al. 2008a, 2008b) can be easily explained (a thinner AT thickness results in decreased velocity of the TFLL), and even non-spreading of the TFLL can be expected to occur in the severest form of ATD. Hence, ATD, depending on its severity, is also accompanied by an evaporative component due to the attenuated recruitment of the TFLL.

Punctal occlusion, to both the upper and the lower puncta, is known to be a very effective treatment for severe ATDDE (Yokoi & Komuro 2004). Prior to treatment, TF is absent on the cornea; as ATs are practically missing ('h' in equation 2 is very low), the TFLL remains unspread. However, after punctal occlusion, the AT accumulates on the cornea and complete spread of the TFLL is recovered. Thus, three of the four mechanisms in ATDDE (i.e. ATD, increased evaporation,

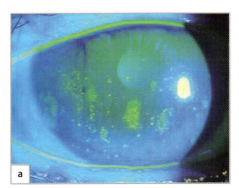
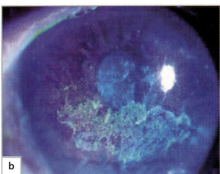
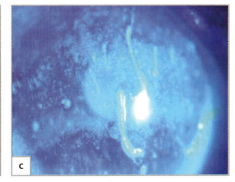

Figure 7.4 Corneal epithelial damage modified by accumulated mucus often seen in aqueous tear-deficient dry eye (ATDDE). In ATDDE, depending on its severity, due to the accumulation of mucus via the possible separation of mucin from the aqueous-mucin gel and delayed tear clearance, possible associated ocular surface inflammation, facilitated evaporation via the restricted upward spread of the tear film lipid layer (TFLL), and increased friction during a blink, corneal epithelial damages are likely to appear as those modified by accumulated mucin (left: patchy pattern; center: mucus plaque; right: corneal filaments).

and increased friction) are completely resolved. This is why severe corneal damage disappears after punctal occlusion. However, delayed tear clearance is rather exacerbated after punctal occlusion, and therefore attention must be paid to the preservative toxicity and the accumulated mucus must be addressed.

In addition to the abnormal dynamics of the TF, in cases with severe ATDDE, the frictional mechanism at the time of blinking is also responsible for increased epithelial damage. In normal eyes, friction is expected to serve to produce epithelial turnover at the time of blinking, but this action is exaggerated in cases with ATDDE and thus results in epithelial damage under the eyelids. In addition, the corneal filament could be related to the friction between the palpebral conjunctiva and the cornea during blinking, and this mechanism is also responsible for the modification of the massive amount of corneal epithelial damage seen in the severest form of ATDDE.

Rheological analysis of the TFLL spread in normal eyes reveals viscoelastic behavior that is well described by the Voigt model (Yokoi et al. 2008a, 2008b). The elasticity of the TFLL is of key importance for ensuring rapid spreading and quick replenishment of TF after eye opening. Human meibum deposited on the air–water surface of the Langmuir trough, in vitro, forms continuous rough viscoelastic multilayers (Georgiev et al. 2011, Leiske et al. 2012, Millar & Mudgil 2011) similar to the thick lipid draperies observed in vivo. The multilayer structure is determined by the very nature of the meibomian lipids; the minor fraction (<5%) of polar lipids (PL) locates at the interface

with aqueous layer, while the abundant non-polar lipids spread over the PL as a 6–20 monomolecular-layer-thick bulk lipid layer (Butovich et al. 2008). When subjected to dynamic area compression–expansion cycling, the lipid film shows (i) high isotherm reversibility indicating instantaneous spread during expansion and (ii) non-collapsibility, that is, no mechanical 'break' of the film at compression, and no loss of lipid molecules between cycles, are registered (**Figure 7.5**, upper row and BAM images).

It can be assumed that at compression, the non-PL ply of the TFLL serves as a reservoir that stores PL at the surface and keeps them ready to immediately return and spread on the surface at expansion (**Figure 7.5**, bottom row). Similar behavior was observed with synthetic multilayer films, with composition partially akin to meibum (Smaby & Brockman 1987). This mechanism avoids loss of lipid between compression–expansion cycles and allows the meibomian multilayer to maintain its function for extended durations without requiring a supply of new lipid material. Thus, the stress on meibomian glands to secrete new lipids is minimized. The proposed mechanism correlates with the in vivo finding of very slow (>8 hours) TFLL turnover in the human eye (Mochizuki et al. 2009). Apart from the functionality described above, the meibomian multilayer will also efficiently suppress evaporation. A pure PL monolayer at the air–tear interface should not maintain the desired material properties, as at compression it will collapse and PL squeezed in AT will be lost due to the rapid AT turnover (**Figure 7.5**, third row).

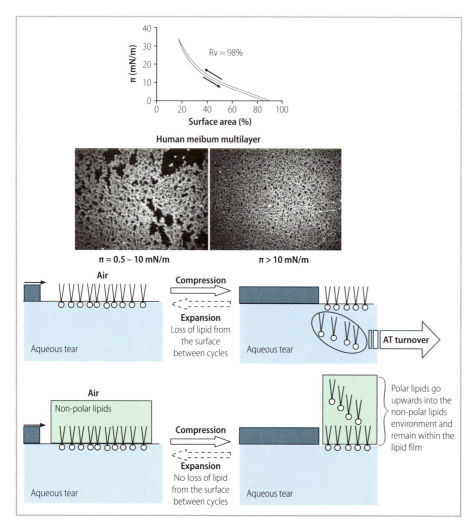

π (mN/m)

Rv = 98%

Surface area (%)

Human meibum multilayer

π = 0.5 – 10 mN/m   π > 10 mN/m

Air   Compression

Expansion
Loss of lipid from
the surface
between cycles

Aqueous tear   Aqueous tear   AT turnover

Air

Non-polar lipids

Compression

Expansion
No loss of lipid
from the surface
between cycles

Aqueous tear   Aqueous tear

Polar lipids go
upwards into the
non-polar lipids
environment and
remain within the
lipid film

Figure 7.5 Material properties of human meibum. Top row: Highly reversible compression–expansion surface pressure (π)/area (A) isocycle of human meibum film that demonstrates the capability of meibum to instantaneously spread on the surface at area expansion. Second row: Brewster angle microscopy images (500 μm × 500 μm) of the meibomian multilayer becoming continuous and rough at higher π [similar to tear film lipid layer (TFLL) draperies observed in vivo]. Third row: The destiny of the pure polar lipid (PL) monolayer. At high compression, the PL monolayer will collapse and a fraction of the PL molecules will be squeezed in aqueous tears (AT) and washed by the rapid AT turnover. Thus, constant and significant lipid loss will take place at every compression. Bottom row: The mechanism of how meibum eventually works is that at compression, PLs, instead of being squeezed in AT, get pushed upward within the bulky non-polar part of the TFLL, and are then ready to be respread over AT at expansion.

The clinical implication of the proposed mechanisms is that the treatment of the ocular surface with pharmaceuticals that facilitate TFLL multilayer properties can be of benefit for DED therapy (particularly for cases of meibomian gland dysfunction), while ingredients disrupting the multilayer integrity bear a risk factor for adverse effects (Georgiev et al. 2011, Holly 1978).

ANOTHER FUNCTION OF THE TEAR MENISCUS

The tear meniscus has a capillary suction effect that supports and holds tears at the meniscus and, as discussed above, plays a key role in the establishment of tear volume. However, capillary suction can cause aqueous TF thinning adjacent to the lower and upper menisci (McDonald & Brubaker 1971, Sharma et al. 1998). When fluorescein staining is applied into the tears, TF thinning can be recognized as a 'black line' (**Figure 7.6**), that is, a darker thinner (~100 nm) line from which fluorescein is excluded along the lower and upper menisci. Then, a three-compartment distribution of tears is achieved at the ocular surface: 3–7 μm thick precorneal TF 'perched' between the thin black lines and tears at the lower and upper menisci (Miller et al. 2002). Tears at the menisci are permitted to flow into the canaliculi through the puncta due to the suction effect of tears within the canaliculus. In contrast, once the 'perched' TF is established, it should not be influenced by the meniscus tear flow. Thus, the direction of movement differs between TF and tears at the meniscus. This may partly support the maintenance of the quality of vision after the eye is opened. The black line affects TF stability because intermolecular forces can initiate TF break-up from this thinnest region at the ocular surface. It is reportedly estimated that it takes 15–40 seconds for TF to break up in normal eyes with a normal tear volume (Creech et al. 1998). On the other hand, this is not true in cases of ATD where

- AT is thinner than normal
- The tear meniscus radius is decreased more than two times (Yokoi et al. 2004) and its capillary suction pressure (equation 1) proportionally increases (the so-called thirsty meniscus)

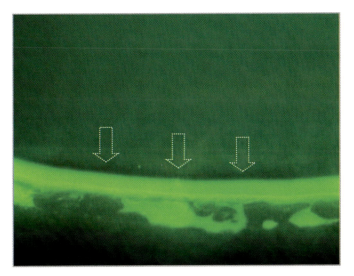

Figure 7.6 Black line distributed at the lower tear meniscus. The black line is a dark fluorescent line seen along the tear meniscus, which corresponds to the thinner aqueous layer induced by the capillary sucking pressure from the meniscus. The black line is physiologically important because it can help to compartmentalize the tears at the meniscus and tear film (TF).

Thus, in ATD, formation of the thin black line is greatly promoted and can take place just within 2 seconds after eye opening (Sharma et al. 1998).

Hence, in cases of DED, more attention should be paid to this line when the fluorescein break-up time is measured.

ECTOPIC TEAR MENISCUS

Since there is an action for the meniscus that makes the neighboring aqueous TF thinner, the tear meniscus produced ectopically is responsible for the focal instability of TF, which results in the epithelial damage. In cases with an ocular surface lesion with a protrusion, which occurs due to rigid contact lens wear (**Figure 7.7**, upper left), pinguecula (**Figure 7.7**, lower left and upper right), and pterygium, the tear meniscus is produced ectopically. For example, in a case with pinguecula, an ectopic meniscus is formed on the temporal side of the pinguecula that leads to meniscus-induced local TF thinning (McDonald & Brubaker 1971), thus resulting in the corneal epithelial damage. Considering that the general non-ectopic tear menisci are also responsible for TF thinning, the triangular region (formed in cases such as pinguecula and rigid contact lens wear) surrounded by the general menisci and ectopic meniscus is very likely to result in TF instability and resultant epithelial damage (**Figure 7.7**, upper right). This mechanism is very useful for understanding the heterogeneous distribution of superficial punctate keratopathy in DED accompanying pinguecula or pterygium. This meniscus-induced TF thinning was previously introduced as the mechanism of 3 o'clock to 9 o'clock corneal staining in rigid contact lens wear (McDonald & Brubaker 1971). From the viewpoint of the ectopic tear meniscus, it is clinically important to find the protruded lesion adjacent to the cornea within the interpalpebral region, which can be responsible for the heterogeneous distribution of corneal epithelial damage. This viewpoint may also provide another clue for the treatment when the eye-drop treatment is ineffective, and such cases are sometimes treated surgically with the resection of the protruding lesion (**Figure 7.7**, lower right).

Dellen (Baum et al. 1968) is also known to be located adjacent to the cornea, and the meniscus-induced TF thinning is related to this mechanism. In dellen, the dehydrated and thinned cornea is generally not seen in the peripheral part of the cornea but adjacent to it, so there must be a protruding lesion of conjunctiva. Ectopic meniscus is formed next to the protruding lesion, and due to its suction effect, aqueous TF adjacent to the ectopic meniscus gets thinner, resulting in the local restricted spread of the TFLL over this thinner aqueous layer. This leads to the facilitated evaporation, and finally, dellen develops. Cases of dellen, such as those produced in relation to postoperative conjunctival edema, massive subconjunctival hemorrhage, or a filtering bleb after trabeculectomy, can be treated by using a temporal eye patch or the topical treatment for DED.

CCh (Meller & Tseng 1998) is another important mechanism that causes disruption of the dynamics of tears and TF, because this is a very common age-related disorder, which is reportedly seen in 98% of subjects older than 60 years (Mimura et al. 2009, Yokoi et al. 2008a, 2008b). CCh is related to the ocular discomfort via: (1) TF instability; (2) increased friction at the time of blinking (**Figure 7.8**); and (3) blockage of tear flow at the meniscus. Hence, it is often seen in CCh that the chief symptom is epiphora caused by the third mechanism, while in some cases, reflex tear secretion due to the first mechanism is responsible for the epiphora. Therefore, the combined mechanism of reflex tear secretion (lacrimation) and blockage of tear flow at the meniscus (epiphora) is important when considering the mechanism of this disorder. In CCh, the meniscus is occupied by the redundant conjunctiva, which is

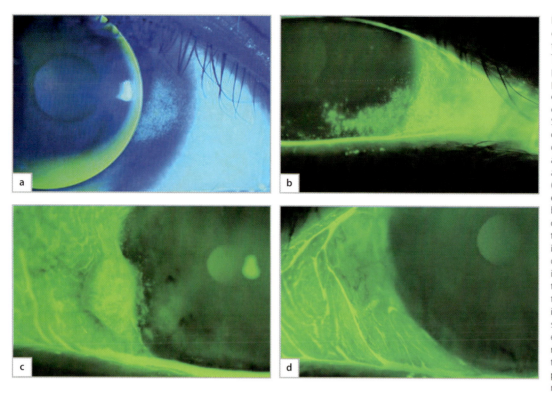

Figure 7.7 Corneal epithelial damage induced by ectopic tear meniscus and its treatment. Tear meniscus ectopically produced in relation to the protrusion adjacent to the cornea is responsible for the corneal epithelial damage. Such corneal epithelial damage can be seen in cases of rigid contact lens wear (upper left) and pinguecula (upper right and lower left), where tear film (TF) instability and resultant epithelial damage are realized based on the mechanism of meniscus-induced TF thinning. In the case shown in the upper-right image, the original lower tear meniscus is also responsible for the TF thinning and, in addition to the ectopic meniscus, it results in a triangular region that is susceptible to the corneal epithelial damage. In cases resistant to the eye-drop treatment, resection of the protrusion may be effective to remove the ectopic meniscus (lower right—also shown as Figure 7.8). This case was treated by the resection of pinguecula, which is replaced by the conjunctival autograft).

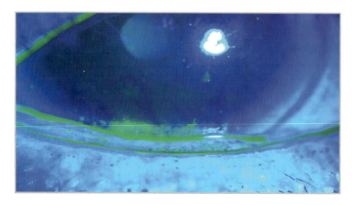

Figure 7.8 Blink-related corneal epithelial damage in a case with conjunctivochalasis (CCh). CCh is responsible for the corneal epithelial damage via the increased friction at the time of a blink. This mechanism may be enhanced in cases with dry eye disease (DED).

responsible for reduction of meniscus tear volume, and also may result in increased friction at blinking. This mechanism of tear deficiency at the lower tear meniscus and increased friction can be related to the increase of the corneal epithelial damage in cases of ATD. However, ectopic meniscus adjacent to the redundant conjunctiva may sometimes be the cause of the epithelial damage via the meniscus-induced tear thinning. In addition, CCh is reportedly related to lymphangiectasia (Watanabe et al. 2004), and this lymphangiectasia-related protrusion may also be responsible for the ectopic meniscus formation. When those mechanisms are involved, the surgical approach may also be effective to obtain a complete resolution.

SUMMARY

The understanding of tear dynamics and TF dynamics is important and useful when looking for a clue to elucidate the mechanism of the clinical manifestation of DED and to consider its treatment. The tear meniscus plays a key role, either positively or negatively, in TF dynamics and knowledge of this role could provide us with a complete understanding of DED.

◼ REFERENCES

Baum JL, Mishima S, Boruchoff SA. On the nature of dellen. *Arch Ophthalmol* 1968; **79**:657–662.

Benedetto DA, Clinch TE, Laibson PR. In vivo observation of tear dynamics using fluorophotometry. *Arch Ophthalmol* 1984; **102**:410–412.

Berger RE, Corrsin S. A surface tension gradient mechanism for driving the pre-corneal tear film after a blink. *J Biomech* 1974; **7**:225–238.

Bron AJ, Yokoi N, Gafney E, Tiffany JM. Predicted phenotypes of dry eye: proposed consequences of its natural history. *Ocul Surf* 2009; **7**:78–92.

Butovich I, Millar TJ, Ham BM. Understanding and analysing meibomian lipids: a review. *Curr Eye Res* 2008; **33**:405–420.

Creech JL, Do LT, Fatt I, Radke CJ. In vivo tear-film thickness determination and implications for tear-film stability. *Curr Eye Res* 1998; **17**:1058–1066.

DEWS. The definition and classification of dry eye disease: report of the Definition and Classification Subcommittee of the International Dry Eye WorkShop. *Ocul Surf* 2007; **5**:75–92.

Georgiev GA, Yokoi N, Koev K, et al. Surface chemistry study of the interactions of benzalkonium chloride with films of meibum, corneal cells lipids, and whole tears. *Invest Ophthalmol Vis Sci* 2011; **52**:4645–4654.

Holly FJ. Surface chemical evaluation of artificial tears and their ingredients. II. Interaction with lipid layer. *Cont Intraoc Lens Med J* 1978; **4**:52–65.

Jones M, Please C, McElwain D, et al. Dynamics of tear film deposition and draining. *Math Med Biology* 2005; **22**:265–288.

Kakizaki H, Zako M, Miyaishi O, et al. The lacrimal canaliculus and sac bordered by the Horner's muscle form the functional lacrimal drainage system. *Ophthalmology* 2005; **112**:710–716.

Kimball SH, King-Smith PE, Nichols JJ. Evidence for the major contribution of evaporation to tear film thinning between blinks. *Invest Ophthalmol Vis Sci* 2010; **51**:6294–6297.

Leiske DL, Leiske CI, Leiske DR, et al. Temperature-induced transitions in the structure and interfacial rheology of human meibum. *Biophys J* 2012; **102**:369–376.

Marangoni CGM. Sul principio della viscosita` superficiale dei liquidi stabilito dal Signor J. Plateau (On the principle of surface viscosity of liquids by Mr. J. Plateau). Il Nuovo Cimento 1871; Ser. 2 5/6:239–273.

McDonald JE, Brubaker S. Meniscus-induced thinning of tear films. *Am J Ophthalmol* 1971; **72**:139–146.

Meller D, Tseng SC. Conjunctivochalasis: literature review and possible pathophysiology. *Surv Ophthalmol* 1998; **43**:225–232.

Millar TJ, Mudgil P. Surfactant properties of human meibomian lipids. *Invest Ophthalmol Vis Sci* 2011; **10**:5445.

Miller KL, Polse KA, Radke CJ. Black-line formation and the "perched" human tear film. *Curr Eye Res* 2002; **25**:155–162.

Mimura T, Yamagami S, Usui T, et al. Changes of conjunctivochalasis with age in a hospital-based study. *Am J Ophthalmol* 2009; **147**:171–177.

Mishima S. Physiology and pathology of tear secretion. *Jpn Rev Clin Ophthalmol* 1970; **64**:89–99.

Mochizuki H. Yamada M, Hatou S, Tsubota K. Turnover rate of tear-film lipid layer determined by fluorophotometry. *Br J Ophthalmol* 2009; **93**:1535–1538.

Nishida K, Yamanishi K, Yamada K, et al. Epithelial hyperproliferation and transglutaminase 1 gene expression in Stevens-Johnson syndrome conjunctiva. *Am J Pathol* 1999; **154**:331–336.

de Paiva CS, Pflugfelder SC. Tear clearance implications for ocular surface health. *Exp Eye Res* 2004; **78**:395–397.

Shanker RM, Ahmed I, Bourassa PA, Carola KV. An in vitro technique for measuring contact angles on the corneal surface and its application to evaluate corneal wetting properties of water soluble polymers. *Int J Pharmaceutics* 1995; **119**:149–163.

Sharma A, Ruckenstein E. Dewetting of solids by the formation of holes in macroscopic liquid films. *J Colloid Interface Sci* 1989; **133**:358–368.

Sharma A, Tiwari S, Khanna R, Tiffany JM. Hydrodynamics of meniscus-induced thinning of the tear film. *Adv Exp Med Biol* 1998; **438**:425–431.

Shen M, Li J, Wang J, et al. Upper and lower tear menisci in the diagnosis of dry eye. *Invest Ophthalmol Vis Sci* 2009; **50**:2722–2726.

Smaby JM, Brockman HL. Acyl unsaturation and cholesteryl ester miscibility in surfaces. Formation of lecithin-cholesteryl ester complexes. *J Lipid Res* 1987; **28**:1078–1087.

Stern ME, Beuerman RW, Pflugfelder SC. The normal tear film and ocular surface. In: Pflugfelder SC, Beuerman RW, Stern ME (eds), Dry eye and ocular surface disorders. *New York: Marcel Dekker,* 2004:41–62. ISBN: 0–8247–4702-X.

Sumiyoshi M, Ricciuto J, Tisdale A, et al. Antiadhesive character of mucin o-glycans at the apical surface of corneal epithelial cells. *Invest Ophthalmol Vis Sci* 2008; **49**:197–203.

Takaoka-Shichijo Y, Nakamura M. Stimulatory effect of diquafosol tetrasodium on the expression of membrane-binding mucin genes in cultured human corneal epithelial cells. Atarashii Ganka (Journal of the Eye) 2011; **28**:425–429.

Takaoka-Shichijo Y, Sakamoto A, Nakamura M. Effect of diquafosol tetrasodium on MUC5AC secretion by rabbit conjunctival tissues. Atarashii Ganka (Journal of the Eye) 2011; **28**:261–265.

Tanioka H, Yokoi N, Komuro A, et al. Investigation of the corneal filament in filamentary keratitis. *Invest Ophthalmol Vis Sci* 2009; **50**:3696–3702.

Urashima H, Okamoto T, Takeji Y, Shinohara H, Fujisawa S. Rebamipide increases the amount of mucin-like substances on the conjunctiva and cornea in the N-acetylcysteine-treated in vivo model. *Cornea* 2004; **23**:613–619.

Watanabe A, Yokoi N, Kinoshita S, et al. Clinicopathologic study of conjunctivochalasis. *Cornea* 2004; **23**:294–298.

Wong H, Fatt I, Radke CJ. Deposition and thinning of the human tear film. *J Colloid Interface Sci* 1996; **184**:44–51.

Yokoi N, Bron AJ, Tiffany JM, et al. Relationship between tear volume and tear meniscus curvature. *Arch Ophthalmol* 2004; **122**:1265–1269.

Yokoi N, Inatomi T, Kinoshita S. Surgery of the conjunctiva. *Dev Ophthalmol* 2008a; **41**:138–158.

Yokoi N, Komuro A. Non-invasive methods of assessing the tear film. *Exp Eye Res* 2004; **78**:399–407.

Yokoi N, Komuro A, Maruyama K, et al. New surgical treatment for superior limbic keratoconjunctivitis and its association with conjunctivochalasis. *Am J Ophthalmol* 2003; **135**:303–308.

Yokoi N, Takehisa Y, Kinoshita S. Correlation of tear lipid layer interference patterns with the diagnosis and severity of dry eye. *Am J Ophthalmol* 1996; **122**:818–824.

Yokoi N, Yamada H, Mizukusa Y, et al. Rheology of tear film lipid layer spread in normal and aqueous tear–deficient dry eyes. *Invest Ophthalmol Vis Sci* 2008b; **49**:5319–5324.

Chapter 8

The role of inflammation, inflammatory cytokines, and ocular surface markers in dry eye disease

Pasquale Aragona, Laura Rania, Domenico Puzzolo

■ INTRODUCTION

The ocular surface is a functional unit that protects eyes from external environment and provides the cornea with an optimal refractive surface by producing an efficient tear film (Gipson 2007). The structures that comprise this functional unit include the epithelia of the cornea, conjunctiva, lacrimal gland, accessory lacrimal glands, meibomian glands (and their basal connective tissue), the eyelashes (and their associated glands of Moll and Zeis), the palpebral muscles responsible for blinking, and the nasolacrimal duct. The activity of all these structures is regulated by the nervous, endocrine, vascular, and lymphatic systems.

The ocular surface acts as an anatomical and functional unit that maintains a controlled immunological protection against antigenic challenges of the external environment (Barabino & Dana 2007). Healthy subjects without ocular surface disease may demonstrate immunological activity, supporting the role of the epithelia in providing an 'immune tone' always present in normal ocular surface.

The malfunctioning of one or more ocular surface structures results in compensatory changes by other members of the functional unit, to maintain efficient tear film production. When a chronic alteration develops, the production of an efficient tear film will be impaired, causing a dysfunctional tear syndrome (**Figure 8.1**). This condition was thoroughly revised by the Dry Eye Workshop report, the results of which were published in 2007 (Lemp et al. 2007). In this workshop, it was stated that dry eye disease (DED), also known as dysfunctional tear syndrome, is an inflammatory condition due to tear hyperosmolarity, which occurs because of either increased tear evaporation [evaporative dry eye (EDE)] or aqueous tear deficiency [aqueous tear-deficient dry eye (ADDE)].

The ocular surface is continuously exposed to external stimuli that may produce a basal level of subclinical tissue response to inflammation. In this way, the inflammatory response of the ocular surface can be considered to be a protective reaction against several stimuli, such as allergens, chemical or physical irritants, traumas, and infections. These stimuli can induce morphological and functional ocular surface changes, which may lead to maintenance of a chronic inflammation if they are not appropriately counterbalanced. Altered conditions at the ocular surface lead to a dysfunctional tear film, due to reduced tear production or increased tear evaporation, both of which increase tear osmolarity, an effect that is responsible for maintaining a chronic proinflammatory stimulus on the ocular surface.

Conditions other than tear hyperosmolarity may also contribute to the activation of the immune system. Both innate and adaptive immunity mechanisms participate in the defensive systems of the ocular surface. Among the innate mechanisms, the aberrant activation of Toll-like receptors (TLRs), due to the modified ocular surface flora, and the increased expression of molecules, such as chitinases [acidic mammalian chitinase (AMCase)], phospholipase A2 (PLA2), and transglutaminase 2 (TG-2), have been described. These molecules have been suggested as possible biomarkers for several inflammatory diseases.

The initiation of innate immunity mechanisms via these molecules results in the activation of the mitogen-activated protein kinase (MAPK) and nuclear factor-κB (NF-κB) signaling pathways, which induce the expression of proinflammatory cytokines such as interleukin (IL)-1α, IL-1β, tumor necrosis factor-α (TNF-α), and matrix metalloproteinases (MMPs) (De Paiva et al. 2006, Li et al. 2004, Luo et al. 2005). The expression of these and other molecules triggers the consequent activation of the adaptive immune pathways and the maintenance of the inflammation on the ocular surface.

Whatever be the initial cause of DED, the chronic irritation caused by the dysfunctional tear film results in an increase in nervous stimulation that aims to induce compensatory responses, in order to achieve a functional recovery. The chronic nervous stimulation is responsible for neurogenic inflammation and T-cell activation with the release of inflammatory cytokines into the lacrimal glands, tear fluid, and ocular surface epithelium. Ocular surface epithelial cells directly participate in the onset and maintenance of the inflammatory process by expressing major histocompatibility complex (MHC)-class II antigens, such as human leukocyte antigen-DR, on their membranes (De Saint Jean et al. 1999, Tsubota et al. 1999), thus acquiring antigen-presenting capability. In this way, epithelial cells either participate in the recruitment of inflammatory cells (dendritic cells, macrophages, and lymphocytes) or become a target for cytotoxic reactions. These activities result in epithelial damage in lacrimal glands, cornea, and conjunctiva.

Inflammatory mediators, which occur as a consequence of the infiltrating activity of inflammatory cells, may result in a dysfunction of ocular surface innervation. Consequently, reduced or absent trophic signals to the lacrimal glands will result in impairment of lacrimal gland function and epithelial damage because of the reduced delivery of trophic molecules, such as epithelial growth factor, by the lacrimal gland. Another consequence of chronic inflammation of the ocular surface is the delivery of proinflammatory molecules in the tear film,

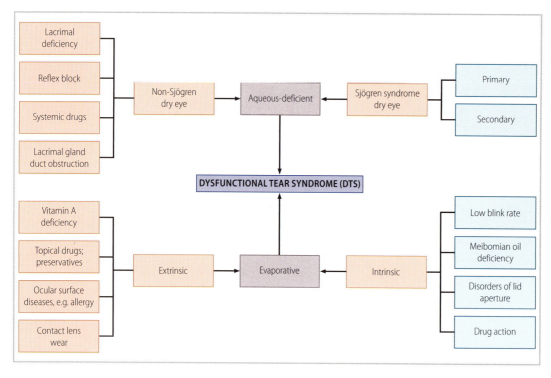

Figure 8.1 Dry eye disease (DED) etiology. DED or dysfunctional tear syndrome can be aqueous tear-deficient or evaporative. The former has two major subgroups: Sjögren's syndrome (SS) DED, either primary or secondary, and non-SS DED. This latter includes those etiologies capable of inducing a failure of lacrimal tear secretion, such as lacrimal gland deficiencies or duct obstruction, reflex hyposecretion, and systemic drug use. Evaporative dry eye (EDE) may be intrinsic, if the regulation of evaporative loss from the tear film is directly affected, owing to meibomian oil deficiency, poor lid congruity and dynamics, low blink rate, and the effects of drugs, such as systemic retinoids. Extrinsic EDE includes those etiologies that increase evaporation by their pathological effects on the ocular surface, such as vitamin A deficiency, toxic topical agents as preservatives, contact lens wear, and a range of ocular surface diseases, including allergic eye disease. Redrawn with modifications from Lemp et al. (2007).

which induces a further expression of HLA-DR on cellular membranes and epithelial cells apoptosis. This epithelial suffering is responsible for altered mucin production, another cause of dysfunctional tear film.

Hormonal dysregulation (even when subclinical), exogenous conditions (such as environmental pollution, infections, and allergies), or iatrogenic reactions can lead to an alteration of the ocular surface homeostasis, contributing to the inflammatory and apoptotic events occurring in the ocular surface in course of DED. Once DED has developed, inflammation becomes the key mechanism of ocular surface injury, being both the origin and the result of cell damage. Therefore, patients with severe DED enter a vicious cycle of inflammation and ocular surface injury (Wakamatsu et al. 2008).

INNATE IMMUNITY: THE MOLECULAR BASIS

Several mechanisms have been identified as promoters for innate immunity. These include the altered production of molecules such as lactoferrin, lysozyme, lipocalin, secretory immunoglobulin A (IgA), AMCase, PLA2, and TG, together with the activation of TLRs.

Lactoferrin

Lactoferrin, also known as lactotransferrin, is an iron-binding globular glycoprotein of the transferrin family that is widely represented in various secretory fluids, such as milk, saliva, tears, and nasal secretions. It is also present in secondary granules of polymorphonuclear leukocyte and secreted by some acinar cells. Lactoferrin exists in two forms: the iron-rich hololactoferrin and the iron-free apolactoferrin. It is a component of the innate immune system, mainly in mucosal cells.

Lactoferrin has several functions, including promotion of cell growth and DNA synthesis, anti-inflammatory effects, antibacterial,

antiviral, antiparasitic, catalytic, antiallergic, and radioprotecting functions, as well as antiangiogenic and antitumoral properties. In fact, lactoferrin can directly inhibit the production of several cytokines, such as TNF-α and IL-1. Antibacterial activity derives from deprivation of the bacterial flora from iron, an element necessary for its growth. In addition, lactoferrin binds to the lipopolysaccharide of bacterial walls and oxidizes bacteria through peroxide formation, thus leading to cell lysis. Lactoferrin's antiviral effect is achieved by affecting natural killer (NK) cells, granulocytes, and macrophages, which play a crucial role in the early stages of viral infection. Moreover, various physiological qualities, including antioxidative activity, have been attributed to this glycoprotein.

Lactoferrin is the main glycoprotein component of tears, mainly secreted from the lacrimal gland acinar cells. It possesses multiple functions including important bacteriostatic activity (Versura et al. 2010) and scavenging of free ions (Ohashi et al. 2003). So, it may attenuate oxidative stress damage and suppress inflammatory mediators in the lacrimal glands, as well as preserve lacrimal gland function. Lactoferrin concentration in tears has been shown to predict tear film stability or volume (Glasson et al. 2003), so it acts as an indicator of lacrimal secretory function. In fact, lactoferrin concentration in tears has been shown to decrease in patients who have DED (Kawashima et al. 2012). Indeed, Versura et al. (2010) showed a low, but significant, lactoferrin decrease in the tears of patients with mild EDE, when compared with controls. In addition, in patients with mild-to-moderate DED, lactoferrin changes occur only in reflex but not in basal tears (Yolton et al. 1991).

Lactoferrin has been considered as a tear-specific biomarker for Sjögren's syndrome (SS) (Karns & Herr 2011). A reduced concentration in tears of non-SS DED patients (Ohashi et al. 2003) and in patients with SS and Stevens–Johnson syndrome (Labbè et al. 2007) has been described. Moreover, it has been demonstrated that the oral administration of lactoferrin improved tear stability and the ocular surface condition in patients with SS who have DED (Dogru et al. 2007, Kawashima et al. 2012). Tear lactoferrin level can be correlated with the severity of corneoconjunctival epithelial lesions in patients with primary and secondary SS and in those with non-SS DED. Furthermore, it has been hypothesized that although lactoferrin is known to be associated with tear lipids and DED symptoms, it is largely related to lacrimal tear function rather than meibomian gland dysfunction (MGD). Therefore, it may contribute to DED pathology via a non-MGD mechanism (Tong et al. 2011).

Lysozyme

Lysozyme, also known as muramidase or N-acetylmuramide glycan-hydrolase, is a glycoside hydrolase that damages bacterial cell walls by attacking their peptidoglycans. It is part of the innate immune system, encoded by the *LYZ* gene, and is abundant in tears, saliva, milk, and mucus. It is also present in the cytoplasmic granules of the polymorphonuclear leukocyte.

Like lactoferrin, lysozyme is produced in the acini of the main lacrimal gland, thus representing an indirect index of its function (Versura et al. 2010). The concentration of lysozyme decreases constantly in DED conditions. Moreover, it can vary according to age and time of day. It is the main protein of reflex tears (Labbè et al. 2007).

Lysozyme, like lactoferrin and tear lipocalin (TLC), performs antimicrobial activity and works synergistically with these molecules to enhance their efficacy. The activity of lysozyme can be inhibited by fatty acids secreted by the meibomian glands and by nucleic acids. However, tear TLC can bind the long-chain fatty acids, whereas lactoferrin binds nucleic acids. These binding patterns can result in an enhancement of lysozyme activity. In addition, TLC, lysozyme, and lactoferrin may directly interact with each other (Dartt 2011).

In addition to the levels of proteins such as lactoferrin and LCN-1, tear lysozyme levels reflect aqueous secretion activity by the lacrimal gland (Zhou et al. 2009). In tears of patients with DED, these three proteins have been shown to be downregulated (Dartt 2011). Additionally, it has been shown in one study that the reduction of tear lysozyme concentration in DED patients was related to the severity of the condition, so that in patients with severe DED the lysozyme concentration falls to zero (Seal et al. 1986), whereas in another study Versura et al. (2010) showed no changes in the lysozyme content in mild EDE patients compared with controls.

Lipocalins

The lipocalins are a broad family of low-molecular-weight proteins that transport small hydrophobic molecules such as steroids, retinoids, and lipids, including vitamin E and A. The lipocalin family is part of a superfamily known as calycins, named so because lipophilic molecules are enclosed within their cup-shaped cavity or calyx. TLC, also known as human tear prealbumin or von Ebner's gland protein, can also bind to macromolecules, including the tear proteins lactoferrin and lysozyme (Dartt 2011). TLCs have been associated with many biological processes, such as the immune response, prostaglandin synthesis, and retinoid binding.

TLC is encoded by the gene *LCN-1* (Glasgow & Gasymov 2011). It is a multifunctional protein, in addition to lysozyme and lactoferrin, mainly secreted from the lacrimal gland into the tear fluid. TLC is the predominant lipid carrier in human tears and is second only to lysozyme as the most concentrated protein. Approximately 15–33% of the tear protein mass is composed of TLC. This protein may regulate the lipid composition of tears by binding lipids from the tear fluid and/or releasing lipids into the tear fluid (Yamada et al. 2005). It scavenges lipids from the cornea, the conjunctiva, and the tear film, as lipids render the corneal surface unwettable. In contrast, it is also able to deliver lipids, which participate in the non-Newtonian behavior of tears (Dartt 2011). Furthermore, TLC may link to meibomian lipids, thus increasing tear film stability and reducing the evaporation rate (Glasgow & Gasymov 2011). TLC may also provide a natural defense against fungal infections by binding to the microbial siderophores (iron-scavenging molecules) (Glasgow & Gasymov 2011). They are also the principal endonuclease in tears responsible for viral DNA inactivation (Dartt 2011).

TLC has been proposed as a biomarker of DED. In fact, it was demonstrated that its concentration is diminished or absent when lacrimal gland mass is reduced, or has disorders causing impaired lacrimal secretion, such as in SS and LASIK-induced DED (Glasgow & Gasymov 2011). Zhou et al. (2009) found a downregulation of TLC, lactoferrin, and lysozyme in tears of DED patients when compared to normal subjects. A similar result was obtained by Caffery et al. (2008): TLC and total tear proteins were decreased in patients with SS compared to those with non-SS DED and controls (patients without DED). Another study (Versura et al. 2010) has shown that TLC-1 is reduced in MGD patients, in correlation with tear stability and subjective symptoms of discomfort but not with tear secretion. Tong et al. (2011) found that TLC-1 was associated with symptoms of eyelid heaviness and tearing.

To date, studies have not been able to demonstrate whether TLC plays a role in the pathogenesis of DED or SS (Dartt 2011). However, Yamada et al. (2005) proposed that a deficiency of TLC may be a predisposing factor for the development of symptoms in MGD.

Immunoglobulin A

IgA is an antibody that plays a critical role in mucosal immunity. IgA exists as two isotypes, IgA1 and IgA2, with the latter isotype being higher in secretions than in serum. IgA can exist in a dimeric form called secretory IgA, which is produced by epithelial cells and represents the main immunoglobulin found in mucous secretions, including tears and saliva. The secretory fragment protects IgA from being degraded by proteolytic enzymes. It has been demonstrated that secretory IgA is the predominant protein in tears obtained from closed eyes, whereas lysozyme is the major protein in tears from open eyes, probably due to reflex tear production (Labbè et al. 2007).

It has been hypothesized that IgA may play a pivotal role in the pathogenesis of SS by representing a link between activated B cells and defective T cells. This interpretation is supported by the high proportion of IgA in immunoglobulin production at the mucosal level (Wehmeyer et al. 1991). It was reported that high levels of serum and secretory IgA, IgA-rheumatoid factor, and IgA-containing circulating immune complexes are present in SS DED. A correlation between disease activity and the latter abnormalities has also been shown (Levy et al. 1994).

Acidic mammalian chitinase

Chitinases are endo-b-1,4-linked b-N-acetyl-glucosaminidase. Recently, two distinct chitinases have been identified in humans: schitotriosidase expressed in phagocytes, and AMCase expressed in allergic diseases of the gastrointestinal tract, lung, and conjunctiva, and in the conjunctiva and tears of DED patients. AMCase activity is required for the production of the chemoattractants monocyte chemotactic protein-1 and 2 (also known as CCL2 and CCL8), macrophage inflammatory protein-1b (MIP-1b, also known as CCL4), eosinophil chemoattractants eotaxin-1 and 2 (CCL11 and CCL24, respectively), and the neutrophil chemoattractant epithelial-derived neutrophil-activating protein 78 (or CXCL5). Increased production of these chemokines may lead to the increased inflammatory infiltrate observed in chronic asthma (Zhu et al. 2004).

AMCase expression has been found in the conjunctival epithelial cells of DED patients, with an increased tear activity of this enzyme. The levels of enzyme expression and the AMCase activity in DED subjects were different in MGD and SS patients (Musumeci et al. 2009). An explanation for this can be found in the different pathogenetic mechanism of the two form of disease. In MGD, the altered tear film is characterized by a primary alteration of the lipid component, which can be accompanied by modification of the bacterial flora on the conjunctiva (Dougherty & McCulley 1984). This might induce a stronger innate response, as demonstrated by the higher AMCase expression level. Moreover, the other chitinase, chitotriosidase, is expressed with lysozyme in the human lacrimal gland (Hall et al. 2008). This expression could be considered as a response to the modified ocular surface flora, which can be responsible for the overinfections associated with chronic MGD.

Phospholipase A2

PLA2 is a superfamily of enzymes that hydrolyze glycerophospholipids to produce lysophospholipids and free fatty acids (Wei et al. 2011). The latter include arachidonic acid, which is the precursor of inflammatory mediators, such as PGE_2, leukotrienes, and eicosanoids (Rosenson & Gelb 2009). Secretory prostaglandin E2 (sPLA2) has been recognized as one of the most important biomarkers of human inflammatory diseases, acting as an inflammation signaling molecule. In ocular terms, it plays a role in the eye's innate immune defenses against Gram-positive bacteria; it has been reported that the level of sPLA2-IIa in normal human tears is at least 10,000 times higher than that in normal human serum (Aho et al. 2002). The human *sPLA2-IIa* gene is expressed approximately 6500 times more in human conjunctiva than in the human cornea, representing the greatest difference in gene expression between the two structures (Turner et al. 2007). It has been documented that both the concentration and enzymatic activity of sPLA2-IIa were elevated twofold in the tears of DED disease patients when compared with the tears of age-matched normal controls (Chen et al. 2009). Furthermore, a role of sPLA2-IIa as an inflammatory mediator on the compromised ocular surface has been suggested.

Transglutaminase-2

TG-2 is a ubiquitous protein, which belongs to a family of calcium-dependent intra- and extracellular cross-linking enzymes. Although TG-2 is found mainly in the cytosol, it can also be found in mitochondria, or imported into the nucleus of the cell. TG-2 is regulated by cellular stress, such as hydrogen peroxide treatment, or by external factors, such as ultraviolet (UV) radiation, and has a role in the induction of cell death (Png et al. 2011). Hyperosmolarity and high intracellular calcium stimulate apoptosis in various cell types and hyperosmolar conditions lead to increased TG-2 activity (Chen et al. 2008). TG-2 plays the main role to ensure that once apoptosis has been initiated, it is completed without causing inflammation and evident tissue injury. TG-2 can promote apoptosis (Tong et al. 2006) either by direct mechanism in certain apoptotic cells or, indirectly, by promoting activation of transforming growth factor (TGF)-b released by macrophages. In apoptotic cells, TG-2 also promotes the formation of chemoattractants, such as the S19 ribosomal protein (Nishiura et al. 1998), and the exposure of phosphatidylserine that enhances the migration of macrophages to the site of the apoptosis and the recognition of apoptotic cells. TG-2-dependent cross-linking of proteins and formation of protective proteinaceous shells prevent the leakage of dangerous cellular products from the apoptotic cells, whereas TG-2

in macrophages promotes the speed of phagocytosis and results in further formation of TGF-b. If necrosis occurs, TG-2 promotes tissue stability and the subsequent repair. In fact, in TG-2-/- animals, all these anti-inflammatory actions are compromised, resulting in the rapid migration of inflammatory cells to the apoptotic sites (Fésüs & Szondy 2005).

FROM INNATE TO ADAPTIVE IMMUNITY

Irritating stimuli, such as hyperosmolar tears, determine, in the epithelial cells, the interaction with receptors that activate response pathways, such as MAPKs, leading to the production of proinflammatory molecules (**Figure 8.2**). These events, occurring in both epithelial and dendritic cells, are responsible for the onset and maintenence of inflammation at the ocular surface (Pan et al. 2011).

Signaling pathways
Toll-like receptors

TLRs are thought to play a role in DED pathogenesis as the consequence of the modified ocular surface flora (Graham et al. 2007, Pflugfelder & Stern 2009). TLRs are type 1 transmembrane glycoproteins, which have two domains: one is leucine-rich extracellular domain and the other is cytoplasmic domain, which is homologous to that of the IL-1 receptor, hence referred to as the Toll/IL-1 receptor domain. This mediates the activation of intracellular signaling pathways, leading to functional changes including cytokines, chemokines, and adhesion molecules expression. To date, 10 functional human TLRs have been identified. TLRs 1, 2, 4, 5, 6, and 10 are located at the cell surface, where they are able to recognize a variety of microbial molecules. TLRs 3, 7, 8, and 9 have an intracellular location on endosomal membranes and recognize nucleic acids from viral or bacterial origin. TLRs are also capable of recognizing endogenous ligands. Many of these molecules are indicative of tissue trauma, such as nucleic acids, heat shock proteins, and extracellular matrix breakdown products, such as hyaluronan fragments, fibrinogen, and high-mobility group box 1 proteins (Kluwe et al. 2009). TLRs primarily activate the innate immune response and mediate neutrophil infiltration to the tissues; most evidences indicate that TLRs activation can determine the phenotype of a T-cell response. TLRs participate in surveillance system to control infection and tissue injury. On the contrary, TLR activation by endogenous ligands is associated with the development of autoimmune disorders, such as human systemic lupus erythematosus (Lamphier et al. 2006). TLRs are key regulators of both innate and adaptive immune responses.

Mitogen-activated protein kinases/ nuclear factor-kB

MAPKs are a family of serine/threonine protein kinases widely conserved among eukaryotes. They play a central role in integrating the signals from a diverse group of extracellular stimuli and proto-oncogenes to the nucleus, which affect cell proliferation, differentiation, movement, and death.

MAPKs signaling pathways are organized into three-tiered hierarchical modules. MAPKs are phosphorylated and activated by MAP kinase kinases, which are phosphorylated and activated by MAP kinase kinase kinases. The MAP kinase kinase kinases are activated by interaction with a family of small GTPases or other protein kinases connecting the MAPK pathway to cell surface receptors and thus to the

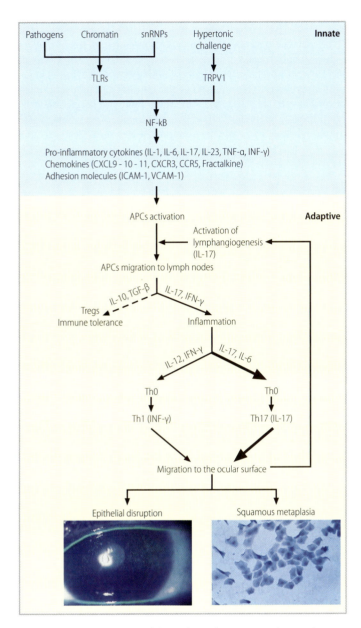

Figure 8.2 Pathophysiology of the ocular surface immune damage. In dry eye disease (DED), the ocular surface epithelium can be stressed by pathogens, postapoptotic fragments of chromatin and small nuclear ribonucleoproteins (snRNPs), or the hypertonic challenge. The former activate Toll-like receptors (TLRs) signaling pathways, the latter the transient receptor potential vanilloid (TRPV) channels; both enhance NF-kB signals, inducing the expression of proinflammatory cytokines, chemokines, and adhesion molecules. Antigen-presenting cells (APCs) are activated on the ocular surface and migrate to the lymph nodes, through newly formed lymphatic vessels. In the regional lymphoid compartment, if IL-10 and TGF-β are expressed, Tregs are able to block any further response, thus inducing immune tolerance. If, on the contrary, other molecules prevail, the activation and the expansion of two subsets of CD4+ T cells occur. When IL-12 and IFN-γ levels are high, T_H1 cells are formed; when IL-6 and IL-17 predominate, T_H17 cells are formed. The latter also seem to be able to antagonize Tregs activity and be the predominant cell type in course of DED. T_H1 and T_H17 migrate, through newly formed IL-17-induced lymphatic vessels, back to the ocular surface, where they both cause the corneal barrier disruption. IFN-γ-producing T_H1 cells are also capable of determining conjunctival metaplasia.

external stimuli. Extracellular signal-regulated kinases (ERK1 and 2) were the first of the ERK/MAP kinase subfamily to be cloned. Other related mammalian enzymes have also been detected, including two ERK3 isoforms, ERK4, Jun N-terminal kinases/stress-activated protein kinases (JNKs/SAPKs), p38/HOG, and p57 MAP kinases. The family of MAPKs (Qi & Elion 2005), therefore, includes the following:

- ERK1 and ERK2, the 'classical' MAPKs, regulate proliferation and differentiation and are activated in response to growth factors and cytokines, which stimulate a variety of receptors and G proteins. A complete pathway from receptor to MAPK has only been fully defined for the ERK1 and ERK2, which have many known targets, including key transcription factors, such as activator protein-1 (AP-1) and NF-kB, and the cell survival regulator Bcl-2
- c-JNKs (MAPK8, MAPK9, MAPK10), also known as SAPKs, play crucial roles in regulating responses to various stresses, in inflammation and apoptosis. They are activated by UV radiation, cytokines, heat shock, and osmotic shock, and by growth factors. JNK1 regulates differentiation of the T helper 2 (T_H2) subset of T cells and T-cell activation, whereas JNK1 and JNK2 are required for control of IL-2 production in T cells and responses to UV radiation
- p38 isoforms [p38-α (MAPK14), p38-β (MAPK11), p38-γ (MAPK12 or ERK6), and p38-δ (MAPK13 or SAPK4)] play an important role in human asthma and autoimmunity and are activated by numerous physical and chemical stresses, including hormones, UV irradiation, cytokines such as IL-1 and TNF, and osmotic and heat shock. Among the targets of p38 MAPKs, there are several important transcription factors, including NF-kB and p53, which modulate the expression of genes encoding for inflammatory cytokines

Other members of the MAPK family are ERK3 (MAPK6), ERK4 (MAPK4), ERK5 (MAPK7), and ERK7/8 (MAPK15), whose role in DED has not been demonstrated.

NF-κB is a pleiotropic transcription factor that plays a critical role in the regulation of the expression of multiple genes involved in inflammatory responses (Zerfaoui et al. 2008). The term NF-κB commonly refers specifically to a p50-RelA heterodimer, whose activity is tightly regulated by the interaction with IκB, which has an inhibitory function.

NF-κB is important in regulating cellular responses because it belongs to the category of 'rapid-acting' primary transcription factors, that is transcription factors that are present in cells in an inactive state and do not require new protein synthesis to be activated. Other members of this family include transcription factors, such as c-Jun, signal transducer and activator of transcriptions (STATs), and nuclear hormone receptors. This allows NF-κB to be the first responder to harmful cellular stimuli. Known inducers of NF-κB activity are highly variable and include reactive oxygen species, TNF-α, IL-1β, and bacterial lipopolysaccharides.

Many bacterial products and a wide variety of cell-surface-receptor stimulation lead to NF-κB activation and fairly rapid changes in gene expression. The identification of TLRs as specific pattern recognition molecules and the finding that stimulation of TLRs leads to activation of NF-κB improved the understanding of how different pathogens activate NF-κB.

■ Proinflammatory proteins
Interleukin-1

IL-1 is a powerful proinflammatory cytokine, which can be produced by many cell types, including macrophages, monocytes, lymphocytes, keratinocytes, and fibroblasts, in response to inflammation, infection, injury, or other environmental stimuli (Dinarello 2011). Two isoforms, a and b, as well as a specific receptor antagonist, have been described. Furthermore, there are two receptors for IL-1, a signaling receptor named IL-1RI and a decoy receptor named IL-1RII (Zouklırı et al. 2007). Activation of the IL-1RI triggers a signaling cascade leading to the transcription of several genes involved in acute and chronic inflammation. IL-1 increases the expression of adhesion molecules, such as intercellular adhesion molecule-1 (ICAM-1) on mesenchymal cells and vascular cell adhesion molecule-1 (VCAM-1) on endothelial cells, leading to the infiltration of inflammatory and immunocompetent cells into the extravascular space (Dinarello 2000).

Both proinflammatory forms of IL-1 (α and β) are multifunctional cytokines that in general produce similar biological effects, although these may vary among different cell types and organ systems. IL-1 has been implicated in the pathogenesis of corneal and ocular surface diseases, such as rosacea, bullous keratopathy, keratoconus, and sterile corneal ulceration. IL-1 is a potent inducer of other inflammatory cytokines such as IL-6 and IL-8, TNF-α, and granulocyte-macrophage colony-stimulating factor. It also stimulates the production of MMP enzymes by epithelial and inflammatory cells.

IL-1α is responsible for causing inflammation, as well as promoting fever and sepsis. It is mainly produced by activated macrophages, as well as by neutrophils, epithelial cells, and endothelial cells. It plays one of the central roles in immune response regulation and binds to the IL-1 receptor. It is on the pathway that activates TNF-α.

IL-1β is produced by activated macrophages as a proprotein, which is proteolytically processed to its active form by the caspase 1 (CASP1/interleukin-1 beta converting enzyme). This cytokine is an important mediator of the inflammatory response, and is involved in a variety of cellular activities, including cell proliferation, differentiation, and apoptosis.

DED is accompanied by an increase in the proinflammatory forms of IL-1 (both IL-1α and mature IL-1β) and a decrease in the biologically inactive precursor IL-1β in tear fluid. Increased protease activity on the ocular surface may be one mechanism by which precursor IL-1β is cleaved to the mature, biologically active form. The tear fluid of DED patients shows an increased concentration of IL-1, also deriving from conjunctival epithelial cells; so IL-1 may play a key role in the pathogenesis of DED (Solomon et al. 2001).

Interleukin-2

IL-2 is a signaling molecule of the immune system that attracts lymphocytes through its receptors (IL-2R), expressed by lymphocytes. Binding of IL-2 activates the Ras/MAPK, Janus Kinase (JAK)/STAT, and PI 3-kinase/Akt signaling modules. Binding of antigens to the T-cell receptor stimulates the secretion of IL-2 and the expression of its receptors, thus leading to the growth, differentiation, and survival of antigen-selected cytotoxic T cells via the activation of the expression of specific genes.

IL-2 is necessary for the development of T-cell immunological memory and the maturation of regulatory T cells (Tregs). In addition, it is required for the discrimination between self and nonself. In fact, the results of a study performed on mice demonstrated that IL-2R is required to maintain homeostasis and prevent autoimmunity (Jabs et al. 2001).

The tears of DED patients contained an increased concentration of IL-2 when compared with normal subjects. This augmentation is because of overproduction, rather than evaporation, which is suggested by an upregulation of its gene in the conjunctiva (Massingale et al. 2009).

Interleukin-6

IL-6 is important for B-cell growth and differentiation. It is thought to induce the production of autoreactive antibodies through infiltration of B cells, via upregulation of specific cytokines, and through its effect on the terminal differentiation of the immunoglobulin-producing plasma B cell. IL-6 acts in T-cell stimulation and recruitment, by promoting the transition of naive T cells to cytotoxic T cells. It also upregulates ICAM-1, which functions as a receptor for activated T cells and, on many cells, as a costimulatory molecule for B cells (Roescher et al. 2009).

Recent reports show increased IL-6 levels in patients with DED, keratoconus, and conjunctivochalasis, for example, in the tears of patients suffering from ADDE when compared with healthy volunteers (Yoon et al. 2007). Similarly, an increase in IL-6 was reported in the tears of patients with mild-to-moderate EDE, thus demonstrating that inflammation plays a role not only in severe DED but also in moderate EDE (Enriquez-de-Salamanca et al. 2010). IL-6 tear levels in DED patients were correlated significantly with tear film break-up time, tear clearance, corneal surface damage, conjunctival goblet cell density, severity of irritation symptoms, Schirmer's score, corneal fluorescein staining, and conjunctival lissamine score (Calonge et al. 2010).

Interleukin-17

IL-17 (or IL-17A) is the founding member of a group of cytokines called the IL-17 family. It is a potent proinflammatory cytokine produced by activated memory T cells (Gurney & Aggarwal 2002) and acts by increasing chemokine production in various tissues to recruit monocytes and neutrophils to the site of inflammation, similar to interferon (IFN)-γ; furthermore, it acts synergistically with TNF and IL-1 (Miossec et al. 2009). In addition to IL-17A, the IL-17 family includes IL-17B, IL-17C, IL-17D, IL-17E (also called IL-25), and IL-17F, all of which have a similar protein structure. IL-17 works by binding to a type 1 cell surface receptor called IL-17R. Transcription factors such as TRAF6, JNK, ERK1/2, p38, AP-1, and NF-κB have been implicated in IL-17-mediated signaling in a stimulation-dependent, tissue-specific manner (Ley et al. 2006).

IL-17 induces the production of many other cytokines (such as IL-6, (G-CSF), granulocyte-macrophage colony-stimulating factor, IL-1β, TGF-β, and TNF-α), chemokines (including IL-8, CXCL1, and CCL2), MMPs, and PGE_2 in different cell types (fibroblasts, endothelial cells, epithelial cells, and macrophages). The increased expression of chemokines attracts other cells, including neutrophils, but not eosinophils. IL-17 function is also essential to a subset of CD4+ T cells called T_H17 cells. As a result of these roles, the IL-17 family has been linked to many immune/autoimmune-related diseases, including rheumatoid arthritis, asthma, lupus, allograft rejection, and antitumour immunity (Kolls & Linden 2004).

The increased presence of tear IL-17 in DED (Chung et al. 2012), along with the presence of T_H17 cells and expression of IL-17R on the ocular surface epithelia, indicates the importance of an IL-17-mediated cytokine cascade in the immunopathogenesis of DED. The constitutive expression of IL-17 receptors by corneal and conjunctival epithelia makes ocular surface more vulnerable to IL-17-mediated inflammation and tissue damage. The presence of proinflammatory cytokines in the milieu may actually favor the generation of autoreactive T cells. For instance, IL-6 in the presence of TGF-β causes differentiation of autoreactive T_H17 cells, which can restrain Treg function and favor autoreactivity.

The functional relevance of T_H17 cells in the immunopathogenesis of DED has been fundamentally confirmed by the finding that in vivo neutralization of IL-17 results in a markedly attenuated induction and severity of the disease, which is paralleled by a reduction in the expansion of T_H17 cells (Kang et al. 2011).

Tumor necrosis factor-α

TNF-α is a cytokine involved in systemic inflammation, and is a member of a group of cytokines that stimulate the acute phase reaction. The primary role of TNF is the regulation of immune cells activity. TNF is primarily produced by macrophages, although, it is also produced by a large variety of other cell types, including lymphoid cells, mast cells, fibroblasts, and epithelial cells. Large amounts of TNF are released in response to lipopolysaccharide, other bacterial products, and IL-1.

The primary form of TNF is a 212-amino-acid-long transmembrane protein arranged in stable homotrimers. This membrane-integrated form undergoes proteolytic cleavage by the action of metalloprotease TNF-a-converting enzyme, and the soluble homotrimeric cytokine (sTNF) is released (Black et al. 1997).

TNF can bind two receptors, TNF-R1 (TNF receptor type 1; CD120a; p55/60) and TNF-R2 (TNF receptor type 2; CD120b; p75/80). TNF-R1 is expressed in most tissues, and can be fully activated by both the membrane-bound and soluble trimeric forms of TNF, whereas TNF-R2 is found only in cells of the immune system, and responds to the membrane-bound form of the TNF homotrimer. This binding causes a conformational change in the receptor, leading to the activation of the adaptor protein Tumor necrosis factor receptor type 1-associated death domain protein (TRADD), which binds to the cellular death domain, and activates three pathways: MAPK, NF-κB, and death signaling.

In the ocular surface, TNF-α is synthetized by mast cells, T lymphocytes, and the majority of epithelial cells, this amplifies the role of these cells in inflammatory, toxic, or degenerative processes. TNF-α interacts with other cytokines, such as Fas ligand, IL-1α and IL-1β, or IFN-γ, thus leading to apoptosis and inflammation (Baudouin & Liang 2005). It has been implicated in the pathogenesis of corneal ulceration, uveitis, and corneal transplant rejection (Goyal et al. 2009). In fact, an increased production and activation of this cytokine has been demonstrated in various ocular surface diseases, including DED (Pflugfelder et al. 1999, VanDerMeid et al. 2011). In the latter condition, the upregulation of *TNF*-α gene in the conjunctiva suggests that the increased concentration in tears is not the result of evaporative effects, but due to overproduction (Massingale et al. 2009). However, it has been shown that TNF-α level, unlike the one of IL-6, is not associated with the severity of the disease and does not correlate with various ocular surface parameters (Yoon et al. 2007).

TNF-α has been found to affect neural sensitivity and cause ocular surface hyperalgesia. In fact, it has been hypothesized that elevated tear cytokine concentrations, especially TNF-α, might be a more sensitive disease marker, than traditional signs, in patients with mild DED who complain of ocular discomfort despite the absence of objective signs (Lam et al. 2009).

Furthermore, differences were noted between ADE and EDDE patients, the latter group presenting a lower TNF-α concentration. This evidence led to the assumption that mechanisms other than inflammation can be responsible for DED in these patients (Boehm et al. 2011).

Interferon-γ

IFN-γ, or type 2 IFN, is a dimerized soluble cytokine encoded by the *IFNG* gene. Unlike INF-α and INF-β, which can be expressed by every cell, IFN-γ is secreted by T_H1 cells, cytotoxic T cells (T_C cells), and NK cells. IFN-γ interactions with a heterodimeric receptor, consisting of IFN-γ receptor 1 and IFN-γ receptor 2, and plays a pivotal role in innate and adaptive immunity against viral and intracellular bacterial infections by direct inhibition of viral replication (Schoenborn & Wilson 2007).

IFN-γ causes a variety of physiological and cellular responses, such as the promotion of NK cell activity, the increase in antigen presentation and lysosomes activity in macrophages, the activation of inducible nitric oxide synthase, and the promotion of T_H1 differentiation by upregulating the transcription factor T-bet. Furthermore, it induces increased expression of class I MHC molecules in normal cells, as well as class II MHC in antigen-presenting cells (APCs). IFN-γ, through the induction of antigen-processing genes, promotes adhesion and binding activity required for leukocyte migration, and induces the expression of intrinsic defense factors. IFN-γ is the primary cytokine that defines T_H1 cells: T_H1 cells secrete IFN-γ, which causes more undifferentiated CD4+ cells (T_H0 cells) to differentiate into T_H1 cells, representing a positive feedback loop, while suppressing T_H2 cell differentiation.

In addition to the crucial role played by IFN-γ in regulating several immune responses (such as delayed-type hypersensitivity, inflammation, and graft rejection), and the pathogenesis of inflammatory diseases (SS, ocular mucous membrane pemphigoid, Stevens–Johnson syndrome, and graft-versus-host disease), it was demonstrated that desiccating stress promoted the migration of CD4+ T cells and IFN-γ-expressing cells into the conjunctiva and increased the concentration of IFN-γ in tears in DED conditions. Increased IFN-γ can lead to conjunctival epithelial squamous metaplasia and pathological apoptosis, characterized by increased T_H1 and T_H17 CD4+ T-cell infiltration on the ocular surface (Zhang et al. 2011).

Transforming growth factor-β

TGF-β is a pleiotropic cytokine that plays a crucial role in the regulation of the cell cycle. In fact, it directs cellular proliferation, differentiation, wound healing, inflammation, and other functions in most cells. Furthermore, it induces apoptosis in numerous cell types. At least three isoforms of TGF-β are known, called TGF-β1, TGF-β2, and TGF-β3. TGF-β1 is the main member of this family. TGF-β acts as an antiproliferative factor in normal epithelial cells. TGF-β1 regulates the expression of many other growth factors through the interaction with its receptors present on various cell types. Some cells that secrete TGF-β1 also have receptors for TGF-β1: this is known as autocrine signaling. Once activated, TGF-β binds a membrane-bound serine/threonine receptor complex (TβRI/TβRII), which phosphorylates various substrates (Dogar et al. 2011).

The functions of TGF-β include promoting the rate of apoptosis, through the induction of TG-2; increasing the efficiency of macrophage phagocytosis; and down-regulating the production of proinflammatory cytokines in macrophages. TGF-β1 is produced by the human lacrimal gland and corneal and conjunctival epithelia and has been detected in tears (Zheng et al. 2010).

TGF-β receptors were detected in epithelial and vascular endothelial cells of conjunctiva (Meyer-Ter-Vehn et al. 2008), and TGF-β in superficial limbal cells was thought to play a role in the transdifferentiation of conjunctival epithelium to corneal epithelium (Pasquale et al. 1993). During corneal wound healing, TGF-β stimulates the synthesis of collagen, as well as hyaluronan, biglycan, and fibronectin, in the fibrotic extracellular matrix (Etheredge et al. 2010).

Because of its diverse functions, regulation of TGF-β activity may be fundamental in the immune system of the ocular surface, where it plays a dual role. The first is the maintenance of homeostasis, by blocking T- and B-cell proliferation and promoting Tregs differentiation and activity, therefore preventing the development of autoimmune reactions. The second is the generation of an immune response to stress, such as desiccation, which induces the generation of pathogenic IL-17-producing effector cells (T_H17) (De Paiva et al. 2011).

Several studies reported increased TGF-β1 protein in tears, or mRNA in conjunctival biopsies, or increased expression of protein in the conjunctival epithelium and salivary gland biopsies, obtained from patients with SS. However, the role of TGF-β1 in the pathogenesis of DED is still not completely understood.

Matrix metalloproteinases

MMPs are a family of zinc- and calcium-dependent enzymes, involved in the breakdown of extracellular matrix in normal physiological processes, such as embryonic development, morphogenesis, reproduction, tissues resorption, and remodeling. Moreover, they play an important role in various pathological processes, such as inflammation, arthritis, cancer, and different autoimmune diseases, including systemic lupus erythematosus, SS, systemic sclerosis, and rheumatoid arthritis. In these diseases they induce extracellular matrix destruction. MMPs, which are released along with the various other molecules during flogosis, play a crucial role in setting and maintenance of ocular surface damage. Most MMPs are secreted as inactive proproteins, which are activated when cleaved by extracellular proteinases.

MMP-9 is the most important gelatinase present on the ocular surface (Meloni et al. 2011), and shows an increased concentration in tears of DED patients, with the highest concentration being observed in SS, corneal epithelial defects, and sterile stromal ulcer. MMP-9 lyses a large number of substrates, including the components of the corneal epithelial basement membrane and the tight junction proteins (ZO-1 and occludin), thus compromising the integrity of the corneal epithelial barrier. Proteolitic cleavage of occludin accelerates loss of superficial corneal epithelium, thus increasing its permeability. MMP-9 appears to play a physiological role in regulating corneal epithelial desquamation. The increased MMP-9 activity in DED may be responsible, in part, for the deranged corneal epithelial barrier function, increased corneal epithelial desquamation, and corneal surface irregularity. Furthermore, MMP-9 has been demonstrated to increase corneal epithelial regeneration by modulating the inflammatory response in the healing cornea (Mohan et al. 2002). Among its various activities, MMP-9 is known to activate precursor IL-1β and latent TGF-1β into their active forms. Therefore, the increase of MMP-9 activity on the ocular surface can amplify the chronic immune-based inflammation in DED (Chotikavanich et al. 2009).

■ Cell-recruiting molecules
HLA-DR

HLA-DR is a MHC class II cell surface receptor encoded by the human leukocyte antigen complex on chromosome 6. It is a a-b heterodimer, cell surface receptor; each subunit contains two extracellular domains, a membrane-spanning domain, and a cytoplasmic tail. Both a and b chains are anchored in the membrane. The primary function of HLA-DR is to present peptide antigens, potentially foreign in origin, to the immune system in order to stimulate or suppress T helper cell responses that eventually lead to the production of antibodies against the same antigens. APCs (macrophages, B cells, and dendritic cells) are those in which DR are typically found. HLA-DR molecules are upregulated in response to signaling. The DR molecule binds antigens to present them to receptors on T helper cells. These cells bind on the surface of B cells stimulating their proliferation.

Like the other molecules in the human MHC class II, HLA-DR plays a critical role in the initiation of the immune response. An overexpression of HLA-DR has been demonstrated in the epithelial cells of both ocular and non-ocular tissues that are affected by inflammatory disorders (Versura et al. 2011); among the former are patients with SS, chronic conjunctivitis, and DED (Mrugacz & Zywalewska 2005). In particular, DED and ocular rosacea were associated with overexpression of inflammatory markers such as HLA-DR and ICAM-1 and a significant decrease in the number of goblet cells (Pisella et al. 2001), whereas, in SS, HLA-DR expression was found at a significantly higher level than in non-SS DED. Similarly, a greater expression of HLA-DR was observed in conjunctival epithelial cells in the different chronic ocular allergic disorders such as vernal keratoconjunctivitis and atopic keratoconjunctivitis. Increased expression of HLA-DR antigen positively correlates with the parameters of DED diagnostic tests, so its measurement might be a useful method for monitoring inflammatory conjunctival changes in this disorder.

Chemokines

Other molecules recently implicated in the ocular surface disorder occurring in DED are chemokines: proteins of low molecular weight, secreted by cells that play important roles in physiological mechanisms and the regulation of inflammatory responses (Barabino & Dana 2007). In fact, some chemokines are considered homeostatic, because of their role in controlling the migration of cells during the normal process of immune surveillance or in angiogenesis during development, whereas others are considered proinflammatory, as they are induced during an immune response to recruit cells of the immune system to the site of inflammation.

Inflammatory chemokines are released from a wide variety of cells in response to bacterial or viral infections, or agents that cause physical damage; their release is often stimulated by proinflammatory cytokines, such as IL-1. They function mainly as chemoattractants for leukocytes, recruiting monocytes, neutrophils, and other cells from the blood to sites of infection or tissue damage, and put forth their biological effects by interacting with transmembrane receptors (chemokine receptors), found on the surface of their target cells. They are released by many different cell types and serve to guide cells of both innate and adaptive immune system.

Members of the chemokine family are divided into four groups depending on the spacing of their first two cysteine residues at the N-terminal region of the protein: CXC (a), CC (b), C (g), and CXXXC (d).

CXC or a chemokines can be further divided into two categories, as ELR+ or ELR-, on the basis of the presence of a specific amino acid sequence of glutamic acid-leucine-arginine (ELR). ELR+ chemokines have high affinity for CXCR1 and CXCR2 receptors on neutrophils; an example of this category is IL-8.

The CXC chemokine IL-8, encoded by the *IL-8* gene, is a potent neutrophil-recruiting and neutrophil-activating factor, produced by macrophages and other cell types, such as epithelial and endothelial cells (Buchholz & Stephens 2007), and is an essential part of the initial innate immune response. Although lipopolysaccharides, IL-1b, and TNF-a are capable of augmenting IL-8 production, IL-10 is a potent inhibitor of its synthesis and appears to play an autoregulatory role. IL-8 production is low in the absence of external stimuli. During stimulation, conserved signaling pathways activate IL-8 expression at the transcriptional and post-transcriptional levels (Hoffmann et al. 2002). Maximal IL-8 amounts can only be generated if the gene promoter is derepressed, NF-kB and JNK pathways are activated to induce transcription, and the resulting mRNA is rapidly stabilized by the p38 MAPK pathway. In this way, cells are able to rapidly increase and, at the same time, fine-regulate the amount of IL-8 secreted and control the quantity of leukocytes attracted to the sites of tissue injury. It is also important to note that this type of signal-dependent gene expression is not restricted to IL-8, but may also be relevant for many other proteins, such as IL-6, expressed during an inflammatory response. IL-8 exerts its effects on neutrophils by strongly binding to two receptors on their surface, the chemokine receptors CXCR1 and CXCR2. In the conjunctival epithelium of patients with SS DED, increased levels of RNA transcripts were detected encoding, among the others, for the inflammatory cytokine IL-8 (Pflugfelder et al. 1999). Furthermore, a study was performed to determine whether there were differences in levels of tear cytokines and chemokines between an asymptomatic control group and DED patients, with and without MGD, which showed that the concentration of IL-8 was higher in all DED groups than in the non-DED group (Lam et al. 2009).

ELRs have a high affinity for the CXCR3 receptor of lymphocytes (activated T cells and NK cells). Members of the ELR category, which are readily induced by IFN-γ, include CXCL9 (MIG or monokine induced by IFN-γ), CXCL10 (IP-10 or IFN-γ-inducible protein, 10 kDa), and CXCL11 (IFN-inducible T-cell chemoattractant or I-TAC).

Among CC or b chemokines, important roles are played by CCL2 (monocyte chemoattractant protein-1), CCL4 (MIP-1b), and CCL5 (regulated upon activation, normal T-cell expressed, and secreted). The first induces monocytes to leave the blood and enter the surrounding tissues to become macrophages; the second and third attract cells such as T cells, eosinophils, and basophils that express the specific receptor.

C or g chemokines have only two cysteines and are called lymphotactin-a and b. Their role in the attraction of T-cell precursors to the thymus has been described.

The only known member of the CXXXC or d chemokine group is called fractalkine (or CX3CL1) and is either secreted or attached to the surface of the cell that expresses it, thereby serving as both a chemoattractant and an adhesion molecule.

As to their behavior in the eye, it was shown that, in tears from healthy subjects (Carreño et al. 2010), RANTES (regulated upon activation, normal T-cell expressed and secreted), IL-8, MIP-1 and fractalkine are normally expressed in a range of concentrations with no differences between males and females.

In DED patients, fractalkine, interferon-gamma-induced protein-10 (IP-10), and IL-8 were the more detected molecules in tear samples and were also the ones with the highest concentration (Enriquez-de-Salamanca et al. 2010). Recently, it has been shown (Choi et al. 2012) that the expression of CCR5 and its ligands CCL3, CCL4, and CCL5 increases in the tear film and on the ocular surface of patients with DED, especially in those with SS, and that CCL5 levels correlate significantly with various tear film and ocular surface parameters. It was also shown that conjunctival epithelial cells of patients with various forms of DED uniformly overexpress CCR5, implicating epithelial cells in the regulation of bone-marrow-derived cell recruitment in DED (Barabino & Dana 2007).

Adhesion molecules (intercellular adhesion molecule-1, vascular cell adhesion molecule-1)

Cellular adhesion molecules play a primary role in cell–cell recognition. They are cell surface proteins that facilitate cellular migration by binding to extracellular matrix components; in DED patients, ICAMs and VCAMs have been identified in the conjunctiva and the lacrimal gland (Turkcapar et al. 2005).

ICAMs are cell surface glycoproteins expressed on leukocytes, epithelial cells, endothelial cells, and fibroblasts. Five ICAMs have been identified, and ICAM-1 (CD54) is the most studied. In normal conditions, ICAM-1 expression is low and, as a ligand for β2 integrins, has a significant role in leukocyte–leukocyte, leukocyte–endothelial, and leukocyte–epithelial interactions and in transendothelial migration (Barreiro et al. 2002; Xu & Li 2009). Stimulation with inflammatory cytokines, such as IL-1, TNF-α, IFN-γ, or with CD40 has been shown to increase ICAM-1 in many cell types. The increased expression of ICAM-1 is dependent on NF-κB (Saito et al. 2007). Either CD40L expressed on CD4+ T cells or sCD40L in serum induces the phosphorylation of inhibitor κB. Then, NF-κB moves from cytoplasm into nucleus and transcription is activated, and ICAM-1 is expressed on the cell surface.

ICAM-1 is not merely an adhesion molecule. As a signaling molecule, it delivers its message through its unique presentation and distribution in various cell types at various locations. ICAM-1 expression is essential in not only promoting infiltrating inflammatory cell homing to the ocular tissues (Goldberg et al. 1994) but also directly and/or indirectly modulating the physiological and functional stage of ocular resident epithelial cells, therefore predisposing them to the immune-mediated ocular inflammation (Gao et al. 2004).

VCAM-1 is a cell surface glycoprotein involved in the recruitment and binding of lymphocytes, monocytes, eosinophils, and basophils to the vascular endothelium (Ley & Huo 2001). It is overexpressed in all DED disorders owing to the presence of lymphocyte activation. VCAM-1 expression is promoted by the nuclear translocation of NF-κB either in cell culture systems or in diseases, such as atherosclerosis, asthma, and autoimmune diseases.

Proinflammatory neurotransmitters, such as substance P, acting via the NF-κB signaling pathway, lead to ICAM-1 and VCAM-1 expression, therefore promoting lymphocyte homing and chemotaxis to sites of inflammation. Many proinflammatory cytokines, including TNF-α and IL-1, not only upregulate ICAM-1 expression but also induce de novo VCAM-1 expression (Nishiyama et al. 2007). VCAM-1 is strongly expressed on vascular endothelial cells, apical duct epithelial cells, and acini in the salivary glands of patients with SS (Mikulowska-Mennis et al. 2001). It is possible that VCAM-1 is an important adhesion molecule (a co-stimulatory molecule) for APCs and CD4+ T cells in SS.

ADAPTIVE IMMUNITY

Once the pathogenic stimulus is prolonged on the ocular surface, the modified epithelial cells and the local immune cells generate systemic responses that are able to recruit specific cells from the immune system. This part of the immune response is called adaptive immunity and follows the innate immunity, which is the non-specific and evolutionarily older response of the immune system. Adaptive immunity is a highly specialized biological answer, aimed to prevent or eliminate a pathogenic stimulus. Through this process, the immune system is not only able to recognize a specific condition and respond stronger each time the pathogenic stimulus is encountered but also generate an autoimmune process that may maintain the inflammatory condition at the ocular surface.

The adaptive immunity is mediated by a cellular response and maintained active by the production of mediators. The final scope of this process is to destroy the target of the immune response. This result can be obtained through the activation of pathways leading to cell damage by either apoptosis or necrosis. In DED, both these pathways have been demonstrated. These processes originate in the site where the innate immune response has developed, stimulating the sentinel cells of the local immune system: the APCs.

Antigen-presenting cells

APCs are sentinel cells that, in presence of external potentially danger-ous signals, internalize, process, and present the antigens on their sur-face. The function of an APC is determined by their state of maturation. APCs are characterized by the expression of MHC molecules on their surfaces; the complex MHC antigen is recognized by T-cell receptors present on their surface. In this way the T cells become activated. Immature APCs express low levels of MHC class II and costimula-tory molecules, so that they are inefficient at presenting antigens and promoting T-cell activation. Inflammatory microenvironments can induce APC maturation via increased expression of MHC class II and costimulatory molecules, rendering APCs efficient at priming T cells. APCs can be distinguished into two categories: professional or non-professional. The former express MHC class II on their surface; among these are dendritic cells, monocytes/macrophages, and Langherans cells (LCs). The latter do not constitutively express the MHC class II necessary for the interaction with naïve T cells, but they can express this protein after stimulation by cytokines, such as INF-γ. Examples of these cells are fibroblasts and activated epithelial cells.

In the cornea (Stevenson et al. 2012), the only cell type that consti-tutively expresses MHC class II antigen on its surface is LC. Peripheral cornea contains both MHC class II-positive and negative cells, while the central cornea just contains MHC class II-negative LCs. In the corneal stroma, APCs derived from monocytic cells are also present (Hattori et al. 2011).

The APCs play a crucial role in the induction of the adaptive (antigen-specific) immune response, as the consequence of a cascade of events culminating in the presentation of the antigens to the T cells by the complex MHC class II and APCs. To better define this process (Dana 2005), six different steps could be identified: (1) infiltration of APCs into the site of antigen challenge and contact with the antigen; (2) pick-up and processing of antigens by APCs; (3) upregulation of MHC class II (Ia/HLA-DR) and costimulatory molecules that lead to mature stimulatory APCs; (4) switch to APC chemokine receptor that allows for the progress of APCs toward lymphatics and lymphatic reservoirs where they can be in contact with naïve T cells; (5) priming of naïve T cells; and (6) expansion and progress toward the periphery of antigen-specific T clones.

Lymphatic immune response

Antigen processing and presentation by ocular surface APCs and migration of antigen-loaded APCs to regional lymph nodes are key events during the afferent immune response. This process is regulated by a variety of cellular factors, such as Tregs, and soluble factors, like TGF-β and IL-1 receptor antagonist, which induce a protective im-munity without causing tissue destruction and autoimmunity. The activation of specific lymphocytic subsets and their homing to the ocular surface contribute to the efferent mechanism of the immune response. The regulation of this phase is fundamental in prevention of the activation of autoreactive lymphocytes during acute inflam-matory responses. In fact, it is of relevant importance to prevent the development of events that may lead to chronic inflammation and tissue damage (**Figure 8.2**).

DED pathogenesis is determined by the activation and the in-filtration of immune competent cells, primarily CD4+ T cells in the conjunctiva and CD11b/CD18+ monocytic cells in the cornea. The hyperosmolar stress that occurs in DED stimulates the ocular surface tissues to secrete inflammatory cytokines, such as IL-1, TNF-a, and IL-6, which facilitate the activation and migration of resident APCs toward the regional draining lymph nodes, where APCs stimulate cognate naïve T cells (T_H0), resulting in the expansion of IL-17-secreting T_H17 cells and INF-γ-secreting T_H1 cells. In the lymph nodes, IL-17 plays a dual action: the antagonization of the Treg function, and T_H17 cells expansion, which may compete with Treg cells for the TGF-β available in the milieu.

Once the effector cells are generated in the lymph nodes, they migrate toward the ocular surface. T-cell infiltration of the ocular surface is a key factor in the pathogenesis of DED. In particular, the T_H17 cells are thought to be the primary effector T cells in DED. In fact, they play a prominent role in DED pathogenesis, through the production of proinflammatory products (such as IL-17, IL-21, IL-22, and IL-23), chemokines (MIP-2, CXCL1, CXCL2, CXCL5), and matrix metalloproteinases (MMP-3, MMP-9, and MMP-13) (Weaver et al. 2007), all actively involved in tissue inflammation. Furthermore, the interaction between IL-17 with its receptors activates chemotactic factors, such as CXCL8, responsible for the recruitment of neutrophils to the site of inflammation.

The T_H1 cells, through the production of INF-γ, play a role in the induction of apoptosis and metaplasia of the ocular surface epithelia; furthermore, they upregulate the expression of receptors for chemo-kine ligands and of adhesion molecules, thus increasing the attraction of immune cells in the ocular surface tissues.

INFLAMMATORY BIOMARKERS IN DED

Both forms of DED, ADDE and EDE, can be considered a model for inflammatory ocular surface disease. Because an overlap of the two forms is often present, it is difficult to differentiate between them. Find-ing biomarkers that could help this differentiation would be of great relevance for the clinical practice. Moreover, diagnostic biomarkers should not only allow a differentiation between patients and controls but also differentiate other diseases with overlapping characteristics, for example, seasonal allergic conjunctivitis. Comparative studies should differentiate affected from unaffected subjects, where the unaffected include both healthy subjects and patients with ocular surface conditions other than DED. For example, a biomarker for DED should achieve a low false-positive rate within an allergic ocular disease population.

Several functions can be attributed to a biomarker: individuate people at risk to develop the disease; screen and diagnose a disease; scale its severity; monitor the progress or the remission phases; predict the response to the therapy; determine the prognosis; and contribute to understanding of the disease pathophysiology. Any measurable, disease-associated, biological parameter can be considered to be a biomarker.

There is no indication for diagnostic DED screening in the general population, but we might have an interest to know about the risk to develop DED in predisposing circumstances. An example of this could be the occurrence of DED in course of both topical or systemic conditions such as contact lens wear; refractive laser surgery; chronic use of preserved eye drops, for example, in glaucoma treatment; postmenopausal estrogen therapy; chronic use of systemic therapies such as antihistamines, b-blockers, diuretics, benzodiazepines, and antidepressants; isotretinoin systemic therapy; connective tissue diseases; graft-versus-host diseases in bone marrow transplantation; androgen deficiency; or androgen receptor blockade.

Individuating a useful biomarker could be of great interest to understand which members of a given population can be considered at risk to develop DED but the task to attain this goal failed to achieve success.

The performance of a biomarker is influenced by the quality of the phenotype. The criteria used to establish the diagnosis of DED, its subtypes (ADE and EDDE), or related diseases (i.e. MGD) are relatively imprecise because of the variance in test measures used. Also, different authors have used different criteria for the same disorder. Furthermore, there is a poor correlation between signs and symptoms, but because DED is a symptomatic disease, an effective therapy must improve or remove symptoms and an ideal therapy should relieve symptoms by targeting the pathogenic mechanisms.

It is unlikely that there is one solitary source of DED symptoms; furthermore, the sources of symptoms could change during the evolution of the disease. For instance, corneal irritation with increased sensitivity may be present at some stage of the disease whereas sensitivity may fall in advanced phases. This is probably why correlations are so poor or variable.

A study of the correlation between biomarker expression on the ocular surface and symptoms would be of interest. Furthermore, biomarkers could be used as indicators of specific pathogenic mechanisms of the disease.

In fact, there are multiple potential sources of symptoms in DED, but their relative contribution could change with the stage of the disease. Symptoms may not be consequent to the most evident cause, but rather the cumulative effect of several causes, that is, inflammation determines alteration of the surface glycocalyx, goblet cell loss, and squamous metaplasia. These alterations are responsible for tear film instability and consequent discomfort symptoms, but the relationship to inflammation as the original cause of the dysfunction is yet to be recognized. In addition, it should be kept in mind that many of the proinflammatory molecules raised in DED are also markers for ocular surface inflammation in seasonal allergic conjunctivitis, vernal keratoconjunctivitis, and atopic keratoconjunctivitis (Tables 8.1–8.3).

Lack of a powerful association between a biomarker and DED symptoms at diagnosis should not discourage its use to track the efficacy of an agent, particularly where it tests a causal hypothesis or could provide proof of principle of drug action.

It is possible to evaluate the expression of ocular surface biomarkers in tears or in corneoconjunctival epithelial cells. The sampling method of the material and the disease stage could interfere with the evaluation of the considered biomarker. In fact, available tear volume varies with disease subtype and stage. In DED, this could affect the difficulty of collection, thus influencing tear biomarker concentration. For example, when testing a tear biomarker in subjects with a low volume of tears (ADDE), a prolonged collection time may increase the reflex lacrimal gland secretion and the risk of epithelial cellular damage, with the consequent contamination of the sample. Furthermore, molecules from the bloodstream may enter the tears causing an increase of their concentration. In general, in ADDE, it should be considered that the tear volume is progressively low, while in EDE it could be normal, so that in ADDE reflex tearing biomarkers deriving from the lacrimal

gland will progressively fall with the increase in lacrimal damage. In EDE, the reflex response of the lacrimal gland can be unimpaired and therefore the sample dilution becomes more likely. In the ocular surface, both vascular and epithelial permeability increase with the severity of the disease and, particularly in the conjunctiva; molecules from vessels and epithelial cells leak out into the tear fluid, thus increasing their concentration. However, the use of small volumes (nL) of tear sampling increases the speed of collection, thus reducing the possible interference due to contamination and dilution. Furthermore, multiplex assays give the opportunity to compare a broad range of key biomarker levels within the same sample.

Although the pathophysiological mechanisms of ocular surface inflammation have been convincingly elucidated, there is a lack of biomarkers representing a specific pattern for each clinical type of DED. Considering this, biomarkers deriving from the inflammatory pathways may be useful in identification of a specific stage of the disease, rather than as an indicator of a specific clinical subtype of DED. The dynamic evolution of ocular surface responses to the various noxae and the peculiar organization of the ocular surface functional unit render the identification of a single biomarker of the disease highly unlikely. Instead, the effort to identify molecules able to indicate a specific stage of a disease and a possible marker of therapeutic response is much more promising.

ACKNOWLEDGMENT

The authors are deeply indebted to Prof. Anthony J. Bron for invaluable suggestions and material provided.

Table 8.1 Expression of cytokines in different forms of ocular surface disorders

Cytokines	SS ADDE	Non-SS ADDE	EDE	Allergies
IL-1α[*]	+		+	
IL-1β	+[*]	+[†]	+[*]	+[‡]
IL-1β precursor[*]	–		–	
IL-1Ra	++[*]		+[§]	
IL-2R				+[‡]
IL-6		+[‖,†]	+[‖]	+[¶]
IL-17[**]	+			
TNF-α		+[‖,†]	+[‖]	+[††]
IFN-γ		+[†]		No[††,‡]

+, increased expression; ++, very increased expression; –, decreased expression; No, not expressed.
ADDE, aqueous tear-deficient dry eye; EDE, evaporative dry eye; IFN, interferon; IL, interleukin; SS, Sjögren's syndrome; TNF, tumor necrosis factor.
[*]Solomon et al. 2001; [†]Boehm et al. 2011; [‡]Leonardi et al. 2009; [§]Enriquez-de-Salamanca et al. 2010 (mild EDE); [‖]Lam et al. 2009; [¶]Irkeç and Bozkurt 2003; [**]Chung et al. 2012; [††]Leonardi 2002.

Table 8.2 Expression of cell-recruiting molecules in different forms of ocular surface disorders

Cell-recruiting molecules	SS ADDE	Non-SS ADDE	EDE	Allergies
CXCL9 (MIG) (tear)*	+			
CXCL10 (IP-10) (tear)	+*		+†	
CXCL11 (I-TAC) (tear)*	+			
CXCR3 (conjunctival cells)*	+*	+*		+‡
CXC (IL-8)		+§,‖	+†,‖	+¶,**
CCL3 (MIP-1α)	++††	+††	+++‖	
CCL4 (MIP-1β)††	++	+++		
CCL5 (RANTES)	+††	++††	+‖	++¶
CX3CL1 (fractalkine)†			+	
HLA-DR		+‡‡		+¶
ICAM		±§§		+¶
VCAM	+¶¶	+¶¶		

±, mild expression; +, increased expression; ++, very increased expression; +++, very high expression.
ADDE, aqueous tear-deficient dry eye; EDE, evaporative dry eye; ICAM, intercellular adhesion molecule; IL, interleukin; I-TAC, interferon-inducible T-cell chemoattractant; MIP, macrophage inflammatory protein; RANTES, regulated upon activation, normal T-cell expressed, and secreted; SS, Sjögren's syndrome; VCAM, vascular cell adhesion molecule.
*Yoon et al. HLA-DR, human leukocyte antigen-DR; MIG, monokine induced by gamma interferon; IP-10, interferon gamma-induced protein 10.; †Enriquez-de-Salamanca et al. 2010 (mild EDE); ‡Kumar 2009; §Boehm et al. 2011; ‖Lam et al. 2009; ¶Hingorani et al. 1998; **Leonardi et al. 2009; ††Choi et al. 2012; ‡‡Versura et al. 2011; §§Narayanan et al. 2006; ¶¶Ciprandi et al. 2002.

Table 8.3 Expression of tear proteins in different forms of ocular surface disorders

Tear proteins	SS ADDE	Non-SS ADDE	EDE	Allergies
EGF	−*		+†	+‡
Lipocalin 1	−§	+‖	−¶,**	+††
Cystatin-1‖		+		
α₁-antitrypsin‖		+		
VEGF			+†	+‡
Lactoferrin	−§		−¶	+††
Lipophillin A-C¶			−	
Albumin			+¶	+††
α-enolase§	+			
α-1 acid glycoprotein§	+			
S 100 A4§	+			
S 100 A8 (calgranulin A)§	+			
S 100 A9 (calgranulin B)§	+			
S 100 A11 (calgizzarin)§	+			
Prolactin-inducible protein§	−			
Lysozime§	−			
MMP-9	+‡‡	+‡‡	+‡‡	+‡‡

+, increased expression; −, decreased expression.
ADDE, aqueous tear-deficient dry eye; EDE, evaporative dry eye; EGF, epithelial growth factor; MMP, matrix metalloproteinases; SS, Sjögren's syndrome; VEGF, vascular endothelial growth factor.
*Lam et al. 2009; †Enriquez-de-Salamanca et al. 2010 (mild EDE); ‡Leonardi et al. 2009; §Zhou et al. 2009; ‖Boehm et al. 2011; ¶Versura et al. 2010; **Yamada et al. 2005; ††Pong et al. 2010; ‡‡Chotikavanich et al. 2009.

■ REFERENCES

Aho VV, Nevalainen TJ, Saari KM. Group IIA phospholipase A2 content of tears in patients with keratoconjunctivitis sicca. *Graefes Arch Clin Exp Ophthalmol* 2002; **240**:521–523.

Barabino S, Dana MR. Dry eye syndromes. *Chem Immunol Allergy* 2007; **92**:176–184.

Barreiro O, Yanez-Mo M, Serrador JM, et al. Dynamic interaction of VCAM-1 and ICAM-1 with moesin and ezrin in a novel endothelial docking structure for adherent leukocytes. *J Cell Biol* 2002; **157**:1233–1245.

Baudouin C, Liang H. Amplifying factors in ocular surface diseases: apoptosis. *Ocul Surf* 2005; **3**:S194–S197.

Black RA, Rauch CT, Kozlosky CJ, et al. A metalloproteinase disintegrin that releases tumour-necrosis factor-alpha from cells. *Nature* 1997; **385**:729–733.

Boehm N, Riechardt AI, Wiegand M, et al. Proinflammatory cytokine profiling of tears from dry eye patients by means of antibody microarrays. *Invest Ophthalmol Vis Sci* 2011; **52**:7725–7730.

Buchholz KR, Stephens RS. The extracellular signal-regulated kinase/mitogen-activated protein kinase pathway induces the inflammatory factor Interleukin-8 following Chlamydia trachomatis infection. *Infect Immun* 2007; **75**:5924–5929.

Caffery B, Joyce E, Boone A, et al. Tear lipocalin and lysozyme in Sjögren and non-Sjögren dry eye. *Optom Vis Sci* 2008; **85**:661–667.

Calonge M, Enríquez-de-Salamanca A, Diebold Y, et al. Dry eye disease as an inflammatory disorder. *Ocul Immunol Inflamm* 2010; **18**:244–253.

Carreño E, Enríquez-de-Salamanca A, Tesón M, et al. Cytokine and chemokine levels in tears from healthy subjects. *Acta Ophthalmol* 2010; **88**:250–258.

Chen D, Wei Y, Li X, et al. sPLA2-IIa is an inflammatory mediator when the ocular surface is compromised. *Exp Eye Res* 2009; **88**:880–888.

Chen Z, Tong L, Li Z, et al. Hyperosmolarity-induced cornification of human corneal epithelial cells is regulated by JNK MAPK. *Invest Ophthalmol Vis Sci* 2008; **49**:539–549.

Choi W, Li Z, Oh HJ, et al. Expression of CCR5 and its ligands CCL3, -4, and -5 in the tear film and ocular surface of patients with dry eye disease. *Curr Eye Res* 2012; **37**:12–17.

Chotikavanich S, de Paiva CS, Li de Q, et al. Production and activity of matrix metalloproteinase-9 on the ocular surface increase in dysfunctional tear syndrome. *Invest Ophthalmol Vis Sci* 2009; **50**:3203–3209.

Chung JK, Kim MK, Wee WR. Prognostic factors for the clinical severity of keratoconjunctivitis sicca in patients with Sjögren's syndrome. *Br J Ophthalmol* 2012; **96**:240–245.

Ciprandi G, Riccio AM, Venturino V, et al. VCAM-1 in conjunctival inflammation. *Allergy* 2002; **57**:961-962.

Dana R. Corneal antigen presentation: molecular regulation and functional implications. *Ocul Surf* 2005; **3**:S169–S172.

Dartt DA. Tear lipocalin: structure and function. *Ocul Surf* 2011; **9**:126–138.

De Paiva CS, Corrales RM, Villarreal AL, et al. Corticosteroid and doxycycline suppress MMP-9 and inflammatory cytokine expression, MapK activation in the corneal epithelium in experimental dry eye. *Exp Eye Res* 2006; **83**:526–535.

De Paiva CS, Volpe EA, Gandhi NB, et al. Disruption of TGF-β signaling improves ocular surface epithelial disease in experimental autoimmune keratoconjunctivitis sicca. *PLoS One* 2011; **6**:e29017.

De Saint Jean M, Brignole F, Feldmann G, et al. Interferon-gamma induces apoptosis and expression of inflammation-related proteins in Chang conjunctival cells. *Invest Ophthalmol Vis Sci* 1999; **40**:2199–2212.

Dinarello CA. Proinflammatory cytokines. *Chest* 2000; **118**:503–508.

Dinarello CA. Interleukin-1 in the pathogenesis and treatment of inflammatory diseases. *Blood* 2011; **117**:3720–3732.

Dogar AM, Towbin H, Hall J. Suppression of latent transforming growth factor (TGF)-beta1 restores growth inhibitory TGF-beta signaling through microRNAs. *J Biol Chem* 2011; **286**:16447–16458.

Dogru M, Matsumoto Y, Yamamoto Y, et al. Lactoferrin in Sjögren's syndrome. *Ophthalmology* 2007; **114**:2366–2367.

Dougherty JM, McCulley JP. Comparative bacteriology of chronic blepharitis. *Br J Ophthalmol* 1984; **68**:524–528.

Enriquez-de-Salamanca A, Castellanos E, Stern ME, et al. Tear cytokine and chemokine analysis and clinical correlations in evaporative-type dry eye disease. *Mol Vis* 2010; **16**:862–873.

Etheredge L, Kane BP, Valkov N, et al. Enhanced cell accumulation and collagen processing by keratocytes cultured under agarose and in media containing IGF-I, TGF-β or PDGF. *Matrix Biol* 2010; **29**:519–524.

Fésüs L, Szondy Z. Transglutaminase 2 in the balance of cell death and survival. *FEBS Lett* 2005; **579**:3297–3302.

Gao J, Morgan G, Tieu D, et al. ICAM-1 expression predisposes ocular tissues to immune-based inflammation in dry eye patients and Sjögrens syndrome-like MRL/lpr mice. *Exp Eye Res* 2004; **78**:823–835.

Gipson IK. The ocular surface: the challenge to enable and protect vision: the Friedenwald lecture. *Invest Ophthalmol Vis Sci* 2007; **48**:4391–4398.

Glasgow BJ, Gasymov OK. Focus on molecules: tear lipocalin. *Exp Eye Res* 2011; **92**:242–243.

Glasson MJ, Stapleton F, Keay L, et al. Differences in clinical parameters and tear film of tolerant and intolerant contact lens wearers. *Invest Ophthalmol Vis Sci* 2003; **44**:5116–5124.

Goldberg MF, Ferguson TA, Pepose JS. Detection of cellular adhesion molecules in inflamed human corneas. *Ophthalmology* 1994; **101**:161–168.

Goyal S, Chauhan SK, Zhang Q, Dana R. Amelioration of murine dry eye disease by topical antagonist to chemokine receptor 2. *Arch Ophthalmol* 2009; **127**:882–887.

Graham JE, Moore JE, Jiru X, et al. Ocular pathogen or commensal: a PCR-based study of surface bacterial flora in normal and dry eyes. *Invest Ophthalmol Vis Sci* 2007; **48**:5616–5623.

Gurney AL, Aggarwal S. IL-17: prototype member of an emerging cytokine family. *J Leukoc Biol* 2002; **71**:1–8.

Hall AJ, Morroll S, Tighe P, et al. Human chitotriosidase is expressed in the eye and lacrimal gland and has an antimicrobial spectrum different from lysozyme. *Microbes Infect* 2008; **10**:69–78.

Hattori T, Chauhan SK, Lee H, et al. Characterization of Langerin-expressing dendritic cell subsets in the normal cornea. *Invest Ophthalmol Vis Sci* 2011; **52**:4598–4604.

Hingorani M, Calder VL, Buckley RJ, Lightman SL. The role of conjunctival epithelial cells in chronic ocular allergic disease. *Exp Eye Res* 1998; **67**:491–500.

Hoffmann E, Dittrich-Breiholz O, Holtmann H, Kracht M. Multiple control of interleukin-8 gene expression. *J Leukoc Biol* 2002; **72**:847–855.

Irkeç M, Bozkurt B. Epithelial cells in ocular allergy. *Curr Allergy Asthma Rep* 2003; **3**:352–357.

Jabs DA, Prendergast RA, Rorer EM, et al. Cytokines in autoimmune lacrimal gland disease in MRL/MpJ mice. *Invest Ophthalmol Vis Sci* 2001; **42**:2567–2571.

Kang MH, Kim MK, Lee HJ, et al. Interleukin-17 in various ocular surface inflammatory diseases. *J Korean Med Sci* 2011; **26**:938–944.

Karns K, Herr AE. Human tear protein analysis enabled by an alkaline microfluidic homogeneous immunoassay. *Anal Chem* 2011; **83**:8115–8122.

Kawashima M, Kawakita T, Inaba T, et al. Dietary lactoferrin alleviates age-related lacrimal gland dysfunction in mice. *PLoS One* 2012; 7:e33148.

Kluwe J, Mencin A, Schwabe RF. Toll-like receptors, wound healing, and carcinogenesis. *J Mol Med* 2009; **87**:125–138.

Kolls JK, Linden A. Interleukin-17 family members and inflammation. *Immunity* 2004; **21**:467–476.

Kumar S. Vernal keratoconjunctivitis: a major review. *Acta Ophthalmol* 2009; **87**:133-147.

Labbé A, Brignole-Baudouin F, Baudouin C. Ocular surface investigations in dry eye. *J Fr Ophtalmol* 2007; **30**:76–97.

Lam H, Bleiden L, de Paiva CS, et al. Tear cytokine profiles in dysfunctional tear syndrome. *Am J Ophthalmol* 2009; **147**:198–205.

Lamphier MS, Sirois CM, Verma A, et al. TLR9 and the recognition of self and non-self nucleic acids. *Ann N Y Acad Sci* 2006; **1082**:31–43.

Lemp MA, Baudouin C, Baum J et al. The definition and classification of dry eye disease: report of the Definition and Classification Subcommittee of the International Dry Eye WorkShop (2007). *Ocul Surf* 2007; **5**:75–92.

Leonardi A. Vernal keratoconjunctivitis: pathogenesis and treatment. *Prog Retin Eye Res* 2002; **21**:319–339.

Leonardi A, Sathe S, Bortolotti M, et al. Cytokines, matrix metalloproteases, angiogenic and growth factors in tears of normal subjects and vernal keratoconjunctivitis patients. *Allergy* 2009; **64**:710–717.

Levy Y, Dueymes M, Pennec YL, et al. IgA in Sjögren's syndrome. *Clin Exp Rheumatol* 1994; **12**:543–551.

Ley K, Huo Y. VCAM-1 is critical in atherosclerosis. *J Clin Invest* 2001; **107**:1209–1210.

Ley K, Smith E, Stark MA. IL-17A-producing neutrophil-regulatory Tn lymphocytes. *Immunol Res* 2006; **34**:229–242.

Li DQ, Chen Z, Song XJ, et al. Stimulation of matrix metalloproteinases by hyperosmolarity via a JNK pathway in human corneal epithelial cells. *Invest Ophthalmol Vis Sci* 2004; **45**:4302–4311.

Luo L, Li DQ, Corrales RM, et al. Hyperosmolar saline is a proinflammatory stress on the mouse ocular surface. *Eye Contact Lens* 2005; **31**:186–193.

Massingale ML, Li X, Vallabhajosyula M, et al. Analysis of inflammatory cytokines in the tears of dry eye patients. *Cornea* 2009; **28**:1023–1027.

Meloni M, De Servi B, Marasco D, Del Prete S. Molecular mechanism of ocular surface damage: application to an in vitro dry eye model on human corneal epithelium. *Mol Vis* 2011; **17**:113–126.

Meyer-Ter-Vehn T, Grehn F, Schlunck G. Localization of TGF-beta type II receptor and ED-A fibronectin in normal conjunctiva and failed filtering blebs. *Mol Vis* 2008; **14**:136–141.

Mikulowska-Mennis A, Xu B, Berberian JM, Michie SA. Lymphocyte migration to inflamed lacrimal glands is mediated by vascular cell adhesion molecule-1/alpha(4)beta(1) integrin, peripheral node addressin/l-selectin, and lymphocyte function-associated antigen-1 adhesion pathways. *Am J Pathol* 2001; **159**:671–681.

Miossec P, Korn T, Kuchroo VK. Interleukin-17 and type 17 helper T cells. *N Engl J Med* 2009; **361**:888–898.

Mohan R, Chintala S, Jung J, et al. Matrix metalloproteinase gelatinase B (MMP-9) coordinates and effects epithelial regeneration. *J Biol Chem* 2002; **277**:2065–2072.

Mrugacz M, Zywalewska N. HLA-DR antigen expression on conjunctival epithelial cells in patients with dry eye. *Klin Oczna* 2005; **107**:278–279.

Musumeci M, Aragona P, Bellin M, et al. Acidic mammalian chitinase in dry eye conditions. *Cornea* 2009; **28**:667–672.

Narayanan S, Miller WL, McDermott AM. Conjunctival cytokine expression in symptomatic moderate dry eye subjects. *Invest Ophthalmol Vis Sci* 2006; **47**:2445–2450.

Nishiura H, Shibuya Y, Yamamoto T. S19 ribosomal protein cross-linked dimer causes monocyte-predominant infiltration by means of molecular mimicry to complement C5a. *Lab Invest* 1998; **78**:1615–1623.

Nishiyama T, Mishima K, Obara K, et al. Amelioration of lacrimal gland inflammation by oral administration of K-13182 in Sjögren's syndrome model mice. *Clin Exp Immunol* 2007; **149**:586–595.

Ohashi Y, Ishida R, Kojima T, et al. Abnormal protein profiles in tears with dry eye syndrome. *Am J Ophthalmol* 2003; **136**:291–299.

Pan Z, Wang Z, Yang H, et al. TRPV1 activation is required for hypertonicity-stimulated inflammatory cytokine release in human corneal epithelial cells. *Invest Ophthalmol Vis Sci* 2011; **52**:485–493.

Pasquale LR, Dorman-Pease ME, Lutty GA, et al. Immunolocalization of TGF-beta 1, TGF-beta 2, and TGF-beta 3 in the anterior segment of the human eye. *Invest Ophthalmol Vis Sci* 1993; **34**:23–30.

Pflugfelder SC, Jones D, Ji Z, et al. Altered cytokine balance in the tear fluid and conjunctiva of patients with Sjögren's syndrome keratoconjunctivitis sicca. *Curr Eye Res* 1999; **19**:201–211.

Pflugfelder SC, Stern ME. Immunoregulation on the ocular surface: 2nd Cullen Symposium. *Ocul Surf* 2009; **7**:67–77.

Pisella PJ, Malet F, Lejeune S, et al. Ocular surface changes induced by contact lens wear. *Cornea* 2001; **20**:820–825.

Png E, Samivelu GK, Yeo SH, et al. Hyperosmolarity-mediated mitochondrial dysfunction requires Transglutaminase-2 in human corneal epithelial cells. *J Cell Physiol* 2011; **226**:693–699.

Pong JC, Chu CY, Chu KO, et al. Identification of hemopexin in tear film. *Anal Biochem* 2010; **404**:82–85.

Qi M, Elion EA. MAP kinase pathways. *J Cell Sci* 2005; **118**:3569–3572.

Roescher N, Tak PP, Illei GG. Cytokines in Sjögren's syndrome. *Oral Diseases* 2009; **15**:519–526.

Rosenson RS, Gelb MH. Secretory phospholipase A2: a multifaceted family of proatherogenic enzymes. *Curr Cardiol Rep* 2009; **11**:445–451.

Saito M, Ota Y, Ohashi H, et al. CD40-CD40 ligand signal induces the intercellular adhesion molecule-1 expression through nuclear factor-kappa B p50 in cultured salivary gland epithelial cells from patients with Sjögren's syndrome. *Mod Rheumatol* 2007; **17**:45–53.

Schoenborn JR, Wilson CB. Regulation of interferon-gamma during innate and adaptive immune responses. *Adv Immunol* 2007; **96**:41–101.

Seal DV, McGill JI, Mackie IA, et al. Bacteriology and tear protein profiles of the dry eye. *Br J Ophthalmol* 1986; **70**:122–125.

Solomon A, Dursun D, Liu Z, et al. Pro- and anti-inflammatory forms of interleukin-1 in the tear fluid and conjunctiva of patients with dry-eye disease. *Invest Ophthalmol Vis Sci* 2001; **42**:2283–2292.

Stevenson W, Chauhan SK, Dana R. Dry eye disease: an immune-mediated ocular surface disorder. *Arch Ophthalmol* 2012; **130**:90–100.

Tong L, Chen Z, De Paiva CS, et al. Transglutaminase participates in UVB-induced cell death pathways in human corneal epithelial cells. *Invest Ophthalmol Vis Sci* 2006; **47**:4295–4301.

Tong L, Zhou L, Beuerman RW, et al. Association of tear proteins with meibomian gland disease and dry eye symptoms. *Br J Ophthalmol* 2011; **95**:848–852.

Tsubota K, Fukagawa K, Fujihara T, et al. Regulation of human leukocyte antigen expression in human conjunctival epithelium. *Invest Ophthalmol Vis Sci* 1999; **40**:28–34.

Turkcapar N, Sak SD, Saatci M, et al. Vasculitis and expression of vascular cell adhesion molecule-1, intercellular adhesion molecule-1, and E-selectin in salivary glands of patients with Sjögren's syndrome. *J Rheumatol* 2005; **32**:1063–1070.

Turner HC, Budak MT, Akinci MA, Wolosin JM. Comparative analysis of human conjunctival and corneal epithelial gene expression with oligonucleotide microarrays. *Invest Ophthalmol Vis Sci* 2007; **48**:2050–2061.

VanDerMeid KR, Su SP, Krenzer KL, et al. A method to extract cytokines and matrix metalloproteinases from Schirmer strips and analyze using Luminex. *Mol Vis* 2011; **17**:1056–1063.

Versura P, Nanni P, Bavelloni A, et al. Tear proteomics in evaporative dry eye disease. *Eye* 2010; **24**:1396–1402.

Versura P, Profazio V, Schiavi C, Campos FC. Hyperosmolar stress upregulates HLA-DR expression in human conjunctival epithelium in dry eye patients and in vitro models. *Invest Ophthalmol Vis Sci* 2011; **52**:5488–5496.

Wakamatsu TH, Dogru M, Tsubota K. Tearful relations: oxidative stress, inflammation and eye diseases. *Arq Bras Oftalmol* 2008; **71**:72–79.

Weaver CT, Hatton RD, Mangan PR, Harrington LE. IL-17 family cytokines and the expanding diversity of effector T cell lineages. *Annu Rev Immunol* 2007; **25**:821–852.

Wehmeyer A, Das PK, Swaak T, et al. Sjögren syndrome: comparative studies in local ocular and serum immunoglobulin concentrations with special reference to secretory IgA. *Int Ophthalmol* 1991; **15**:147–151.

Wei Y, Epstein SP, Fukuoka S, et al. sPLA2-IIa amplifies ocular surface inflammation in the experimental dry eye (DE) BALB/c mouse model. *Invest Ophthalmol Vis Sci* 2011; **52**:4780–4788.

Xu, Y, Li, S. Blockade of ICAM-1: a novel way of vasculitis treatment. *Biochem Biophys Res Commun* 2009; **381**:459–461.

Yamada M, Mochizuki H, Kawai M, et al. Decreased tear lipocalin concentration in patients with meibomian gland dysfunction. *Br J Ophthalmol* 2005; **89**:803–805.

Yolton DP, Mende S, Harper A, Softing A. Association of dry eye signs and symptoms with tear lactoferrin concentration. *J Am Optom Assoc* 1991; **62**:217–223.

Yoon KC, Jeong IY, Park YG, Yang SY. Interleukin-6 and tumor necrosis factor alpha levels in tears of patients with dry eye syndrome. *Cornea* 2007; **26**:431–437.

Zerfaoui M, Suzuki Y, Naura AS, et al. Nuclear translocation of p65 NF-kappaB is sufficient for VCAM-1, but not ICAM-1, expression in TNF-stimulated smooth muscle cells: differential requirement for PARP-1 expression and interaction. *Cell Signal* 2008; **20**:186–194.

Zhang X, Chen W, De Paiva CS, et al. Interferon-g exacerbates dry eye-induced apoptosis in conjunctiva through dual apoptotic pathways. *Invest Ophthalmol Vis Sci* 2011; 52:6279–6285.

Zheng X, De Paiva CS, Rao K, et al. Evaluation of the transforming growth factor-beta activity in normal and dry eye human tears by CCL-185 cell bioassay. *Cornea* 2010; **29**:1048–1054.

Zhou L, Beuerman RW, Chan CM, et al. Identification of tear fluid biomarkers in dry eye syndrome using iTRAQ quantitative proteomics. *J Proteome Res* 2009; **8**:4889–4905.

Zhu Z, Zheng T, Homer RJ, et al. Acidic mammalian chitinase in asthmatic Th2 inflammation and IL-13 pathway activation. *Science* 2004; **304**:1678–1682.

Zoukhri D, Macari E, Kublin CL. A single injection of interleukin-1 induces reversible aqueous-tear deficiency, lacrimal gland inflammation, and acinar and ductal cell proliferation. *Exp Eye Res* 2007; **84**:894–904.

Chapter 9

The effect of dry eye disease on vision and its implications for cataract and refractive surgery

Richard Chu, Mujtaba A. Qazi, Jay S. Pepose

■ INTRODUCTION

Real-world functional vision requires the recognition of objects comprising various sizes, contrasts, luminosities, wavelengths, and spatial frequencies. This is a complex process that has many contributing factors and progressive levels of processing, such as the tear film and focusing elements of the eye, the neurosensory retina, optic nerve, lateral geniculate, visual cortex, and related visual pathways. Traditional Snellen acuity is a measure of vision in an ideal high-contrast setting and, therefore, is often a poor measure of true visual function. This is evident in some postcataract and refractive surgery patients who complain about fogginess, glare, and poor night vision despite a 20/20 vision according to the Snellen chart. Many tests and devices have been designed to quantify and provide metrics of visual quality. Different characteristics of the retinal image can be measured by double-pass devices or wavefront aberrometers, whereas contrast-sensitivity testing, functional visual acuity (FVA) testing, and driving simulations can be used to subjectively measure both neural and optical performance (Kaido et al. 2011).

These tools become especially useful when evaluating visual impairment from dry eye disease (DED). Patients with DED often complain of transient blur, ocular fatigue, irritation, redness, as well as many other symptoms. The negative impact of DED and fluctuating vision on quality of life (QoL) is profound (Friedman 2010). Utility analysis of mild and severe DED patients showed a reduced QoL, similar to that experienced by patients with mild psoriasis and class III/IV (moderate-to-severe) angina, respectively (Miljanović et al. 2007). In 2007, the International Dry Eye Workshop amended their definition of DED to include 'visual disturbance' and 'tear film instability,' thus highlighting the dynamic role of the tear film in visual function (DEWS 2007).

■ DRY EYE DISEASE AND REAL-WORLD VISION

The performance of many crucial daily activities, such as reading, computer use, driving, and video terminal display use, becomes more difficult in DED patients by three- to fivefold (Miljanović et al. 2007). These subjective complaints show little correlation ($p > 0.05$) to clinical signs such as Schirmer's and van Bijsterveld scores, and thus are difficult to reproduce or measure (García-Catalán et al. 2009). Various patient questionnaires have been studied to quantify the effect of DED on vision and QoL, for example, the Short Form-12 Health Status Questionnaire, the McMonnies Dry Eye Questionnaire, the Ocular Surface Disease Index (OSDI), the National Eye Institute Visual Functioning Questionnaire (NEI VFQ-25), and the Impact of Dry Eye on Everyday Life. Of these, the OSDI and the Impact of Dry Eye on Everyday Life are the least generic and most specific to DED (Friedman 2010).

OSDI vision-related function subscale scores in patients with severe DED were 3.5 times greater than controls, and about two times greater in patients with mild-to-moderate DED. The sensitivity and specificity of this subscale were 0.47 and 0.77, respectively (Schiffman et al. 2000). This OSDI subscale was found to be significantly correlated ($r > 0.42$) to NEI VFQ-25 vision-related questions of general vision, near vision, far vision, work capacity, and driving dependency (Vitale et al. 2004). It is of interest to note that the NEI VFQ-25 vision subscale was not statistically significantly correlated to either binocular high-contrast visual acuity (VA) ($z = -0.30$) or contrast sensitivity ($z = 0.38$) (Richman et al. 2010). These findings suggest that some vision-related survey instruments may offer unique insights with regard to 'real-world' vision and QoL loss in DED patients that may not be accurately reflected by other measures.

■ SUBJECTIVE TESTING IN DRY EYE DISEASE

Daily tasks such as recognizing faces, reading the newspaper, and driving at night require the ability to see details at low contrast levels. Contrast is created by the difference in luminance, that is, the amount of reflected light of two adjacent surfaces. A greater ratio of luminance between the darker versus the lighter surface equates to a greater contrast. By multiplying the ratio by 100, we can express contrast as a percentage. The maximum contrast is thus 100% contrast.

Contrast-sensitivity testing measures the relation between the optical efficiency of the eye and the minimum retinal threshold for pattern detection, across a range of spatial frequencies, and has been shown as a good measure of visual function (Packer et al. 2003). Rolando et al. (1998) reported a 35–70% reduction of contrast sensitivity in DED patients, which improved following instillation of artificial tears. This improvement was observed for both low and high spatial frequencies of contrast sensitivity (Akin et al. 2006).

FVA testing was developed to detail temporal changes in vision. Goto et al. (2002) measured FVA by instructing the patients to blink normally while responding to a constantly changing Landolt optotype. By monitoring user response and blink rate, FVA can be utilized to measure changes in VA over the time course of a blink and calculate a visual maintenance ratio (VMR) for comparison (Goto et al. 2002). The VMR is an objective index that evaluates vision over time. It is calculated by dividing the logMAR values of the FVA scores over the time frame of testing by the logMAR baseline VA score: VMR = (lowest logMAR VA score - FVA at 60 seconds)/(lowest logMAR VA score - baseline VA). LogMAR FVA and VMR scores were consistently worse in DED patients when compared to normal subjects. These were significantly correlated with an increase in corneal staining and blink rate, as well as a decrease in Schirmer's scores and tear film break-up times . When blink rate is suppressed by topical anesthetics in healthy eyes, there is a worsening of FVA, which further emphasizes the importance of tear film stability and regularity (**Figure 9.1**) (Kaido et al. 2011). When treated with punctal plugs, both FVA and VMR improved significantly (P < 0.005) (Kaido et al. 2008).

Tear film and the corneal surface

The tear film is the most anterior refractive surface of the eye. A good-quality tear film serves to mask and soften the optical impact of the irregularities of the corneal epithelium. With a radius of approximately 7.8 mm, a refractive index of 1.336, and a thickness that ranges from 6 to 20 μm, the tear film optical power can be estimated mathematically to be 48.35 D alone or 42.36 D when coupled with the cornea (Albarrán et al. 1997). A local change in radius to 7.6 mm would theoretically create a 1.3 D change in power. As the tear film evaporates and thins between blinks, the surface becomes irregular, producing local variations that cause higher order aberrations (HOA) (**Figure 9.2**) (Montés-Micó 2007, Montés-Micó et al. 2004).

Serial corneal topographies taken after a blink show significant worsening of both the surface regularity index and surface asymmetry index in DED patients when compared to normal subjects (**Figure 9.3**). Degradation of surface irregularity indices positively correlated with increased fluorescein staining, increased astigmatism, and decreased potential VA (Liu & Pflugfelder 1999). Increased irregularity indices were also associated with a decrease in spatial contrast sensitivity below 15 cycles per degree (Huang et al. 2002). It was shown in these studies that instillation of artificial tears improved surface regularity as well as contrast sensitivity (Akin et al. 2006, Huang et al. 2002, Liu & Pflugfelder 1999). Tear film break-up (TFBU) can be directly observed with the instillation of fluorescein dye or with the use of retroillumination. Tutt et al. (2000) observed TFBU to be a direct cause of reduced quality in retinal imaging, which correlated to a 20–40% decrease in subjective contrast sensitivity.

Tear film and optical quality

Optical quality can be measured objectively with instruments to obtain the modulation transfer function (MTF). MTF describes the efficiency of the optical system in transferring the contrast of an object to an image as a function of spatial frequency. It is the ratio of the modulation in image-to-object contrast defined over a range of spatial frequencies. One method of measuring optical quality is a double-pass technique that captures the spatial distribution of the retinal point spread function (Benito et al. 2011). A temporal analysis of double-pass images at 0.5-second intervals over the course of a blink can provide information about ocular scatter and image quality caused by changes in the tear film (**Figure 9.4**). Image quality measured at the beginning of the blink and after the tear film break-up

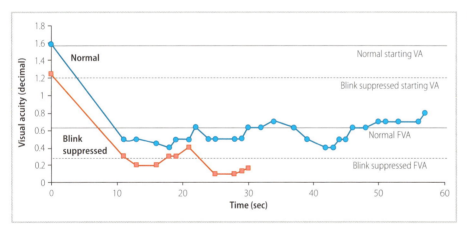

Figure 9.1 Example of functional visual acuity (FVA) testing of patients with a normal blink state (solid line) and blink suppressed with topical anesthesia (dash line). FVA, starting visual acuity (VA) score, and VA change with time are shown.

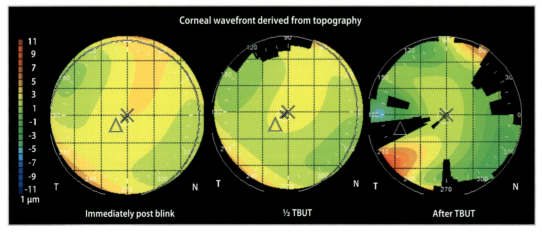

Figure 9.2 Changes in corneal wavefront measurements of a normal patient during tear film break-up.

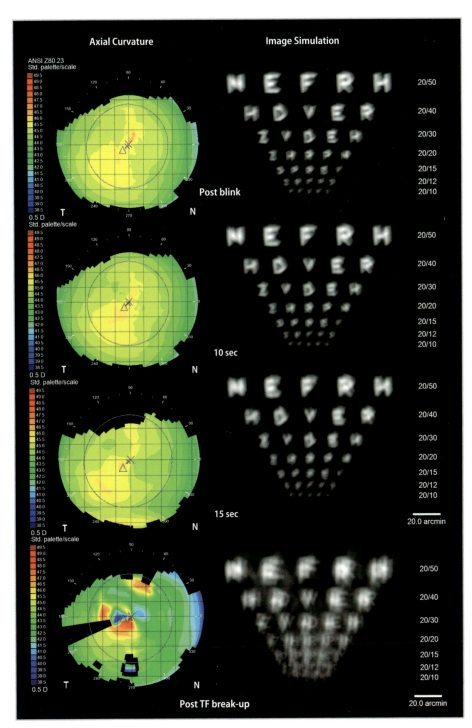

Figure 9.3 Humphrey Atlas corneal topographic maps and image simulation immediately after blink, 10 seconds after blink, 15 seconds after blink, and after tear film break-up (TFBU). Astigmatism increased from 0.58 D pre-TFBU to 1.74 D.

time (TFBUT) showed about a 20% decrease ($p < 0.01$) in MTF and subjective optical quality (Schiffman et al. 2000).

The HD Analyzer (Visiometrics, Terrassa, Spain) is a commercially available double-pass device that has been applied to quantify the differences in temporal changes of image quality between DED subjects and normal subjects. A threshold estimating the probable TFBUT in DED subjects was found to be in good agreement with the clinical break-up time (BUT) (objective BUT of 7.1 ± 2.7 versus clinical BUT of 6.2 ± 2.8) (Benito et al. 2011).

Tear film and wavefront

Local variations of tear film are thought to contribute to HOAs. Corneal wave aberrations can be derived from topography, whereas total ocular aberrations have been most commonly measured with a Hartmann–Shack aberrometer. Small local variations in the surface regularity in DED patients may distort individual points in the Hartmann–Shack centroid pattern, inducing lower order aberrations and HOAs. When comparing DED patients with normal subjects, coma-like (S3) and spherical-like aberrations were 2.29–2.70 times higher in DED patients, in case of both 4

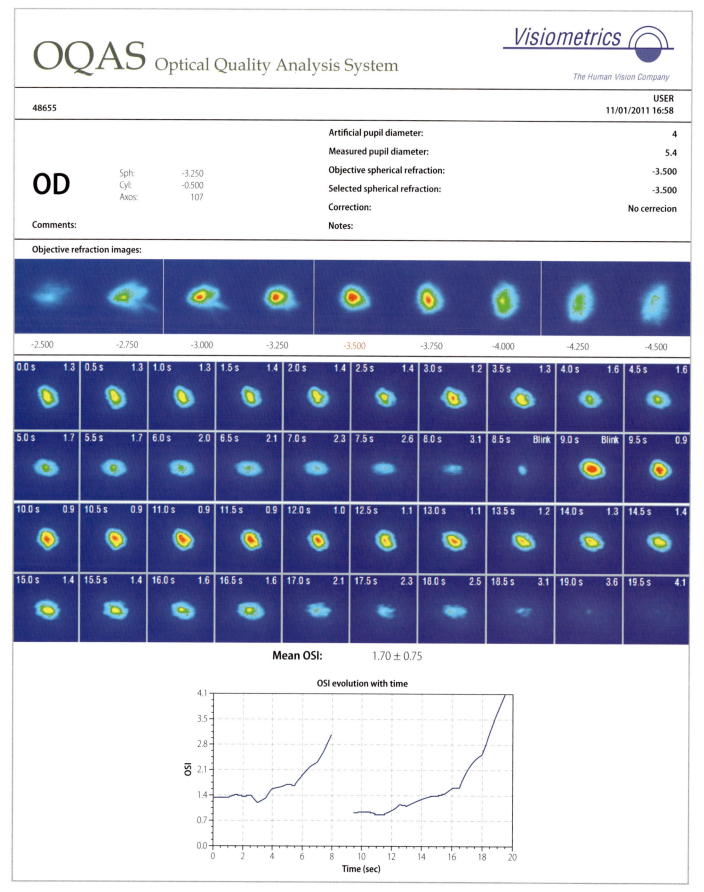

Figure 9.4 A series of double-pass images from a dry eye disease patient showing increasing scatter. Time and intensity distribution index value are recorded, right and left, respectively.

and 6 mm pupils. DED patients had a larger ratio of vertical to horizontal coma compared with normal subjects. This is thought to be related to the impact of gravity on tear film irregularity (Montés-Micó et al. 2004).

During the TFBU, HOAs, including coma, trefoil, third, fourth, and fifth order, gradually increase after a blink (**Figure 9.5**) (Koh & Maeda 2007). An analysis of normal eyes led to the classification of HOA change after a blink into four patterns: stable, small fluctuations, sawtooth, and others (Koh & Maeda 2007). In both dry and normal eyes, HOAs were found to increase by a similar factor, but occurred sooner in DED patients (Lin et al. 2005).

Instillation of artificial tears improved HOA by 2.5 times in DED patients (Montés-Micó et al. 2004, 2010). Daily use of artificial tears improved total aberrations and contrast sensitivity by 35% (Ridder et al. 2009). Punctal occlusion in the post-LASIK DED patients significantly reduced total, lower, and higher order wavefront aberrations by 47–63%. In one study, there were significant reductions in coma and spherical aberration among HOAs, but not in trefoil (Huang et al. 2004).

IMPLICATIONS OF DRY EYE DISEASE ON REFRACTIVE SURGERY

It is estimated that 50% of LASIK patients suffer from DED symptoms. This is partially attributed to patients who seek refractive surgery secondary to DED-related contact lens intolerance (Tanaka et al.

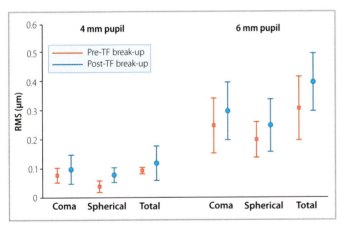

Figure 9.5 Changes in higher order aberration pre- and post-tear film break-up. Adapted from Koh & Maeda 2007.

2004). Preexisting DED is a risk factor for severe postoperative DED, with lower tear function, more vital staining of the ocular surface, and more severe symptoms (Toda et al. 2002). DED has been associated with regression following laser vision correction (Albietz et al. 2004). Nevertheless, in a series of Sjögren's patients, a group of patients with severe DED, who underwent aggressive pretreatment, refractive surgery has been shown to be safe and effective (Toda et al. 2004).

Preoperative optimization of the ocular surface becomes especially important when taking wavefront measurements (Montés-Micó 2007). Although, changes in HOA caused by the tear film become cloaked by those induced by LASIK treatments (**Figure 9.6**) (Lin et al. 2005), the use of irregular, poor-quality Hartmann–Shack images to drive wavefront-guided treatments may induce unwanted aberrations. Thus, one must be careful to select wavefront maps that are taken prior to TFBU (**Figure 9.7**).

Increased corneal irregularity decreases TFBUTs after LASIK and can limit visual improvement. A real-time video technique has demonstrated that tear film coating does little to smoothen corneal irregularities after refractive surgery (Campbell 2005). Irregular interference fringes observed during post-LASIK tear layer interferometry suggest that irregular epithelium and irregular local topography cause tear film instability and reduced TFBUTs (Szczesna et al. 2009). Decreased 1-day post-LASIK FVAs have been correlated to an increase in the surface regularity index. Although both corneal regularity and VA return to normal by 1 week, initial decreased FVA may influence patient confidence and satisfaction (Tanaka et al. 2004).

Decreased Schirmer's value, TFBUT, and increased corneal staining after LASIK and photorefractive keratectomy (PRK) have all been well studied (Toda et al. 2001). Postrefractive patients with DED that lasted >6 months after myopic correction had a higher risk of regression, 27 versus 7% ($p < 0.0001$). The factors associated with chronic DED are: female sex, higher refractive correction, and greater ablation depth; the following pre-LASIK variables are also associated with chronic DED: increased ocular surface staining; lower tear volume, tear stability, and corneal sensation; and DED symptoms before LASIK (Albietz et al. 2004).

IMPLICATIONS OF DRY EYE DISEASE ON CATARACT SURGERY

Accurate diagnosis and aggressive treatment of early signs and symptoms of dry eyes are especially important to meet the high expectations of today's cataract patients. Recent studies estimate that 4.91 million

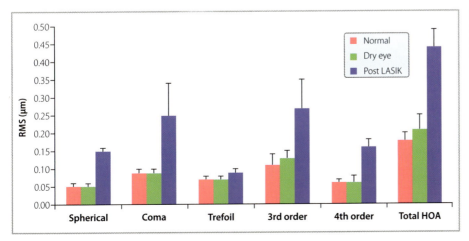

Figure 9.6 Increasing higher order aberrations of the anterior cornea immediately after blink in normal eyes, dry eyes, and post-LASIK. Adapted from Lin et al. 2005.

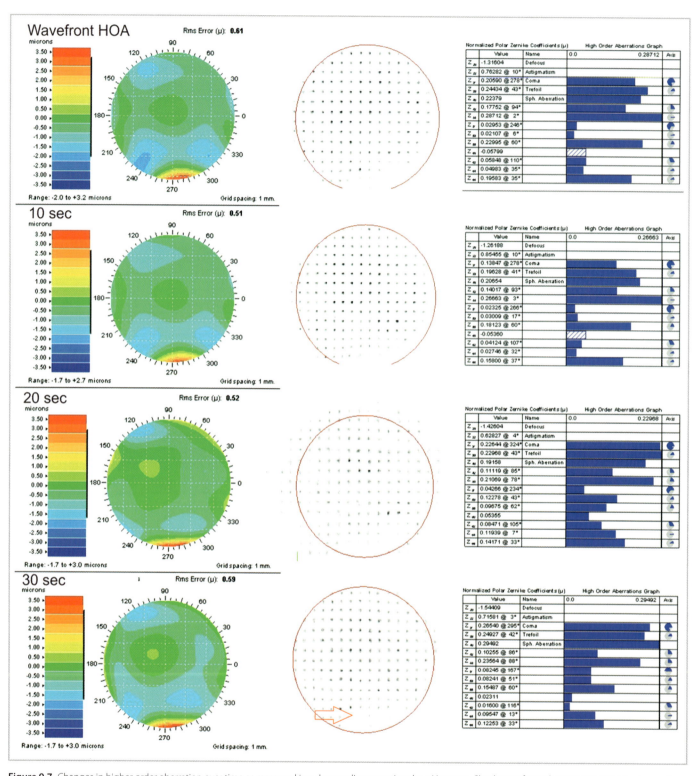

Figure 9.7 Changes in higher order aberration over time as measured in a dry eye disease patient by a Hartman–Shack wavefront aberrometer. Note the increasing coma post-tear film break-up. Arrow shows centroid drop out in area of punctate keratopathy.

people older than 50 years experience DED in the United States (DEWS 2007). As this population ages, the overlap of patients needing cataract surgery and patients with DED increases. In a small prospective study of patients, at least 55 years old, undergoing cataract surgery, 25.9% of the surveyed patients had been diagnosed with DED, but up to 76.8% of patients showed clinical signs of DED (Trattler et al. 2011).

Although cataract surgery has been shown to be safe for DED patients, evaluation and treatment of DED are crucial for accurate surgical planning, especially with the increasing popularity of presbyopia-correcting and toric intraocular lenses (IOLs). It is important to note that keratometry performed on DED patients may be an inaccurate reflection of astigmatism and show more irregularity, thus making proper planning and alignment of toric IOLs and limbal relaxing incisions less exact. Other measures used in lens power calculations, such as ultrasound-measured axial length and anterior chamber depth, appeared to be unaffected by DED (Sanchis-Gimeno et al. 2006).

DED symptoms worsen after cataract surgery (Li et al. 2007). Decreased corneal sensitivity and goblet cell density, and increased tear evaporation, tear turnover rate, and tear osmolarity have all been found in postcataract patients (Li et al. 2007, Ram et al. 2002). This may be attributed to the preservatives in topical antibiotic and anti-inflammatory eye drops used postoperatively, as well as reduced feedback from corneal nerve desensitization (Khanal et al. 2008, Li et al. 2007). Tear turnover rate and osmolarity improved by 2 weeks after surgery, whereas corneal sensitivity took up to 3 months to recover (Khanal et al. 2008).

■ CONCLUSION

The tear film is a dynamic structure that plays an important role in visual function. The aberrations induced by irregularities of the ocular surface are correlated with a decrease in contrast sensitivity and VA. Objective testing of tear film quality, quantity, and composition is important when diagnosing and treating subjective visual complaints of DED patients. The number of DED patients needing cataract and refractive surgery as well as their expectations is increasing; thus, early and aggressive treatment of DED becomes even more crucial toward achieving patient satisfaction. Future research may be directed toward using new technologies, such as tear osmolarity and interferometry, to respectively measure the severity of DED and dysfunction of individual tear film components and the characteristics and frequency of blinking, thereby helping clinicians to better target treatment strategies.

■ REFERENCES

Akin T, Karadayi K, Aykan U, Certel I, Bilge AH. The effects of artificial tear application on contrast sensitivity in dry and normal eyes. *Eur J Ophthalmol* 2006; **16**:785–790.

Albarrán C, Pons AM, Lorente A, Montés R, Artigas JM. Influence of the tear film on optical quality of the eye. *Cont Lens Anterior Eye* 1997; **20**:129–135.

Albietz JM, Lenton LM, McLennan SG. Chronic dry eye and regression after laser in situ keratomileusis for myopia. *J Cataract Refract Surg* 2004; **30**:675–684.

Benito A, Pérez GM, Mirabet S, et al. Objective optical assessment of tear-film quality dynamics in normal and mildly symptomatic dry eyes. *J Cataract Refract Surg* 2011; **37**:1481–1487.

Campbell C. The effect of tear film on higher order corrections applied to the corneal surface during wavefront-guided refractive surgery. *J Refract Surg* 2005; **21**:S519–S524.

DEWS. 2007 Report of the International Dry Eye WorkShop (DEWS). *Ocul Surf* 2007; **5**:163–178.

Friedman NJ. Impact of dry eye disease and treatment on quality of life. *Curr Opin Ophthalmol* 2010; **21**:310–316.

García-Catalán MR, Jerez-Olivera E, Benítez-Del-Castillo-Sánchez JM. Dry eye and quality of life. *Arch Soc Esp Oftalmol* 2009; **84**:451–458.

Goto E, Yagi Y, Matsumoto Y, Tsubota K. Impaired functional visual acuity of dry eye patients. *Am J Ophthalmol* 2002; **133**:181–186.

Huang B, Mirza MA, Qazi MA, Pepose JS. The effect of punctal occlusion on wavefront aberrations in dry eye patients after laser in situ keratomileusis. *Am J Ophthalmol* 2004; **137**:52–61.

Huang F, Tseng S, Shih M, Chen F. Effect of artificial tears on corneal surface regularity, contrast sensitivity, and glare disability in dry eyes. *Ophthalmology* 2002; **109**:1934–1940.

Kaido M, Ishida R, Dogru M, Tamaoki T, Tsubota K. Efficacy of punctum plug treatment in short break-up time dry eye. *Optom Vis Sci* 2008; **85**:758–763.

Kaido M, Ishida R, Dogru M, Tsubota K. The relation of functional visual acuity measurement methodology to tear functions and ocular surface status. *Jpn J Ophthalmol* 2011; **55**:451–459.

Khanal S, Tomlinson A, Esakowitz L, et al. Changes in corneal sensitivity and tear physiology after phacoemulsification. *Ophthalmic Physiol Opt* 2008; **28**:127–134.

Koh S, Maeda N. Wavefront sensing and the dynamics of tear film. *Cornea* 2007; **26**:S41–S45.

Lin YY, Carrel H, Wang IJ, Lin PJ, Hu FR. Effect of tear film break-up on higher order aberrations of the anterior cornea in normal, dry, and post-LASIK eyes. *J Refract Surg* 2005; **21**:S525–S529.

Liu Z, Pflugfelder SC. Corneal surface regularity and the effect of artificial tears in aqueous tear deficiency. *Ophthalmology* 1999; **106**:939–943.

Li XM, Hu L, Hu J, Wang W. Investigation of dry eye disease and analysis of the pathogenic factors in patients after cataract surgery. *Cornea* 2007; **26**:S16–S20.

Miljanović B, Dana R, Sullivan DA, Schaumberg DA. Impact of dry eye syndrome on vision-related quality of life. *Am J Ophthalmol* 2007; **143**:409–415.

Montés-Micó R. Role of the tear film in the optical quality of the human eye. *J Cataract Refract Surg* 2007; **33**:1631–1635.

Montés-Micó R, Cáliz A, Alió JL. Changes in ocular aberrations after instillation of artificial tears in dry-eye patients. *J Cataract Refract Surg* 2004a; **30**:1649–1652.

Montés-Micó R, Cáliz A, Alió JL. Wavefront analysis of higher order aberrations in dry eye patients. *J Refract Surg* 2004b; **20**:243–247.

Montés-Micó R, Cerviño A, Ferrer-Blasco T, García-Lázaro S, Ortí-Navarro S. Optical quality after instillation of eyedrops in dry-eye syndrome. *J Cataract Refract Surg* 2010; **36**:935–940.

Packer M, Fine IH, Hoffman RS. Functional vision, contrast sensitivity, and optical aberrations. *Int Ophthalmol Clin* 2003; **43**:1–3.

Ram J, Gupta A, Brar G, Kaushik S, Gupta A. Outcomes of phacoemulsification in patients with dry eye. *J Cataract Refract Surg* 2002; **28**:1386–1389.

Richman J, Lorenzana LL, Lankaranian D, et al. Relationships in glaucoma patients between standard vision tests, quality of life, and ability to perform daily activities. *Ophthalmic Epidemiol* 2010; **17**:144–151.

Ridder WH 3rd, LaMotte J, Hall JQ Jr, et al. Contrast sensitivity and tear layer aberrometry in dry eye patients. *Optom Vis Sci* 2009; **86**:E1059–E1068.

Rolando M, Lester M, Macrı´ A, Calabria G. Low spatial contrast sensitivity in dry eyes. *Cornea* 1998; **17**:376–379.

Sanchis-Gimeno J, Herrera M, Sanchez-del-Campo F. Differences in ocular dimensions between normal and dry eyes. *Surg Radiol Anat* 2006; **28**:267–270.

Schiffman RM, Christianson MD, Jacobsen G, Hirsch JD, Reis BL. Reliability and validity of the Ocular Surface Disease Index. *Arch Ophthalmol* 2000; **118**:615–621.

Szczesna DH, Kulas Z, Kasprzak HT, Stenevi U. Examination of tear film smoothness on corneae after refractive surgeries using a noninvasive interferometric method. *J Biomed Opt* 2009; **14**:064029.

Tanaka M, Takano Y, Dogru M, et al. Effect of preoperative tear function on early functional visual acuity after laser in situ keratomileusis. *J Cataract Refract Surg* 2004; **30**:2311–2315.

Toda I, Asano-Kato N, Hori-Komai Y, Tsubota K. Laser-assisted in situ keratomileusis for patients with dry eye. *Arch Ophthalmol* 2002; **120**:1024–1028.

Toda I, Asano-Kato N, Hori-Komai Y, Tsubota K. Ocular surface treatment before laser in situ keratomileusis in patients with severe dry eye. *J Refract Surg* 2004; **20**:270–275.

Toda I, Asano-Kato N, Komai-Hori Y, Tsubota K. Dry eye after laser in situ keratomileusis. *Am J Ophthalmol* 2001; **132**:1–7.

Trattler W, Reilly C, Goldberg D, et al. Cataract and dry eye: Prospective Health Assessment of Cataract Patients Ocular Surface Study. http://ascrs2011. abstractsnet.com/handouts/000269_PHACO_eposter_ASCRS_2011.ppt. (Last accessed on 19 September 2011.)

Tutt R, Bradley A, Begley C, Thibos LN. Optical and visual impact of tear break-up in human eyes. *Invest Ophthalmol Vis Sci* 2000; **41**:4117–4123.

Vitale S, Goodman LA, Reed GF, Smith JA. Comparison of the NEI-VFQ and OSDI questionnaires in patients with Sjögren's syndrome-related dry eye. *Health Qual Life Outcomes* 2004; **2**:44.

Chapter 10

Contact lens-related dry eye disease

Heiko Pult, Jason J. Nichols

INTRODUCTION

Many soft contact lens wearers experience symptoms of dryness in contact lens wear, even if they are asymptomatic without lens wear (Nichols & Sinnott 2006, Sindt & Longmuir 2007). This is generally referred to as contact lens-related dry eye (CLDE), or contact lens-induced dry eye (CLIDE) (referred to as CLDE hereafter). The frequency of CLDE occurrence is about 50% (Begley et al. 2000b, Nichols & Sinnott 2006, Nichols et al. 2002) and it is associated with altered visual performance, decreased wearing comfort, as well as an increased risk of ocular surface alterations (Pritchard et al. 1999). Ocular surface symptoms such as discomfort and dryness during contact lens wear are the major causes of discontinuation (Richdale et al. 2007). Approximately 50% of patients who drop out from contact lens wear in the United Kingdom and 75% in the United States do so because of discomfort related to lens wear (Pritchard 2001).

CONTACT LENS WEAR

Epidemiology of lens wearers

It is difficult to estimate the number of contact lens wearers in the United States and worldwide, but it is generally considered at about 35 and 120–140 million, respectively. Overall, about 11–13% of lens fits are with rigid lens materials, with the remaining market comprising soft lens materials (Morgan et al. 2012). At present, within the soft lens materials, silicone hydrogel materials dominate most major contact lens markets, with an average worldwide usage at about 50% (Morgan et al. 2012). About two thirds of lens wearers are female, and the average age of contact lens wearers is 31.2 ± 13.9 years (Morgan et al. 2012).

Contact lens polymers

Many types of contact lens materials are available in the market, and they differ in parameters such as optical design, water content, wettability, oxygen permeability, surface friction, deposit resistance, durability, and modulus (Sindt & Longmuir 2007). Contact lens materials may be categorized as rigid gas-permeable and hydrogels and silicone hydrogels (**Table 10.1**). All contact lens materials are made of polymers that give them their individual material properties.

Polymers are macromolecular substances made of numerous repeated constitutive units. Many gas-permeable or hydrogel contact lenses contain esters of methacrylic acid. Esterification of methacrylic acid with methyl ester results in methyl methacrylate (MMA), hydroxylation results in hydroxyethyl methacrylate (HEMA), and esterification with glycerol results in glycerol methacrylate (GMA). Breaking down the CH2=C– double bond enables polymerization, resulting in the formation of polymethyl methacrylate (PMMA), polyhydroxyethyl methacrylate (pHEMA), or polyglycerol methacrylate (pGMA) (Müller-Treiber 2009).

Additional monomers can be included to improve water binding, including agents such as N-vinyl pyrrolidone (NVP), polyvinylpyrrolidone (PVP), dimethylacrylamide, polyvinylalcohol, phosphorylcholine, and the ionic contact lens components sulfobetaine methacrylate and amino acids (Müller-Treiber 2009).

Using monomer reactants in silicone hydrogel contact lenses is a more complex process because of the difficulty in obtaining an optimized mixture of the hydrophobic silicone monomers and the hydrophilic monomers, resulting in a copolymer. Examples of such agents include trimethylsiloxy silyl propyl vinyl carbamate and flou flourodimethylsiloxane.

In rigid gas-permeable materials, copolymers of methyl methacrylate (PolyMMA), silicone alkyl methacrylate (silicone acrylates), and fluorosilicone alkyl methacrylate (fluorosilicone acrylates) are commonly used. The latter two provide a higher permeability to oxygen.

In hydrogel and silicone hydrogel contact lens materials, the water content, oxygen permeability, mechanical properties, and water binding properties depend upon the different monomer combinations utilized and the cross-linking of the polymers used. Ionicity of a material is essential in the interaction between the tear film and the contact lens surface. A biofilm quickly forms around the lens when the lens encounters the lipid-protein-mucin-rich environment of the ocular surface, sometimes potentially helping in the improvement of the wettability (Sindt & Longmuir 2007). Theoretically, non-ionic materials do not attract protein to the surface of the lens as much as ionic materials; however, it has been demonstrated that both ionic and non-ionic materials attract and bind proteins to the surface of the lens (Guillon et al. 1997). A related concern is that ionic materials continue to accumulate more protein. The amount of protein deposited after 1 month of lens wear is positively correlated with degree of iconicity (Maissa et al. 1998). Even though this biofilm can, at first, improve the lens wettability, it can later lead to discomfort and giant papillary

Table 10.1 Categories established for contact lenses

Group	Rigid gas-permeable lenses	Soft contact lenses*
1.	Does not contain either silicone or fluorine	<50% water content, non-ionic
2.	Contains silicone but not fluorine	≥50% water content, non-ionic
3.	Contains both silicone and fluorine	<50% water content, ionic
4.	Contains fluorine but not silicone	≥50% water content, ionic
5.	Silicone hydrogels 5-1 5-2 5-3 5-4	 <50% water content, non-ionic ≥50% water content, non-ionic <50% water content, ionic ≥50% water content, ionic
*FDA grouping		

conjunctivitis (GPC). Although ionic materials are more likely to deposit increased amounts of protein, non-ionic polymers [particularly from Food and Drug Administration (FDA) Group 2] can deposit more lipid (Jones et al. 1996). Regular replacement, in addition to appropriate lens hygiene, will result in improved clinical performance (Sindt & Longmuir 2007).

Oxygen permeability

A sufficient level of available oxygen is fundamental for a healthy ocular surface and successful contact lenses wear (Dillehay 2007). In the absence of a contact lens, the oxygen required for the aerobic metabolism of the cornea comes primarily from the atmosphere. The peripheral cornea also receives some oxygen supply from the limbal vasculature, while the posterior cornea is supplied oxygen from the tear film (French 2005b). For many years, soft contact lens dehydration was considered to be the primary source of discomfort in contact lens wear. However, although lens dehydration may play a role in discomfort, research studies have been unable to prove that theory (Dillehay 2007, Gispets et al. 2000, Nichols & Sinnott 2006). Conversely, literature and current clinical research have established that clinical signs of hypoxia improve concurrently with improvements in patient comfort and symptoms of dryness with silicone hydrogel lenses (Dillehay 2007). Low Dk soft contact lens wearers are assumed to experience an increase in corneal touch thresholds with reduced corneal sensitivity (Liesegang 2002). High Dk soft and rigid gas-permeable lenses are suggested to be less associated with decreased corneal sensation (Liesegang 2002). It is believed that decreased corneal sensitivity interferes with the normal neural feedback loop (Bourcier et al. 2005). Even though a decrease in corneal sensation may reduce lens awareness, long-term hypoaesthesia may affect the lacrimal system, leading to significant symptoms of dry eye disease (DED).

Modulus

A contact lens is subject to physical interactions with the ocular surface and eyelids when on the eye. The success of a contact lens material and the impact of these physical interactions depend on the mechanical properties of the material (French 2005a). In general, higher water-content contact lenses are of lower modulus. The modulus of the contact lens is the material's resistance to deformation under tension: the higher the modulus, the stiffer the lens. Silicone hydrogel materials vary in modulus (Sindt & Longmuir 2007). Higher modulus lenses can result in edge lift-off or fluting because of the inability to achieve contact lens–cornea alignment with an appropriate sagittal depth, resulting in foreign body sensation. In addition to edge fluting, high-modulus lenses are associated with general lens awareness, mechanically induced GPC, conjunctival flaps (Sindt & Longmuir 2007), and superior epithelial arcuate defects, all of which lead to symptoms of discomfort (Sindt & Longmuir 2007). A high degree of flexibility can also be a disadvantage when trying to achieve optimum vision (French 2005a). Many questions remain to be answered regarding lens modulus and its relationship to DED (e.g. how do modulus complications affect goblet cell density and, in the long term, the 'core mechanism' of DED?) (Sindt & Longmuir 2007). The further development of silicone hydrogels to allow a reduced modulus while still maintaining excellent oxygen permeability, now considered as the third generation of silicone hydrogels materials, continues to maintain this trend.

Water content

Contact lens materials go through phases of dehydration during lens wear. The amount of initial water fluctuation is related to the lens thickness, osmolarity of the storage solution, and the temperature of the lens upon application to the ocular surface (Sindt & Longmuir 2007). After the initial phase of dehydration, bulk water content remains fairly stable throughout the wearing period.

Lenses with higher nominal water content have been associated with CLDE (Nichols & Sinnott 2006). Low-water-content materials have approximately the same amount of bound water as materials with higher water content, but the higher water content lenses have more free water that is not bound to the material (Tranoudis & Efron 2004). Lenses with higher ratios of free to bound water content show rapid initial dehydration (Maldonado-Codina & Efron 2005), irrespective of the water content.

However, water lost through lens material dehydration is relatively minor compared to water evaporated from the anterior lens surface (Cedarstaff & Tomlinson 1983). In prelens tear film (PLTF) rupture, an evaporative dehydration process draws water through the lens and possibly out of the postlens tear film, leading to ocular surface desiccation (e.g. conjunctival and corneal staining) (Fonn 2007). A reflex blink spreads a new PLTF on the contact lens surface and the soft contact lens partially rehydrates, which is repeated upon each blink. In this way, the contact lens reaches a steady state of hydration (Nichols et al. 2005). Therefore, lens surface dehydration is more important than overall bulk dehydration (Sindt & Longmuir 2007). The cycle is more applicable in case of traditional HEMA-based materials rather than silicone hydrogel materials (Fonn 2007).

Lens dehydration can reduce the oxygen transmission through HEMA-based materials, because hydrogel lenses depend on water for their oxygen transmissibility. However, it is difficult to attribute DED symptoms associated with lens dehydration to any one factor, such as free lens-water content, lens fit, or oxygen permeability. Nevertheless, dehydration changes the flexibility of the contact lens, as well as oxygen transmission and lens fit, which can affect lens comfort, visual quality, and the ocular surface more indirectly (Dillehay 2007).

Wettability

Surface wettability determines how the tear film spreads across the material during a blink. It can be measured as contact angle or clinically evaluated by the prelens break-up time. In vivo wettability may be different from in vitro or ex vivo wettability because of the different contact angles created by standard tear film components and biofilm, regardless of the material (Cheng et al. 2004). However, wettability is a more complex issue than just the surface contact angle, since, for new lens materials, it can be influenced by factors such as leaching of solution from lenses or ambient conditions. A lower contact angle (<90°) indicates an increased wettability of the material (Sindt & Longmuir 2007). Symptoms of dryness may be related to the surface wettability of a contact lens (Tonge et al. 2001). Increasing wettability of the lens surface might enhance lens wear comfort because wettability affects the interaction of the lid with the lens and the deposition of the lens (Tonge et al. 2001). Also, rewetting drops and care regimes with appropriate surfactants are thought to potentially improve lens wettability (Sindt & Longmuir 2007).

Hydrogels are made of complex polymeric matrices containing hydrophobic and hydrophilic ends. The hydrophobic ends are oriented toward the inside of the lens matrix, while the hydrophilic ends are on the lens surface. When a contact lens surface dries, the hydrophilic ends might retreat inward, toward the center of the material matrix, to seek moisture and the hydrophobic ends move outward toward the dehydrated surface.

A dry ocular surface or surface of a contact lens can lead to increased friction with the leading edge of the eyelid (lid wiper). Korb et al. (2002) showed a positive correlation between the presence of superior lid margin staining and symptoms of DED. Discomfort caused by lid friction may not be sufficient to adequately increase reflex tearing, which might relieve the symptoms of dryness (McMonnies 2007). It has been reported that lid wiper symptoms can decrease blink frequency and increase the number of incomplete blinks (McMonnies 2007). Prolonged interblink intervals result in faster evaporation and thinner tear films with reduced lubricating properties, which, in turn, leads to further increased friction (McMonnies 2007).

Silicone hydrogels in general have had little success in reducing the frequency of CLDE. Second- and third-generation silicone hydrogel materials were invented to alleviate the symptoms of CLDE by providing surface chemistries that allow better wettability or reduced friction, but the actual reduction in the problem has still not been realized.

Biocompatibility represents a relatively new concept in contact lenses. The aim is to use biomimetic materials, which are less likely to disturb the normal ocular surface. Goda and Ishihara (2006) have proposed improving silicone hydrogel lenses by coating them with biomimetic phospholipid polymers, such as 2-methacryloyloxyethyl phosphorylcholine. The combination of high oxygen permeability provided by silicone-containing lenses and biomimetic material used to increase hydrophilic properties and decrease protein or lipid build-up may result in improved comfort (Sindt & Longmuir 2007). First-generation silicone hydrogel lenses require surface treatments to keep the lens wettable. In case of balafilcon A (Purevison, Bausch & Lomb, Rochester, NY, USA), plasma oxidation converts surface silicone [trimethylsilyl (TRIS) molecules] to islands of glassy silicate. Lotrafilcon A and B (O2Optix; Alcon Laboratories, Forth Worth, TX, USA) are treated with a chemically uniform, dense, high-refractive-index plasma coating (Sindt & Longmuir 2007). Later generation of silicone hydrogel materials are not surface treated. Some of these newer materials contain PVP, a long-chain, high-molecular-weight, flexible, humectant molecule, which functions as an internal wetting agent (Sindt & Longmuir 2007). PVP produces a hydrophilic layer on the outside lens surface by sequestering the silicone within the center of the lens. Other later-generation silicone hydrogel materials contain no TRIS- or PVP-based chemistry. The material is inherently wettable through hydrogen bonding internally and does not require surface treatment.

Contact lens designs

The design of the back surface of a contact lens defines fitting behavior of lenses and depends on corneal topography, optical aspects, and, especially in soft contact lenses, the corneal–scleral profile and bulbar conjunctiva's curvature.

There are two principal back-surface designs: rotation symmetric design or non-rotation symmetric designs, known as toric and/or asymmetric lenses. The back surface can be spherical (one curvature, two curvatures, three curvatures, or multiple curvatures) or aspheric (continuous aspheric vs. progressive aspheric). The proper combination of front-surface and back-surface design, and lens thickness, defines lens optic fitting criteria, as well as the stiffness of the lens, especially in silicone hydrogel materials.

There is evidence that edge design, thickness, and lubrication of contact lenses are related to conjunctival changes (Shen et al. 2011), lid wiper epitheliopathy (LWE) (Pult et al. 2008), drop-out of meibomian glands (Arita et al. 2009), and, consequently, contact lens wearing comfort.

Contact lens wear options

A variety of contact lens materials are used in various wearing modalities. In gas-permeable lenses, usually there is no strict recommendation on how often the lens material needs to be replaced; however, many practitioners recommend replacement every 12 months. Soft contact lenses are commonly worn on a 2- or 4-week replacement modality. Particularly special soft contact lenses are worn on a 12-month replacement schedule. Lens age is significantly related to wearing comfort. During the last decade, daily disposable lenses are growing in the market to overcome the need for lens cleaning. Contact lens materials with higher Dk allow for the option of continuous wear (Efron et al. 2010). This is thought to be more convenient for patients and is restricted to 4-week continuous wear (Sindt & Longmuir 2007). Replacing a contact lens more frequently can improve comfort (Ehlers et al. 2003, Malet & Schnider 2002).

Contact lens care systems and regimens

Choosing a contact lens care system with regard to action, cytotoxicity, and biocompatibility may be as important to comfortable lens wear as is the lens itself. Contact lens solutions remove debris from contact lenses by using surfactants that solubilize the debris, removing it from the lens surface. Alternatively, a lens may be protected from deposition by enhancing the surface wettability (Sindt & Longmuir 2007).

Surfactant wetting agents have a hydrophilic and a hydrophobic end to their structures, whereby the hydrophobic end clusters around debris to form micelles. The hydrophilic end is able to react with water, and the micelles can be washed off the lens surface. Surfactant wetting agents also improve lens hydrophilicity; the hydrophobic end of the agent interacts with the dry hydrophobic lens surface, exposing the hydrophilic end of the lens polymer on the lens surface. The newest generations of contact lens care products address surface wettability through the addition of increased surfactants or humectants (Sindt & Longmuir 2007).

To increase lens wettability and prevent the lens from sticking to the package or itself, surfactant agents are added to the contact lens packaging solution. Many newer lens care solutions contain lubricating agents and surfactants specifically formulated to promote comfort upon application and to maintain wettability throughout the day. Some contain hyaluronan, a conditioning agent that forms a hydrating network on the lens surface; others contain HydraGlyde, a moisture matrix, to enhance surface hydrophilicity and supply a continuous shield of moisture to the lens surface. Removing the lens from the packaging and soaking it in a contact lens solution may further increase the initial lens wettability (Sindt & Longmuir 2007). However, solution-related cytotoxic biguanide (poly-hexylmethyl biguanide or PHMB) disinfecting agents are related to contact lens dryness (Lievens et al. 2006). Significantly more corneal staining has been shown with PHMB than with hydrogen peroxide and polyquaternarium-based solutions. Andrasko et al. (2006) reported that PHMB solutions cause different cytotoxicity in different lenses, and therefore not all solutions are compatible with all contact lens materials. Garofalo et al. (2005) reported an increased corneal staining with the combination of FDA group II lenses and biguanide-based systems. As a result of their recent study of preserved multipurpose care solutions, Choy et al. (2012) suggested that practitioners should advise patients using these products to rinse their soaked lenses with saline before applying them in order to avoid the potential for cytotoxic effects. However, even though the impact of preservatives and disinfecting agents on the tear film stability and DED is obvious, a clear relation between different multipurpose contact lens care systems and CLDE is not generally confirmed in literature (Ramamoorthy et al. 2008, Sindt & Longmuir 2007). For example, Ramamoorthy et al. (2008) reported that there is no effect of care solutions on CLDE. Nevertheless, preservative-free care solutions or a one-step peroxide system can be useful for patients who do not find multipurpose care solutions suitable. Even though peroxide-based systems are used less frequently (Efron & Morgan 2008), they might cause fewer solution-related DED symptoms, are not toxic once neutralized, and are compatible with most soft contact lens materials (Carnt et al. 2007, Dalton et al. 2008, Dursun et al. 2002). For some materials, however, additional surface cleaners should be considered to improve initial wettability.

CONTACT LENSES AND THE OCULAR SURFACE

Tear film structure with contact lens on eye

Contact lenses impact tear film stability, which affects the ocular surface and, in turn, the contact lens itself (Foulks 2003). Quality and quantity of the precorneal tear film are significantly related to contact lens wearing comfort. Both the mucin layer and the lipid layer are vital to obtain a stable tear film.

Since contact lenses rest within the tear film, the tear film is subdivided into the PLTF and postlens tear films. The PLTF is less than half the thickness of the normal precorneal tear film (Nichols et al. 2005). The lipid tear film layer, mostly anterior to the PLTF layer, is disrupted by a contact lens (Nichols et al. 2005). Without contact lenses, the membrane-associated mucins lubricate and anchor the tear film to surface epithelia (Berry et al. 2004). However, they are not able to do so sufficiently on contact lens material. The mechanism of tear break-up on the surface of contact lenses is different from that on the surface of the eye, due to the absence of properly formed lipid or mucous layers on the lens surface.

Along with material factors, enzymatic degradation and oxidation of lipids are considered to be the two major pathways that result in the breakdown of lipid species and production of different intermediates and end products of lipid oxidation (Glasson et al. 2002). For example, phospholipids can undergo enzymatic degradation. Increased levels of phospholipases have been seen in contact lens-intolerant patients (Glasson et al. 2002). Phospholipids are assumed to act as surfactant in the tear film and degradation of these lipids can result in tear film instability. Phospholipases can degrade phospholipids leading to the production of diacylglycerides and lysophospholipids. Lipids with higher levels of unsaturation are more unstable and susceptible to auto-oxidation. The more unsaturated the fatty acids, the quicker the rate of oxidation (Glasson et al. 2002).

Deposit formation on contact lenses

Lens materials, surface characteristics, surfactant use, and environment, all affect lens deposition. Deposits may come from the tears, the environment, or even from handling of the contact lens. Deposition of proteins, lipids, and mucins occurs relatively quickly after lens insertion. Lens deposits can decrease the prelens break-up time, and consequently can lead to symptoms of dryness.

Adsorption of protein

In lens dehydration, the internal hydrophobic regions of tear proteins (including lactoferrin, albumin, and lysozymes) bind to the hydrophobic regions of the material. The water content and the surface charge (ionicity) influence the rate of deposit absorption and adsorption to the contact lens (Sindt & Longmuir 2007).

Lysozyme accounts for a substantial portion of the total lens protein deposits. In its natural state, lysozyme is a bacteriolytic enzyme that plays an important role in the eye's defense against pathogens. Unfortunately, these proteins get denatured if deposited on the contact lens surface, and are likely to cause immunological responses (Senchyna et al. 2004). Lysozyme is a very small, positively charged protein that gets adsorbed to negatively charged materials with a relatively large pore size. Increased lysozyme deposition has been measured on conventional hydrogel materials, particularly FDA group IV materials. It has been reported that HEMA/GMA lenses absorb the least amount of protein among the pHEMA lenses, which indicates that carboxymethylation (increasing the negative charge) is probably a more significant factor than high water content in protein spoliation (Maldonado-Codina & Efron 2004). However, increasing charge density often leads to an increase in effective pore size, which may promote diffusive penetration of lysozyme (Garrett et al. 2000). Silicone hydrogel lenses show reduced protein deposition, but they have a greater percentage of denatured lysozyme. The difference in deposition can be attributed to the hydrophobic nature and small pore size of silicone hydrogel materials (Senchyna et al. 2004). Denatured proteins are related to contact lens complications, such as GPC and inflammation, both of which are associated with symptoms of DED (Sindt & Longmuir 2007).

Lipid deposition

Numerous lipids classes and species are secreted from the meibomian glands to create the lipid layer, however the composition varies between individuals and in terms of deposition on contact lenses (Lorentz & Jones 2007). Lipids attach to the hydrophobic areas of the lens surface. Increased lipid depositions are related to decreased lens wettability (Sindt & Longmuir 2007). Higher levels of NVP result in increased levels of lipid deposition (Maissa et al. 1998), because of the amphiphilic nature of NVP (hydrophilic groups are sandwiched between hydrocarbon domains and the methylene groups). Organic silicone is more hydrophobic than the hydrocarbon domains in NVP, which causes silicone hydrogel contact lenses to show higher levels of lipid deposition (Lorentz & Jones 2007). Some patients who previously wore hydrogel lenses may experience more lipid deposition with silicone hydrogel lenses. However, not all lipids deposited on lenses cause complications. The lipid layer is vital in lubrication of the anterior eye as well as in contact lens wear. The problem occurs when deposited lipids become dominated by hydrophobic lipids, and they undergo structural changes, such as oxidation and cross-linking. Lipids can diffuse into the lens material; the clinical consequence of cross-linking is that the lipids are not extractable by care solution. This fails to fulfill the function of native lipids, resulting in a new local environment with numerous problems. Individual tear film composition, contact lens wearing schedule, and lens material influence lipid deposition, which is most pronounced in uncoated silicone hydrogels (Lorentz & Jones 2007).

Subjective findings in contact lens dry eye

Since DED symptoms are more distinct than ocular signs, a good medical history is crucial in the diagnosis of CLDE (**Figure 10.1**). Many questionnaires are frequently utilized, including the Contact Lens Dry Eye Questionnaire (CLDEQ) (Begley et al. 2000b, Nichols et al. 2002), Dry Eye Questionnaire (DEQ) (Begley et al. 2001), CLDEQ-8 (Chalmers et al. 2010), Impact of Dry Eye on Everyday Life Questionnaire (Rajagopalan et al. 2005), McMonnies Dry Eye Index (McMonnies) (McMonnies 1986, McMonnies & Ho 1987), and Ocular Surface Disease Index (OSDI) (Schiffman et al. 2000).

The McMonnies is probably the most noted questionnaire. Epidemiological risk factors, the frequency of symptoms of ocular irritation, and sensitivity to environmental triggers are considered. Even though the questionnaire was developed for non-contact lens wearers, it was suggested to be useful for contact lens wearers as well (sensitivity = 66.7%, specificity = 72.4%) (Michel et al. 2009). However, the McMonnies may be more useful for assisting with diagnosis of DED, than as a measurement of DED symptoms (Gothwal et al. 2010).

Although the OSDI was developed more recently to grade the severity of DED as well as act as a diagnostic aid in non-contact lens wearers, it was also used in many contact lens studies {sensitivity = 76.9%, specificity = 90.0% [naïve lens wearers (Pult et al. 2009)]}. It is notable among other questionnaires related to ocular surface disease for having undergone psychometric testing and having been accepted by the U.S. FDA as an outcome measure for use in DED trials. This instrument has three subscales that sequentially ask for symptoms of ocular irritation, the impact on vision-related functioning, and environmental triggers of DED.

The CLDEQ assists in diagnosis of DED in contact lens wearers by providing a dichotomous outcome (sensitivity = 61%, specificity = 83%)

(Nichols et al. 2002). This questionnaire focuses on ocular surface symptoms rather than presumed risk factors for DED. There are nine symptom subscales, and each subscale asks about the frequency of the symptom, followed by three questions concerning the intensity of the symptom at different times of day, to examine diurnal fluctuations in symptoms (Nichols et al. 2002). The difference in CLDEQ (companion to the DEQ) is that it anchors to the overall DED status via the question 'do you think you have dry eyes?' and uses that to stratify. Most of the other DED questionnaires do not have this internal anchor. The CLDEQ is also available in a short form (three questions plus subscales).

To measure contact lens-related symptoms that differentiate between wearers who report varying overall opinion of their contact lens performance, the CLDEQ-8 was developed by anchoring responses against the question on 'overall opinion' (Chalmers et al. 2012). A subset of eight questions from the longer CLDEQ was selected that reflected the wearer's overall opinion and thus gave a quantitative CLDEQ-8 score that reflected baseline status and change of overall opinion regarding contact lens performance after refitting. The CLDEQ-8 score could be an efficient outcome measure in clinical trials and practice (Chalmers et al. 2012).

Objective findings in contact lens dry eye

Even though DED has been intensely investigated over the past decade, the effectiveness of common DED tests in the prediction of CLDE is still disputed (Pult et al. 2008). However, a good slit-lamp biomicroscope examination, with and without contact lenses, is vital. The eyelids, lid margin, and blink behavior need to be observed carefully, as well as the tear film (quantity and quality) and integrity of the ocular surface (**Figure 10.2**).

While the tear film can easily be evaluated at the first visit of new lens wearers, experienced lens wearers present with worn lenses. In the latter, tear film measurements can often not be fully applied in normal routine of contact lens after care, since lenses have to be removed for some time prior to measurements (Johnson & Murphy 2005). Therefore, an extra appointment in the CLDE assessment for symptomatic contact lens wearers seems to be reasonable. However, the measure-

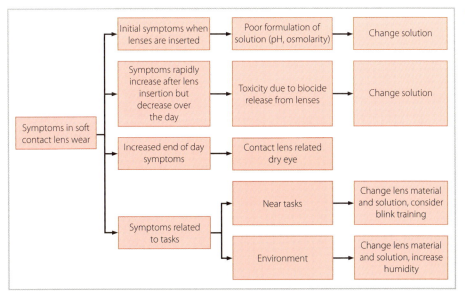

Figure 10.1 Symptoms in contact lens wear. From Pult (2011).

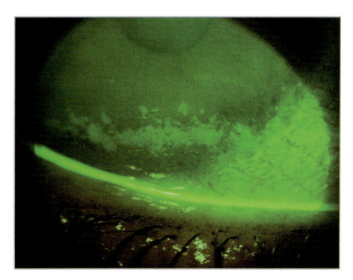

Figure 10.2 Significant smiley-like corneal staining in contact lens dry eye.

ment of the PLTF thinning may be a good option in experienced lens wearers. While Hom and Bruce (2009) found good relations between CLDE symptoms and PLTF thinning (using specular reflection), as so did Nichols and Sinnott (2006) (using a thickness-dependent fringe imaging interferometer), others suggested that PLTF thinning is not a good predictor of CLDE (using the TearScope Plus (Keeler Ltd, Windsor, UK) (Pult et al. 2008).

Inflammatory processes in DED affect the mucin layer and corneal and conjunctival epithelial cells (Nelson et al. 2011). Additionally, contact lenses as well as contact lens care regimes can induce corneal staining (Sindt & Longmuir 2007).

Tear hyperosmolarity is a central mechanism associated with ocular surface inflammation, damage, and DED symptoms, and the initiation of compensatory events in DED. Tear hyperosmolarity, defined by a reference of 308 mOsmol/L, is superior in overall accuracy to any other single test for DED diagnosis [sensitivity = 73%, specificity = 92% (Lemp et al. 2011)]. The TearLab (TearLab Cooperation, San Diego, CA, USA) has enabled a possibility of measuring tear film osmolarity in clinical practice. Numerous studies have been published discussing its value in the DED diagnosis (Benelli et al. 2010, Messmer et al. 2010, Sullivan et al. 2010, Tomlinson et al. 2010, Versura et al. 2010). The 'TearLab Research Guide' recommends the measurement of osmolarity 10–15 minutes before insertion or after removal of the contact lenses and measurement of the effect of lens wear with the lens in the eye. However, cut-off values of osmolarity in CLDE have not been fully investigated yet.

Many objective tests are used in clinical practice; however, their efficacy in the prediction of CLDE is still under discussion (Nichols et al. 2004, Pult et al. 2008). Some DED studies demonstrate the correlation between tear meniscus height, tear film break-up time, and symptoms of dryness (Glasson et al. 2003). A lipid layer thickness of <30 nm may represent a contact lens contraindication (Guillon 1998).

The investigation of less commonly performed tests, such as lid-parallel conjunctival folds (LIPCOF) (Höh et al. 1995, Pult et al. 2008, 2009, Sickenberger et al. 2000), LWE (Korb et al. 2002), and test combinations, showed promising results.

The combined LIPCOF score (LIPCOF Sum) were reported to be significant discriminators of CLDE (Pult et al. 2008, 2009). LIPCOF (**Figure 10.3**) are subclinical folds in the lateral, lower quadrant of the bulbar conjunctiva, parallel to the lower lid margin (Höh et al. 1995),

which are easily observed by the slit-lamp examination. LIPCOF are evaluated in the area perpendicular to the temporal and nasal limbus on the bulbar conjunctiva, above the lower lid with a slit-lamp microscope using 18–27´ magnification as necessary, and classified by the number of folds (Pult et al. 2008). The sum of temporal and nasal LIPCOF has a higher predictive value than regional LIPCOF scores (new contact lens wearers (Pult et al. 2009): sensitivity = 69.2%, specificity = 90.0%; experienced contact lens wearers (Pult et al. 2008): sensitivity = 82.6%, specificity = 84.1%). The LIPCOF Sum is calculated by adding the temporal LIPCOF grade and nasal LIPCOF grade (Pult et al. 2008). Care must be taken to differentiate between parallel, permanent conjunctival folds (LIPCOF) and disrupted microfolds, and to utilize the correct technique (no fluorescein, no lens, primary gaze) of observation (Pult et al. 2008).

LIPCOF are assumed to be caused by mechanical forces in blinks in DED patients, since LWE and LIPCOF are significantly correlated and LWE and LIPCOF are related to mucin quantity (Berry et al. 2008). Both tests can be performed immediately after lens removal (Korb et al. 2002, Pult et al. 2008).

LWE is a clinically observable alteration in the epithelium of the advancing lid margin, the lid wiper (**Figure 10.4**). In patients with DED, the tear film is insufficient to separate the ocular surface and lid wiper (Korb et al. 2005); hence, the lid wiper is subjected to trauma during the entire lid movement (Korb et al. 2002, 2005). LWE is a significant discriminator of CLDE (sensitivity = 87.0%, specificity = 42.1%) in experienced lens wearers (Pult 2008, Pult et al. 2008)

LWE is visible following instillation of a combination of 1% lissamine green (or Rose Bengal) and 2% fluorescein, and evaluation of the upper lid. A second instillation of both dyes should be carried out aftewr 5 minutes (Korb et al. 2006). LWE is classified by width and length (Korb et al. 2002, 2005). Care must be taken to differentiate between staining associated with Marx's line (Korb & Blackie 2010, Pult et al. 2010a) and that of the lid wiper (Korb et al. 2002, 2005).

Combining different tests has been shown to increase predictive ability of DED (Begley et al. 2000a, Glasson et al. 2003, Sullivan et al. 2010). The Contact Lens Dry Eye Index (CLIDE-Index), a combination of temporal and nasal LIPCOF with the patient's symptoms [CLDEQ questions 2–5 (dryness minus grittiness)], was suggested to be able to screen and measure DED state of experienced contact lens wearers

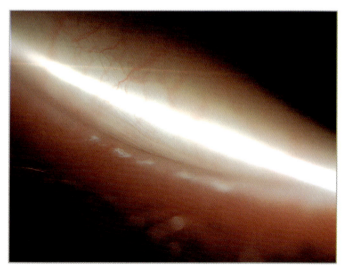

Figure 10.3 Lid-parallel conjunctival folds.

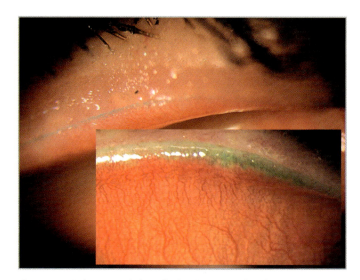

Figure 10.4 Lid wiper epitheliopathy (LWE). (a) Marx's line. (b) LWE. From Pult (2011).

(sensitivity = 87%, specificity = 87%) (Pult et al. 2010b). Glasson et al. (2003) suggested a combination of the McMonnies DED questionnaire with tear film stability and tear film volume to detect symptomatic lens wearers (sensitivity = 87%, specificity = 50%). The combination of the OSDI with temporal and nasal LIPCOF and non-invasive break-up time [known as the Contact-Lens-Predicting-Test (P-Test)] showed good discrimination (sensitivity = 92.3%, specificity = 90.0%) of later CLDE symptoms in naïve lens wearers. Nevertheless, sensitivity and specificity figures should be regarded as estimates as they depend on the standard against which they are being measured.

Systemic correlates (systemic disease, medications)

Most symptomatic lens wearers may have some degree of preexisting DED (Pult et al. 2009). Therefore, a good medical history is essential. The composition of the tear film is suggested to be related to diet (including amounts of protein, alcohol, and fat), systemic medications (including diuretics, anticholinergics, or sympathomimetic drugs), age, gender, and environment, as well as contact lens wear (Lorentz & Jones 2007, Miljanovic et al. 2005, Yamada et al. 2006). Besides lipid anomalies and primary aqueous tear deficiency (Sjögren's and non-Sjögren's syndrome), ocular allergies must be addressed, as they overlap with DED symptoms (Sindt & Longmuir 2007). Unfortunately, the role of the lid margin is often underestimated (Knop et al. 2010). A dysfunction of the meibomian glands [meibomian gland dysfunction (MGD)] should be considered since MGD can be considered the most common cause of DED (Foulks & Bron 2003, Knop et al. 2009, Lemp et al. 2012).

TREATMENTS FOR CONTACT LENS DRY EYE

Materials and designs

Even though not all lens characteristics of silicone hydrogels are superior to those of hydrogel lenses, refitting hydrogel lens wearers into silicone hydrogel lenses is worth a try, since they usually improve CLDE

symptoms (Schafer et al. 2007). Changing the lens design in terms of diameter, edge design, back-surface design, and lens thickness can be beneficial (Dumbleton et al. 2002, Santodomingo-Rubido & Rubido-Crespo 2008). Large-diameter gas-permeable lenses (≥11 mm) often seem to be more comfortable than small gas-permeable lenses; however, there is no magic rule to improve CLDE. Improvement of wetting criteria and affinity to deposits should be considered, especially if there are differences between a fresh and a worn lens. Many clinicians offer a right versus left comparison to let the contact lens wearer experience which type of lens provides better comfort.

Rewetting drops

Artificial tears containing hyaluronic acid (Johnson & Murphy 2006) [or surrogates (Springs 2010)], trehalose (Luyckx & Baudouin 2011), hypo-osmotic eye drops (Stahl et al. 2010), or liposomal eye sprays (Craig et al. 2010, Pult et al. 2012) can improve symptoms, ocular signs, and the tear film; therefore, their recommendation may be beneficial for the patient.

Hypo-osmotic eye drops are considered to 'neutralize' hyperosmolarity of the tear film to prevent epithelium damage (Stahl et al. 2010). Hyaluronic acids, with similar characteristics as mucins, are directly focused on treating epithelium damage (Johnson & Murphy 2006). Additionally, they can improve wettability and protect lenses against hydrophobization. Trehalose is a naturally occurring disaccharide widespread in many species of plants and animals. Trehalose has the ability to protect cellular membranes and labile proteins against damage and denaturation that occurs as a result of desiccation and oxidative stress. This natural disaccharide is assumed to improve cell water management, avoid cell membrane lipid oxidation and protein denaturation, and preserve epithelial cell life in dry conditions (Luyckx & Baudouin 2011).

In all the three types of eye drops, the epithelium is assumed to recover, and consequently the mucin layer and cornea wettability improves, which results in a more stable tear film. Tear hyperosmolarity results from water evaporation in situations of a low aqueous tear flow, as a result of excessive evaporation, or a combination of these events. Hyperosmolarity stimulates a cascade of inflammatory events in the epithelial surface cells involving the generation of inflammatory cytokines [interleukin (IL)-1α, IL-1β, tumor necrosis factor α)] and matrix metalloproteinases (e.g. MMP-9) (De Paiva et al. 2006), which arise from or activate inflammatory cells on the ocular surface (Baudouin 2001). These inflammatory events lead to apoptosis of surface epithelial cells including goblet cells (Yeh et al. 2003); thus, goblet cell loss may be directly related to chronic inflammation. Epithelial cell loss is a feature of every form of DED, and the demonstration of reduced levels of mucins is consistent with this. Finally, this loss of mucin results in tear film instability. This is named the core mechanism of DED (Nelson et al. 2011). Since the hyperevaporative DED is the most common DED type, liposomal eye sprays are an effective option in preventing the development of this core mechanism of DED by improving the lipid layer (Schaumberg et al. 2011).

Care solutions

The choice of contact lens cleaning solutions with regard to action, cytotoxicity, and biocompatibility is as important as the choice of the lens itself (**Figure 10.5**). The avoidance of preservatives and considering wetting agents may be beneficial. Solution-related cytotoxic biguanide (PHMB) disinfecting agents are related to contact lens

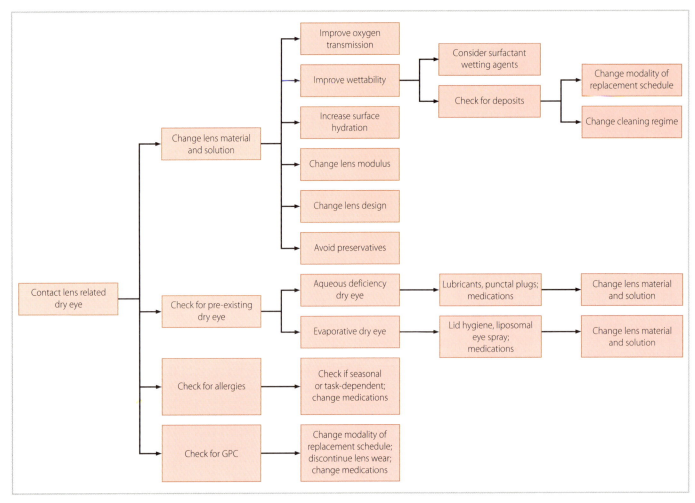

Figure 10.5 Management of contact lens discomfort. GPC, giant papillary conjunctivitis. From Pult (2011).

dryness (Lievens et al. 2006). As a result, peroxide-based systems are in revival (Carnt et al. 2007). However, with some lenses, additional surface cleaners are important to deal with deposits. Since lipids attach to the hydrophobic areas of the lens surface, some patients who previously wore hydrogel lenses may experience more lipid deposition with silicone hydrogel lenses (Lorentz & Jones 2007). Rubbing and rinsing the lenses has been shown to be effective in removing the lipids and proteins from the lens surface, since lipids are not soluble in water-based cleaners (Sindt & Longmuir 2007).

Meibomian glands

DED symptoms in contact lens wearers are multifactorial. However, some state of preexisting DED is common and should be addressed in the management of CLDE. MGD is one of the most common causes of evaporative DED, and consequently of DED (Schaumberg et al. 2011).

MGD is a chronic, diffuse abnormality of the meibomian glands, commonly characterized by terminal duct obstruction and/or qualitative or quantitative changes in the glandular secretion (Nelson et al. 2011). This may result in alteration of the tear film, symptoms of eye irritation, clinically apparent inflammation, and ocular surface disease (Nelson et al. 2011).

Meibomian gland drop-out is significantly correlated to lipid layer thickness, non-invasive break-up time, and DED symptoms (Pult &

Riede-Pult 2012). Since the lipid layer is an important component in stabilization of the tear film (King-Smith et al. 2009), especially in contact lens wear, a correlation between meibomian gland drop-out and contact lens wearing comfort is obvious.

Contact lens wearers show higher scores of meibomian gland drop-out than non-lens wearers (Arita et al. 2009). Therefore, it is important to address MGD in daily contact lens practice.

Daily application of warm and moist compresses, followed by appropriate lid hygiene, improves MGD (Geerling et al. 2011, Spiteri et al. 2007).

Omega three fatty acids

Essential fatty acids (EFAs) have been more and more recognized to have anti-inflammatory properties, which are important in mediating the underlying pathology of diverse diseases (Rosenberg & Asbell 2010). Fats can be divided into two categories 'saturated' and 'unsaturated.' No double bonds exist in the saturated fats molecule, but in unsaturated fats, at least one double bond exists in the carbon chain (Rosenberg & Asbell 2010). Unsaturated fats are further subdivided into 'mono-' or 'poly-'unsaturated, which depends on the number of double bonds that are present. Even though there are two groups of EFAs, the omega-6 (n-6) and omega-3 (n-3) families, most investigation has been conducted on the n-3 fats. N-3 fats are assumed to have an anti-inflammatory mechanism of action (Rosenberg & Asbell 2010).

Even though current data related to the treatment of DED with EFAs remain unclear (Rosenberg & Asbell 2010), it may be a promising additional option in ocular surface therapeutics (Rosenberg & Asbell 2010).

CONCLUSIONS

CLDE is a major subclassification of DED (Foulks 2003). DED symptoms in contact lens wearers are multifactorial. Preexisting DED states are obvious and should be addressed in the management of CLDE. New objective tests such as LWE and LIPCOF may be useful in clinical routine, as they can be performed easily, without additional equipment, and immediately after lens removal. The best evaluation method for the DED status of new and experienced contact lens wearers is a combination of objective tests and questionnaires. Refitting symptomatic hydrogel contact lens wearers with silicone hydrogels has been shown to be effective in reducing DED symptoms in most patients. Also, the avoidance of preservatives and use of wetting agents to provide continuous lubrication of the ocular surface may be beneficial.

REFERENCES

Andrasko GJ, Ryen KA, Garofalo RJ, Lemp JM. Compatibility of silicone hydrogel lenses with multi-purpose solutions. *Invest Ophthalmol Vis Sci* 2006; **47**:2392.

Arita R, Itoh K, Inoue K, et al. Contact lens wear is associated with decrease of meibomian glands. *Ophthalmology* 2009; **116**:379–384.

Baudouin C. The pathology of dry eye. *Surv Ophthalmol* 2001; **45**:S211–S220.

Begley C, Caffery B, Nichols K, et al. Results of a dry eye questionnaire from optometric practices in North America. Survey of preferred tests for diagnosis of the tear film and dry eye. *Cornea* 2000a; **19**:75.

Begley CG, Caffery B, Nichols KK, Chalmers R. Responses of contact lens wearers to a dry eye survey. *Optom Vis Sci* 2000b; **77**:40–46.

Begley CG, Chalmers RL, Mitchell GL, et al. Characterization of ocular surface symptoms from optometric practices in North America. *Cornea* 2001; **20**:610–618.

Benelli U, Nardi M, Posarelli C, Albert TG. Tear osmolarity measurement using the TearLab Osmolarity System in the assessment of dry eye treatment effectiveness. *Cont Lens Anterior Eye* 2010; **33**:61–67.

Berry M, Ellingham RB, Corfield AP. Human preocular mucins reflect changes in surface physiology. *Br J Ophthalmol* 2004; **88**:377–383.

Berry M, Pult H, Purslow C, Murphy PJ. Mucins and ocular signs in symptomatic and asymptomatic contact lens wear. *Optom Vis Sci* 2008; **85**:E930–E938.

Bourcier T, Acosta MC, Borderie V, et al. Decreased corneal sensitivity in patients with dry eye. *Invest Ophthalmol Vis Sci* 2005; **46**:2341–2345.

Carnt N, Jalbert I, Stretton S, et al. Solution toxicity in soft contact lens daily wear is associated with corneal inflammation. *Optom Vis Sci* 2007; **84**:309–315.

Cedarstaff TH, Tomlinson A. A comparative study of tear evaporation rates and water content of soft contact lenses. *Am J Optom Physiol Opt* 1983; **60**:167–174.

Chalmers R, Begley C, Moody K, Hickson-Curran S. Contact Lens Dry Eye Questionnaire-8 and overall opinion of contact lenses. *Optom Vis Sci* 2012; **89**:1435–1442.

Chalmers RL, Moody K, Young G, et al. Contact Lens Dry Eye Questionnaire-8 (CLDEQ-8) reflects status of and responds to change in overall opinion of CL performance. *Cont Lens Anterior Eye* 2010; **33**:E-abstract:256–300.

Cheng L, Muller SJ, Radke CJ. Wettability of silicone-hydrogel contact lenses in the presence of tear-film components. *Curr Eye Res* 2004; **28**:93–108.

Choy CK, Cho P, Boost MV. Cytotoxicity and effects on metabolism of contact lens care solutions on human corneal epithelium cells. *Clin Exp Optom* 2012; **95**:198–206.

Craig JP, Purslow C, Murphy PJ, Wolffsohn JS. Effect of a liposomal spray on the pre-ocular tear film. *Cont Lens Anterior Eye* 2010; **33**:83–87.

Dalton K, Subbaraman LN, Rogers R, Jones, L. Physical properties of soft contact lens solutions. *Optom Vis Sci* 2008; **85**:122–128.

De Paiva CS, Corrales RM, Villarreal AL, et al. Corticosteroid and doxycycline suppress MMP-9 and inflammatory cytokine expression, MAPK activation in the corneal epithelium in experimental dry eye. *Exp Eye Res* 2006; **83**:526–535.

Dillehay SM. Does the level of available oxygen impact comfort in contact lens wear? A review of the literature. *Eye Contact Lens* 2007; **33**:148–155.

Dumbleton KA, Chalmers RL, Mcnally J, et al. Effect of lens base curve on subjective comfort and assessment of fit with silicone hydrogel continuous wear contact lenses. *Optom Vis Sci* 2002; **79**:633–637.

Dursun D, Wang M, Monroy D, et al. Experimentally induced dry eye produces ocular surface inflammation and epithelial disease. *Adv Exp Med Biol* 2002; **506**:647–655.

Efron N, Morgan, P. Soft contact lens care regimens in the UK. *Cont Lens Anterior Eye* 2008; **31**:283–284.

Efron N, Morgan PB, Helland M, et al. Daily disposable contact lens prescribing around the world. *Cont Lens Anterior Eye* 2010; **33**:225–227.

Ehlers WH, Donshik PC, Suchecki JK. Disposable and frequent replacement contact lenses. *Ophthalmol Clin North Am* 2003; **16**:341–352.

Fonn D. Targeting contact lens induced dryness and discomfort: what properties will make lenses more comfortable. *Optom Vis Sci* 2007; **84**:279–285.

Foulks GN. What is dry eye and what does it mean to the contact lens wear? *Eye Contact Lens* 2003; **29**:S96–S100; discussion S115–S108, S192–S104.

Foulks GN, Bron AJ. Meibomian gland dysfunction: a clinical scheme for description, diagnosis, classification, and grading. *Ocul Surf* 2003; **1**: 107–126.

French K. Contact lens material properties. Part 2—mechanical behaviour and modulus. Optician ; **230**:29-34.

French K. Contact lens material properties. Part 3—oxygen performance. Optician; **230**:16-20.

Garofalo RJ, Dassanayake N, Carey C, et al. Corneal staining and subjective symptoms with multipurpose solutions as a function of time. *Eye Contact Lens* 2005; **31**:166–174.

Garrett Q, Laycock B, Garrett RW. Hydrogel lens monomer constituents modulate protein sorption. *Invest Ophthalmol Vis Sci* 2000; **41**:1687–1695.

Geerling G, Tauber J, Baudouin C, et al. The international workshop on meibomian gland dysfunction: report of the subcommittee on management and treatment of meibomian gland dysfunction. *Invest Ophthalmol Vis Sci* 2011; **52**:2050–2064.

Gispets J, Sola R, Varon C. The influence of water content of hydrogel contact lenses when fitting patients with 'tear film deficiency.' *Cont Lens Anterior Eye* 2000; **23**:16–21.

Glasson MJ, Stapleton F, Keay L, et al. Differences in clinical parameters and tear film of tolerant and intolerant contact lens wearers. *Invest Ophthalmol Vis Sci* 2003; **44**:5116–5124.

Glasson M, Stapleton F, Willcox M. Lipid, lipase and lipocalin differences between tolerant and intolerant contact lens wearers. *Curr Eye Res* 2002; **25**:227–235.

Goda T, Ishihara K. Soft contact lens biomaterials from bioinspired phospholipid polymers. *Expert Rev Med Devices* 2006; **3**:167–174.

Gothwal VK, Pesudovs K, Wright TA, Mcmonnies CW. McMonnies questionnaire: enhancing screening for dry eye syndromes with Rasch analysis. *Invest Ophthalmol Vis Sci* 2010; **51**:1401–1407.

Guillon JP. Use of the Tearscope Plus and attachments in the routine examination of the marginal dry eye contact lens patient. *Adv Exp Med Biol* 1998; **438**:859–867.

Guillon M, Mcgrogan L, Guillon JP, et al. Effect of material ionicity on the performance of daily disposable contact lenses. *Cont Lens Anterior Eye* 1997; **20**:3–8.

Höh H, Schirra F, Kienecker C, Ruprecht KW. Lid-parallel conjunctival folds are a sure diagnostic sign of dry eye. *Ophthalmologe* 1995; **92**:802–808.

Hom MM, Bruce AS. Prelens tear stability: relationship to symptoms of dryness. *Optometry* 2009; **80**:181–184.

Johnson ME, Murphy PJ. The effect of instilled fluorescein solution volume on the values and repeatability of TBUT measurements. *Cornea* 2005; **24**:811–817.

Johnson ME, Murphy PJ, Boulton M. Effectiveness of sodium hyaluronate eyedrops in the treatment of dry eye. *Graefes Arch Clin Exp Ophthalmol* 2006; **244**:109–112.

Jones L, Franklin V, Evans K, et al. Spoilation and clinical performance of monthly vs three monthly group II disposable contact lenses. *Optom Vis Sci* 1996; **73**:16–21.

King-Smith PE, Fink BA, Nichols JJ, et al. The contribution of lipid layer movement to tear film thinning and breakup. *Invest Ophthalmol Vis Sci* 2009; **50**:2747–2756.

Knop E, Knop N, Brewitt H, et al. Meibomian glands: part III. Dysfunction— argument for a discrete disease entity and as an important cause of dry eye. *Ophthalmologe* 2009; **106**:966–979.

Knop E, Korb DR, Blackie CA, Knop N. The lid margin is an underestimated structure for preservation of ocular surface health and development of dry eye disease. *Dev Ophthalmol* 2010; **45**:108–122.

Korb DR, Blackie CA. Marx's line of the upper lid is visible in upgaze without lid eversion. *Eye Contact Lens* 2010; **36**:149–151.

Korb DR, Greiner JV, Herman JP, et al. Lid-wiper epitheliopathy and dry-eye symptoms in contact lens wearers. *CLAO J* 2002; **28**:211–216.

Korb DR, Herman JP, Greiner JV, et al. Lid wiper epitheliopathy and dry eye symptoms. *Eye Contact Lens* 2005; **31**:2–8.

Korb DR, Herman JP, Solomon JD, et al. Lid wiper staining and sequential fluorescein instillation. *Invest Ophthalmol Vis Sci* 2006; **47**:ARVO E-abstract:242.

Lemp MA, Bron AJ, Baudouin C, et al. Tear osmolarity in the diagnosis and management of dry eye disease. *Am J Ophthalmol* 2011; **151**:792–798; e791.

Lemp MA, Crews LA, Bron AJ, et al. Distribution of aqueous-deficient and evaporative dry eye in a clinic-based patient cohort: a retrospective study. *Cornea* 2012; **31**:472–478.

Liesegang TJ. Physiologic changes of the cornea with contact lens wear. *CLAO J* 2002; **28**:12–27.

Lievens CW, Hakim N, Chinn A. The effect of multipurpose solutions on the ocular surface. *Eye Contact Lens* 2006; **32**:8–11.

Lorentz H, Jones L. Lipid deposition on hydrogel contact lenses: how history can help us today. *Optom Vis Sci* 2007; **84**:286–295.

Luyckx J, Baudouin C. Trehalose: an intriguing disaccharide with potential for medical application in ophthalmology. *Clin Ophthalmol* 2011; **5**:577–581.

Maissa C, Franklin V, Guillon M, Tighe B. Influence of contact lens material surface characteristics and replacement frequency on protein and lipid deposition. *Optom Vis Sci* 1998; **75**:697–705.

Maldonado-Codina C, Efron N. Impact of manufacturing technology and material composition on the clinical performance of hydrogel lenses. *Optom Vis Sci* 2004; **81**:442–454.

Maldonado-Codina C, Efron N. An investigation of the discrete and continuum models of water behavior in hydrogel contact lenses. *Eye Contact Lens* 2005; **31**:270–278.

Malet F, Schnider CM. Influence of replacement schedule and care regimen on patient comfort and satisfaction with daily wear frequent-replacement contact lenses. *CLAO J* 2002; **28**:124–127.

McMonnies CW. Key questions in a dry eye history. *J Am Optom Assoc* 1986; **57**:512–517.

McMonnies CW. Incomplete blinking: exposure keratopathy, lid wiper epitheliopathy, dry eye, refractive surgery, and dry contact lenses. *Cont Lens Anterior Eye* 2007; **30**:37–51.

McMonnies CW, Ho A. Responses to a dry eye questionnaire from a normal population. *J Am Optom Assoc* 1987; **58**:588–591.

Messmer EM, Bulgen M, Kampik A. Hyperosmolarity of the tear film in dry eye syndrome. *Dev Ophthalmol* 2010; **45**:129–138.

Michel M, Sickenberger W, Pult H. The effectiveness of questionnaires in the determination of contact lens induced dry eye. *Ophthalmic Physiol Opt* 2009; **29**:479–486.

Miljanovic B, Trivedi KA, Dana MR, et al. Relation between dietary n-3 and n-6 fatty acids and clinically diagnosed dry eye syndrome in women. *Am J Clin Nutr* 2005; **82**:887–893.

Morgan PB, Woods CA, Tranoudis IG, et al. International contact lens prescribing in 2011. *CL Spectrum* 2012; **27**:26–31.

Müller-Treiber A. Kontaktlinsen Know-how.Heidelberg: DOZ Verlag, 2009.

Nelson JD, Shimazaki J, Benitez-Del-Castillo JM, et al. The international workshop on meibomian gland dysfunction: report of the definition and classification subcommittee. *Invest Ophthalmol Vis Sci* 2011; **52**:1930–1937.

Nichols JJ, Mitchell GL, King-Smith PE. Thinning rate of the precorneal and prelens tear films. *Invest Ophthalmol Vis Sci* 2005; **46**:2353–2361.

Nichols JJ, Mitchell GL, Nichols KK, et al. The performance of the contact lens dry eye questionnaire as a screening survey for contact lens-related dry eye. *Cornea* 2002; **21**:469–475.

Nichols JJ, Sinnott LT. Tear film, contact lens, and patient-related factors associated with contact lens-related dry eye. *Invest Ophthalmol Vis Sci* 2006; **47**:1319–1328.

Nichols KK, Nichols JJ, Mitchell GL. The lack of association between signs and symptoms in patients with dry eye disease. *Cornea* 2004; **23**:762–770.

Pritchard N. How can we avoid CL drop-outs? *Optician* 2001; **222**:14–18.

Pritchard N, Fonn D, Brazeau D. Discontinuation of contact lens wear: a survey. *Int Contact Lens Clin* 1999; **26**:157–162.

PhD Thesis. The predictive ability of clinical tests for dry eye in contact lens wear. Cardiff: Cardiff University, 2008.

Pult H. Dry eye in soft contact lens wearers. *Contact Lens Spectrum* 2011; **07**:26–53.

Pult H, Gill F, Riede-Pult BH. Effect of three different liposomal eye sprays on ocular comfort and tear film. *Cont Lens Anterior Eye* 2012; **35**:203–207.

Pult H, Korb DR, Blackie CA, Knop E. About vital staining of the eye and eyelids. I. the anatomy, physiology, and pathology of the eyelid margins and the lacrimal puncta by E. Marx. *Optom Vis Sci* 2010a; **87**:718–724.

Pult H, Murphy PJ, Purslow C. A novel method to predict dry eye symptoms in new contact lens wearers. *Optom Vis Sci* 2009; **86**:E1042–E1050.

Pult H, Murphy PJ, Purslow, C. Clide-index: a novel method to diagnose and measure contact lens induced dry eye. *Cont Lens Anterior Eye* 2010b; **33**:E-abstract:256–300.

Pult H, Purslow C, Berry M, Murphy PJ. Clinical tests for successful contact lens wear: relationship and predictive potential. *Optom Vis Sci* 2008; **85**:E924–E929.

Pult H, Riede-Pult BH. Non-contact meibography: keep it simple but effective. *Cont Lens Anterior Eye* 2012; **35**:77–80.

Rajagopalan K, Abetz L, Mertzanis P, et al. Comparing the discriminative validity of two generic and one disease-specific health-related quality of life measures in a sample of patients with dry eye. *Value Health* 2005; **8**:168–174.

Ramamoorthy P, Sinnott LT, Nichols JJ. Treatment, material, care, and patient-factors in contact lens related dry eye. *Invest Ophthalmol Vis Sci* 2008; **49**:ARVO E-abstract:4862.

Richdale K, Sinnott L, Skadahl E, Nichols JJ. Frequency of and factors associated with contact lens dissatisfaction and discontinuation. *Cornea* 2007; **26**:168–174.

Rosenberg ES, Asbell PA. Essential fatty acids in the treatment of dry eye. *Ocul Surf* 2010; **8**:18–28.

Santodomingo-Rubido J, Rubido-Crespo MJ. The clinical investigation of the base curve and comfort rate of a new prototype silicone hydrogel contact lens. *Eye Contact Lens* 2008; **34**:146–150.

Schafer J, Mitchell GL, Chalmers RL, et al. The stability of dryness symptoms after refitting with silicone hydrogel contact lenses over 3 years. *Eye Contact Lens* 2007; **33**:247–252.

Schaumberg DA, Nichols JJ, Papas EB, et al. The international workshop on meibomian gland dysfunction: report of the subcommittee on the epidemiology of, and associated risk factors for, MGD. *Invest Ophthalmol Vis Sci* 2011; **52**:1994–2005.

Schiffman RM, Christianson MD, Jacobsen G, et al. Reliability and validity of the ocular surface disease index. *Arch Ophthalmol* 2000; **118**:615–621.

Senchyna M, Jones L, Louie D, et al. Quantitative and conformational characterization of lysozyme deposited on balafilcon and etafilcon contact lens materials. *Curr Eye Res* 2004; **28**:25–36.

Shen M, Cui L, Riley C, et al. Characterization of soft contact lens edge fitting using ultra-high resolution and ultra-long scan depth optical coherence tomography. *Invest Ophthalmol Vis Sci* 2011; **52**:4091–4097.

Sickenberger W, Pult H, Sickenberger B. LIPCOF and contact lens wearers—a new tool of forecast subjective dryness and degree of comfort of contact lens wearers. *Contactologia* 2000; **22**:74–79.

Sindt CW, Longmuir RA. Contact lens strategies for the patient with dry eye. *Ocul Surf* 2007; **5**:294–307.

Spiteri A, Mitra M, Menon G, et al. Tear lipid layer thickness and ocular comfort with a novel device in dry eye patients with and without Sjögren's syndrome. *J Fr Ophtalmol* 2007; **30**:357–364.

Springs CL. Novel hydroxypropyl-guar gellable lubricant eye drops for treatment of dry eye. *Adv Ther* 2010; **27**:681–690.

Stahl U, Willcox M, Stapleton F. Role of hypo-osmotic saline drops in ocular comfort during contact lens wear. *Cont Lens Anterior Eye* 2010; **33**:68–75.

Sullivan BD, Whitmer D, Nichols KK, et al. An objective approach to dry eye disease severity. *Invest Ophthalmol Vis Sci* 2010; **51**:6125–6130.

Tomlinson A, Mccann LC, Pearce EI. Comparison of human tear film osmolarity measured by electrical impedance and freezing point depression techniques. *Cornea* 2010; **29**:1036–1041.

Tonge S, Jones L, Goodall S, Tighe B. The ex vivo wettability of soft contact lenses. *Curr Eye Res* 2001; **23**:51–59.

Tranoudis I, Efron N. Water properties of soft contact lens materials. *Cont Lens Anterior Eye* 2004; **27**:193–208.

Versura P, Profazio V, Campos EC. Performance of tear osmolarity compared to previous diagnostic tests for dry eye diseases. *Curr Eye Res* 2010; **35**:553–564.

Yamada MMD, Mochizuki HMD, Kawashima MMD, Hata SMD. Phospholipids and their degrading enzyme in the tears of soft contact lens wearers. *Cornea* 2006; **25**:S68–S72.

Yeh S, Song XJ, Farley W, et al. Apoptosis of ocular surface cells in experimentally induced dry eye. *Invest Ophthalmol Vis Sci* 2003; **44**:124–129.

Chapter 11 · Dry eye disease and glaucoma

Christophe Baudouin

■ INTRODUCTION

For the large majority of patients with primary open-angle glaucoma, medical management represents first-line therapy. Thus, most patients receive long-term medical treatment, often for several decades and some for the greater part of their lifetimes, since even surgical patients often require adjunctive medical therapy. There has been mounting evidence recently, from both basic science and clinical research, demonstrating that long-term eye drop use may induce frequent and significant ocular surface changes (Baudouin et al. 2010). In patients treated with long-term topical glaucoma medications, numerous signs of low-grade chronic inflammation have been described. Such medications, which are often used for decades in clinical practice, may alone cause chronic inflammation and/or may exacerbate preexisting ocular surface disease, such as dry eye, meibomian gland dysfunction, or chronic allergy. The safety profiles of topical medications, which are determined by short-term clinical trials as monotherapy in otherwise healthy eyes, may therefore not correlate satisfactorily with the safety of these formulations used in clinical practice.

In most cases, randomized clinical trials actually demonstrate satisfactory tolerability, with only a small minority of patients having to discontinue the medication due to local intolerance or allergy. However, it is important to note several major differences between clinical trials of glaucoma medications and actual clinical practice. First, since toxic compounds may take years or even decades to cause identifiable signs and symptoms, typical 6- to 12-month clinical trials may grossly underestimate the incidence of such effects over the long term. Second, research subjects typically receive only one trial medication or control eye drops, while in clinical practice, topical medications are frequently combined, leading to possible additive toxic interactions, which could not have been observed in, nor predicted by, these clinical trials. Due to additivity between side effects of each individual drug and preservative, and/or drug–drug interactions, multiple drug therapy is likely to increase the incidence of adverse events. This may be especially true with preservatives, which may be instilled four to five times per day, leading to accumulation of high tissue levels. In addition, clinical practitioners may have to prescribe topical glaucoma medications despite known or unknown hypersensitivity to the drug and/or preservative or despite the presence of established ocular surface disease. For ethical reasons, these types of patients are excluded from clinical trials, thus creating a selection bias and likely overestimating the ocular surface tolerability of the study medications relative to their eventual safety in actual practice. Since the prevalence of dry eye disease (DED) in patients over 65 is as high as 15–34% (Dry Eye Workshop 2007), and since dry eye may reduce the resistance of the cornea and conjunctiva to toxic or irritating compounds, a vicious cycle may ensue, whereby ocular surface disease and drug toxicity continue to exacerbate each other's deleterious effects.

■ PREVALENCE OF OCULAR SURFACE DISEASE IN GLAUCOMATOUS PATIENTS

Several observational studies have reported a much higher percentage of patients with signs and symptoms of ocular surface disease than that found in prospective clinical trials and than expected from the known prevalence of such diseases. Some of these observational studies impart undeniable clinical relevance due to their large sample sizes. Pisella et al. (2002) conducted an epidemiological survey of 4107 patients with glaucoma to determine the rate of ocular symptoms and conjunctival, corneal, and palpebral signs in a routine clinical practice. Among patients using preserved drops, the prevalence of symptoms was found to be as high as 43% with discomfort upon instillation, 40% with burning or stinging, 31% with foreign body sensation, 23% with dry eyes, 21% with tearing, and 18% with itching. The incidence of signs and symptoms correlated with the number of preserved drops used and was found to be significantly lower, with regard to all study criteria, in a group of patients treated with unpreserved beta-blockers, and lowered when switching to unpreserved eye drops or when diminishing the number of eye drops containing benzalkonium chloride (BAK) (Pisella et al. 2002). Similar studies have been conducted in Italy, Belgium, and Portugal—all with quite similar results. Pooled data from 9658 patients revealed an incidence of ocular symptoms ranging from 30 to 50% (Jaenen et al. 2007).

Similarly, one observational study of prevalence of DED in glaucoma was conducted in Germany, including a total of 20,506 patients from 900 centers. Each center recruited its first 30 consecutive glaucoma patients. According to the registry data, more women develop (DED) and glaucoma than men (56.9% vs. 45.7%), an association that was not significantly found in our current study. The more severe glaucoma cases, requiring three or more glaucoma drugs, exhibited more frequent (DED), particularly as the duration of glaucoma increased (Erb et al. 2008). Another recent European observational study confirmed the correlation between the number of eye drop use and the high prevalence of (DED) in patients with glaucoma: 11% with one drop, 39% with two drops, and 43% with three drops. With regard to surface symptoms, 8.7% of patients on two eye drops and 15% of those on three drops were found to have severe (DED) (Rossi et al. 2009).

In the United States, a similar cross-sectional study evaluated the impact of the ocular surface on glaucoma management in 101 patients with open-angle glaucoma or ocular hypertension. Fifty-nine percent of patients reported symptoms of (DED) in at least one eye, with 27% qualifying as severe, as defined by the Ocular Surface Disease Index (OSDI). Sixty-one percent of patients exhibited decreased tear production in at least one eye by Schirmer's testing, with 35% severely affected. Positive lissamine green staining of the cornea and conjunctiva was found in 22% of cases, whereas 78% of patients exhibited decreased tear break-up time, with 65% qualifying as severe (Leung et al. 2008). Another recent observational study of 630 patients in the United States, using the OSDI to record symptom prevalence and severity, found mild (21.3%), moderate (13.3%), or severe (13.8%) ocular surface disease symptoms. Significantly, more severe OSDI scores have been found in patients using multiple intraocular pressure-lowering medications and in those with dry eye syndrome or treatment at inclusion (Fechtner et al. 2010). All these studies concluded that glaucoma medication-related ocular surface symptoms substantially impacted the patients' quality of life.

CLINICAL MANIFESTATIONS OF DRUG INTOLERANCE

Allergic reactions

The symptoms of conjunctival allergy induced by the instillation of eye drops may widely vary, including congestion, tearing, photophobia, burning, or stinging sensations. Allergic manifestations are often spectacular (**Figure 11.1**), occurring a few days after treatment initiation, and recover rapidly when treatment is stopped. However, delayed allergic reactions may occur months or years after starting the treatment, often mimicking blepharitis with low-grade inflammation (**Figure 11.2**). In this condition, the relationship between the eye drops and ocular inflammation is often difficult to assess, especially when the treatment is mandatory for a severe sight-threatening condition.

Dry eye disease

In contrast to data obtained from prospective clinical trials, the real world shows a much larger proportion of patients suffering from symptoms and signs related to the DED, as assessed by observational surveys (**Figure 11.3**). As mentioned previously, dry eye symptoms are much more frequent in patients with glaucoma than expected from the prevalence of DED in the general population. Signs and symptoms of ocular surface disease have been observed in 15–50% of glaucoma patients, which is substantially more common than in normal controls.

Additionally, a number of studies have documented a correlation of these signs and symptoms with the presence of BAK (Jaenen et al. 2007, Pisella et al. 2002) and the number of concomitantly used eye drops containing BAK (Leung et al. 2008). These signs and symptoms significantly improved upon discontinuation of the BAK-preserved drops or substitution with unpreserved drops (Pisella et al. 2002, Uusitalo et al. 2010). The need for sterility in multidose eye drops requires the inclusion of an antimicrobial preservative in these solutions, most frequently the quaternary ammonium BAK. BAK toxicity for eye structures has been reported since the 1940s, and many studies in experimental or cell models have consistently and reliably shown its toxic effects (reviewed in Baudouin et al. 2010). Conversely, BAK is a hapten causing relatively few short-term allergic reactions, but it has been shown to destroy goblet cells and disrupt the lipid layer of tear film—two major components of tear film stability (Herreras et al. 1992, Labbé et al. 2012, Rolando et al. 1991). A clear correlation has recently been shown between tear hyperosmolarity, as a marker

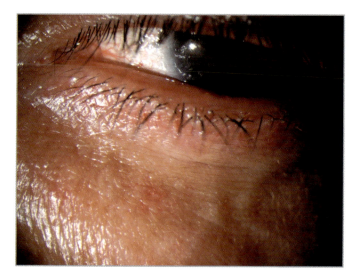

Figure 11.2 Chronic blepharitis due to the long-term use of antiglaucoma eye drops.

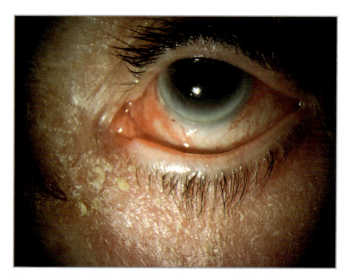

Figure 11.1 Drug-induced allergic reaction occurring 2 days after initiating the treatment.

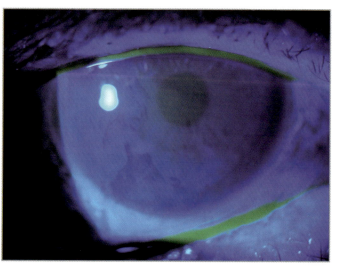

Figure 11.3 Decreased break-up time in a glaucomatous patient treated over the long term.

for DED, and the number of BAK-containing medications in patients with glaucoma (Labbé et al. 2012).

Severe ocular surface diseases

Chronic inflammation may result in more severe complications, with keratoconjunctivitis and alterations of the limbus (**Figure 11.4**). The development of subconjunctival fibrosis has been reported in patients treated with antiglaucoma medications for a long period, most likely resulting from an increase in fibroblast density in the subepithelial substantia propria, related to an increase in inflammatory cells (Baudouin et al. 1999, Broadway et al. 1994a, Sherwood et al. 1989). The use of long-term antiglaucoma medications has been shown to cause conjunctival foreshortening and shrinkage, which may be associated with an ocular pemphigoid-like condition or evolve into severe scarring conjunctivitis, with definitive corneal opacities (Schwab et al. 1992). In a series of 145 patients, Thorne et al. (2004) showed that exposure to antiglaucoma eye drops was the primary cause of toxic pseudopemphigoid. Almost all the cases reported (97.4%) involved an association of antiglaucoma medications (Thorne et al. 2004).

SUBCLINICAL CHANGES IN THE OCULAR SURFACE

Because clinical data and observations often lack specificity, numerous reports have investigated the ocular surface of patients with glaucoma by means of histopathological techniques. They have clearly demonstrated that, even without evident symptoms or clinical manifestations, inflammation is abnormally observed in the conjunctival epithelium and substantia propria. In most cases, conjunctival biopsies have been taken at the time of glaucoma surgery and examined using immunohistological techniques. Infiltration of immune cells in the conjunctiva has therefore been consistently reported. A significant increase in the number of macrophages, lymphocytes, mast cells, and fibroblasts in the conjunctiva and the Tenon capsule and a significant decrease in the number of epithelial goblet cells have been observed in patients undergoing surgery compared to a primary surgery group (Sherwood et al. 1989). In another study, conducted on 124 conjunctival biopsy specimens from patients undergoing filtration surgery, Broadway et al. (1994a) found that administration of topical medication, irrespective of type, for ≥3 years induced a significant degree of subclinical inflammation in the conjunctiva. Associations of two or more medications thus induced a significant decrease in goblet cells, an increase in pale cells, macrophages, and lymphocytes within the epithelium, and an increase in fibroblasts, macrophages, mast cells, and lymphocytes in the substantia propria. In addition, administration of one topical medication for >3 years was found to be associated with similar inflammatory and fibroblast infiltration. These data were directly correlated to risk of surgical failure (Broadway et al. 1994b). Similarly, in medium- and long-term therapy patients, Nuzzi et al. (1995) confirmed significant increases in the thickness and number of epithelial cell layers, in the fibroblast density in both subepithelial and deep connective tissues, and a more compact connective tissue, richer in collagen fibers arranged in whirls, with some inflammatory elements and increased expression of inflammatory markers (HLA-DR, CD1a, CD4, CD8, IL-2, and C3b).

Using impression cytology specimens, several reports also showed consistent ocular surface changes in glaucomatous patients (**Figure 11.5**). Brandt et al. (1991) showed statistically significant degrees of metaplasia in 72 patients treated over the long term and

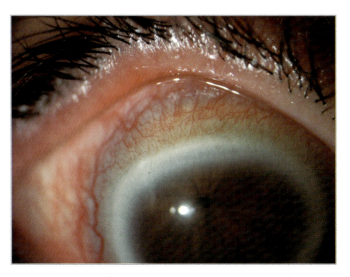

Figure 11.4 Chronic inflammation with keratoconjunctivitis and inflammatory pseudogerontoxon.

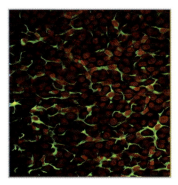

Figure 11.5 Impression cytology: infiltration of the conjunctiva by inflammatory dendritiform cells.

associated with the number of medications. Clinical impairment of the tear film and a rapid decrease of goblet cell density have also been demonstrated after starting treatment with preserved timolol (Herreras et al. 1992). The Schirmer's test and break-up time were significantly altered already in the first month of treatment compared to the basal control. Similarly, impression cytology showed a progressive decrease in goblet cell density that was also significant at the first month.

Using immunocytological and flow cytometry methods, HLA-DR expression can be measured, and it has become a very reliable marker for demonstrating inflammation in ocular surface diseases and for quantifying the level of inflammation. High rates of HLA-DR were found in patients treated with BAK-containing eye drops compared to normal eyes and a group receiving chlorhexidine-containing eye drops, for the first time highlighting a possible role played by BAK in conjunctival changes in patients with glaucoma (Baudouin et al. 1994). The flow cytometry technique has been further developed in impression cytology and repeatedly demonstrated that glaucoma patients, even though clinically asymptomatic, exhibit significant overexpression of HLA-DR class II antigens, ICAM-1, interleukins (IL)-6, IL-8, and IL-10, as well as CCR4 or CCR5 in the epithelium. Preserved drugs and multiple treatments reliably showed higher levels of inflammatory markers or cytokines compared to patients receiving unpreserved eye drops and normal control eyes in patients of the same age (Baudouin et al. 2004, 2008).

Another group similarly investigated HLA-DR in patients with glaucoma and the expression of trefoil factor family 1, MUC5AC, and HLA-DR, which were significantly higher in patients than in controls (Souchier et al. 2006). However, most interestingly, a higher MUC5AC expression and a lower HLA-DR expression were observed in patients with further successful glaucoma surgeries than in failures. Surface marker expression could therefore become a predictive factor for successful glaucoma surgery.

CLINICAL EVIDENCE OF PRESERVATIVE INVOLVEMENT

Few prospective studies have addressed the question of the deleterious role of the preservative, in part because of the current lack of preservative-free compounds and to a large extent because a normal ocular surface will experience weak toxic effects after a short duration of treatment, especially with a monotherapy, that is at a low BAK exposure rate. Nevertheless, in healthy volunteers Ishibashi et al. (2003) demonstrated that preserved timolol caused significantly higher tear film instability and disruption of corneal barrier function than preservative-free timolol. Similar results were also found in healthy volunteers when comparing preservative-free and BAK-containing carteolol (Baudouin & de Lunardo 1998). The tear break-up time was significantly lower in volunteers receiving BAK. Considering that both studies were conducted in young subjects with a fully normal ocular surface, these results may help better understand the high rate of dry eye symptoms and signs in patients with glaucoma who accumulate a long duration of treatment, a higher number of medications, and an increased risk of impaired ocular surface. Indeed, one study was conducted in healthy volunteers prospectively evaluating various concentrations of BAK in tear substitutes, given eight times a day for 7 days. Even a low concentration of BAK induced goblet cell loss and increased cytoplasmic–nucleus ratio, two characteristics of dry eye disease (Rolando et al. 1991).

Another recent study used impression cytology and the in vivo confocal microscopy (IVCM) technique to prospectively investigate the effects of preserved or unpreserved levobunolol on the conjunctival epithelium in 27 eyes of 27 patients. The patients were naive of previous antiglaucoma treatment. IVCM and impression cytology were performed before and after 6 months of therapy, and this showed significant differences from baseline in both groups and between the two groups. The IVCM analysis showed 61% and 17% of goblet cell density reduction from baseline, respectively, in patients receiving preserved levobunolol compared to unpreserved levobunolol ($p < 0.001$). Similarly, using the Nelson score, the grading of impression cytology parameters was found to be significantly higher in the preserved group (Ciancaglini et al. 2008).

Likewise, in order to evaluate the long-term effects of preservative-free and preservative-containing antiglaucoma eye drops on the ocular surface, a total of 84 patients were evaluated using the sophisticated method of IVCM, with respect to their treatment. Significant differences were found between groups on topical BAK-containing therapy, namely preserved beta-blocker, preserved prostaglandin, fixed or unfixed combinations of both drugs, and a preservative-free beta-blocker group. In particular, the density of superficial epithelial cells and the number of sub-basal nerves were reduced in all preservative-containing groups, whereas the basal epithelial cell density, stromal keratocyte activation, and bead-like nerve shape were higher in the glaucomatous preservative therapy groups (Martone et al. 2009). Moreover, this study evidenced decreased corneal sensitivity, based

on esthesiometry, in all groups with preservative (ranging from 39.1 in the unfixed combination group to 49.4 in the fixed combination group) compared to control or unpreserved eye drops (58.2 ± 1.7 and 55.8 ± 4.3, respectively, $p < 0.05$). These results were recently confirmed in another study measuring corneal sensitivity, which was consistently reduced in patients who were using BAK-containing eye drops (Van Went et al. 2011). This property of BAK could therefore participate in the overall good comfort of patients receiving preserved therapy.

At a larger scale, in the above-mentioned epidemiological survey conducted in 2002 in 4107 patients with glaucoma (Pisella et al. 2002), all ocular symptoms were significantly more prevalent (about twice as much) in patients using preserved drops compared with those on preservative-free treatment. Likewise, the similarly conducted European survey also demonstrated that the incidence of ocular signs and symptoms was higher in patients receiving preserved eye drops (Jaenen et al. 2007), and Leung et al. (2008) found a clear relationship between ocular surface involvement and the number of BAK-containing medications.

Mechanisms of preservative toxicity

Several different mechanisms contribute to the cytotoxicity of preservatives, in part dependent on the concentration used (Baudouin et al. 2010). First, the quaternary ammoniums, like most preservatives, are detergents. They have a positively charged hydrophilic head and an uncharged hydrophobic tail, which enables the molecules to insert into membranes, creating gaps that allow ionic or aqueous substances to penetrate into the intracellular or intercellular spaces. At high concentrations of quaternary ammoniums (0.01–0.05%, namely those mostly used in eye drops), proapoptotic or necrotic cytotoxic effects can be seen. At lower BAK concentrations, cell growth is inhibited and a process of programmed cell death starts. This includes morphological and metabolic changes typical of apoptosis, namely cell retraction, chromatin condensation, DNA fragmentation, and the expression of apoptosis markers. BAK is also known to cause oxidative stress, as eye drops containing quaternary ammoniums (0.01%) generate significantly more superoxide anions than preservative-free eye drops, and these levels have been shown to correlate with the loss of membrane integrity and apoptosis in the presence of BAK. In addition, there is strong evidence to support a role played by preservatives in the perpetuation of an immunoinflammatory reaction and onset of subconjunctival fibrosis: inflammatory cells, especially Langerhans cells, have been observed to infiltrate the conjunctiva and trabeculum following instillations of timolol-containing preservatives for 1 month, which was not seen with use of preservative-free timolol (Pisella et al. 2000).

In a sophisticated model of 3D reconstructed human corneal epithelial cells, consistent with what was previously observed in monolayer cell models, BAK was confirmed to have a dose-dependent response, with significant toxic effects at concentrations as low as 0.005% (Pauly et al. 2009). The most superficial cell layer, namely the cells mostly exposed to the toxic effect, showed high terminal deoxynucleotidyl transferase nick end labeling (TUNEL) positivity, quite consistent with apoptotic and cell death features observed in the monolayer model, whereas deeper cell layers, which received much lower doses of toxic compounds, showed the activation of caspase-3, consistent with the early stage of apoptosis and demonstrating the range of effects that BAK may cause in a multilayered epithelium. At the same time, BAK increased ICAM-1 expression in the corneal epithelium, an adhesion molecule related to inflammation and inflammatory cell recruitment. Indeed, overexpression of ICAM-1 by conjunctival cells has been observed in patients with glaucoma treated over the long term (Pisella et al. 2004). BAK also induced a dose-dependent disruption of the epithelial tight junctions in the superficial cells. As a possible compensatory mechanism, BAK stimulated the expression of Ki67, a cell marker of proliferation, most likely to replace dead cells and increase epithelial turnover. These results illustrate the tissue-level response to a toxic environment, most likely on stimulatory and inflammatory modes, in contrast to the cell-level response, which mainly responds in a binary cell death mode. They are fully in agreement with the histopathological findings in humans.

EXPERIMENTAL EVIDENCE OF PRESERVATIVE TOXICITY IN ANIMAL MODELS

The assessment of the acute eye irritation, potential of chemicals, cosmetics, and pharmaceuticals, is still based on the Draize rabbit test, proposed in 1944, a method widely criticized by animal welfare advocates and whose relevance, validity, and precision have been challenged because of the variability and low predictiveness of the human response. The rabbit model showed weaknesses in assessing non-severe irritants and low concentrations of toxic compounds. Histological models in rats have also been further developed. To overcome the natural resistance of healthy rats and the high variability of ocular behavior in these animals, higher concentrations are often required for toxicological purposes. Concentrations of 0.25% and 0.5% caused epithelial denudation as well as major damage to the deep structures, such as stromal inflammation and neovascularization, as well as loss of endothelial visibility and fibrosis, with incomplete corneal recovery even long after toxic substance removal (Pauly et al. 2007). At lower concentrations, ocular lesions resulting from a short duration of treatment in healthy animals are mild and more difficult to identify. Nevertheless, histological analyses, comparing BAK-containing and BAK-free compounds, consistently favored BAK-free compounds (Baudouin et al. 1999).

In order to improve the reliability of standard clinical assessment and postmortem histology, the use of in vivo corneal confocal microscopy now allows non-traumatic investigations of the ocular surface, by providing histological-like levels of resolution, close to 1 μm. Various applications have been developed in human diseases, and the technique has been further adapted to animal use. A scoring system was proposed to assess mild toxic changes in the ocular surface, today available for routine use (Pauly et al. 2007). However, as rat models are poorly reliable, and despite the improvement provided by confocal microscopy, other attempts have been made using animal models closer to human eyes, especially in rabbits.

Ichijima and colleagues developed an acute stress mode protocol, suitable for mimicking the effects of long-term use of low-toxicity compounds over a short period, and used confocal microscopy to assess the toxicological profiles of BAK and antiglaucomatous drugs,

further confirming the corneal toxicity of even low concentrations of BAK (Ichijima et al. 1992). Combined with clinical assessment, impression cytology, and immunohistology, new-generation confocal microscopy recently confirmed the overall toxicity of BAK and BAK-containing eye drops, in a dose-dependent manner. The absence of toxicity of preservative-free prostaglandins was also clearly demonstrated, and, interestingly, excipients based on cationic emulsions were found to decrease BAK toxicity (Liang et al. 2008a, 2008b). In addition, in these experiments, it was possible to identify, in vivo in rabbits, the conjunctiva-associated lymphoid tissue (CALT) and a major inflammatory infiltration after an acute challenge, with BAK or BAK-containing eye drops (Liang et al. 2010). This finding demonstrated immunoinflammatory involvement that was not only restricted to the conjunctiva but also extended toward deep structures and most likely the immune system distant from the instillation site, as was found in animal models of DED, another closely related ocular surface disease (Chauhan et al. 2009). Additionally, as in DED, another major finding in animals challenged with BAK was a dramatic decrease in goblet cells. Similarly, Kahook and Noecker found significantly lower densities of goblet cells in animals receiving BAK-containing latanoprost compared to preservative-free artificial tears (Kahook & Noecker 2008). Such findings are clearly in line with human findings of reduced goblet cell densities in patients treated with BAK-containing eye drops.

CONCLUSIONS

There is a large body of evidence showing that long-term administration of antiglaucomatous drugs may cause adverse events, most visible at the ocular surface, consisting of chronic irritation, dry eye, allergy, subconjunctival fibrosis, or increased risk of glaucoma surgery failure. Ocular surface symptoms most certainly have a substantial impact on patients' quality of life, as is well known in DED irrespective of the cause. An impact on compliance is very likely, although more difficult to assess. In an observational study conducted in 204 patients, the high rate of symptoms—with 25.4% experiencing burning sensation, 20.8% blurred vision, and 20.2% tearing—led to poor patient satisfaction and reduced adherence. Dissatisfied patients also visited their ophthalmologists more frequently (Nordmann et al. 2003). In a survey conducted in the United States between 2001 and 2004, based on the refilling rate of initial therapy in 300 patients, adverse effects were found to be the second most common reasons noted by physicians for switching medications after lack of efficacy (19% vs. 43%, respectively) (Zimmerman et al. 2009).

A large share of these effects could be due to the preservative, whose toxic, proinflammatory, and detergent effects have extensively been shown experimentally and largely suggested in clinical studies. Therefore, in patients with glaucoma it is advisable to use preservative-free medications, or alternatively eye drops with 'soft' preservatives—all solutions that should become the new gold standards of glaucoma therapy in the near future.

REFERENCES

Baudouin C, de Lunardo C. Short-term comparative study of topical 2% carteolol with and without benzalkonium chloride in healthy volunteers. *Br J Ophthalmol* 1998; **82**:39–42.

Baudouin C, Garcher C, Haouat N, Bron A, Gastaud P. Expression of inflammatory membrane markers by conjunctival cells in chronically treated patients with glaucoma. *Ophthalmology* 1994; **101**:454–460.

Baudouin C, Hamard P, Liang H, et al. Conjunctival epithelial cell expression of interleukins and inflammatory markers in glaucoma patients treated over the long term. *Ophthalmology* 2004; **111**:2186–2192.

Baudouin C, Labbé A, Liang H, et al. Preservatives in eyedrops: the good, the bad and the ugly. *Prog Retin Eye Res* 2010; **29**:312–334.

Baudouin C, Liang H, Hamard P, et al. The ocular surface of glaucoma patients treated over the long term expresses inflammatory markers related to both T-helper 1 and T-helper 2 pathways. *Ophthalmology* 2008; **115**:109–115.

Baudouin C, Pisella PJ, Fillacier K, et al. Ocular surface inflammatory changes induced by topical antiglaucoma drugs: human and animal studies. *Ophthalmology* 1999; **106**:556–563.

Brandt JD, Wittpenn JR, Katz LJ, Steinmann WN, Spaeth GL. Conjunctival impression cytology in patients with glaucoma using long-term topical medication. *Am J Ophthalmol* 1991; **112**:297–301.

Broadway DC, Grierson I, O'Brien C, Hitchings RA. Adverse effects of topical antiglaucoma medication. I. The conjunctival cell profile. *Arch Ophthalmol* 1994a; **112**:1437–1445.

Broadway DC, Grierson I, O'Brien C, Hitchings RA. Adverse effects of topical antiglaucoma medication. II. The outcome of filtration surgery. *Arch Ophthalmol* 1994b; **112**:1446–1454.

Chauhan SK, El Annan J, Ecoiffier T, et al. Autoimmunity in dry eye is due to resistance of Th17 to Treg suppression. *J Immunol* 2009; **182**:1247–1252.

Ciancaglini M, Carpineto P, Agnifili L, et al. An in vivo confocal microscopy and impression cytology analysis of preserved and unpreserved levobunolol-induced conjunctival changes. *Eur J Ophthalmol* 2008; **18**:400–407.

Dry Eye WorkShop. The epidemiology of dry eye disease: report of the Epidemiology Subcommittee of the International Dry Eye WorkShop. *Ocul Surf* 2007; **5**:93–107.

Erb C, Gast U, Schremmer D. German register for glaucoma patients with dry eye. I. Basic outcome with respect to dry eye. *Graefes Arch Clin Exp Ophthalmol* 2008; **246**:1593–1601.

Fechtner RD, Godfrey DG, Budenz D, et al. Prevalence of ocular surface complaints in patients with glaucoma using topical intraocular pressure-lowering medications. *Cornea* 2010; **29**:618–621.

Herreras JM, Pastor JC, Calonge M, Asensio VM. Ocular surface alteration after long-term treatment with an antiglaucomatous drug. *Ophthalmology* 1992; **99**:1082–1088.

Ichijima H, Petroll WM, Jester JV, Cavanagh HD. Confocal microscopic studies of living rabbit cornea treated with benzalkonium chloride. *Cornea* 1992; **11**:221–225.

Ishibashi T, Yokoi N, Kinoshita S. Comparison of the short-term effects on the human corneal surface of topical timolol maleate with and without benzalkonium chloride. *J Glaucoma* 2003; **12**:486–490.

Jaenen N, Baudouin C, Pouliquen P, et al. Ocular symptoms and signs with preserved and preservative-free glaucoma medications. *Eur J Ophthalmol* 2007; **17**:341–349.

Kahook MY, Noecker R. Quantitative analysis of conjunctival goblet cells after chronic application of topical drops. *Adv Ther* 2008; **25**:743–751.

Labbé A, Terry O, Brasnu E, Van Went C, Baudouin C. Tear film osmolarity in patients treated for glaucoma or ocular hypertension. 2012; **31**:994–999.

Leung EW, Medeiros FA, Weinreb RN. Prevalence of ocular surface disease in glaucoma patients. *J Glaucoma* 2008; **17**:350–355.

Liang H, Baudouin C, Dupas B, Brignole-Baudouin F. Live conjunctiva-associated lymphoid associated tissue (CALT) analysis using in vivo confocal microscopy (IVCM) under inflammatory stimuli. *Invest Ophthalmol Vis Sci* 2010; **51**:1008–1015.

Liang H, Baudouin C, Pauly A, Brignole-Baudouin F. Conjunctival and corneal reactions in rabbits following short- and repeated exposure to preservative-free tafluprost, commercially available latanoprost and 0.02% benzalkonium chloride. *Br J Ophthalmol* 2008a; **92**:1275–1282.

Liang H, Brignole-Baudouin F, Rabinovich-Guilatt L, et al. Reduction of quaternary ammonium-induced ocular surface toxicity by emulsions: an in vivo study in rabbits. *Mol Vis* 2008b; **14**:204–216.

Martone G, Frezzotti P, Tosi GM, et al. An in vivo confocal microscopy analysis of effects of topical antiglaucoma therapy with preservative on corneal innervation and morphology. *Am J Ophthalmol* 2009; **147**:725–735.

Nordmann JP, Auzanneau N, Ricard S, Berdeaux G. Vision related quality of life and topical glaucoma treatment side effects. *Health Qual Life Outcomes* 2003; **1**:75.

Nuzzi R, Vercelli A, Finazzo C, Cracco C. Conjunctiva and subconjunctival tissue in primary open-angle glaucoma after long-term topical treatment: an immunohistochemical and ultrastructural study. *Graefes Arch Clin Exp Ophthalmol* 1995; **233**:154–162.

Pauly A, Brignole-Baudouin F, Labbe A, et al. New tools for the evaluation of toxic ocular surface changes in the rat. *Invest Ophthalmol Vis Sci* 2007; **48**:5473–5483.

Pauly A, Meloni M, Brignole-Baudouin F, et al. Multiple endpoint analysis of the 3D-reconstituted corneal epithelium after treatment with benzalkonium chloride: early detection of toxic damage. *Invest Ophthalmol Vis Sci* 2009; **50**:1644–1652.

Pisella PJ, Debbasch C, Hamard P, et al. Conjunctival proinflammatory and proapoptotic effects of latanoprost and preserved and unpreserved timolol: an ex vivo and in vitro study. *Invest Ophthalmol Vis Sci* 2004; **45**:1360–1368.

Pisella PJ, Fillacier K, Elena PP, et al. Comparison of the effects of preserved and unpreserved formulations of Timolol on the ocular surface of albino rabbits. *Ophthalmic Res* 2000; **32**:3–8.

Pisella PJ, Pouliquen P, Baudouin C. Prevalence of ocular symptoms and signs with preserved and preservative free glaucoma medication. *Br J Ophthalmol* 2002; **86**:418–423.

Rolando M, Brezzo V, Giordano G, et al. The effect of different benzalkonium chloride concentrations on human normal ocular surface. In: Van Bijsterveld O, Lemp M, Spinelli D (eds), The Lacrimal System. Amsterdam, Berkely, Milano: Kugler and Ghedini Publications, 1991.

Rossi GC, Tinelli C, Pasinetti GM, et al. Dry eye syndrome-related quality of life in glaucoma patients. *Eur J Ophthalmol* 2009; **19**:572–579.

Schwab IR, Linberg JV, Gioia VM, Benson WH, Chao GM. Foreshortening of the inferior conjunctival fornix associated with chronic glaucoma medications. *Ophthalmology* 1992; **99**:197–202.

Sherwood MB, Grierson I, Millar L, Hitchings RA. Long-term morphologic effects of antiglaucoma drugs on the conjunctiva and Tenon's capsule in glaucomatous patients. *Ophthalmology* 1989; **96**:327–335.

Souchier M, Buron N, Lafontaine PO, et al. Trefoil factor family 1, MUC5AC and human leucocyte antigen-DR expression by conjunctival cells in patients with glaucoma treated with chronic drugs: could these markers predict the success of glaucoma surgery? *Br J Ophthalmol* 2006; **90**:1366–1369.

Thorne JE, Anhalt GJ, Jabs DA. Mucous membrane pemphigoid and pseudopemphigoid. *Ophthalmology* 2004; **111**:45–52.

Uusitalo H, Chen E, Pfeiffer N, et al. Switching from a preserved to a preservative-free prostaglandin preparation in topical glaucoma medication. *Acta Ophthalmol* 2010; **88**:329–336.

Van Went C, Alalwai H, Brasnu E, et al. Corneal sensitivity in patients treated medically for glaucoma or ocular hypertension. *J Fr Ophtalmol* 2011; **34**:684–690.

Zimmerman TJ, Hahn SR, Gelb L, Tan H, Kim EE. The impact of ocular adverse effects in patients treated with topical prostaglandin analogs: changes in prescription patterns and patient persistence. *J Ocul Pharmacol Ther* 2009; **25**:145–152.

Chapter 12

Sjögren's syndrome and other causes of cicatrizing conjunctivitis

Saaeha Rauz, Geraint P. Williams, Valerie P. Saw

INTRODUCTION

Immune-mediated systemic disease is frequently associated with ocular surface disorders. The underlying etiopathogenesis can emanate from the full spectrum of immunologically classified 'hypersensitivity' reactions that lead to autoimmune disease. One of the key features of the ocular manifestations of these systemic diseases is an inflammatory dry eye disease, occurring either as primary aqueous deficiency due to infiltration of the lacrimal gland, such as in primary or secondary Sjögren's syndrome, or tear film abnormalities due to mucocutaneous syndromes that cause cicatrizing conjunctivitis, including ocular mucous membrane pemphigoid (OcMMP) and Stevens–Johnson syndrome (SJS)/toxic epidermal necrolysis (TEN). Multidisciplinary input in managing these complex diseases is often required. Patient engagement with regard to the chronic and debilitating nature of their disease is essential, ideally with help from patient support groups.

SJÖGREN'S SYNDROME

Sjögren's syndrome (SS) is a multisystem disorder with significant morbidity. First described in 1892 as a case of parotid gland swelling with histological features it is now confirmed to be consistent with primary Sjögren's syndrome (pSS); it wasn't until in 1933 that Henrik Sjögren (a Swedish ophthalmologist), in his postdoctoral thesis, went on to describe 19 female patients with arthritis, associated with symptoms of dryness, and termed the ocular features as keratoconjunctivitis sicca. This condition is characterized by anti-Ro (SS-A) and anti-La (SS-B) antibodies with or without the HLA-D3 haplotype. Secondary Sjögren's syndrome (sSS) relates to the late presentation of sicca features in the natural history of diseases such as rheumatoid arthritis (RA), systemic lupus erythematosus, scleroderma, or other connective tissue disorders, but rather confusingly, systemic diseases such as primary biliary cirrhosis or scleroderma may also evolve in patients with existing pSS.

Epidemiology and classification

pSS appears to have no specific geographical distribution, but it has a strong female preponderance (13:1), typically presenting in the fifth or sixth decades of life. The recent acceptance of the American European Consensus Group criteria, summarized in **Table 12.1**, has enabled both a more robust system for confirming diagnosis and an estimation of prevalence of 0.1–0.5% in women, which had not been possible previously due to the absence of accepted diagnostic criteria (Vitali et al. 2002). Additionally, a number of activity and damage indices have been validated to facilitate research-driven registries to provide a basis for translational research and clinical trials for emerging disease therapies (Barry et al. 2008, Bowman et al. 2007).

Table 12.1 American European Consensus Group Criteria for Sjögren's syndrome*

Criteria	1. Symptomatic dry mouth for >3 months as demonstrated by a positive response to at least one of the oral screening questions 2. Symptomatic dry eyes for >3 months as demonstrated by a positive response to at least one of the ocular screening questions 3. A reduced Schirmer-1 test (<5 mm/5 min) without anesthetic† or Rose Bengal or equivalent score, that is, lissamine green 4. A labial gland biopsy demonstrating at least one focal periductal aggregation of 50 or more lymphocytes in a high-powered field 5. Reduced unstimulated whole salivary flow rate of ≤1.5 mL in 15 minutes, or abnormal parotid sialography, or salivary gland scintigraphy 6. Antibodies to Ro (SS-A) and/or La (SS-B) antigens
Ocular screening questions	Have you had daily, persistent, troublesome dry eyes for >3 months? Do you have a recurrent sensation of sand or gravel in the eyes? Do you use tear substitutes more than three times a day?
Oral screening questions	Have you had a daily feeling of dry mouth for >3 months? Have you had recurrent or persistent swelling of the salivary glands as an adult? Do you frequently drink liquids to aid swallowing dry food?
Exclusions	Head and neck radiation therapy Hepatitis C infection Acquired immunodeficiency syndrome Preexisting lymphoma Sarcoid Graft-versus-host disease Use of anticholinergic drugs

Adapted from Vitali et al. (2002).
*Primary Sjögren's syndrome is defined as either (i) four out of the six listed items, provided that one of these includes item 4 (histological evidence) and/or item 6 (autoantibodies), or (ii) three out of the four objective criteria (items 3–6) are present. By contrast, secondary Sjögren's syndrome is defined as an autoimmune disease, usually a mixed connective tissue disease and either symptomatic dry eyes or dry mouth (or both), with at least two out of items 3–5, generally with late onset of sicca symptoms.
†Not stated in the criteria, which is usually taken to be the average of the measurement in the two eyes.

Pathogenesis

The pathogenesis of SS is not fully understood. The dry eye disease (DED) is primarily an aqueous tear-deficient dry eye resulting from lacrimal infiltration and destruction. A similar process occurs in the salivary glands with consequent xerostomia. Lacrimal and salivary glands are infiltrated by activated T cells as a result of an autoimmune process, possibly triggered by the expression of epithelial cell autoantigens, such as fodorin, SS-A, and SS-B, with consequent acinar and ductular destruction resulting in glandular hyposecretion. Approximately two-thirds of patients with pSS are positive for anti-Ro antibodies, of whom one-third have anti-La antibodies. Very few patients have anti-La in the absence of anti-Ro. Other autoantibodies have been linked with SS, and these have been associated with a number of specific clinical features. For example, antimuscarinic M3 receptor antibodies may have a role in potentially reversible glandular neurosecretory block; anticarbonic anhydrase with renal tubular acidosis; antiaquaporin 4 with neuromyelitis optica; and anticentromere with Raynaud's phenomenon and overlap with scleroderma.

What initiates the autoimmune acinar damage is unresolved. Based upon case reports and small-scale twin studies, the estimated concordance rate for SS is low, suggesting that environmental factors are key (Anaya et al. 2006). An androgen-depleted inflammatory environment, exposure to environmental agents such as viruses or pollution, and nutritional deficiency in omega-3 or other unsaturated fatty acids, together with unsupplemented vitamin C intake, may have a role in the development of the sicca features of SS. Although the genetic predisposition appears not to be fundamental in the pathogenesis of SS, HLA haplotypes have been linked to Ro and La autoantibodies (HLA DR3 DQ2 haplotype with positive anti-Ro and anti-La antibodies; HLA DR2*15 and DQ6 with positive anti-Ro but negative anti-La in pSS; HLA-DR4 with sSS in RA). A viral trigger has also been postulated as there appears to be an overexpression of IFN-γ-inducible genes, including Toll-like receptor 3 (TLR 3) and STAT4 in salivary epithelial cells, or TLR 7 and TLR 9 in B cells (Low & Witte 2011). Conversely, there are several viruses that masquerade as SS, including hepatitis C virus, HIV, human T-lymphotropic virus type 1, Epstein–Barr virus, cytomegalovirus, and human herpes virus 6, which should all be excluded at the time of diagnosis.

Regardless of the trigger, an autoimmune process is apparent. Once initiated, the innate immune signaling cascade is activated through non-specific mediators such as TLRs with IFN-γ production. Additionally, epithelial apoptosis and subsequent expression of Ro and La autoantigens result in the synthesis of Ro and La autoantibodies, with consequent CD4+ T-cell and B-cell infiltration of the gland (Stern et al. 2010). Upregulation of endothelial adhesion molecules and recruitment of immune cells into the tissues, together with the release of a number of immunomodulators, including IL-6, IL-10, TNF-α, IL-17, IL-23, and B-cell-activating factor/B-lymphocyte stimulator, are thought to be critical in the formation of lymphoid structures that are pivotal to perpetuating the inflammatory immune response, leading not only to glandular dysfunction and destruction but also to potentially life-threatening lymphomatous change. While transportation of the inflammatory mediators to the ocular surface contributes to ocular surface inflammation, reduced lacrimal tear secretion is compounded by aqueous evaporation, with resultant tear film and ocular surface epithelial cell hyperosmolarity. This in turn stimulates mitogen activated protein (MAP) kinase and nuclear factor kappa beta (NFκB) pathways, with further production of proinflammatory cytokines (e.g. IL-1α, IL-1β, and TNF-α) and MMP-9, leading to conjunctival goblet cell loss and squamous metaplasia.

Experimental murine models of dry eye, based on a desiccating stress environment, have revealed the importance of antigen-presenting cells in initiating and maintaining the recruitment of autoreactive T cells. A CD4+ infiltrate has been recognized in the conjunctiva of patients with pSS, and evidence points to the importance of the role of IFN-γ-producing CD4+ T cells and Th17 subsets in the pathogenesis of the disease with IL-17, detected in the tears of patients with pSS. In murine models, there appears to be a defective suppressor function by T-regulatory cells on Th17 cells. The inflammatory cascade of DED is discussed in Chapter 8.

■ Clinical features
Ocular manifestations

Why symptoms occur in dry eyes is not fully understood, but it is thought to be a combination of decreased lubrication (e.g. rapid tear film break-up, increased mechanical shear stresses between the lids and globe, and reduced expression of mucins) and alteration of tear film composition (e.g. hyperosmolarity and presence of inflammatory mediators), together with hypersensitivity of the nociceptive sensory nerves, subserving the ocular surface. The latter frequently results in symptomatology disproportionate to the clinical signs, necessitating treatments with drugs such as tramadol, gabapentin, and pregabalin (although some of these have the potential to compound sicca symptoms) (Rosenthal et al. 2009). Typically, patients complain of ocular discomfort, described as dry, gritty, or burning of varying degrees of severity, from mild and/or episodic discomfort triggered by environmental stress to severe constant, visually debilitating symptomatology profoundly affecting the quality of life. The detailed grading of symptoms, clinical features of DED, and how these provide a guide for therapeutic strategies are discussed extensively elsewhere in this book. Slowly progressive cicatrizing conjunctivitis (PCC) may also be a feature particularly in sSS, which is discussed later in this chapter. Uveitis and orbital lymphoma, although rare, are more common in patients who are seropositive. Specifically, uveitis is characterized by bilateral or unilateral chronic intraocular inflammation, typified by keratic precipitates in association with pars planitis in the absence of chorioretinitis. High erythrocyte sedimentation rate (ESR) and positive anti-nuclear antibody (ANA) serology in a speckled pattern, with high titers of anti SS-A and anti-SS-B, are common. Systemic steroid-sparing agents necessitating consolidation of inflammation, with intravenous cyclophosphamide and high-dose oral prednisone, followed by long-term maintenance with oral cyclosporin A may be required (Bridges & Burns 1992).

Oral manifestations

It is imperative that ophthalmologists recognize relevant oral symptoms and implement appropriate first-line therapeutic strategies while a referral is made to an oral medicine colleague. Dry mouth (xerostomia) (**Figure 12.1**) and non-painful swelling of the parotid and/or submandibular salivary glands are by far the most common oral features of pSS. Xerostomia is frequently associated with general oral discomfort due to inadequate mucous lubrication compounding speech and swallowing, altering taste perception, increasing the rate of dental decay, and periodontal disease. Clinical examination is typified by angular cheilitis, dry flaky lips, associated with a dry dorsal tongue with absence of a saliva pool in the floor of the mouth. Of note, smooth surface and cervical dental caries are the hallmark of longstanding disease. The assessment of salivary gland enlargement should be tailored to determining whether the swelling is diffuse or nodular, or whether there is accompanying inflammatory change in the overlying skin or VII nerve motor weakness. Gentle milking of the glands may reveal thick mucoid saliva, but frank glandular pain

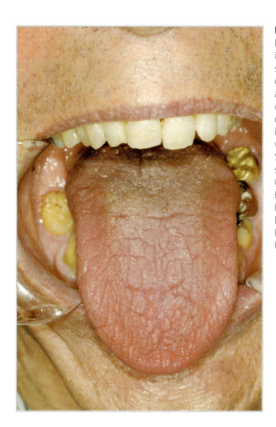

Figure 12.1 Dry mouth in Sjögren's syndrome: glossitis and a severely desiccated dorsal tongue in a patient with primary Sjögren's syndrome. Courtesy of J. Hamburger, Birmingham Dental Hospital, Birmingham, UK.

is rare. Blood-stained pus discharge should raise suspicion of infection, while intermittent pain exacerbated at mealtimes is suggestive of obstructive etiology such as SS-related ductal stenosis, salivary calculi, or neoplastic change.

Investigations for oral Sjögren's syndrome

Salient investigations consist of monitoring the salivary flow rate, salivary gland imaging, and minor salivary gland biopsy. Salivary flow rates are usually measured in the clinic as unstimulated whole salivary flow over a 15-minute interval, with <0.1 mL/min being considered abnormal. From an imaging perspective, high-resolution ultrasonography defines characteristic and probably diagnostic hypoechoic regions in a heterogeneous salivary gland tissue mass. Sialography visualizes the extent of sialectasis but the 'gold standard' diagnostic tool remains labial gland biopsy, but not without risk (false-negatives, mental nerve damage, etc.). While biopsy is generally reserved for cases that are anti-SS-A and anti-SS-B negative, emerging evidence suggests that certain histological features may provide prognostic information. Detection of myoepithelial sialadenitis or the presence of germinal center-like structures may represent predictors of lymphomatous change, whereas a typical diagnostic biopsy shows features of focal, periductal lymphocytic foci at a minimum density of 1 focus/4 mm², accompanied by sialadenitis, acinar atrophy, and ductal hyperplasia.

Management of the oral Sjögren's syndrome

The management of xerostomia is largely symptomatic, but preventative measures are essential to maintain dentition and periodontal tissues.

Limiting sugary food substances is essential, and a minimum delay of 30 minutes between eating and brushing teeth is advised to minimize damage to the surface enamel, which can occur as a result of acidic softening after food intake. Manual toothbrushes should be used with care so the gums are not traumatized, and attention to interdental cleaning is critical. Daily hygiene practices should be supplemented, with professional dental hygiene performed at least on a 6-monthly basis. Although commercially available alcohol-free fluoride mouthwashes that promote dental mineralization are easily accessible to patients, higher concentration fluoride toothpastes and mouth rinses can be prescribed by a dentist for at-risk patients. Chlorhexidine-containing substances may aid oral hygiene, particularly where arthritis curbs dexterity, but use is restricted due to mucosal and dental staining. Adjunctive treatment with saliva replacement preparations, providing chiefly symptomatic relief, can be helpful and include a range of substances, such as carboxymethyl cellulose, glycerin, sodium hyaluronate, mucin-based compounds, or oils, and for those who have some retained salivary gland function, sialogogues in the form of sugar-free chewing gum, pastilles, or lozenges. Muscarinic agonists (pilocarpine or cevimeline—not available in Europe) may also be useful. To build up tolerance to systemic muscarinic effects, pilocarpine is typically initiated at a low dose of 2.5 mg per day, increasing gradually up to a maximum dose of 20 mg per day. Future horizons in the management of oral SS include B-cell-directed therapy, glandular electrostimulation, transplantation of ex vivo tissue-engineered salivary gland-like structures, and gene therapy for aquaporin 1.

Systemic features

Three quarters of the patients with pSS have extraglandular features of disease, particularly those who have positive serology to anti-SS-A/SS-B antibodies (**Table 12.2**). These patients have the highest risk of systemic, hematological, or immunological complications, Raynaud's phenomenon, respiratory tract and gastrointestinal involvement, peripheral neuropathy, thyroid disease, and lymphoma. Neonatal complications are also higher in mothers with pSS sero-positive for anti-SS-A and SS-B. It is important to recognize 'at-risk' patients and adopt a multidisciplinary approach to management, with the tripartite liaison between rheumatologists, oral medicine physicians, and ophthalmologists generally representing the helm.

Hematological and immunological complications

Lymphadenopathy is reported in about 30% of anti-SS-A/SS-B positive patients. A spectrum of hematological abnormalities are more prevalent in pSS and these include leukopenia, neutropenia, lymphopenia, a normochromic normocytic anemia, or thrombocytopenia, possibly related to the presence of anti-neutrophil, anti-CD4, or anti-RBC antibodies. A positive Coombs test is common in pSS, and formal autoimmune hemolytic anemia is relatively rare but amenable to steroid therapy. Hypocomplementemia is seen in a subgroup of patients and is associated with a higher frequency of vasculitis, lymphoma, leukopenia, and cryoglobulinemia, and is strongly associated with the presence of extraglandular manifestations in seropositive patients. It is also an independent risk factor for the development of lymphoma.

A low-grade fever and weight loss may be suggestive of an underlying malignancy. The risk of B-cell-derived mucosa-associated lymphoid tissue lymphoma is increased in seropositive patients and

Table 12.2 Systemic features of Sjögren's syndrome and management strategies*

	Systemic feature	Reported Prevalence (%)	Management
Constitutional	Fatigue	75–90	Exclude secondary causes: fibromyalgia, anemia, celiac disease, depression, hypothyroidism, etc. DMARDs: hydroxychloroquine Biologics: rituximab
	Pyrexia, malaise, weight loss	–	Exclude lymphoma or other malignancies NSAIDs Hydroxychloroquine, prednisolone
Thyroid	Hypothyroidism	20	Thyroxine
	Autoimmune thyroiditis	–	NSAIDs
Musculoskeletal	Arthralgia, arthritis, synovitis	33	NSAIDs DMARDs: hydroxychloroquine, methotrexate or sulfasalazine Local or oral glucocorticoids
	Myositis	–	As arthritis but pulsed IV methylprednisolone or cyclophosphamide if severe
Skin	Raynaud's	80	Gloves and hand heating devices Calcium antagonists: nifedipine or ACE inhibitors
	Cutaneous	50	Dryness: avoid perfumed products and use emollients Vasculitis: hydroxychloroquine Lupus: sun protection factor screens and hydroxychloroquine Cryoglobulinemia: pulsed IV methylprednisolone and cyclophosphamide, IV Ig, plasmaphoresis, or rituximab
Solid organ	Respiratory	–	Dry cough: saline inhalers and/or pilocarpine Interstitial lymphocytic pneumonitis: NSAIDs or prednisolone
	Cardiac	–	Pericarditis: analgesia, NSAIDs, or prednisolone Pulmonary hypertension: antihypertensives
	Celiac disease	12	Biopsy and avoid gluten-containing products
	Primary biliary cirrhosis		Ursodeoxycholic acid Cholecystectomy
	Hepatitis and pancreatitis		Asymptomatic or mild
	Renal impairment	50	Mild or asymptomatic
	Renal tubular acidosis	33	Bicarbonate or potassium citrate
	Urinary symptoms/ sterile cystitis	66	Simple analgesia, antihistamines or cimetidine Intrabladder therapy: DMSO or sodium hyaluronate
Neurological	Neuropathy/trigeminal neuralgia	5–10	Hydroxychloroquine
	Mononeuritis multiplex/myelopathy	5/3	Corticosteroids and cyclophosphamide
	Autonomic neuropathy	3	Support stockings Fluid-retaining drugs
Neoplasia	Lymphoma	10	Asymptomatic: watch With enlarged parotid glands: radiotherapy With active SS: IV rituximab, cyclophosphamide, and methylprednisolone

DMARDs, disease-modifying antirheumatic drugs; DMSO, dimethyl sulfoxide; IV, intravenous; IV Ig, intravenous immunoglobulin; NSAIDs, non-steroidal anti-inflammatory drugs.
*Systemic features are most common and severest in patients who are seropositive for SS-A and SS-B autoantibodies.

those with neutropenia, lymphadenopathy, and low C4 levels. Classically affecting the parotid gland, other sites include the orbit, stomach, thyroid, and respiratory tract. Confirmatory diagnostic tissue biopsy followed by a combination of surgical excision, radiotherapy, or chemotherapy is frequently required. Chemoreduction with rituximab, delivered with cyclophosphamide and methylprednisolone, affords in >90% 5-year disease-free survival, dependent on the stage of disease at the time of diagnosis.

Pregnancy and the neonate

Persistent vaginal dryness predisposes to candidiasis, and treatment is predominantly symptomatic with short-acting lubricants, longer-acting gels, and muscarinic agonists. Although fertility is normal in pSS, there is an increased risk of recurrent miscarriage in women who are seropositive. Neonatal cutaneous lupus is seen around 6 weeks in approximately 5% of births and lasts around 17 weeks before fading spontaneously. In some children, residual depigmentation or telangiectasia may persist. Congenital heart block occurs in up to 2% of first pregnancies, but the frequency increases to 17% of subsequent pregnancies. First- and third-degree blocks can be detected in utero from around the 16th week and progression may be prevented by the use of dexamethasone, but third-degree heart block is irreversible. Almost 70% of these affected children survive, but nearly all require pacemakers in early life.

CICATRIZING CONJUNCTIVITIS AND IMMUNOBULLOUS DISEASES

Cicatrizing conjunctivitis

Cicatrizing conjunctivitis (conjunctival inflammation associated with scarring) is a rare, usually bilateral, sight-threatening group of disorders for which early diagnosis and appropriate treatment are essential (**Table 12.3**). The conjunctival inflammation that underlies the disease process may cause ocular surface failure, as a result of chronic limbitis and limbal stem cell deficiency (LSCD), leading to blinding keratopathy in addition to causing progressive conjunctival scarring that is the hallmark of the disease. The molecular processes of conjunctival scarring and chronic inflammation disrupt not only the intricate immunoprotective ocular surface microenvironments but also the protective action of the eyelids and tear film, leading to DED and ocular surface damage. The compromised ocular surface is predisposed to corneal ulceration, complicated by infectious keratitis and corneal scarring, which is another route to blindness in this disease. Both surface changes and the inflammation result in discomfort, which is often unremitting and severe. The differential diagnosis of cicatrizing conjunctivitis is detailed in **Table 12.3**, and it may be classified into PCC or slowly progressive or static.

Immunobullous disease

Many of the disorders causing PCC fall under the category of mucocutaneous syndromes or immunobullous disease, where the key target for pathology is the basement membrane zone (BMZ) **Figure 12.2**. The ocular surface epithelial BMZ is composed of an extracellular matrix of proteins, which bind the epithelium to the underlying stroma. The BMZ itself can be subdivided into the lamina lucida, lamina densa, and an underlying fibroreticularis. An understanding of the components of cell–matrix adhesion (hemidesmosomes and basement membrane) and cell–cell adhesion (desmosomes) molecular structures is fundamental to not only understanding the pathophysiological processes that underpin immunobullous diseases but also classifying the disease. Using this concept, the major groups of autoimmune diseases that affect the basal epithelial cells and dermal–epidermal junction of the skin and mucous membranes include (i) pemphigus diseases, (ii) pemphigoid diseases, (iii) epidermolysis bullosa acquisita (EBA), and (iv) dermatitis herpetiformis (Mihai & Sitaru 2007), summarized in **Table 12.4** and **Figure 12.2**. This classification is not all inclusive, and several other disease entities should also be considered that is paraneoplastic cicatrizing conjunctivitis, drug-induced cicatrizing conjunctivitis (DICC), PCC associated with linear IgA disease, and EBA.

Paraneoplastic pemphigus, as the name suggests, is a paraneoplastic syndrome associated most often with hematological (lymphoid) malignancy. Around 66% of cases involve the eye, with cicatrizing conjunctivitis and epitheliopathy. The diagnosis is confirmed by direct immunofluorescence (DIF), showing intraepithelial blistering due to IgG and C3 deposition on the surface of epithelial cells (Ahuero et al. 2010). The condition responds to systemic immunosuppression, but the prognosis is guarded.

DICC (Broadway 1997), cutaneous linear IgA disease, or EBA with associated PCC (Chan et al. 2002) may all be clinically and pathologically indistinguishable from OcMMP (discussed in detail later this chapter). DICC represents a spectrum of disease, ranging from a self-limiting toxic form to a progressive immunological form (called 'drug-induced OcMMP'). Management involves drug cessation or substitution where possible, with a non-preserved preparation, DIF biopsy to investigate immunologically driven disease, and careful monitoring, instituting immunosuppression if necessary.

Monitoring disease activity, damage, and progression

Inflammation of the conjunctiva may be induced by a large variety of exogenous and endogenous infectious and toxic agents. The speed of onset (acute or subacute), type of exudate, laterality, drug use, affected contacts, and associated systemic involvement can help differentiate the type of inflammation. The majority of physical signs are a poor discriminator of acute or chronic disease (**Table 12.5**). The pattern of conjunctival fibrosis, however, may provide helpful information in the assessment of PCC. Fibrosis may be classified as superficial (involving the epithelial structures) or deep (involving the subepithelial layers), although distinction is not always possible and most patients show a combination of both; that is, subepithelial fibrosis, without obvious involvement of the conjunctival epithelial layer, is characteristic of OcMMP, whereas superficial scarring is typically seen after membranous conjunctivitis.

Conjunctiva

Conjunctival cicatrization, inflammatory disease activity, damage, and corneal changes are important indices that should be assessed and documented at each clinic visit by accurate clinical drawings and photography. There are no validated and accepted grading systems, defining activity and damage in PCC as a whole, but systems exist (albeit with limitations) for specific diseases such as OcMMP (Foster 1986, Mondino & Brown 1981, Tauber et al. 1992) or SJS–TEN (Power et al. 1995, Sotozono et al. 2007). The 'proposed' system, described by Tauber, incorporates the Mondino and Foster systems. The advantage of combining both systems is that the scale allows for a simpler and, it is argued, more sensitive system of recording damage, but this scale requires documentation of both the number and involvement of symblephara. The mechanism for objectively enumerating these parameters was not described in the original system, which has limited its use in daily clinical practice. Development of prototype tools to objectively quantify conjunctival shrinkage has the potential to foster accurate documentation to enable detection of disease progression, including the use of fornix depth measurers (**Figure 12.3**) (Schwab et al. 1992, Williams et al. 2011b).

Cornea

While conjunctival fibrotic changes could historically be considered primary outcome measures of disease damage, they are not the terminal event as far as vision is concerned. Corneal scarring, including vascularization, ultimately results in the sight-threatening manifestations of disease (Elder & Bernauer 1997). A simple schema for corneal

Table 12.3 Summary of the differential diagnosis for cicatrizing conjunctivitis*

Etiology		Progression	Immunobullous disease	Ocular involvement in systemic disease
Physical	Heat	SSP	–	–
	Ionizing radiation	SSP	–	–
Chemical	Alkali	SSP	–	–
	Acid	SSP	–	–
Infection	Trachoma	SSP	–	Common
	Membranous conjunctivitis (i.e. streptococcus and adenovirus)	SSP	–	–
	Corynebacterium diphtheria	SSP	–	Rare
	Chronic mucocutaneous candidiasis	SSP	–	Rare
Oculocutaneous disorders	OcMMP	Prog	Yes	Common
	Bullous pemphigoid	SSP	Yes	Rare
	Linear IgA disease	SSP or Prog	Yes	
	Dermatitis herpetiformis	SSP	Yes	Rare
	Pemphigus	Prog	Yes	Rare
	Systemic lupus erythematosus	SSP		Rare
	Epidermolysis bullosa acquisita	Prog	Yes	Common
	Ectodermal dysplasia	SSP or Prog	Yes	Rare
	Stevens–Johnson syndrome and toxic epidermal necrolysis	SSP or Prog†	Yes†	Common
	Lichen planus	Prog		Common
	Chronic atopic keratoconjunctivitis	SSP		Rare
Other associated systemic disorders	Rosacea	SSP		Rare
	Sjögren's syndrome	SSP		Common
	Inflammatory bowel disease	SSP		Rare
	Graft-versus-host disease	SSP		Common
	Immune complex diseases	SSP		Rare
	Paraneoplastic syndromes	SSP or Prog		Common
	Sarcoid	SSP		Rare
	Porphyria	SSP		Rare
Drug induced	Drug-induced cicatrizing conjunctivitis (antiglaucoma medication)	SSP or Prog		Common
Neoplasia	Ocular surface squamous neoplasia (squamous cell or sebaceous cell carcinoma)	Prog	–	–
	Lymphoma	SSP	–	Rare

Adapted from Wright (1986), Bernauer et al. (1997), Saw et al 2008b, and Williams et al. (2011a).

OcMMP; mucous membrane pemphigoid; Prog, progressive; SSP, static/slowly progressive.

*Slowly progressive or static cases include a history of trachoma and an acute infectious membranous conjunctivitis or trauma (e.g. chemical, radiation, heat, mechanical, and surgical). Progressive cases show an increase in the extent or severity of conjunctiva.

†A subset may develop autoantibody-positive progressive scarring akin to OcMMP.

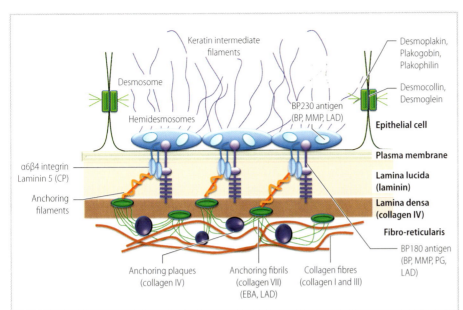

Figure 12.2 The basement membrane zone (BMZ). Epithelial cells are held together by desmosomes and anchored to the underlying lamina lucida of the BMZ by hemidesmosomes. The lamina lucida and lamina densa are composed of type IV collagen and laminin, which in turn are attached to the underlying fibroreticularis of the anterior stroma via anchoring filaments (composed of Type VII collagen) to anchoring plaques.

Table 12.4 Immunopathological features of autoimmune bullous diseases

Disease	Immunofluorescence	Autoantigens	Location of BMZ antigen
Pemphigus diseases			
Pemphigus vulgaris	Intercellular IgG and C3	Dsg3, Dsg1	Desmosome
Pemphigus foliaceus	Intercellular IgG and C3	Dsg1	Desmosome
Paraneoplastic pemphigus	IgG and C3 intercellularly and at the dermal–epidermal junction	Dsg3, Dsg1, plakines	Desmosome
IgA pemphigus	Intercellular IgA and C3	Dsc1, Dsg3	Desmosome
Pemphigoid diseases			
Bullous pemphigoid	Linear C3 and IgG at the dermal–epidermal junction	BP180, BP230	Hemidesmosome
Pemphigoid gestationis	Linear C3 at the dermal–epidermal junction	BP180, BP230	Hemidesmosome
Mucous membrane pemphigoid	Linear IgG, IgA, and C3 at the dermal–epidermal junction	Epiligrin (subunit of laminin 5) BP180 BP230 α6 integrin β4 integrin Laminin 5 (laminin 332) Collagen VII 45 kDa protein 168 kDa protein	Ligand for α6β4 integrin Role in hemidesmosomal assembly and formation; located in inner plate of Hd Transmembrane molecules and part of Hd anchoring filament complex Heterodimeric molecules associated with Hd Heterodimeric molecules associated with Hd Adhesion molecules associated with anchoring filaments in the lamina lucida and densa Fibroreticularis Implicated in pure ocular disease (identity unclear) Implicated in pure oral disease (identity unclear)
Linear IgA disease	Linear IgA (and C3) at the dermal–epidermal junction	LAD-1 type VII collagen	Fibroreticularis
Other diseases			
Epidermolysis bullosa acquisita	Linear IgG, IgA, and C3 at the dermal–epidermal junction	Type VII collagen	Fibroreticularis
Dermatitis herpetiformis	Granular IgA deposits in the dermal papillae	Transglutaminase*	–

Adapted from (Mihai & Sitaru 2007).
BMZ, basement membrane zone; Dsc, desmocollin; Dsg, desmoglein; Hd, hemidesmosomes.
*Not a BMZ Ag, but part of the immunobullous disease spectrum.

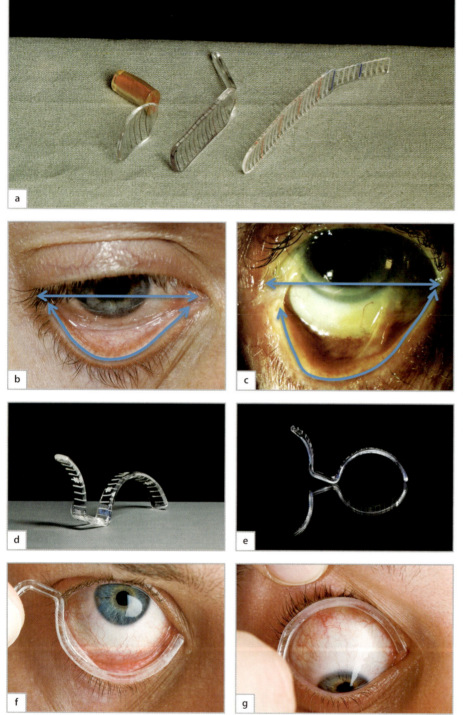

Figure 12.3 Objective measurement of conjunctival scarring. (a) The evolution of our fornix depth measurer (FDM). From left to right: an adaptation of an FDM originally described by Schwab et al. (1992), an FDM constructed at Moorfields Eye Hospital, which is an elongated polymethylmethacrylate modification of the Schwab FDM using a hand-made plaster cast (specifically to facilitate upper fornix depth measurement for use in a clinical trial), and a computer-designed bespoke FDM prototype (Williams et al. 2011b). This is an elongated, biconcave design with engraved markings to a precision of 2 mm/step, and increments expressed at 2 mm intervals on both the main body of the FDM and the narrower 'handle'. The markings on the handle facilitate upper fornix measurement and the ability to measure the fornix in the presence of symblephara. The accuracy and reproducibility of the computer-generated design and jewelry precision engraving provides the potential for commercial manufacture. (b and c) Measurement of symblephara extent and number depends on the ability to enumerate objectively. Currently, no accepted system exists for this purpose. The curved distance from canthus to canthus can be measured, inferiorly (lower) and superiorly (upper), thereby circumventing an underestimation taken with a straight-line measurement (b and c) using an enhanced FDM. The symblephara can be measured and subtracted from the total fornix intercanthal distance (d), (e) the short (conventional FDM for lower and upper fornix measurement) and the curved, extended arm for intercanthal measurement, demonstrated in (f) and (g). Courtesy of Jonas Brane, Birmingham, and Midland Eye Center, Birmingham, UK.

drawings was originally described by Bron in 1973, but quantification of the extent of corneal damage has only really been attempted in relation to SJS–TEN by Sotozono et al. (2007). The scoring system for chronic SJS–TEN—defined as >12 months since disease onset—discussed later in this chapter, may possibly serve as a template for documenting corneal damage to OcMMP and other PCC.

Inflammation

No universally agreed grading system exists for the quantification of clinically manifest ocular mucosal inflammation in PCC. A simple four-step ordinal scale has been proposed by Elder and colleagues (none, absence of conjunctival inflammation; mild +, conjunctival hyperemia and mild stromal edema; moderate ++, extensive or marked

Table 12.5 Classification of conjunctivitis based on speed of onset and principal clinical signs

Time course	Principal signs	Classification	Examples
Acute (<3 weeks)	Papillae prominent	Acute mucopurulent	Bacterial conjunctivitis, staphylococcal lid disease
	Associated skin rash	Oculocutaneous	Atopy, acne rosacea, HZO, OcMMP, SJS
	Follicles prominent	Acute follicular	EKC, pharyngoconjunctival fever, primary HSK
Chronic (>3 weeks)	Papillae prominent	Chronic papillary	AKC, PAC, SAC, GPC, VKC, floppy eyelid syndrome
	Follicles prominent	Chronic follicular	Rosacea keratitis, staphylococcal hypersensitivity, molluscum contagiosum, toxic drug reactions
	Localized or generalized hyperaemia	Chronic hyperemic	Local: SLK, limbal vernal, artefacta General: DED, ocular irritation
	Conjunctival fornix shortening	Cicatricial	OcMMP, SJS–TEN, SS, GVHD, chemical injury, trauma, infection, toxic, EBA

AKC, atopic keratoconjunctivitis; DED, dry eye disease; EBA, epidermolysis bullosa acquisita; EKC, epidemic keratoconjunctivitis; GPC, giant papillary conjunctivitis; GVHD, graft-versus-host disease; HSK, herpes simplex keratitis; HZO, herpes zoster ophthalmicus; OcMMP, ocular mucous membrane pemphigoid; PAC, perennial allergic conjunctivitis; SAC, seasonal allergic conjunctivitis; SJS–TEN, Stevens–Johnson syndrome/toxic epidermal necrosis; SLK, superior limbic keratoconjunctivitis; SS, Sjögren's syndrome; VKC, vernal keratoconjunctivitis.

conjunctival hyperemia with stromal edema and significant tissue thickening; severe +++, inflammation in all quadrants with severe ocular edema together with limbitis and/or conjunctival ulceration) (Elder & Bernauer 1997). Alternatively, a five-step system graded on a scale from 0 (absent) to 4+ (severe) has been described for OcMMP (Foster 1986, Thorne et al. 2008). A consensus to determine a robust schema for grading inflammation, together with a non-invasive method for quantifying cellular infiltrate or inflammatory cytokines that could deliver putative biomarkers of inflammation, is required to aid measurement of secondary outcomes (i.e. progression of conjunctival scarring, keratopathy). This will enable accurate monitoring of occult (clinically undetectable) and manifest (clinically observed) inflammation.

Documenting disease

The corneal drawing schemas, described by Bron, were initially adapted to include conjunctival shrinkage, superficial scarring, subepithelial fibrosis, and keratinization by Elder and Bernauer (1997). Clinical examples of this type of documentation are shown in **Figure 12.4**. We are currently building upon this clinical data collection form, by grading inflammation, and conjunctival and corneal involvement to develop scales for defining activity and damage to PCC in our respective centers. It is hoped that with consensus building and validation, these types of activity and damage tools can not only assist a better monitoring of disease progression in a clinical setting but also unify data capture for comparative clinical trials and for trailing emerging therapies. A prototype clinical record form for grading of disease is illustrated in **Figure 12.5**.

■ OCULAR MUCOUS MEMBRANE PEMPHIGOID

OcMMP, previously known as ocular cicatricial pemphigoid, is an autoimmune bullous disease characterized by recurrent blistering of mucous membranes and the skin, and healing with excessive scar tissue formation. Mucous membranes involved include the mouth, conjunctiva, laryngopharynx, esophagus, nose, genitalia, and rectum, although healing of blisters or ulcers without scar formation is the norm in oral mucosa (**Figure 12.6**). Isolated ocular disease, which may occur in up to 50% of cases, referred to ophthalmologists, while ocular involvement in systemic OcMMP occurs in around 70% of cases, and blindness in 27%. OcMMP is a rare disorder with a minimum incidence around 0.8–1.6 per million per year in the United Kingdom (Radford BJO et al. 2012), with a mean age of onset of 65 years, but it may occur in children, with a more aggressive phenotype in younger patients (Rauz et al. 2005).

■ Immunopathogenesis

The pathogenesis of OcMMP is believed to involve an as-yet unknown trigger, often in a genetically susceptible individual, which initiates a loss of tolerance to one or more components of the BMZ (Kasperkiewicz et al. 2011) (**Figure 12.7**). In particular, expression of HLA-DQB*0301 allele, which is involved in antigen presentation to T cells, predisposes to OcMMP (Zakka et al. 2011). Autoreactive T cells generate specific B-cell clones, which produce circulating autoantibodies (IgG and IgA) that bind to the BMZ components, initiating a type II hypersensitivity reaction. This leads to subepithelial bullae and inflammatory infiltration of the substantia propria, which, in the acute stage, comprises neutrophils, macrophages, and antigen-presenting cells, together with an increase in T cells, resulting in granulation tissue formation and fibrosis.

T-cell infiltration of the conjunctival stroma (with a CD4:CD8 ratio of 0.5 in clinically mildly inflamed eyes) increases in severe conjunctival inflammation, with a threefold increase in neutrophils and dendritic cells compared with controls, a twofold increase in macrophages, and an increase in CD4:CD8 ratio to 1.0 (Bernauer et al. 1997). Neutrophils normally exert an immediate innate response, and their removal relies upon apoptosis and phagocytosis by macrophages. Given the short lifespan of neutrophils, a process is therefore required to maintain turnover, which may also be a feature of chronic disease: a persistent neutrophil infiltrate is evident in RA joints. The autoantibodies activate the complement cascade (presumably this involves the classical pathway via IgG binding to C1q, resulting in the BMZ being coated in C3b), which in turn maintains neutrophil recruitment. Activated neutrophils not only destroy pathogens via their azurophilic granules but also have the potential to cause collateral tissue damage and modulate the local immune response, releasing proinflammatory cytokines such as TNF-α that promotes further inflammatory cell infiltration (Witko-Sarsat et al. 2011). The persistent inflammatory infiltrate may contribute to the progressive fibrotic damage seen in OcMMP.

Profibrogenic factors involved include TGF-β, IL-13, connective tissue growth factor, heat shock protein, and IL-4 (Razzaque et al. 2004, Saw et al. 2009). While systemic immunosuppression decreases

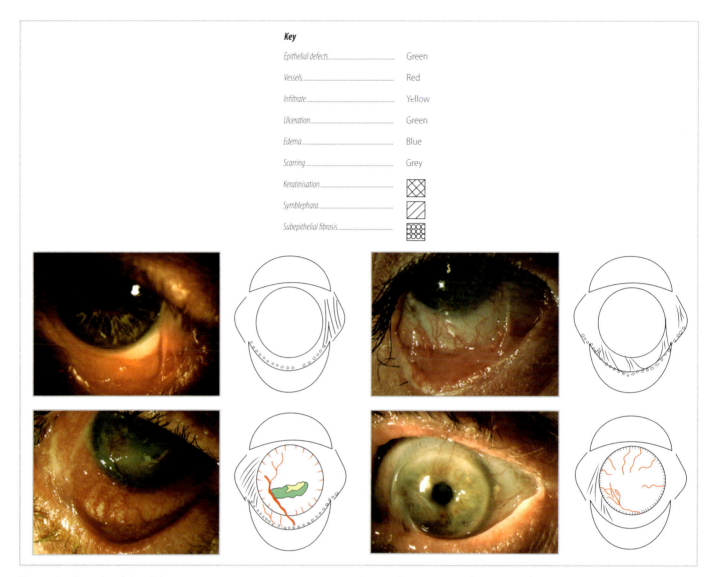

Figure 12.4 Examples of clinical drawings in progressive cicatrizing conjunctivitis. Accurate documentation of conjunctival fibrosis, symblephara, together with corneal scarring, neovascularization, and keratinization, is of paramount importance. The eyes of patients with ocular mucous membrane pemphigoid are shown here. Schema from Elder and Bernauer (1997), Bernauer et al. (1997); courtesy of G. Holloway.

conjunctival levels of IL-13 and other cytokines, residual levels of cytokines persist in clinically uninflamed conjunctiva. Moreover, conjunctival fibroblasts from OcMMP patients appear to be transformed into an activated phenotype, behaving independent of cytokine influences (Saw et al. 2011). It is probable that both subclinical inflammation and altered fibroblast gene expression are also responsible for progressive fibrosis despite clinical control of inflammation.

■ Clinical features

The clinical hallmark of OcMMP is chronic autoimmune PCC, during the course of which intermittent acute episodes of conjunctival inflammation may occur, or slowly progressive conjunctival scarring with subacute inflammation.

Symptoms and signs

Delayed or missed diagnosis for many months is typical in OcMMP (Radford et al. 2012). A high index of suspicion for cicatrizing conjunc-

tival disease is imperative when a patient presents with an entropion, chronic conjunctivitis or recurrent red sticky eye, recurrent entropion, and trichiasis despite surgery or ptosis.

The majority of patients present with subacute or chronic inflammation with progressive scarring, although this is more common in those with early-onset disease. The earliest clinical sign in subacute OcMMP disease is typically flattening of the medial canthus, with loss of the plica and caruncle. This, in combination with horizontal scarring at the upper tarsal marginal sulcus, is almost diagnostic. Other signs include subepithelial sheet fibrosis, inflammatory infiltration of the tarsal and bulbar conjunctiva, forniceal shortening, symblepharon, cicatricial entropion, ankyloblepharon, and finally, in late disease a dry keratinized ocular mucosa (**Figures 12.8** and **12.9**). This disfigured ocular surface is susceptible to not only corneal ulceration due to lash trauma, epithelial instability, sicca, lagophthalmos, and exposure, but also bacterial and fungal infections.

About 10% of patients present with acute disease, with limbitis leading to rapidly progressive scarring, LSCD, and corneal vascularization.

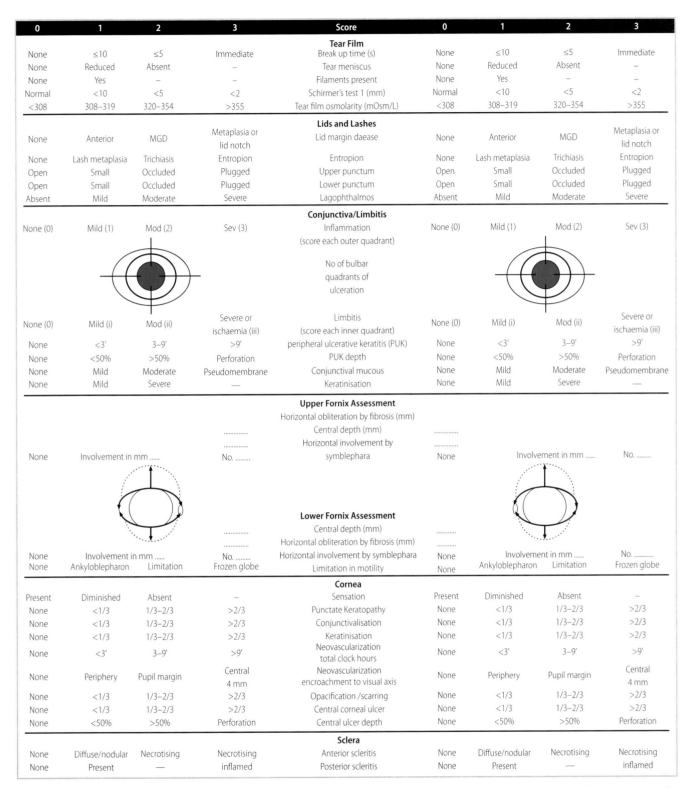

0	1	2	3	Score	0	1	2	3
				Tear Film				
None	≤10	≤5	Immediate	Break up time (s)	None	≤10	≤5	Immediate
None	Reduced	Absent	–	Tear meniscus	None	Reduced	Absent	–
None	Yes	–	–	Filaments present	None	Yes	–	–
Normal	<10	<5	<2	Schirmer's test 1 (mm)	Normal	<10	<5	<2
<308	308–319	320–354	>355	Tear film osmolarity (mOsm/L)	<308	308–319	320–354	>355
				Lids and Lashes				
None	Anterior	MGD	Metaplasia or lid notch	Lid margin daease	None	Anterior	MGD	Metaplasia or lid notch
None	Lash metaplasia	Trichiasis	Entropion	Entropion	None	Lash metaplasia	Trichiasis	Entropion
Open	Small	Occluded	Plugged	Upper punctum	Open	Small	Occluded	Plugged
Open	Small	Occluded	Plugged	Lower punctum	Open	Small	Occluded	Plugged
Absent	Mild	Moderate	Severe	Lagophthalmos	Absent	Mild	Moderate	Severe
				Conjunctiva/Limbitis				
None (0)	Mild (1)	Mod (2)	Sev (3)	Inflammation (score each outer quadrant)	None (0)	Mild (1)	Mod (2)	Sev (3)
				No of bulbar quadrants of ulceration				
None (0)	Mild (i)	Mod (ii)	Severe or ischaemia (iii)	Limbitis (score each inner quadrant)	None (0)	Mild (i)	Mod (ii)	Severe or ischaemia (iii)
None	<3'	3–9'	>9'	peripheral ulcerative keratitis (PUK)	None	<3'	3–9'	>9'
None	<50%	>50%	Perforation	PUK depth	None	<50%	>50%	Perforation
None	Mild	Moderate	Pseudomembrane	Conjunctival mucous	None	Mild	Moderate	Pseudomembrane
None	Mild	Severe	—	Keratinisation	None	Mild	Severe	—
				Upper Fornix Assessment				
			....	Horizontal obliteration by fibrosis (mm)				....
			....	Central depth (mm)				....
None	Involvement in mm		No.	Horizontal involvement by symblephara	None	Involvement in mm		No. ....
None	Ankyloblepharon	Limitation	Frozen globe		None	Ankyloblepharon	Limitation	Frozen globe
				Lower Fornix Assessment				
			....	Central depth (mm)				....
			....	Horizontal obliteration by fibrosis (mm)				....
None	Involvement in mm		No.	Horizontal involvement by symblephara	None	Involvement in mm		No. ....
None	Ankyloblepharon	Limitation	Frozen globe	Limitation in motility	None	Ankyloblepharon	Limitation	Frozen globe
				Cornea				
Present	Diminished	Absent	–	Sensation	Present	Diminished	Absent	–
None	<1/3	1/3–2/3	>2/3	Punctate Keratopathy	None	<1/3	1/3–2/3	>2/3
None	<1/3	1/3–2/3	>2/3	Conjunctivalisation	None	<1/3	1/3–2/3	>2/3
None	<1/3	1/3–2/3	>2/3	Keratinisation	None	<1/3	1/3–2/3	>2/3
None	<3'	3–9'	>9'	Neovascularization total clock hours	None	<3'	3–9'	>9'
None	Periphery	Pupil margin	Central 4 mm	Neovascularization encroachment to visual axis	None	Periphery	Pupil margin	Central 4 mm
None	<1/3	1/3–2/3	>2/3	Opacification /scarring	None	<1/3	1/3–2/3	>2/3
None	<1/3	1/3–2/3	>2/3	Central corneal ulcer	None	<1/3	1/3–2/3	>2/3
None	<50%	>50%	Perforation	Central ulcer depth	None	<50%	>50%	Perforation
				Sclera				
None	Diffuse/nodular	Necrotising	Necrotising inflamed	Anterior scleritis	None	Diffuse/nodular	Necrotising	Necrotising inflamed
None	Present	—		Posterior scleritis	None	Present	—	

Figure 12.5 Prototype tool for scoring the clinical features of cicatrizing conjunctivitis. Consensus building and validation are required to define specific indices for activity and damage. The captured data include the scoring system for clinical conjunctival inflammation in ocular mucous membrane pemphigoid, described by Elder and Bernauer (1997). The division of conjunctival and limbal hyperemia into quadrants is utilized at the Birmingham and Midland Eye Centre and Moorfields Eye Hospital and this provides a platform for future validation studies. In order to calculate primary outcome measures of conjunctival fibrosis, based upon the proposed system described by Tauber, measurement of upper and lower fornix depth, number and extent of symblephara between the medial and lateral canthi, and the intercanthal distance is incorporated into the tool (Foster 1986, Mondino & Brown 1981, Tauber et al. 1992). The scoring system, described by Sotozono and colleagues, is adapted for measurement of disease damage to the cornea. Indices relevant to the tear film, eyelids, conjunctiva, and sclera are also considered for completion, including those described in the Delphi report on dry eyes; the Dry Eye Workshop, eyelid and corneal changes described for the chronic ocular manifestations of Stevens–Johnson syndrome (Behrens et al. 2006, Dry Eye Workshop 2007, Sotozono et al. 2007), and scleritis using standardized International Uveitis Study Group criteria. Forniceal shrinkage and involvement by symblephara are measured in millimeters, using a fornix depth measurer, and quantified according to the scale described by Tauber (currently not enumerated).

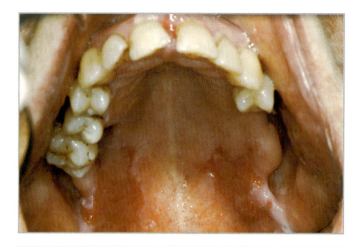

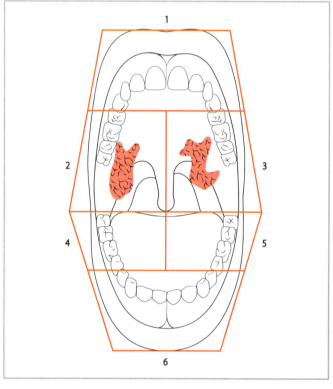

Segment key		
1	Upper anterior segments: Incisors to canines	
2 and 3	Upper posterior segments: Canines to anterior pillars of fauces	
4 and 5	Lower posterior segments: Canines to anterior pillars of fauces; Anterior two-thirds of tongue (dorsal, lateral and ventral aspects to circumvallate papillae)	
6	Lower anterior segments: Incisors to canines	
Assessment (Circle appropriate grade)				
Caries	None		Few		Excessive
Dentures	None	Partial	<1/2	>1/2	Full
Ulceration score (Circle score)	
0	Nil
1	Minimal (<1 segment*)
2	1–2 segments* involved or 2 ulcerated
3	3–4 segments* involved or 2 ulcerated
4	5–6 segments* ulcerated
5	Severe generalised ulcerative desquamative gingivits

Figure 12.6 Scoring of oral disease associated with cicatrizing conjunctivitis. This patient has active oral mucous membrane pemphigoid, scored according to that originally proposed by Setterfield et al. (1998). Note: the adaptation to include the presence of excessive caries and dentures is to enable capture of the spectrum of diseases that are associated with a dry mouth, that is, Sjögren's syndrome. Two ulcerated areas reveal a score of 3.

Conjunctival blisters are rarely seen. OcMMP usually affects both eyes, but the signs can be very asymmetric. Unilateral conjunctival scarring should therefore raise a high suspicion of a masquerade such as ocular surface squamous neoplasia.

Immunohistology and diagnosis

A biopsy from at least one site (skin or mucosa) positive on DIF, showing linear deposition of IgG, IgA, and/or complement along the BMZ, has been recommended as a requirement for the diagnosis of OcMMP (Chan et al. 2002). Nevertheless, conjunctival DIF is positive in around 60–86% cases of OcMMP, and if sequential biopsies are undertaken during the course of disease, the results can be positive on the initial biopsy and then subsequently negative, or vice versa, and this switch is apparently unrelated to disease activity or treatment. Additionally, severe inflammation may disrupt the anatomy of the BMZ, which may also give rise to a false-negative biopsy. As such, OcMMP cannot be excluded by a negative DIF alone if typical clinical characteristics are

evident (Bernauer et al. 1994, Radford et al. 2012, Saw et al. 2009). Indirect immunofluorescence (IIF) is not an absolute criterion for diagnosis in the consensus document, but patients with negative DIF from any site and positive serology (using IIF or other methods), provided they have a typical progressive conjunctival scarring and other diseases have been excluded, can be diagnosed as having Oc-MMP. Nonetheless, approximately 50% of systemic OcMMP sera and <50% OcMMP sera have positive IIF performed on salt-split skin or monkey esophagus, indicating that sensitivity of current methodology is poor. This is particularly important for the subset of patients who are both DIF and IIF negative (Kasperkiewicz et al. 2011), but have clinical disease indistinguishable from OcMMP. We therefore propose a revision to the diagnostic criteria for OcMMP (**Table 12.6**) and encourage current research programs to develop protocols to improve the sensitivity of IIF, or to evaluate alternative techniques such as enzyme-linked-immunosorbent serologic assay and Western blotting to detect autoantibodies for clinical practice.

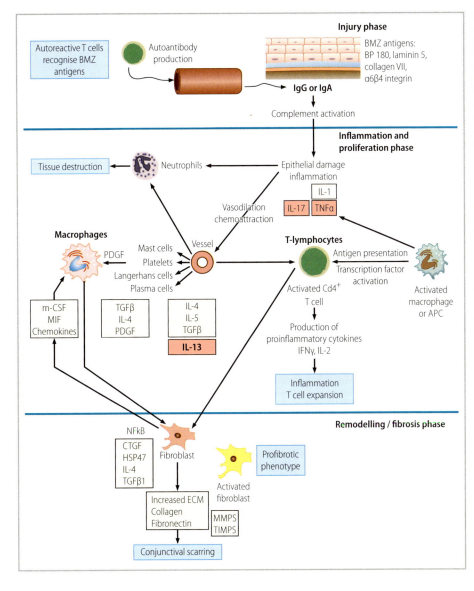

Figure 12.7 Proposed immunopathogenesis of ocular mucous membrane pemphigoid. Injury phase: antibasement membrane zone (anti-BMZ) antibodies (Ab) are directed against conjunctival BMZ antigens, such as BP180 bullous pemphigoid 180 kDa antigen, laminin 5 (laminin 332), collagen VII, and α6β4 integrin, causing B cells in germinal centers to produce autoantibodies immunoglobulin G (IgG) and IgA. These bind to the BMZ and initiate a type II hypersensitivity reaction, activating the complement cascade. Inflammation and proliferation phase: complement-mediated BMZ, epithelial and connective tissue damage causes vasodilation and release of blood cells and plasma proteins into the damaged site, and attracts an acute inflammatory cell infiltrate, consisting of neutrophils, which may release proteinases and reactive oxygen species (ROS), activated macrophages, mast cells, platelets, Langerhans cells, and lymphocytes (B cells and T cells although the phenotypes are poorly defined), as well as acute inflammatory cytokine interleukin-1 (IL-1), IL-17, and necrosis factor-alpha (TNF-α) production. TNF-α has profibrotic and proinflammatory effects on conjunctival fibroblasts. T-cell activation and proliferation characteristic of a type 1 helper T-cell (Th1) response occurs, with interferon-gamma (IFN-γ) and IL-2 production. Type 2 helper T-cell cytokines IL-4, IL-5, and IL-13 are also synthesized. IL-13 has a strong profibrotic and proinflammatory effect on conjunctival fibroblasts. Macrophages proliferate and play an important role in scar tissue formation, and contribute to the production of the fibrogenic cytokines, transforming growth factor-beta (TGF-β) and platelet-derived growth factor (PDGF). Fibrosis phase: fibroblasts become activated, proliferate, and synthesize increased extracellular matrix, connective tissue growth factor (CTGF), TGF-β, and other cytokines, for example, heat shock protein 47 (HSP47), and macrophage inhibitory factor (MIF). Endothelial cells may proliferate, forming fibrovascular granulation tissue. The scar tissue is then remodeled, becoming less cellular, and the final result is subconjunctival scarring. The roles of matrix metalloproteinases (MMPs), their inhibitors (TIMPs), vascular endothelial growth factor (VEGF), and fibroblast growth factors (FGFs) have yet to be defined.

APC, antigen-presenting cell; ECM, extracellular matrix; m-CSF, macrophage colony-stimulating factor; TIMPs, tissue inhibitors of matrix metalloproteinases.

Table 12.6 Proposed revised immunopathology criteria for the diagnosis of ocular mucous membrane pemphigoid

Consensus criteria*	Direct immunofluorescence—presence of BMZ deposits of IgG, IgA, IgM, and/or C3
	Detection of one or combination of the above linear epithelial BMZ immune deposits establishes the diagnosis of autoimmune OcMMP
	Patients with clinical manifestations similar or identical to OcMMP but in whom epithelial BMZ immune deposits have not been demonstrated; these patients may be drug induced or the pathogenesis of the disease needs to be further elucidated
	Indirect immunofluorescence—presence of IgG and IgA autoantibodies binding to skin BMZ on salt-split epithelial substrate
	Not all patients with OcMMP have detectable circulating autoantibodies to the BMZ; the consensus does not consider these findings to be an absolute criterion
Proposed revised criteria†	Patients with positive conjunctival direct immunofluorescence or positive direct immunofluorescence from any other site (e.g. oral mucosa and skin) that meet the current consensus criteria
	Patients with negative direct immunofluorescence from any site and positive indirect immunofluorescence can be diagnosed as having OcMMP
	Patients with negative immunofluorescence studies (direct or indirect) can be diagnosed with ocular mucous membrane pemphigoid, provided that they have a typical ocular phenotype of progressive conjunctival scarring, and that other diseases that may cause this phenotype have been excluded

*Chan et al. (2002).
†Radford et al. (2012).
BMZ, basement membrane zone; OcMMP; ocular mucous membrane pemphigoid.

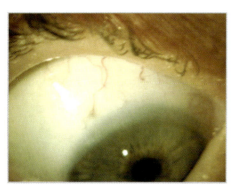

None

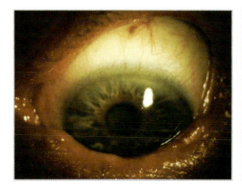

Mild

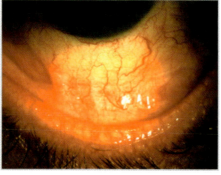

Moderate

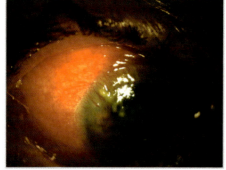

Severe

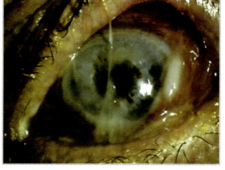

Limbitis

Grade	Description
None	**Absence** of conjuctival inflammation
Mild	**Mild inflammation:** Conjuctival hyperaemia and mild stromal oedema
Moderate	**Moderate inflammation:** extensive or marked conjuctival hyperaemia with stromal oedema and significant tissue thickening
Severe	**Severe inflammation:** inflammation in all quadrants with severe ocular oedema; limbitis, conjuctival ulceration may be present.

Figure 12.8 Disease activity in ocular mucous membrane pemphigoid. This is currently determined by clinically identifiable conjunctival inflammation. The simple ordinal 4-point scale described by Elder and Bernauer (1997) is supplemented by an additional 'minimal' stage in the alternative 5-point scale, originally described by Foster (Foster 1986, Thorne et al. 2008).

Bulbar conjunctival biopsy is a simple and safe procedure, provided the fornix and temporal regions are avoided, combined with a 4-week course of non-preserved topical steroids, and systemic immunosuppression commenced the same day if there is a high clinical suspicion of active disease. It is recommended that both conjunctival and buccal and oral mucosal biopsies (buccal and oral biopsies are occasionally positive in patients without oral symptoms when conjunctival biopsies are negative) are also taken and processed in an experienced laboratory. Conventional histopathology is essential to exclude ocular surface neoplasia, and it can help exclude atopic disease or sarcoid.

Management

The primary goals of treatment of OcMMP are to control inflammation, arrest fibrosis, and prevent keratopathy, thus preventing progression to

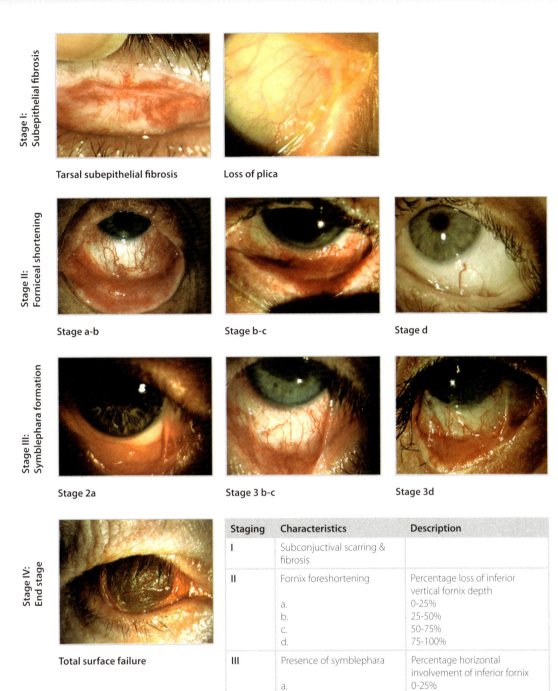

Figure 12.9 Disease damage and conjunctival scarring in ocular mucous membrane pemphigoid. Disease damage is according to Tauber's proposed staging systems. This incorporates the staging systems of Mondino and Foster and quantifies the percentage horizontal involvement and number of symblephara.

Staging	Characteristics	Description
I	Subconjuctival scarring & fibrosis	
II	Fornix foreshortening	Percentage loss of inferior vertical fornix depth
	a.	0-25%
	b.	25-50%
	c.	50-75%
	d.	75-100%
III	Presence of symblephara	Percentage horizontal involvement of inferior fornix
	a.	0-25%
	b.	25-50%
	c.	50-75%
	d.	75-100%
IV	Ankyloblepharon, frozen globe	

more advanced stages and blindness. An ideal management algorithm for OcMMP includes early diagnosis and identifying active disease (both discussed earlier in this chapter) together with lid surgery and visual rehabilitation.

Preventing progression of disease

Disease progression is multifactorial, and a result of a combination of (1) local ocular surface disease, (2) microbial infection, (3) toxicity due to topical medications, and (4) underlying immune-mediated inflammation, each of which perpetuates inflammation leading to (5) progressive scarring. The management of ocular surface disease in OcMMP is summarized in **Table 12.7**. It is imperative that inflammation due to local ocular surface disease, microbial infection, and toxicity is treated and excluded, before grading the clinically manifest inflammation due to the underlying autoimmune disease. The use of non-preserved tear substitutes with cytoprotective properties is

Table 12.7 Ocular surface clinical features and diseases to treat and exclude prior to systemic immunosuppression in OcMMP

	Clinical features	Management
1.	Blepharitis and evaporative dry eyes	Lid hygiene and hot compresses, oral doxycycline, ocular lubricants, topical cyclosporine*
2.	Dry eyes—aqueous deficient	Exclude concomitant Sjögren's syndrome, ocular lubricants, topical acetylcysteine, punctal occlusion if patent and no blepharitis, autologous serum, RGP contact lenses, oral pilocarpine, topical cyclosporine*
3.	Trichiasis, entropion, lagophthalmos, exposure keratopathy	Electrolysis, entropion surgery (which does not require increased immunosuppression providing it does not incise conjunctiva), ocular lubricants, consider fornix reconstruction with immunosuppression cover for lagophthalmos in 'wet' eyes (i.e. non-anesthetized Schirmer >5 mm at 5 minutes)
4.	Filamentary keratopathy	Treatment of dry eye disease and blepharitis, topical acetylcysteine, therapeutic silicone hydrogel contact lenses
5.	Punctate epithelial keratopathy	Treat lid margin disease, conjunctival inflammation; exclude topical toxicity, tear deficiency; ocular lubricants
6.	Persistent epithelial defect and corneal perforation	Exclude and treat bacterial, herpes, atypical infection; exclude and treat inturned lashes, exposure, dry eye disease; 1- to 2-hourly ointment; bandage contact lens if 'wet' eyes; temporary central tarsorrhaphy; control inflammation; autologous serum; amniotic membrane graft; lamellar corneal graft; conjunctival flap or buccal mucosal graft Treat perforation with glue and/or bandage contact lens; tectonic patch lamellar graft if necessary; penetrating keratoplasty only if unavoidable, usually with a buccal mucosal graft
7.	Keratinization	Topical retinoic acid, mechanical removal, contact lenses
8.	Toxicity	Avoid unnecessary topical treatment, use unpreserved topical medications where possible and practical, avoid aminoglycosides
9.	Microbial keratitis	High index of suspicion in any corneal ulcer, often no infiltrate if on topical steroids or systemic immunosuppressants, always scrape for microscopy and culture to exclude fungi and resistant bacteria in compromised ocular surface, consider PCR for herpes, intensive fluoroquinolones first-line empiric, modify according to culture results, repeat scrape or biopsy if inconclusive results

Adapted from Saw and Dart (2008b).
PCR, polymerase chain reaction; RGP, rigid gas permeable.
*Topical cyclosporine is best used as an adjunctive measure for persistent conjunctival inflammation despite systemic immunosuppression, in order to avoid masking underlying systemic autoimmune activity.

paramount, together with long-term topical and systemic modulators of matrix metalloproteinases (these therapeutic strategies are covered elsewhere in this book).

Inflammation due to autoimmune disease activity

Persistent conjunctival inflammation due to underlying autoimmune disease requires systemic disease-modifying agents such as immunosuppression. As discussed earlier, this represents a key clinical challenge; inflammation is clinically undetectable in up to 50% of patients who demonstrate disease progression, and to date, there are no biomarkers to non-invasively gauge whether disease activity is ongoing or whether it is immunologically quiescent. For clinically apparent inflammation, this is best evaluated by examining the upper bulbar conjunctiva for evidence of inflammation, which is least likely to be affected by exposure, trichiasis, and lid margin disease.

For end-stage 'burnt-out' disease, immunosuppression may be unnecessary because treatment can only arrest scarring, not reverse it. If conjunctival incision surgery is contemplated, such as fornix reconstruction or glaucoma tube surgery, then immunosuppression is instigated as part of the preoperatively conditioning regimen to prevent exacerbations of disease in the postoperative period, which could lead to disease progression and poor surgical outcome.

Topical immunosuppressive therapy

Historical evidence suggests that topical therapy does not alter the natural history of the disease (Foster 1986), offering only variable symptomatic relief. But in patients who are intolerant to

immunosuppression or where it is not safe to administer immunosuppression, topical steroids combined with systemic matrix metalloproteinase inhibitors (tetracyclines) are a useful alternative. Subconjunctival steroids, such as triamcinolone, may provide temporary benefit, but relapses may occur, together with cataract, glaucoma, or localized scleral thinning. Topical cyclosporin A has been used in isolated cases with limited response.

Systemic immunosuppression

The gold standard is either the 'stepladder' approach to systemic immunosuppression detailed in **Figure 12.10**) (Rauz et al. 2005, Saw & Dart 2008a, 2008b, Williams et al. 2011a) or aggressive 'myeloablation' with primary use of oral cyclophosphamide (Thorne et al. 2008). Oral corticosteroids are a useful adjunct in acutely inflamed eyes for a period of 12 weeks or so, while inducing remission with steroid-sparing immunosuppressive agents. Generally, if there are no adverse effects, treatment is continued, and if the disease has been severe and resulted in loss of useful vision in one eye, long-term therapy is also advised. Relapse following withdrawal of therapy is common, possibly due to 'white inflammation' discussed later.

Biological therapies

Biological therapies have been sought where OcMMP is resistant to treatment, or in patients who have been unable to tolerate conventional immunosuppression. A few isolated case reports and series indicate that 'biological' agents, such as rituximab (anti-CD20) or infliximab (anti-TNF-α), may be beneficial in some of these patients, but in the absence of randomized trials, funding for such treatment may prohibit regular use (Canizares et al. 2006, Ross et al. 2009, Segura et al. 2007).

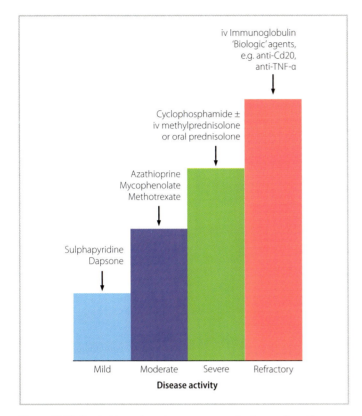

Figure 12.10 Stepladder regimen immunosuppressive therapy in ocular mucous membrane pemphigoid. Step-up or step-down treatment, with agents having the fewest side effects, is undertaken for ocular mucous membrane pemphigoid (Rauz et al. 2005, Saw & Dart 2008b, Williams et al. 2011a). Disease activity (mild, moderate, or severe) is used to guide therapy. Dapsone (25–50 mg twice a day) and sulfapyridine (500 mg twice a day) are used for mild inflammation; azathioprine (1.0–2.5 mg/kg per day) or mycophenolate mofetil (500–1000 mg twice a day if intolerant to azathioprine) is added or substituted for recalcitrant disease. Severe inflammatory disease is treated with cyclophosphamide (1–2 mg/kg per day). Adjuvant prednisolone (1 mg/kg per day with or without a maximum of three supplementary loading doses of 1 g intravenous methylprednisolone preceding oral therapy) tapering over 3 months until the optimal effects is frequently required for moderate or severe inflammation, while the myelosuppressives take full effect. It is imperative that appropriate prophylaxis against adverse effects of steroids is done, including bisphosphonates, calcium and vitamin D3 supplements, proton pump inhibitors, and baseline bone density scans for the patients older than 60 years. Because treatment with cyclophosphamide is limited due to an increased risk of hemorrhagic cystitis and squamous cell carcinoma of the bladder, immunosuppression is stepped down to less toxic agents, such as azathioprine, mycophenolate mofetil, methotrexate, or dapsone, after a maximum of 14-month therapy. Refractory disease is managed through combination therapy of a sulfa-based agent (dapsone or sulfapyridine), with a myelosuppressive agent (e.g. cyclophosphamide, azathioprine, mycophenolate and methotrexate) and corticosteroids. If this fails, intravenous immunoglobulin or biologics such as anti-CD 20 (rituximab) or anti-TNF-α therapy should be considered.

Does systemic immunosuppression prevent fibrosis?

With conventional immunosuppression, progression of cicatrization has still been observed in 10–53% of OcMMP patients, including up to 50% who appear to have ongoing conjunctival fibrosis without obvious clinical signs of inflammation, related to persistent inflammatory cellular infiltrate within the conjunctival tissues ('white inflammation'). Currently, the only demonstrated means of slowing the progression of scarring is good control of inflammation with systemic immunosuppression. Given that progression occurs in the apparent absence of clinically identifiable inflammation, a means of detecting these changes non-invasively needs to be established. Then we may target therapy better according to specific cellular infiltrates or cytokines, and this may actually involve escalating to more potent specific immunosuppression in apparently uninflamed eyes.

Therapy specifically targeting fibrosis in OcMMP includes mitomycin C, delivered either subconjunctivally or applied intraoperatively, following division of symblephara for asymmetrical disease or those intolerant to systemic immunosuppression. Adverse effects include ischemia and LSCD. No currently available medical intervention is able to reverse the process of cicatrization or ocular surface damage, once they have developed.

Surgery and visual rehabilitation

Provided conjunctival inflammation is controlled for a minimum of 3 months, both clear corneal incision cataract surgery and entropion surgery that does not involve conjunctival incision (anterior lamellar reposition, retractor plication surgery) are safe and do not require specific increased perioperative immunosuppression. Fornix reconstruction surgery is indicated for corneal exposure, but this carries a high risk of a severe disease exacerbation if undertaken without increased systemic immunosuppression. Usually cyclophosphamide is introduced to induce a lymphopenia without neutropenia, which takes around 2–3 months, combined with perioperative oral corticosteroids. Frequent monitoring after oculoplastic surgery, to identify and manage the corneal epithelial defects that may complicate the surgery, is critical.

Rigid contact lenses can be useful not only for comfort but also as treatment for irregular astigmatism in scarred corneas; OcMMP eyes are usually too dry for soft lens use.

Due to the difficulties with access and compromised view during surgery, cataract surgery is best performed when the density is mild to moderate, rather than advanced under either general or peribulbar local anesthesia but not subtenon anesthesia. Because of fornix contracture, an eyelid speculum may not be easily inserted and eyelid retraction using silk sutures through the gray line is occasionally required. Use of hydroxypropyl methylcellulose intraoperatively is essential to prevent corneal ulceration, possibly combined with therapeutic contact lenses or amniotic membrane grafting to minimize postoperative ocular surface breakdown; oral or intravenous glucocorticoids to prevent or treat inflammation are a useful adjunct. Close postoperative follow-up is mandatory.

Keratoplasty and ocular surface reconstruction are usually contraindicated in dry eyes and result in poor outcomes, due to the suboptimal corneal microenvironment, causing poor epithelialization, melt, infection, corneal vascularization, and disease reactivation. Keratoprosthesis surgery involves high risk and complications are frequent, but with rigid selection criteria, good visual outcomes can be achieved with the osteo-odonto keratoprosthesis (OOKP) for bilaterally blind patients. Nonetheless, the harvest of oral mucosa may exacerbate oral disease, and a healthy molar tooth is also required.

Management of glaucoma

In addition to cicatricial complications of antiglaucoma medication resulting in DICC, glaucoma itself presents a challenge in PCC. Ocular surface inflammation and the use of topical and systemic steroids may increase the risk of glaucoma in OcMMP. Glaucoma may also be compounded by the use of preserved antiglaucoma medication, through exacerbation of ocular surface disease including DED, meibomian gland dysfunction, and conjunctival inflammation. The complex nature of diseases causing PCC requires early referral to glaucoma specialists for advice on managing high pressure. Preserved topical antiglaucoma medication or filtering procedures may be precluded in the scarred conjunctiva, and therefore approaches such as SLT laser or I-stents may be more appropriate in controlling concomitant or iatrogenic high intraocular pressure. Any tube surgery will require will require aggressive perioperative prophylaxis with potent immunosuppression, usually cyclophosphamide.

STEVENS–JOHNSON SYNDROME/ TOXIC EPIDERMAL NECROLYSIS

SJS and TEN are reaction patterns that have the potential to cause a life-threatening mucocutaneous blistering disease (**Figure 12.11**). TEN is a severe manifestation of SJS in which keratinocyte cell death results in subepidermal separation of varying proportions of the body surface area (BSA) (SJS <10% BSA detachment; SJS–TEN overlap 10–30% BSA; TEN >30% BSA), which can be classified systemically by scales such as the SCORTEN (Bastuji-Garin et al. 2000). SCORTEN is a predictor of mortality, which in turn is dependent on the extent of skin sloughing and organ failure in the acute stages of disease. One point is assigned for each of the risk factors—age >40 years, presence of malignancy, heart rate >120/min, BSA >10%, serum urea >10 mmol/L (28 mg/dL), serum glucose >14 mmol/L (252 mg/dL), and serum bicarbonate <20 mmol/L (20 mEq/L)—and expected mortality is based upon total score: 0–1 (3.2%), 2 (12.1%), 3 (35.3%), 4 (58.3%), and >5 (90%) (although this cannot be used to predict long-term ocular sequelae, as discussed later).

Typically the disease is an acute, self-limiting condition of the skin and mucous membranes. A prodrome of fever and malaise is usually followed by a vesiculobullous eruption, whereby stroking on the skin induces epidermal separation (Nikolsky sign). Despite a high prevalence of the causative factors, the current estimated annual incidence of SJS and TEN ranges from 0.4 to 7.0 per million population. Erythema multiforme is a separate disease entity, characterized by target lesions as opposed to macular changes and an extensive dermal cellular infiltrate compared to SJS–TEN (discussed later) and with <10% BSA involvement.

Immunopathology

TEN and SJS are severe blistering diseases with resultant apoptotic keratinocyte cell death that results in the separation of large areas of skin at the dermoepidermal junction, producing the appearance of scalded skin. The underlying etiology is usually attributed to pharmacological agents including antibiotics (in particular sulfonamides but also penicillin, cephalosporins, and tetracyclines), non-steroidal anti-inflammatory drugs, and anticonvulsants, less commonly to infections such as mycoplasma, although the exact agent often remains unknown, malignancy or be idiopathic. Drugs may activate T cells by behaving as haptens, fusing endogenous proteins following metabolic breakdown to form antigens, or by direct interaction with the MHC molecule and T-cell receptor (TCR), resulting in activation of the T cell.

Little is known about the ocular surface inflammatory process in SJS-TEN. The mechanism by which keratinocyte death occurs has

been attributed to ligation of various cell surface death receptors, including TNF and Fas, triggering activation of the caspase system, causing DNA disassembly and cell death. Additionally, it has been proposed that death receptor-independent mechanisms, such as cytotoxic T cells, can induce apoptosis via either caspase-dependent or caspase-independent mechanisms, mediated by expression and release perforin and granzyme B, with consequent epidermal cell death leading to the epidermal sloughing seen in TEN. More recently however, keratinocyte death in cutaneous SJS-TEN has been shown to be induced by blister fluid granulysin rather than by granzyme B and FasL, secreted by CD8+ cytotoxic T cells and CD56+ natural killer cells, explaining why the tissue destruction may appear out of keeping with the lymphocytic cellular infiltrate, which may be modest (Chung et al. 2008). There is evidence for the presence of CD8+ cytotoxic T cells in the cornea during the acute stages of TEN (Williams et al. 2007), but detailed knowledge of the cellular profile during the acute and chronic stages of the disease in the

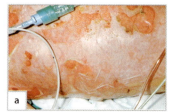
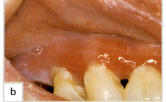
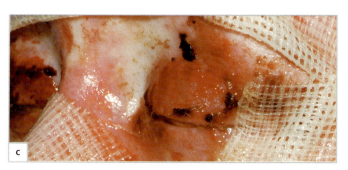
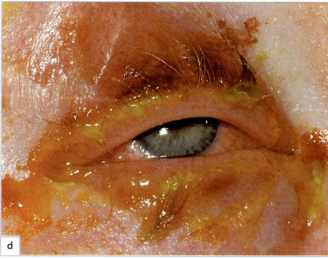

Figure 12.11 Acute sequelae of Stevens–Johnson syndrome/toxic epidermal necrolysis. (a) Severe cutaneous, (b) oral, and (c) eyelid desquamation is observed in a patient with acute Stevens–Johnson syndrome/toxic epidermal necrolysis. (d) Conjunctival hyperemia and temporal symblephara can be seen in the right eye of a patient with ocular toxic epidermal necrolysis.

conjunctival mucosa is unknown. Furthermore, how acute ocular SJS–TEN converts to a chronic condition in some patients remains unresolved. There is evidence for a role for disordered innate immune responses in ocular SJS–TEN, including the presence of TLR 3 polymorphisms in a cohort of Japanese patients with SJS–TEN (Ueta et al. 2007). Disruption of the innate immune responses in genetically susceptible individuals has been postulated as one reason for abnormal drug reactions in some individuals and a predisposition to SJS (Ueta 2008, Ueta et al. 2011).

Ocular grading of disease and classification of different disease entities

From an ophthalmic perspective, 50% of patients with SJS–TEN experience ocular complications, ranging from minimal (i.e. mild conjunctival hyperemia) to very severe (i.e. corneal melting and perforation). Contrary to a popular belief, inflammation and epithelial erosion of the ocular surface often persist beyond the acute stage of the disease, that is, beyond the resolution of skin eruptions. Severe ocular surface disease arising from SJS encompasses a spectrum of ocular manifestations and complications that are often associated with significant visual morbidity (**Figure 12.12**). Visual impairment and ocular discomfort continue throughout life, and patients usually require long-term medication for disease control.

Acute and chronic distinctions

The distinction between the acute and chronic stages of ocular SJS–TEN is a moot point (Fu et al. 2010). Power and colleagues suggested that this period was up to 6 weeks after onset (Power et al. 1995). By 6 weeks the systemic disease may have completely resolved, and in this respect, it can be argued that this period is too long to be truly considered as the acute phase. Conversely, the only definition suggested

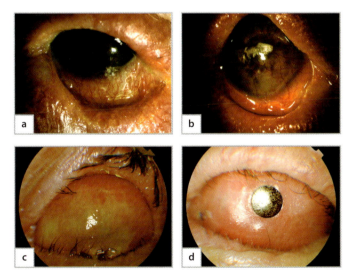

Figure 12.12 Chronic sequelae of Stevens–Johnson syndrome/toxic epidermal necrolysis. (a and b) Conjunctival inflammation, lower fornix foreshortening, symblephara, and extensive corneal neovascularization in chronic Stevens–Johnson syndrome/toxic epidermal necrolysis. (c and d) A patient with end-stage disease after stage 1 odontokeratoprosthesis (note the oral mucous membrane graft) and after stage 2. This patient achieved a visual acuity of 6/5 in this eye, with a +6 corrective lens.

for chronic ocular SJS–TEN is >12 months (Sotozono et al. 2007). There is, therefore, a discord between the acute systemic and chronic ocular diseases. The process by which this switch occurs is not established, and understanding how the initial disease alters to one that has a phenotype resembling OcMMP is not clear. There may be important similarities or indeed differences in the ocular surface cell populations of SJS–TEN in the acute or chronic phases, which may help us to understand how this disease can contribute to the scarring process and behave like OcMMP in some individuals.

Discriminating acute and chronic ocular features of SJS–TEN is challenging because of the absence of a universally agreed grading system or indeed one that discriminates markers of activity and damage. These limitations mean that two current scoring systems to classify acute and chronic disease, respectively, are employed. The grading system for the evaluation of acute disease, described by Power and colleagues, considers disease grading as mild, moderate, or severe. Mild disease is characterized by lid edema, conjunctival injection, and injection; moderate disease by conjunctival membrane and cornea epithelial defect >30%, ulceration or infiltrates; and severe as conjunctival fornix foreshortening, symblepharon formation, and non-healing corneal epithelial defect. Prognosis is determined as full or near-complete resolution before hospital discharge for mild and moderate disease, respectively, while severe disease is sight-threatening with ongoing ocular inflammation. Chronic ocular manifestations of patients with SJS–TEN have been proposed and are summarized in **Table 12.8** (Sotozono et al. 2007). This detailed system takes the form of a 39-point scale, assessing criteria involving the eyelid, conjunctiva, tear film, and cornea, and has been shown to correlate with visual acuity, but may present challenges in the very acute stages of severe disease, for example, ascertaining meibomian gland secretion by manual expression due to the friable nature of eyelid skin in severe acute disease. Nonetheless, the other parameters allow for a systematic determination of eyelid, conjunctival, and corneal disease severity. The chronic disease entities associated with SJS disease have also been classified by De Rojas and colleagues as mild SJS or severe SJS sequelae, resulting from conjunctival scarring, ocular surface failure (SJS-OSF), recurrent inflammation (SJS-RI), scleritis (SJS-S), and ocular mucous membrane pemphigoid (SJS-OcMMP) (De Rojas et al. 2007).

Management strategies

It is imperative that ophthalmologists recognize the importance of prompt and close supervision of care in patients with SJS–TEN. This often presents a challenge because these patients may be cared for in intensive care facilities, including burns units, and ophthalmic intervention may understandably come second to initial life-preserving intervention. Nevertheless, the potential for long-term complications demands full attention to their ocular surface health as soon as possible. This requires a close multidisciplinary approach with intensivists, burns specialists, and other acute care physicians and/or pediatricians. Close input in constructing referral pathways and management protocols should take place, not least as eye drop application will often have to be delegated to medical and nursing staff that may not have ophthalmic training and may not understand the need for intensive topical therapy.

Acute ocular Stevens–Johnson syndrome/toxic epidermal necrolysis

The approach to managing systemic disease has classically been supportive, including the use of intravenous immunoglobulin (IV Ig), while

Table 12.8 Sotozono scoring system for the chronic ocular features in SJS–TEN

Score	0	1	2	3
Corneal complications				
Superficial punctate keratopathy (corneal area)	No staining	<1/3	1/3–2/3	>2/3
Superficial punctate keratopathy (density)	No staining	Sparse	Moderate	High
Corneal epithelial defect (corneal area)	No defect	<1/4	1/4–1/2	>1/2
Loss of palisades of Vogt (circumference)	No loss	<1/2	>1/2	Total loss
Conjunctivalization (corneal area)	Absent	<1/4	1/4–1/2	>1/2
Corneal neovascularization (radial involvement)	Absent	Periphery	Pupil margin	Center
Corneal keratinization (corneal area)	Absent	<1/4	1/4–1/2	>1/2
Corneal opacification	Clear cornea	Partial obscuration of iris details	Iris details poorly defined	No iris or pupil details
Conjunctival complications				
Conjunctival hyperemia (vessel engorgement)	Absent	Mild	Moderate	Severe
Symblepharon formation	Absent	Involving conjunctival surface	Involving <1/2 of corneal surface	Involving >1/2 of corneal surface
Eyelid complications				
Trichiasis (lid margin)	Absent	<1/4	1/4–1/2	>1/2
Mucocutaneous junction involvement (irregularity)	Normal	Mild	Moderate	Severe
Meibomian gland involvement (expressed secretion)	Clear oily	Yellowish-white oily	Cheesy material	Total stagnation
Punctal involvement	Normal	Iatrogenic punctal occlusion	Either upper or lower scarred occlusion	Scared occlusion of all puncta

Adapted from Sotozono et al. (2007).

systemic steroids have been controversial because of fears regarding systemic infection. Recent data have indicated a role in improving visual outcome (Araki et al. 2009), and early, aggressive intervention by ophthalmologists may help prevent blinding sequelae of the disease (Fu et al. 2010). Intensive topical non-preserved lubrication, steroids, and autologous serum drops may all play a role in the management of DED and ocular surface inflammation, but critically early use of amniotic membrane transplantation (AMT) for acute SJS–TEN has been advocated to minimize ocular morbidity. This may take the form of sutured integration or through the use of Prokera devices or AMT associated with conformers (Gregory 2011, John et al. 2002, Shay et al. 2010). Injection of intraforniceal slow-release steroids (triamcinolone), combined with AMT and conformers in a 'triple-TEN' protocol (Tomlins et al 2013), may also be a useful adjunct. Therapeutic contact lenses, including gas-permeable scleral contact lenses, have also been advocated. The use of glass rods to break forniceal adhesions is an approach that should only be used with caution and should not be performed by a non-ophthalmic trained individual due to inadvertent traumatic sloughing of the friable ocular surface epithelium. Formal surgical division of symblephara, using curved microscissors and gentle removal of fibrinous membranes, is preferred. The use of topical or local fibrinolytics, such as tissue plasminogen activator or heparin, in the acute setting remains unknown. The key message is that supportive measures must include control of ocular surface inflammation, prevention of damage by progressive scarring, maintenance of ocular surface lubrication, and prevention of secondary infections due to ocular surface breakdown.

In the absence of clinical trials, this demanding disease requires an aggressive early approach, close monitoring of changes that can occur within hours, and ensuring that all prescribed regular medications such as topical lubrication are applied religiously by attending staff.

Chronic ocular Stevens–Johnson syndrome/toxic epidermal necrolysis

Management strategies for ocular SJS–TEN are similar to OcMMP. Conjunctival inflammation secondary to external triggering factors, such as trichiasis or severe DED, should be addressed before endogenous inflammation is graded and treated (recurrent or persistent inflammation). The use of systemic immunosuppression with corticosteroids and/or steroid-sparing agents must be considered; treatment guidelines are similar to those for other autoimmune bullous disorders such as OcMMP, except that the use of sulfonamides and dapsone should be avoided, as these may precipitate keratinocyte apoptosis. As with the OcMMP cohort of patients, cataract, glaucoma, and oculoplastic surgery should be avoided until the disease is controlled by systemic immunosuppressive therapy for a minimum of 3 months.

■ FUTURE DIRECTIONS IN OCMMP AND SJS–TEN

As can be seen from this review, the major issues in the management of OcMMP and SJS–TEN are several:

- Diagnosis is often delayed due to clinicians failing to recognize early signs of what is a rare disease. Current studies of the autoantibody response to BMZ epitopes in OcMMP are likely to lead to improvements both in diagnosis and to our understanding of disease pathogenesis
- Without robust activity and damage scoring systems, it will be impossible to trial new diagnostic tools or therapeutic interventions
- A non-invasive ocular or peripheral blood biomarker of disease activity and damage based upon underlying inflammatory cellular infiltrates or cytokines requires further exploration

- The multidisciplinary nature of management needs to be established early and extensively. This may include a multidisciplinary team clinic and ward rounds in the intensive therapy environment, including colleagues such as ocular surface specialists, optometrists, low-vision team, glaucoma and oculoplastic specialists, rheumatologists, dermatologists, oral medicine physicians, and close liaison with the patients' primary care physicians. In complex disease, communication is the key
- Management of the inflammation in many patients requires toxic systemic therapies. The success of newer approaches using more targeted biological drugs may reduce toxicity and potentially provide local ocular therapies as opposed to systemic treatment. A better understanding of the pathogenesis of inflammation in this disease is key to making use of available biologics and identifying potential new therapies
- There have been very few treatments directed against the problem of scarring, which probably progresses independently of inflammation, once the disease has started. Developing antiscarring therapies is an area that is likely to progress rapidly within the next decade

- Engaging with patients is vital to encourage research; management and therapeutics need to be directed to patient needs

◼ ACKNOWLEDGMENTS

The authors thank (1) Mr Peter McDonnell, FRCP, FRCS, FRCOphth, Consultant Ophthalmologist and Honorary Senior Clinical Lecturer, University of Birmingham; Birmingham and Midland Eye Center, City Hospital, Birmingham and Queen Elizabeth Hospital Birmingham; and (2) Professor Peter Shah, BSc (Hons), MBChB, FRCOphth, FRCP Edin, University Hospitals Birmingham NHS Foundation Trust, Birmingham, UK; UCL Partners Academic Health Science Center 'Eyes & Vision' Theme, London, UK; NIHR Biomedical Research Center for Ophthalmology, Moorfields Eye Hospital NHS Foundation Trust and UCL Institute of Ophthalmology, London, UK; and Center for Health and Social Care Improvement, School of Health and Well-being, University of Wolverhampton, UK, for reviewing this chapter.

◼ REFERENCES

Ahuero AE, Jakobiec FA, Bhat P, Ciralsky JB, Papaliodis GN. Paraneoplastic conjunctival cicatrization: two different pathogenic types. *Ophthalmology* 2010; **117**:659–664.

Anaya JM, Tobon GJ, Vega P, Castiblanco J. Autoimmune disease aggregation in families with primary Sjögren's syndrome. *J Rheumatol* 2006; **33**:2227–2234.

Araki Y, Sotozono C, Inatomi T, et al. Successful treatment of Stevens-Johnson syndrome with steroid pulse therapy at disease onset. *Am J Ophthalmol* 2009; **147**:1004–1011.

Barry RJ, Sutcliffe N, Isenberg DA, et al. The Sjögren's Syndrome Damage Index—a damage index for use in clinical trials and observational studies in primary Sjögren's syndrome. *Rheumatology (Oxford)* 2008; **47**:1193–1198.

Bastuji-Garin S, Fouchard N, Bertocchi M, et al. SCORTEN: a severity-of-illness score for toxic epidermal necrolysis. *J Invest Dermatol* 2000; **115**:149–153.

Behrens A, Doyle JJ, Stern L, et al. Dysfunctional tear syndrome: a Delphi approach to treatment recommendations. *Cornea* 2006; **25**:900–907.

Bernauer W, Elder MJ, Dart JK. Introduction to Cicatrising conjunctivitis. In: Bernauer W., Dart JKG, Elder MJ (eds), Cicatrising conjunctivitis. Basel, Switzerland: Karger, 1997.

Bernauer W, Elder MJ, Leonard JN, Wright P, Dart JK. The value of biopsies in the evaluation of chronic progressive conjunctival cicatrisation. *Graefes Arch Clin Exp Ophthalmol* 1994; **232**:533–537.

Bowman SJ, Sutcliffe N, Isenberg DA, et al. Sjögren's Systemic Clinical Activity Index (SCAI)—a systemic disease activity measure for use in clinical trials in primary Sjögren's syndrome. *Rheumatology (Oxford)* 2007; **46**:1845–1851.

Bridges AJ, Burns RP. Acute iritis associated with primary Sjögren's syndrome and high-titer anti-SS-A/Ro and anti-SS-B/La antibodies. Treatment with combination immunosuppressive therapy. *Arthritis Rheum* 1992; **35**:560–563.

Broadway D. Drug-induced conjunctival cicatrisation. *Dev Ophthalmol* 1997; **28**:86–101.

Canizares MJ, Smith DI, Conners MS, Maverick KJ, Heffernan MP. Successful treatment of mucous membrane pemphigoid with etanercept in 3 patients. *Arch Dermatol* 2006; **142**:1457–1461.

Chan LS, Ahmed AR, Anhalt GJ, et al. The first international consensus on mucous membrane pemphigoid: definition, diagnostic criteria, pathogenic factors, medical treatment, and prognostic indicators. *Arch Dermatol* 2002; **138**:370–379.

Chung WH, Hung SI, Yang JY, et al. Granulysin is a key mediator for disseminated keratinocyte death in Stevens-Johnson syndrome and toxic epidermal necrolysis. *Nat Med* 2008; **14**:1343–1350.

De Rojas MV, Dart JK, Saw VP. The natural history of Stevens Johnson syndrome: patterns of chronic ocular disease and the role of systemic immunosuppressive therapy. *Br J Ophthalmol* 2007; **91**:1048–1053.

Dry Eye Workshop. The definition and classification of dry eye disease: report of the Definition and Classification Subcommittee of the International Dry Eye WorkShop. *Ocul Surf* 2007; **5**:75–92.

Elder MJ, Bernauer W. Monitoring of activity and progression in cicatrising conjunctivitis. In: Bernauer W, Dart JKG, Elder MJ (eds), Cicatrising conjunctivitis. Basel, Switzerland: Karger, 1997.

Foster CS. Cicatricial pemphigoid. *Trans Am Ophthalmol Soc* 1986; **84**:527–663.

Fu Y, Gregory DG, Sippel KC, Bouchard CS, Tseng SC. The ophthalmologist's role in the management of acute Stevens-Johnson syndrome and toxic epidermal necrolysis. *Ocul Surf* 2010; **8**:193–203.

Gregory D G. Treatment of acute Stevens-Johnson syndrome and toxic epidermal necrolysis using amniotic membrane: a review of 10 consecutive cases. *Ophthalmology* 2011; **118**:908–914.

John T, Foulks GN, John ME, Cheng K, Hu D. Amniotic membrane in the surgical management of acute toxic epidermal necrolysis. *Ophthalmology* 2002; **109**:351–360.

Kasperkiewicz M, Zillikens D, Schmidt E. Pemphigoid diseases: Pathogenesis, diagnosis, and treatment. *Autoimmunity* 2012; **45**:55-70.

Low HZ, Witte T. Aspects of innate immunity in Sjögren's syndrome. *Arthritis Res Ther* 2011; **13**:218.

Mihai S, Sitaru C. Immunopathology and molecular diagnosis of autoimmune bullous diseases. *J Cell Mol Med* 2007; **11**:462–481.

Mondino BJ, Brown SI. Ocular cicatricial pemphigoid. *Ophthalmology* 1981; **88**:95–100.

Power WJ, Ghoraishi M, Merayo-Lloves J, Neves RA, Foster CS. Analysis of the acute ophthalmic manifestations of the erythema multiforme/Stevens-Johnson syndrome/toxic epidermal necrolysis disease spectrum. *Ophthalmology* 1995; **102**:1669–1676.

Radford CF, Rauz S, Williams GP, Saw VP, Dart JKG. Incidence, presenting features and diagnosis of cicatrising conjunctivitis in the United Kingdom. *Eye* 2012; **26**:1199–208.

Rauz S, Maddison PG, Dart JK. Evaluation of mucous membrane pemphigoid with ocular involvement in young patients. *Ophthalmology* 2005; **112**:1268–1274.

Razzaque MS, Foster CS, Ahmed AR. Role of macrophage migration inhibitory factor in conjunctival pathology in ocular cicatricial pemphigoid. *Invest Ophthalmol Vis Sci* 2004; **45**:1174–1181.

Rosenthal P, Baran I, Jacobs DS. Corneal pain without stain: is it real? *Ocul Surf* 2009; **7**:28–40.

Ross AH, Jaycock P, Cook SD, Dick AD, Tole DM. The use of rituximab in refractory mucous membrane pemphigoid with severe ocular involvement. *Br J Ophthalmol* 2009; **93**:421–422, 548.

Saw VP, Dart JKG. Author reply to ocular cicatricial pemphigoid. *Ophthalmology* 2008a; **115**:1640–1641.

Saw VP, Dart JK. Ocular mucous membrane pemphigoid: diagnosis and management strategies. *Ocul Surf* 2008b; **6**:128–142.

Saw VP, Schmidt E, Offiah I, et al. Profibrotic phenotype of conjunctival fibroblasts from mucous membrane pemphigoid. *Am J Pathol* 2011; **178**:187–97.

Saw VPJ, Offiah I, Dart RJ, et al. Conjunctival interleukin-13 expression in mucous membrane pemphigoid and functional effects of interleukin-13 on conjunctival fibroblasts in vitro. *Am J Pathol* 2009; **175**:2406–2415.

Schwab IR, Linberg JV, Gioia VM, et al. Foreshortening of the inferior conjunctival fornix associated with chronic glaucoma medications. *Ophthalmology* 1992; **99**:197–202.

Segura S, Iranzo P, Martínez-DE Pablo I, et al. High-dose intravenous immunoglobulins for the treatment of autoimmune mucocutaneous blistering diseases: evaluation of its use in 19 cases. *J Am Acad Dermatol* 2007; **56**:960–967.

Setterfield J, Shirlaw PJ, Kerr-Muir M, et al. Mucous membrane pemphigoid: a dual circulating antibody response with IgG and IgA signifies a more severe and persistent disease. *Br J Dermatol* 1998; **138**:602–610.

Shay E, Khadem JJ, Tseng SC. Efficacy and limitation of sutureless amniotic membrane transplantation for acute toxic epidermal necrolysis. *Cornea* 2010; **29**:359–361.

Sotozono C, Ang LP, Koizumi N, et al. New grading system for the evaluation of chronic ocular manifestations in patients with Stevens-Johnson syndrome. *Ophthalmology* 2007; **114**:1294–1302.

Stern ME, Schaumburg CS, Dana R, et al. Autoimmunity at the ocular surface: pathogenesis and regulation. *Mucosal Immunol* 2010; **3**:425–442.

Tauber J, Jabbur N, Foster CS. Improved detection of disease progression in ocular cicatricial pemphigoid. *Cornea* 1992; **11**:446–451.

Thorne JE, Woreta FA, Jabs DA, Anhalt GJ. Treatment of ocular mucous membrane pemphigoid with immunosuppressive drug therapy. *Ophthalmology* 2008; **115**:2146–2152.

Tomlins PJ, Parulekar MV, Rauz S. 'Triple-TEN' in the treatment of acute ocular complications from toxic epidermal necrolysis. *Cornea* 2013; **32**:365–369.

Ueta M. Innate immunity of the ocular surface and ocular surface inflammatory disorders. *Cornea* 2008; **27**:S31–S40.

Ueta M, Sotozono C, Inatomi T, et al. Toll-like receptor 3 gene polymorphisms in Japanese patients with Stevens-Johnson syndrome. *Br J Ophthalmol* 2007; **91**:962–965.

Ueta M, Sotozono C, Yokoi N, Inatomi T, Kinoshita S. Prostaglandin E receptor subtype EP3 expression in human conjunctival epithelium and its changes in various ocular surface disorders. *PLoS One* 2011; **6**:e25209.

Vitali C, Bombardieri S, Jonsson R, et al. Classification criteria for Sjögren's syndrome: a revised version of the European criteria proposed by the American-European Consensus Group. *Ann Rheum Dis* 2002; **61**: 554–558.

Williams GP, Mudhar HS, Leyland M. Early pathological features of the cornea in toxic epidermal necrolysis. *Br J Ophthalmol* 2007; **91**:1129–1132.

Williams GP, Radford C, Nightingale P, Dart JK, Rauz S. Evaluation of early and late presentation of patients with ocular mucous membrane pemphigoid to two major tertiary referral hospitals in the United Kingdom. *Eye (Lond)* 2011a; **25**:1207–1218.

Williams GP, Saw VP, Saeed T, et al. Validation of a fornix depth measurer: a putative tool for the assessment of progressive cicatrising conjunctivitis. *Br J Ophthalmol* 2011b; **95**:842–847.

Witko-Sarsat V, Pederzoli-Ribeil M, Hirsch E, Sozzani S, Cassatella MA. Regulating neutrophil apoptosis: new players enter the game. *Trends Immunol* 2011; **32**:117–124.

Wright P. Cicatrizing conjunctivitis. *Trans Ophthalmol Soc U K* 1986; **105**:1–17.

Zakka LR, Reche P, Ahmed AR. Role of MHC class II genes in the pathogenesis of pemphigoid. *Autoimmun Rev.* 2011; **11**:40–47.

Chapter 13 Graft-versus-host disease

Hasanain Shikari, Reza Dana

INTRODUCTION

Despite being an established and potentially curative treatment for both malignant and benign hematological diseases, use of allogeneic hematopoietic stem cell transplantation (allo-HSCT) is limited due to graft-versus-host disease (GVHD), which is a major cause of morbidity and non-relapse mortality following allogeneic HSCT.

Though covered under an umbrella term—bone marrow transplantation (BMT)—the type of transplantation would depend on the source of donor cells. These include autologous (self), syngeneic (identical), and allogeneic (other individual). The donor cells can now be harvested not only from bone marrow but also from peripheral blood and placental cord blood.

The efficacy of allo-HSCT is dependent on the critically important donor-derived, immunologically driven, graft-versus-leukemia or graft-versus-tumor effect, which improves the graft uptake (engraftment) and reduces the risk of relapse, but can cause GVHD-type morbidity. The occurrence of GVHD is correlated with a positive graft-versus-tumor effect. GVHD is mediated by donor-derived T cells, and its incidence varies in literature, from 20% to 60% of patients receiving the BMT (Ferrara et al. 2009, Filipovich et al. 2005).

The incidence of GVHD varies greatly with the source of the donor tissue, such as bone marrow or peripheral blood stem cells (Ferrara et al. 2009, Filipovich et al. 2005). GVHD is an immune response by the donor cells (graft) against the recipient (host), resulting in an immunological attack against organ systems (e.g. skin, gastrointestinal system, liver, mouth and eyes) (Ferrara et al. 2009).

There are several established risk factors associated with the development of GVHD that affect the severity of presentation. These include human leukocyte antigen (HLA) mismatch between the donor and the recipient, gender disparity (male donor for female recipient and vice versa), advanced recipient and donor age, source of the stem cells and the type of prophylaxis or conditioning regimen undertaken, and a history of acute GVHD (in cases of chronic GVHD) (McGuirk & Weiss 2011). However, optimally HLA-matched transplant recipients also present with GVHD mainly due to the mismatch of many potential minor histocompatibility antigens, which are not accounted for in routine HLA typing (McGuirk & Weiss 2011).

Traditionally GVHD has been described as acute or chronic, based on a temporal classification, with all cases occurring within 100 days post-transplant labeled 'acute' and those occurring after as 'chronic.' This 3-month (100 days) separation point held true in the myeloablative era, but it was observed that non-myeloablative allo-HSCT and reduced-intensity conditioning were associated with a 2-month delay in onset of acute GVHD (Westeneng et al. 2010), while acute and chronic GVHDs were found to present simultaneously in patients treated with, for example, donor lymphocyte infusions. The importance of GVHD grading in determining the prognosis in relation to morbidity and mortality has been realized, and the current grading systems for acute GVHD have been updated. The classification of GVHD has also been updated, factoring in clinical presentation, mandated by the above-mentioned findings.

Hence, by current consensus, it is primarily the clinical manifestations and not the time to onset of symptoms after transplant that determines the classification of GVHD as acute or chronic.

The National Institutes of Health (NIH) Consensus reports on criteria for clinical trials in chronic GVHD have published the requisites, composed of criteria (e.g. diagnostic and distinctive), histopathology, and management, relevant to a diagnosis of chronic systemic and chronic ocular GVHD (Couriel et al. 2006a, 2006b, Filipovich et al. 2005, Pavletic et al. 2006, Shulman et al. 2006). To establish a diagnosis of chronic GVHD requires the presence of one diagnostic sign or one distinctive sign (confirmed by biopsy and/or laboratory test) and/or the involvement of another organ or system. This formed the basis for the addition of two new categories to the existing classification of GVHD: persistent, recurrent, or late-onset acute GVHD (>3 months) and overlap syndrome (no temporal relation) in which features of acute and chronic GVHD appear together (Filipovich et al. 2005).

PATHOPHYSIOLOGY

The pathogenesis of GVHD is multifactorial. It is established that donor T cells derived from the graft tissue mainly cause it. However, recent animal studies suggest that B cells are also involved in the pathogenesis, and this is based on circumstantial evidence of successful treatment of GVHD by anti-CD20 B-cell depletion. Based on various studies, researchers have now concluded that chronic GVHD is associated with disturbed B-cell homeostasis, with a relative reduction in naïve B cells and a relative increase in the number of activated memory-type B cells. Elevated levels of B-cell activation factor (BAFF) have been correlated with the development and severity of chronic GVHD. High levels of BAFF in the presence of lower numbers of naïve B cells might thus foster the survival of activated alloreactive and autoreactive B cells, resulting in immune pathology (Ferrara et al. 2009, Shimabukuro-Vornhagen et al. 2009).

Based largely on experimental murine and canine models, the development of acute GVHD can be envisaged as a three-step 'cytokine storm' reaction with fulminant systemic disease (Ferrara et al. 2009). The first is the activation of the antigen-presenting cells (APCs), followed by donor T-cell activation, proliferation, differentiation, and migration, which are subsequently followed by target tissue destruction (**Figure 13.1**).

Phase 1—activation of APCs

The underlying disease process or the conditioning regimen (e.g. irradiation) leads to activation of the APCs with consequent host tissue damage and resultant liberation of 'danger' signals, such as proinflammatory cytokines (e.g. TNF-α), chemokines, and increased expression of ICAM-1, major histocompatibility complex antigens, and costimulatory molecules on host APCs (Ferrara et al. 2009).

Damage to the gastrointestinal (GI) mucosa from the conditioning regimen leads to a damaged barrier, allowing ease of systemic

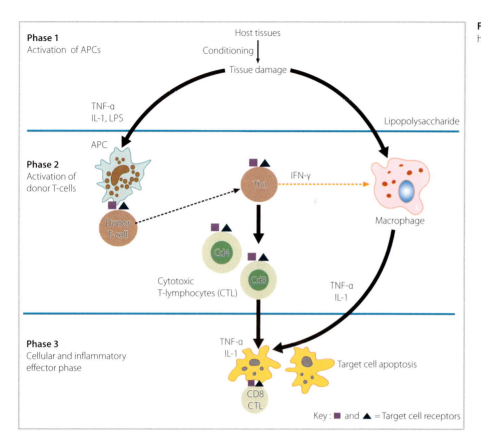

Figure 13.1 Pathophysiology of acute graft-versus-host disease.

translocation of microbial gut pathogen-associated inflammatory stimuli such as lipopolysaccharides or other molecules, consequently also leading to APC activation (Ferrara et al. 2009).

Phase 2—activation of donor T cells

This phase forms the crux of the graft-versus-host reaction in which the host APCs cause the proliferation and differentiation of donor T cells. This proliferation is amplified partly by the 'danger' signals, released in phase 1, due to upregulation of expression of costimulatory molecules (Dustin 2001).

In acute GVHD, the principal T-cell response is a helper T-cell type 1 (Th1)-mediated inflammatory response, with production of large amounts of Th1 cytokines (IFN-γ, IL-2, and TNF-α). The majority of present clinical therapies and prophylactic regimens are targeted at the IL-2 production by donor T cells (e.g. cyclosporine, tacrolimus, and monoclonal antibodies directed against IL-2 and its receptor) (Loiseau et al. 2007).

Phase 3—cellular and inflammatory effector phase

This phase encompasses a complex cascade involving the release of cellular and soluble mediators of inflammation, which in turn harmonize, to cause gross local tissue injury and promote inflammation and target tissue destruction. Examples of the cellular mediators include cytotoxic T lymphocytes and natural killer cells and soluble mediators, including IFN-γ, IL-1, TNF-α, and nitric oxide (Ferrara et al. 2009). TNF-α causes greater tissue damage in the GI tract and plays a major role in the augmentation and spread of the 'cytokine storm.'

CLINICAL MANIFESTATIONS OF SYSTEMIC GVHD

Clinical manifestations of systemic GVHD are seen mainly in the skin, GI tract, and liver. Martin et al. (1990), in an exhaustive review, demonstrated characteristics of initial presentation of patients with acute GVHD and found that 81% of patients had skin involvement (pruritic maculopapular rash sparing the scalp, with blistering and ulceration in severe cases), 54% GI involvement (presenting with voluminous, secretory diarrhea, vomiting, anorexia, and/or abdominal cramping), and 51% liver involvement (associated with raised conjugated bilirubin and alkaline phosphatase levels). Cooke et al. (1996) have also demonstrated pulmonary involvement in experimental GVHD models.

OCULAR GVHD

The incidence of ocular GVHD has been reported to be 40–60% in patients receiving allo-HSCT (Franklin et al. 1983, Hirst et al. 1983). Ocular GVHD encompasses a variety of eye disorders, including but not limited to, the ocular surface and lacrimal glands. Inflammation and cicatricial scarring of the conjunctiva, keratoconjunctivitis sicca (KCS) due to dysfunction of the lacrimal gland, and meibomian gland dysfunction (MGD)—all lead to ocular surface disease. Ocular involvement, though rare in systemic acute GVHD, is considered a poor prognostic factor for mortality caused by systemic acute GVHD (Holler 2007, Saito et al. 2002). Though known to impair the quality of life and activities of daily living, ocular GVHD usually does not lead to permanent visual loss (Westeneng et al. 2010).

High-risk factors for development of ocular GVHD include patients with skin and mouth involvement (Westeneng et al. 2010) as well as patients with allo-HSCT from related donors (as opposed to those receiving donor tissue from matched-unrelated donors) (Westeneng et al. 2010).

Clinical features of ocular GVHD

Manifestations of ocular GVHD involve all layers of the eye, including the eyelids, lacrimal gland, conjunctiva, cornea, uveal tract, vitreous, retina, and optic nerve. The ocular surface and lacrimal gland tend to be affected in higher frequency than other parts of the eye (with the posterior segment involvement being extremely rare). The ocular manifestations, though mostly similar in acute and chronic GVHD, differ immunopathologically.

ACUTE OCULAR GVHD

In general, ocular manifestations are uncommon in acute GVHD (Arocker-Mettinger et al. 1991). Conjunctival and corneal findings have been described in patients with acute GVHD, with severity of ocular signs correlating with severity of systemic disease (Hirst et al. 1983, Janin et al. 1996). Researchers have demonstrated that the cornea and conjunctiva are immunological targets in GVHD, and histological findings similar to those seen in cutaneous GVHD have been demonstrated (Jabs et al. 1989). Conjunctival symptom staging by Jabs et al. has been summarized in **Table 13.1** as stage 0–4. Other authors have reported similar findings (Hirst et al. 1983).

Subtle conjunctival hyperemia (stage 1) in the presence of systemic GVHD, having ruled out infectious etiology, should arouse suspicion of ocular GVHD, if accompanied by symptoms as well as evidence of aqueous deficiency (**Figure 13.2**). Conjunctival

hyperemia associated with chemosis (ranging from moderate to frank serosanguinous exudation) is seen in stage 2. The cause of chemosis may be attributed to fluid imbalance (due to concurrent systemic fluid overload in patients immunosuppressed with steroids) or ocular GVHD. A careful review of systems and evaluation of medication history, as well as ruling out hyponatremia and hypoalbuminemia, help to clinch the diagnosis of ocular GVHD and can be confirmed by conjunctival biopsy. Pseudomembranous conjunctivitis (stage 3) has been reported in 12–17% of patients with acute GVHD (Hirst et al. 1983, Jabs et al. 1989, Janin et al. 1996). Its presence has been considered a marker for systemic involvement (Jabs et al. 1989) and is associated with a poor prognosis (Janin et al. 1996). Conjunctival hyperemia with epithelial sloughing gives rise to pseudomembranous changes and subsequent scarring. In severe cases, corneal epithelial sloughing accompanies the pseudomembranous changes (stage 4), and may be seen in up to a third of the patients with pseudomembranes (Jabs et al. 1989).

Routine conjunctival biopsies are considered to be unnecessary for early GVHD (Hirst et al. 1983, Jabs et al. 1983). Histological features, similar to those seen in the skin, liver, and GI, can be encountered and include dyskeratosis with loss of epithelium, lymphocyte exocytosis, satellitosis, and epithelial cell necrosis, with apoptotic bodies in the epithelium. These findings are characteristic of GVHD. Immunochemistry of one acute conjunctival GVHD specimen shows the presence of CD4+ T-helper cells (Jabs et al. 1989), with Saito et al. showing them to be mainly donor-derived (Saito et al. 2002). Histological findings, studied for the first time in murine models of GVHD, demonstrated epithelial atrophy and cellular vacuolization of basal and medium layers of the cornea. This was also associated with diffuse stromal edema with neovascularization and inflammatory infiltrate. No significant endothelial changes were noted (Perez et al. 2011).

Conjunctival involvement in acute systemic GVHD has been shown to have a prognostic role. It is associated with a higher mortality in those with a similar grade of acute GVHD than in those without. Clinical experience dispels the long-held belief that conjunctival ocular GVHD occurs only in the presence of systemic GVHD. Conjunctival acute GVHD has been shown to be the initial presentation of GVHD in some post-BMT patients, presenting at Massachusetts Eye and Ear Infirmary, Boston (Balaram et al. 2005).

Table 13.1 Staging of ocular symptoms in GVHD

Scoring of dry eyes in GVHD - NIH Eye Score (organ scoring of chronic GVHD)
0 No dry eye symptoms
1 Dry eye symptoms not affecting ADL (eye drops ≤3 × per day) or asymptomatic signs of KCS
2 Dry eye symptoms partially affecting ADL (eye drops >3 × per day or punctual plugs) without vision impairment
3 Dry eye symptoms, significantly affecting ADL (special eye wear to relieve pain) or unable to work because of ocular symptoms or loss of vision caused by KCS

Staging of conjunctivitis in acute GVHD
0 None
1 Hyperemia
2 Hyperemia with serosanguinous discharge
3 Pseudomembranous conjunctivitis
4 Pseudomembranous conjunctivitis with corneal epithelial sloughing

Staging of conjunctivitis in chronic GVHD
0 None
1 Hyperemia
2 Palpebral conjunctival fibrovascular changes with or without epithelial sloughing
3 Palpebral conjunctival fibrovascular changes, involving 25–75% of total surface area
4 Involvement of >75% of total surface area with or without cicatricial entropion

ADL, activities of daily living; GVHD, graft-versus-host disease; KCS, keratoconjunctivitis sicca.

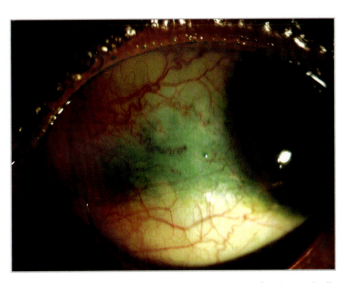

Figure 13.2 Lissamine green staining of conjunctiva: areas of conjunctival cell death and degeneration and goblet cell loss.

Dry eye syndrome/KCS remains the most common ocular complication after BMT (Martin et al. 2006), and most of the other ocular complications, such as persistent corneal epitheliopathy, resulting in infected/non-infected stromal ulceration can be attributed to dry eye disease (DED) (**Figure 13.3**). Clinical studies have demonstrated a strong association between development of DED (decreased clinical tear function) and acute GVHD (Hirst et al. 1983). Histopathological studies of lacrimal glands in patients with acute GVHD showed the presence of 'lacrimal gland stasis' with PAS-positive material accumulation in the acini and distended ductules, with obliteration of the lumen.

CHRONIC OCULAR GVHD

Ocular manifestations occur in a large percentage of chronic systemic GVHD patients and may have severe visual consequences (Arocker-Mettinger et al. 1991).

Cicatricial conjunctival changes and superior limbic keratoconjunctivitis (accompanied with a Schirmer's test <5 mm) are quite commonly seen in chronic ocular GVHD, with associated symblepharon in the palpebral and forniceal conjunctivae and consequent lid scarring and disturbed lid anatomy (e.g. ectropion, entropion, meibomian gland atrophy, and punctal stenosis). Immunochemistry analysis of conjunctival biopsy specimen shows mainly suppressor and cytotoxic T-lymphocytes (Bhan et al. 1982). There is also increased expression of inflammatory marker ICAM-1 associated with decreased Schirmer's scores and decreased goblet cell density (Aronni et al. 2006). Secondary epithelial changes, such as punctate keratopathy, develop with the formation of corneal filaments and painful erosions with resultant secondary infections, non-healing ulcerations, and corneal perforations. All these changes compound the dysfunctional tear film and ocular surface disorder (**Figure 13.4**) (Balaram et al. 2005).

KCS has been observed in 69–77% of patients with chronic systemic GVHD. It is also considered to be an early sign of systemic involvement in extensive chronic GVHD. Tichelli et al. have reported that KCS occurs more frequently in patients with chronic GVHD than in those with acute GVHD, with an incidence of 80% in patients with chronic GVHD (Tichelli et al. 1996), and aqueous tear dysfunction in most patients with sicca does not resolve (Hirst et al. 1983). Development of KCS has been attributed to a cause beyond a simple alloreactive immune reaction. This has been substantiated by demonstration of KCS in patients receiving autologous or syngeneic transplants and who are consequently not at risk for development of GVHD. The primary etiology of DED in chronic GVHD has been ascribed to the extensive fibrotic destruction of tubuloalveolar glands by a subset of fibroblasts CD4+ and CD8+ T-cell expression (Ogawa et al. 2001a, 2001b). This is associated with a rise in the stromal CD34+ fibroblasts (nearly half are donor origin), accompanied by mild lymphocytic infiltration (Ogawa et al. 2001a, 2001b).

Total body irradiation (TBI) administered in single, rather than fractionated dose, ocular toxicity of chemotherapy, infections, immunosuppressive therapy, and MGD may also contribute to the sicca syndrome (Tichelli et al. 1996). However, Perez et al., using murine models to study histopathological findings in ocular GVHD, were unable to demonstrate external or histopathological findings of inflammatory cell infiltration and fibrosis among control mice receiving TBI and bone marrow cells. Hence, they were able to conclude that stress, TBI, and other non-specific causes were not involved (Perez et al. 2011). Patients with KCS present with complaints such as ocular irritation, foreign body sensation, grittiness, redness, intermittent blurring of vision, photophobia, discharge, and pain (Balaram et al. 2005).

The Schirmer's test assists in diagnosis of lacrimal function in chronic ocular GVHD by proxy. New-onset KCS with Schirmer's score of 6–10 mm or a symptomatic patient with Schirmer's score of ±5 mm in presence of other organ involvement forms the criteria for diagnosis of chronic ocular GVHD. The ocular surface disease index (OSDI) has been shown to be statistically higher in patients with chronic ocular GVHD than in pretransplant or post-transplant patients without ocular GVHD (Agomo et al. 2008). Another modality that may be used in evaluation of patients is the videokeratoscope, with higher aberrations of indices in patients of chronic ocular GVHD than in those without (Chang-Strepka 2009).

Cataract formation, though technically a complication of BMT and GVHD, is nowadays less frequently observed due to conditioning regimens as well as GVHD prophylaxis relying less on prolonged systemic corticosteroids. Rarely, patients present with uveitis, which

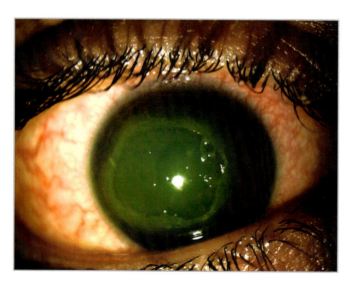

Figure 13.3 Corneal epithelial defect. Flourescein staining of epithelial defect secondary to dry eye disease (DED) in a patient with ocular graft-versus-host disease.

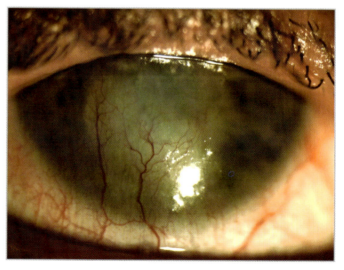

Figure 13.4 Severe ocular surface damage. Prolonged and extensive dry eye resulting in corneal opacification secondary to limbal stem cell involvement and neovascularization leading to reduced visual acuity.

is thought to be a result of direct immunological attack of donor lymphocytes against host incompatibility antigens (Franklin et al. 1983). Retinal findings comprise cotton-wool spots, retinal hemorrhages, lipid deposits, and even infectious retinitis (Arocker-Mettinger et al. 1991).

The NIH Health Consensus Development Project defined findings of new-onset dry, gritty, or painful eyes, cicatricial conjunctivitis, KCS, and confluent areas of punctate keratopathy, as well as periorbital hyperpigmentation, difficulty in opening the eyes in the morning because of dried mucoid secretions, and blepharitis as 'distinctive signs' (seen in chronic GVHD but insufficient, alone, to establish a diagnosis of chronic GVHD). As per the report, a diagnosis of chronic GVHD could be made in the presence of one diagnostic sign or the presence of a distinctive sign confirmed by biopsy and laboratory testing and/or distinctive signs in one other organ system. Chronic GVHD based only on ocular findings (presence of one distinctive sign) can be confirmed on the basis of biopsy proof of KCS or Schirmer's test and if accompanied by distinctive manifestations in at least one other organ (Filipovich et al. 2005). Routine screening biopsy is generally believed to serve little benefit for early detection of ocular GVHD. Lacrimal gland biopsy is invasive and risks decreasing the gland's functional capacity.

It needs to be emphasized that chronic GVHD-related severe OSD can occur with absolutely no evidence of systemic GVHD—a finding that has important implications for the monitoring of these patients post allo-BMT. This was noted in a series where a small subgroup of eight patients had isolated ocular GVHD disease, manifesting as moderate to severe chronic OSD in the absence of systemic GVHD (Balaram et al. 2005). Hence, the ocular surface can be an isolated target tissue of chronic GVHD many months post-BMT (West et al. 1991).

CARE FOR GVHD PATIENTS

The two principal approaches to managing GVHD include prevention and treatment.

Systemic GVHD prophylaxis

Strategies for prevention include optimal HLA-matched donors (MHC class I and II loci between the donor and the recipient).

Based on findings of a T-cell-mediated response being central to the pathogenesis of acute and chronic GVHD, many clinical studies have evaluated the role of T-cell depletion (TCD) as a prophylactic measure for GVHD. The three strategies employed were negative selection of T-cells ex vivo, positive selection of CD34+ stem cells ex vivo, and anti-T-cell antibodies in vivo (Ferrara et al. 2009). However, it was observed that a decrease in both acute and chronic GVHDs (with TCD) (Ferrara et al. 2009) was offset by an increase in the rates of graft failure, relapse of malignancy, infections, and Epstein–Barr virus-associated lymphoproliferative disorders. Other strategies for prevention and prophylaxis are enlisted in **Table 13.2**.

Treatment of acute systemic GVHD

The initial treatment choice remains steroids. Steroid therapy results in complete remission in <50% of the patients (Ferrara et al. 2009), and severe cases are less likely to respond to steroid therapy alone (Ferrara et al. 2009). Steroid-resistant GVHD usually implies a poor prognosis, with very low 5-year survival rates. The therapeutic modalities used in cases of steroid resistance are enlisted in **Table 13.3**.

Table 13.2 GVHD prophylaxis and mechanism of action

Cyclosporine	Calcineurin inhibitor → blockade of T-cell activation
FK506	Calcineurin inhibitor → blockade of T-cell activation
Methotrexate	Antimetabolite, folic acid analog
Prednisone	Receptor-mediated lympholysis and additional mechanisms
Antithymocyte globulin	Rabbit or equine antibodies against human T cells; pretransplant ATG protected against extensive chronic GVHD and chronic lung dysfunction
MMF	Inhibition of DNA synthesis → lymphocyte apoptosis
Alemtuzumab	Humanized monoclonal antibody to CD52; depletes donor T cells and targets host dendritic cells
Reduced-intensity conditioning	Non-myeloablative; suppression of the host immune system, allowing donor T cells to engraft followed by lymphohematopoietic ablation of the recipient; causes less tissue damage → reduced intensity 'cytokine storm'; may delay acute GVHD onset to beyond 100 days after the transplant and may present simultaneously with chronic GVHD (overlap syndrome)

GVHD, graft-versus-host disease; MMF, mycophenolate mofetil.

Table 13.3 Treatment modalities in acute GVHD

Frontline therapy	
Methylprednisolone	Receptor-mediated lympholysis and additional mechanisms
Salvage therapy	
Antithymocyte globulin	Rabbit or equine antibodies against human T cells
Pentostatin	Adenosine deaminase inhibitor
Extracorporeal photopheresis	Ex vivo apoptosis of donor lymphocytes by UVA irradiation; induction of T-cell apoptosis, monocyte differentiation into dendritic cells, and antigen-specific T_{Reg} cells with anti-inflammatory effects and prevention of solid-organ graft rejection
Daclizumab	Humanized monoclonal IL-2 receptor antagonist
Infliximab	Humanized monoclonal TNF-α antibody
Mesenchymal stem cells	Immunosuppressive cells from unrelated donor that can be given across MHC barriers
Etanercept	Solubilized TNFR II (decoy receptor) → TNF inhibition; TNF-α blockade → discontinuity in the activation of APCs and effector cell recruitment → decreased direct tissue damage; significant benefit in conjunction with systemic steroids, as a primary therapy for acute GVHD

APCs, antigen-presenting cells; GVHD, graft-versus-host disease.

Treatment of chronic systemic GVHD

Corticosteroids, as in acute GVHD, remain the mainstay of therapy in chronic GVHD. Siadak et al. showed that the addition of cyclosporine orally in high-risk GVHD patients (those with thrombocytopenia) appeared to improve survival (Siadak & Sullivan 1994) and reduce steroid complications, without a beneficial effect on mortality or survival rates.

Various other therapeutic agents, ranging from azathioprine, alternating cyclosporine and prednisolone, high-dose pulse methyl prednisolone, tacrolimus, and thalidomide, have been tried and no superiority of one over the other has been seen in patients showing a failure to steroid response (Browne et al. 2000, Carnevale-Schianca et al. 2000, Mookerjee et al. 1999, Sullivan et al. 1992). Others have studied and shown the activity of daclizumab (anti-IL-2 receptor monoclonal antibody) and etanercept (anti-TNF antibody) in patients refractory to steroid therapy (Chiang et al. 2002) as also with mycophenolate mofetil and hydroxychloroquine (Lopez et al. 2001). Extracorporeal photopheresis has also shown promise in high-risk patients with significant response rates. The best responses have been demonstrated in the liver, skin, oral mucosa, eye, and lung (Couriel et al. 2006a, 2006b).

Supportive care, which includes infection (fungal and viral) prevention, prophylaxis, and treatment, forms an important part of management of GHVD patients. Non-infectious complications such as diabetes, avascular necrosis, muscle weakness, osteoporosis, and cushingoid features may develop with chronic steroid use. Calcineurin inhibitors may cause renal impairment, hypertension, and neurological paresthesias, and may, to some extent, be prevented by intense oral outpatient hydration (Ferrara et al. 2009).

Ocular GVHD—treatment strategies

The approach advocated is organ-specific in cases of organ-specific GVHD. Increasing the systemic immunosuppression with steroids or other agents is not considered an optimal approach for ocular GVHD, especially since the graft-versus-tumor effect needed for disease remission may be affected by systemic pharmacotherapy as well as the associated risks of long-term immunosuppression.

The treatment strategies for ocular GVHD are based on four main principles—lubrication and tear preservation, prevention of evaporation, decrease in inflammation, and epithelial support.

In both acute and chronic ocular GVHDs with severe aqueous-deficient dry eyes, topical lubrication with artificial non-preserved phosphate-free tears is usually accompanied by other therapeutic modalities. In a systematic review of various lubricants used in all cases of DED by Doughty et al., no difference in the results was found between specific products used (Doughty & Glavin 2009). Frequent use of artificial drops is beneficial not only in terms of lubrication but also theoretically in terms of diluting the local inflammatory mediators present on the ocular surface. Oral secretagogues such as selective muscarinic agonists (Pilocarpine or Cevimeline) may be beneficial in stimulating aqueous tear flow, but in our clinical experience, they are not of much clinical benefit in patients with sicca symptoms secondary to ocular GVHD. The concern for adverse drug interactions and toxicities in these patients already on a multitude of systemic medications also limits their use.

Punctal occlusion remains the mainstay of tear preservation and may be achieved by use of silicone plugs or thermal cauterization of punctum. The decision on how many punctae need occlusion is based on the Schirmer's test and patient symptom severity. At Massachusetts Eye and Ear Infirmary, Boston, we maintain a low symptom threshold for punctal occlusion, with a high percentage of patients having plugs inserted in each clinic. In a retrospective record review of dry eye patients in our clinic, it was found that there was a reduced dependency on artificial lubricants as well as relief from symptoms of DED after punctal plugs (Balaram et al. 2001). However, spontaneous plug loss does occur in a substantial minority of patients.

Autologous serum eye drops are used quite extensively in our patients and are a safe and effective modality to treat severe dry eye syndrome associated with chronic GVHD. The beneficial effect of autologous serum tears in chronic GVHD has been shown by clinical studies as well (Ogawa et al. 2003). Autologous serum contains vitamin A, epidermal growth factor, fibronectin, and TGF-b, which are essential for the integrity of the corneal and conjunctival surfaces. Yoon and colleagues published data from 12 patients with GVHD DED who showed significant improvement in dry eye symptoms and signs with the use of 20% umbilical cord serum eye drops (Yoon et al. 2007).

Topical cyclosporine eye drops have been used with success in patients with chronic ocular GVHD and KCS who were refractory to conventional lubrication and steroid drops. Topical cyclosporine acts by the inhibition of T-lymphocyte proliferation and the production and release of lymphokines from activated T cells in the conjunctiva. CsA has also been shown to increase the goblet cell density and epithelial cell turnover in conjunctiva. Dastjerdi et al. have reported improved symptoms, corneal flourescein staining, and basal tear secretion in ocular GVHD patients on off-label high-frequency (greater than bid) 0.05% cyclosporine eye drops (Dastjerdi et al. 2009).

The anti-inflammatory properties of topical steroids have been employed in treatment of acute ocular GVHD. There have been conflicting reports with regards to its beneficial effects, with older studies demonstrating no effects (Hirst et al. 1983, Jabs et al. 1989). However, Kim et al. (2006) have demonstrated its beneficial effects in this setting. The use of steroids in chronic ocular GVHD has been indicated in patients presenting with cicatricial changes. Raised intraocular pressure and posterior subcapsular cataracts remain the most common complications of long-term topical steroid therapy. Topical steroids are contraindicated in patients with corneal epithelial defects, stromal thinning, or infiltrates.

The use of tetracycline antibiotics (doxycycline or minocycline) and macrolides (azithromycin) is indicated in meibomian gland disorders (MGD) (**Figure 13.5**), contributing to ocular surface disease, usually in concert with warm compresses and lid hygiene. Doxycycline has been shown to have an anti-inflammatory role in addition to its antibiotic capacity by inhibiting matrix metalloproteinase (MMP) activity and both MMP and IL-1 syntheses (Smith et al. 2008). Nutritional supplements such as omega-3 fatty acids and flax seed oil also have an anti-inflammatory effect (Couriel et al. 2006a, 2006b). These result in increased tear film stability as well as decreased inflammation.

Tacrolimus (FK506), a macrolide antibiotic, has been shown to have a mechanism of action and pharmacokinetics, similar to cyclosporin A (Kino et al. 1987) albeit with a much higher immunosuppressive potency in vitro. Systemic tacrolimus has been found to be of beneficial effect in ocular GVHD (Ogawa et al. 2001a, 2001b) probably by an improved tear production. There are, however, no data available on its topical use.

Topical tranilast (Rizaben, antiallergic) inhibits the production and/or release of ocular inflammatory mediators and cytokines and inhibits collagen synthesis as well as TGF-b-induced matrix production. Though not extensively studied, its investigational use has been found to improve reflex tearing and Rose Bengal scores in a small group of patients with GVHD (Ogawa et al. 2010).

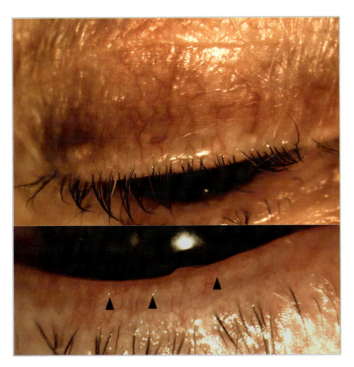

Figure 13.5 Meibomian gland dysfunction (MGD). Upper lid shows evidence of telangiectasia with engorged vessels running parallel to meibomian glands. Lower lid shows lid margin telangiectasia with viscous meibomian gland secretions causing meibomian capping (black arrows).

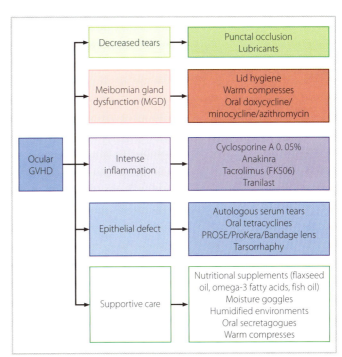

Figure 13.6 Treatment options available for ocular graft-versus-host disease.

Topical IL-1 receptor antagonist (IL-1Ra) has been used to control inflammation in DED. Clinical experience from off-label use of 2.5% IL-1Ra (Kineret) in patients with ocular GVHD shows promising results.

Contact lenses have been used in ocular surface disorders in order to stabilize the tear film and to restore normal cell turnover (Russo et al. 2007). The most commonly used lenses include scleral lens (PROSE—prosthetic replacement of ocular surface ecosystem) and the bandage contact lens (BCL). The liquid layer provided by the fluid-ventilated, gas-permeable scleral lens helps overcome the symptoms and aids in resurfacing the damaged corneal epithelium in patients with ocular GVHD-induced dry eyes in a small group, with improvement in the OSDI scores in patients refractory to other forms of therapy (Takahide et al. 2007). The use of BCL is advocated under physician supervision and with judicious follow-up. In acute stage 5 GVHD, however, their use is contraindicated due to concern for causing infection, hypoxia, and other contact lens-related pathologies. The suture-less amniotic membrane has also been used in patients with ocular surface disorders with positive outcomes and has also been described in patients with ocular GVHD (Kim et al. 2008).

Severe cases of ocular surface disruption warrant surgical intervention. Balaram et al. have documented treatment of large non-healing epithelial defects with BCL and the use of tarsorraphy in patients with severe DED associated with corneal thinning. Multilayer amniotic membrane transplantation has been used to treat corneal perforation. Also, limbal stem cell transplantation and penetrating keratoplasty may be employed to treat severe OSD. Our approach to treatment is depicted in **Figure 13.6.**

■ CONCLUSION

The spectrum of chronic OSD after allo-BMT varies from dry-eye to vision-threatening surface inflammation, which may present many months after the BMT. Notably, severe OSD occurs even in the absence of systemic GVHD. Although ocular GVHD is very common, it is often overlooked because of the grave systemic manifestations. Early diagnosis and intervention is necessary for a good visual outcome.

A combined effort of the oncologist, ophthalmologist, and primary care physician may prove effective, and an ocular surveillance protocol (pre- and post-BMT) including patient education and periodic eye evaluations must be incorporated in the long-term follow-up to facilitate the prompt diagnosis and treatment of the ocular surface complications of bone marrow transplant.

■ REFERENCES

Agomo E, Tan A, Champlin R, et al. Role of ocular surface disease index (OSDI) in chronic ocular graft vs. host disease (OGVHD). *Invest Ophthalmol Vis Sci* 2008; **49S**:2369.

Arocker-Mettinger E, Skorpik F, Grabner G, et al. Manifestations of graft-versus-host disease following allogenic bone marrow transplantation. *Eur J Ophthalmol* 1991; **1**:28–32.

Aronni S, Cortes M, Sacchetti M, et al. Upregulation of ICAM-1 expression in the conjunctiva of patients with chronic graft-versus-host disease. *Eur J Ophthalmol* 2006; **16**:17–23.

Balaram M, Rashid S, Dana R. Chronic ocular surface disease after allogeneic bone marrow transplantation. *Ocul Surf* 2005; **3**:203–211.

Balaram M, Schaumberg DA, Dana MR. Efficacy and tolerability outcomes after punctal occlusion with silicone plugs in dry eye syndrome. *Am J Ophthalmol* 2001; **131**:30–36.

Bhan AK, Mihm MC, Jr, Dvorak HF. T cell subsets in allograft rejection. In situ characterization of T cell subsets in human skin allografts by the use of monoclonal antibodies. *J Immunol* 1982; **129**:1578–1583.

Browne PV, Weisdorf DJ, DeFor T, et al. Response to thalidomide therapy in refractory chronic graft-versus-host disease. *Bone Marrow Transplant* 2000; **26**:865–869.

Carnevale-Schianca F, Martin P, Sullivan K, et al. Changing from cyclosporine to tacrolimus as salvage therapy for chronic graft-versus-host disease. *Biol Blood Marrow Transplant* 2000; **6**:613–620.

Chang-Strepka J. Videokeratoscopic indices in chronic ocular graft versus host disease (OGVHD). *Invest Ophthalmol Vis Sci* 2009; 50S:2610.

Chiang KY, Abhyankar S, Bridges K, et al. Recombinant human tumor necrosis factor receptor fusion protein as complementary treatment for chronic graft-versus-host disease. *Transplantation* 2002; **73**:665–667.

Cooke KR, Kobzik L, Martin TR, et al. An experimental model of idiopathic pneumonia syndrome after bone marrow transplantation: I. The roles of minor H antigens and endotoxin. *Blood* 1996; **88**:3230–3239.

Couriel D, Carpenter PA, Cutler C, et al. Ancillary therapy and supportive care of chronic graft-versus-host disease: national institutes of health consensus development project on criteria for clinical trials in chronic Graft-versus-host disease: V. Ancillary Therapy and Supportive Care Working Group Report. *Biol Blood Marrow Transplant* 2006a; **12**:375–396.

Couriel D, Hosing C, Saliba R, et al. Extracorporeal photopheresis for acute and chronic graft-versus-host disease: does it work? *Biol Blood Marrow Transplant* 2006b; **12**:37–40.

Dastjerdi MH, Hamrah P, Dana R. High-frequency topical cyclosporine 0.05% in the treatment of severe dry eye refractory to twice-daily regimen. *Cornea* 2009; **28**:1091–1096.

Doughty MJ, Glavin S. Efficacy of different dry eye treatments with artificial tears or ocular lubricants: a systematic review. *Ophthalmic Physiol Opt* 2009; **29**:573–583.

Dustin ML. Role of adhesion molecules in activation signaling in T lymphocytes. *J Clin Immunol* 2001; **21**:258–263.

Ferrara JL, Levine JE, Reddy P, et al. Graft-versus-host disease. *Lancet* 2009; **373**:1550–1561.

Filipovich AH, Weisdorf D, Pavletic S, et al. National institutes of health consensus development project on criteria for clinical trials in chronic graft-versus-host disease: I. diagnosis and staging working group report. *Biol Blood Marrow Transplant* 2005; **11**:945–956.

Franklin RM, Kenyon KR, Tutschka PJ, et al. Ocular manifestations of graft-vs-host disease. *Ophthalmology* 1983; **90**:4–13.

Hirst LW, Jabs DA, Tutschka PJ, et al. The eye in bone marrow transplantation. I. Clinical study. *Arch Ophthalmol* 1983; **101**:580–584.

Holler E. Risk assessment in haematopoietic stem cell transplantation: GvHD prevention and treatment. *Best Pract Res Clin Haematol* 2007; **20**:281–294.

Jabs DA, Hirst LW, Green WR, et al. The eye in bone marrow transplantation. II. Histopathology. *Arch Ophthalmol* 1983; **101**:585–590.

Jabs DA, Wingard J, Green WR, et al. The eye in bone marrow transplantation. III. Conjunctival graft-vs-host disease. *Arch Ophthalmol* 1989; **107**:1343–1348.

Janin A, Facon T, Castier P, et al. Pseudomembranous conjunctivitis following bone marrow transplantation: immunopathological and ultrastructural study of one case. *Hum Pathol* 1996; **27**:307–309.

Kim SKC, D. Ghosh, S. Champlin, R. Ocular graft vs. host disease experience from MD Anderson Cancer Center: Newly described clinical spectrum and new approach to the management of stage III and IV ocular GVHD. *Biol Blood Marrow Transplant* 2006; **12**:49–50.

Kim SK, J. Couriel, D. Champlin, R. Surgical management of ocular graft vs. host disease. *Invest Ophthalmol Vis Sci* 2008; **49**:819 (supp).

Kino T, Hatanaka H, Miyata S, et al. FK-506, a novel immunosuppressant isolated from a Streptomyces. II. Immunosuppressive effect of FK-506 in vitro. *J Antibiot (Tokyo)* 1987; **40**:1256–1265.

Loiseau P, Busson M, Balere ML, et al. HLA Association with hematopoietic stem cell transplantation outcome: the number of mismatches at HLA-A, -B, -C, -DRB1, or -DQB1 is strongly associated with overall survival. *Biol Blood Marrow Transplant* 2007; **13**:965–974.

Lopez F, Parker P, Nademanee A, et al. Efficacy of Mycophenolate mofetil (MMF) in the treatment of chronic graft-versus-host disease. *Blood* 2001; **98**:398a.

Martin PJ, Schoch G, Fisher L, et al. A retrospective analysis of therapy for acute graft-versus-host disease: initial treatment. *Blood* 1990; **76**:1464–1472.

Martin PJ, Weisdorf D, Przepiorka D, et al. National institutes of health consensus development project on criteria for clinical trials in chronic graft-versus-host disease: VI. Design of clinical trials working group report. *Biol Blood Marrow Transplant* 2006; **12**:491–505.

McGuirk JP, Weiss ML. Promising cellular therapeutics for prevention or management of graft-versus-host disease (a review). *Placenta* 2011; **32**:S304–S310.

Mookerjee B, Altomonte V, Vogelsang G, Salvage therapy for refractory chronic graft-versus-host disease with mycophenolate mofetil and tacrolimus. *Bone Marrow Transplant* 1999; 24:517–520.

Ogawa Y, Dogru M, et al. Topical tranilast for treatment of the early stage of mild dry eye associated with chronic GVHD. *Bone Marrow Transplant* 2010; **45**:565–569.

Ogawa Y, Okamoto S, Uchino M, et al. Successful treatment of dry eye in two patients with chronic graft-versus-host disease with systemic administration of FK506 and corticosteroids. *Cornea* 2001a; **20**:430–434.

Ogawa Y, Okamoto S, Mori T, et al. Autologous serum eye drops for the treatment of severe dry eye in patients with chronic graft-versus-host disease. *Bone Marrow Transplant* 2003; **31**:579–583.

Ogawa Y, Yamazaki K, Kuwana M, et al. A significant role of stromal fibroblasts in rapidly progressive dry eye in patients with chronic GVHD. *Invest Ophthalmol Vis Sci* 2001b; **42**:111–119.

Pavletic SZ, Martin P, Lee SJ, et al. Measuring therapeutic response in chronic graft-versus-host disease: National Institutes of Health Consensus Development Project on Criteria for Clinical Trials in Chronic Graft-versus-Host disease: IV. Response Criteria Working Group report. *Biol Blood Marrow Transplant* 2006; **12**:252–266.

Perez RL, Perez-Simon JA, Caballero-Velazquez T, et al. Limbus damage in ocular graft-versus-host disease. *Biol Blood Marrow Transplant* 2011; **17**:270–273.

Russo PA, Bouchard CS, Galasso JM. Extended-wear silicone hydrogel soft contact lenses in the management of moderate to severe dry eye signs and symptoms secondary to graft-versus-host disease. *Eye Contact Lens* 2007; **33**:144–147.

Saito T, Shinagawa K, Takenaka K, et al. Ocular manifestation of acute graft-versus-host disease after allogeneic peripheral blood stem cell transplantation. *Int J Hematol* 2002; **75**:332–334.

Shimabukuro-Vornhagen A, Hallek MJ, Storb RF, et al. The role of B cells in the pathogenesis of graft-versus-host disease. *Blood* 2009; **114**:4919–4927.

Shulman HM, Kleiner D, Lee SJ, et al. Histopathologic diagnosis of chronic graft-versus-host disease: National Institutes of Health Consensus Development Project on Criteria for Clinical Trials in chronic graft-versus-host disease: II. Pathology Working Group Report. *Biol Blood Marrow Transplant* 2006; **12**:31–47.

Siadak M, Sullivan KM. The management of chronic graft-versus-host disease. *Blood Rev* 1994; **8**:154–160.

Smith VA, Khan-Lim D, Anderson L, et al. Does orally administered doxycycline reach the tear film? *Br J Ophthalmol* 2008; **92**:856–859.

Sullivan KM, Mori M, Sanders J, et al. Late complications of allogeneic and autologous marrow transplantation. *Bone Marrow Transplant* 1992; **10**: 127–134.

Takahide K, Parker PM, Wu M, et al. Use of fluid-ventilated, gas-permeable scleral lens for management of severe keratoconjunctivitis sicca secondary to chronic graft-versus-host disease. *Biol Blood Marrow Transplant* 2007; **13**:1016–1021.

Tichelli A, Duell T, Weiss M, et al. Late-onset keratoconjunctivitis sicca syndrome after bone marrow transplantation: incidence and risk factors. European Group or Blood and Marrow Transplantation (EBMT) Working Party on Late Effects. *Bone Marrow Transplant* 1996; **17**:1105–1111.

West RH, Szer J, Pedersen JS. Ocular surface and lacrimal disturbances in chronic graft-versus-host disease: the role of conjunctival biopsy. *Aust N Z J Ophthalmol* 1991; **19**:187–191.

Westeneng AC, Hettinga Y, Lokhorst H, et al. Ocular graft-versus-host disease after allogeneic stem cell transplantation. *Cornea* 2010; **29**:758–763.

Yoon KC, Jeong IY, Im SK, et al. Therapeutic effect of umbilical cord serum eyedrops for the treatment of dry eye associated with graft-versus-host disease. *Bone Marrow Transplant* 2007; **39**:231–235.

Chapter 14　Computer vision syndrome

David E. Wang, John D. Awad, Richard W. Yee

■ INTRODUCTION

The advent of desktops, laptops, tablet computers, and even smartphones has revolutionized the workplace and our work habits. Office work had involved a range of activities including typing, filing, reading, and writing. Each activity was adequately varied in the requirements of posture and vision, posing a natural 'break' from the previous activity. The introduction of computers, however, has combined these tasks to where most can be performed without moving from the desktop, thereby improving quality, production, and efficiency. In fact, it is estimated that 75% of all jobs in the year 2000 involved computer usage (Costanza 1994). The popularity and affordability of personal computers with the Internet capabilities at home have introduced even more computer users. In 1990, about 15% of US households owned a computer, a number that has now increased to 50% of all households (Samuelson 1999).

Because of this extensive use of computers, many studies have been conducted in an attempt to address questions concerning safety and health for video display terminal (VDT) users. The large majority of research has addressed the question of radiation levels from VDTs, known to emit many types of radiation, including X-radiation, optical radiation, radiofrequency radiation, very low frequency radiation, and extremely low frequency radiation. Studies have not clearly indicated a negative effect on the computer user. During the late 1980s and early 1990s, concern of possible reproductive effects from using VDTs arose following reports of adverse pregnancy outcomes among groups of women computer users. Most women in modern offices, who work with VDTs, do not increase their risk of miscarriage. One study has revealed that somatic disorders, depression, and obsession are increased with computer usage, especially when operating times are >30 h/week and usage of >10 years (Wang et al. 1998).

Studies have shown, however, that vision problems and symptoms associated with the use of the eyes are the most frequently occurring health problems among VDT users (Thomson 1998). The main visual symptoms reported by VDT users include eyestrain, tired eyes, irritation, burning sensation, redness, blurred vision, and double vision, thus termed the phrase 'computer vision syndrome' (CVS). CVS not only causes pain and discomfort to the individual, but also reduces overall efficiency by reducing the time that a person can effectively work and concentrate while using a computer. Thus, CVS represents a drain on productivity and serves to increase medical expenses associated with treating ocular complaints.

In 1992, a total of 1307 surveys were completed by optometrists who reported that the majority of VDT patients had symptoms that were different than other near-point workers, especially as related to glare, lighting, unique viewing conditions, and spectacle requirements. Greater frequency and severity of symptoms were also noted (Sheedy 1992). It is estimated that the diagnosis and treatment of these symptoms cost almost US$2 billion each year (Abelson 1999). One recent study shows that there is a significantly higher degree of meibomian gland dysfunction (MGD) in symptomatic computer users than in computer users who have lesser degrees of ocular surface complaints (Yee et al. 2007). As computer users become more aware of CVS, it is important that ophthalmologists are attentive to this rapidly evolving disorder, as we could be facing a possible epidemic of the twenty-first century. If 90% of the 70 million US workers, who use computers for >3 h/day, experience CVS in some form, that equates to at least 63 million sufferers who are in need of an effective remedy. This chapter examines the epidemiology, causes, associations, and current treatments of CVS.

■ DIAGNOSIS

■ CVS and asthenopia

It is quite clear that use of a VDT creates asthenopia or a feeling of ocular discomfort or tiredness. In fact, visual complaints were reported by 75% of VDT operators working 6–9 hours in front of their screens compared to 50% of the other workers (Mutti & Zadnik 1996). Surveys of optometrists in the United States and the UK indicate that 12.4% and 9.0% of their patients, respectively, are examined primarily because of visual or ocular problems associated with using a computer. The eye-related problems are largely symptomatic.

Many individuals have marginal vision disorders, such as difficulties with accommodation, or binocular vision problems that do not cause symptoms when performing less demanding visual tasks. After working with the monitor, the most important changes are the following: diminished power of accommodation, removal of the near point of convergence, and deviation of phoria for near vision. These results suggest that the weakness of important visual functions could be the cause of eyestrain in computer operators (Trusiewicz et al. 1995). In another study subjects overaccommodated by an average of –0.50 to –0.75 D when stimuli were at 40 cm, and by –0.75 D to colored letters on a colored background. Prolonged work at a VDT has been reported to result in changes in both relative accommodation and vergence. Gur and Ron evaluated the prevalence of vision problems in VDT workers as well as the effect of 4 days of VDT use on near-point accommodation (NPA). They measured NPA for VDT users and non-users at the beginning of the day at the start of the workweek, and again at the end of the day, 4 days later. Interestingly, a high prevalence of exophoria, convergence insufficiency, and low fusional convergence was found among VDT workers. They also found that the accommodative amplitude decreased significantly more for VDT users (by 0.69 D) than for non-users (0.18 D) between the first examination and the second one, 4 days later (Mutti & Zadnik 1996).

In another longitudinal study, Yeow and Taylor reported that subjects younger than 40 years who used VDTs lost more accommodative amplitude than who did not.

In summary, changes in accommodative and vergence functions have been reported to occur after work periods at a VDT, and these changes have been proposed as objective indicators of subjective visual fatigue. They are also most likely transient, with workers returning to baseline values by the end of the workday or week. If not, substantial losses in these functions would be expected in long-term studies.

Such studies have not found any difference, at least in NPA and near-point of convergence (NPC), between VDT users and non-users. VDTs are a major source of near work for many adults, but do not appear to result in losses of accommodative and vergence function beyond the ordinary effects of age.

CVS and transient myopia

Accommodative effort during near work is thought to be a causative factor in the development of myopia. While it is questionable whether VDTs are associated with a risk of myopic progression in adults compared to paperwork, it is clear that near work with VDTs results in a small, temporary myopic shift. In a cross-sectional comparison of VDT users and typists, VDT users experienced a myopic shift of about −0.12 D after the work period, while the refractive error of typists was unchanged (Laubli & Grandjean 1981). The shifts were too small to affect distant visual acuity.

There is no compelling evidence in the literature that there is a significant increase in the risk of myopia onset or progression from the use of VDTs by adults compared to other forms of near work. A small, transient myopic shift appears to occur after VDT use, but its significance to creating permanent myopic change is unknown.

Computer vision syndrome and MGD: a working hypothesis

The rate at which people blink decreases by >60% when they stare at a computer screen, suggesting that the acute decrease in blinks can acutely increase symptoms of dry eye disease (DED) (Freudenthaler et al. 2003). Computer users often report that their eyes feel dry, burning, gritty, or heavy after an extended period at the terminal. Their eyes may even reflexively tear in an attempt to restore the proper chemical balance and to properly lubricate and rewet the front surface of the eye. DED may be a primary cause of ocular fatigue, such as experienced when using a VDT, where the blink rate is decreased and the exposed ocular surface area is increased, causing desiccation of the eye. It has been postulated that the blink rate is decreased further in a dark setting where it is difficult to read, and that accelerated desiccation may be responsible for the fatigue (Wallin et al. 1994).

The tear film, which overlies and protects the cornea, consists of, from anterior surface inward, a lipid layer, an aqueous gel layer, and a mucin layer. DED results from evaporation of the aqueous component. The lipid surface layer protects the aqueous layer from too-rapid evaporation. It is secreted as meibum by the meibomian glands embedded in the eyelids. The normal physiological mechanism of meibum secretion is associated with the eye blink. The normal full eye blink expresses meibum from the glands and spreads it evenly on top of the aqueous layer over the cornea. Several studies have shown that computer use, significantly more than other visual tasks, such as reading and watching television, produces considerable reduction of the spontaneous blink rate. Hence, our current observations suggest that computer use reduces meibum secretion and exposes the tear film to increased aqueous evaporation, increasing the risk of DED signs and symptoms. Because the tear film is maintained by a balance of secretion of the lipid meibum layer by the meibomian glands and the aqueous layer by the lacrimal and auxiliary lacrimal glands, reduction of secretion of either results in a tear film imbalance that can lead to symptoms and, if severe enough, signs of DED. If loss of meibum is unavoidable with aging, it would seem that reducing evaporation of aqueous by other methods should effectively restore the normal balance. Although

there is a significantly high association of moderate-to-severe MGD with computer use, one can only speculate that computer use may increase the occurrence of and possibly play a role in the progression and pathogenesis of MGD.

An immediate reduction in blink rate will acutely alter the ocular surface because it causes poor tear spreading and dessication. Longer term reduction of blinking may alter meibomian gland secretion not directly related to the gland's natural course, leading to chronic changes in the muscles involved in secretion (Riolan's and orbicularis muscles) and possibly the secretion itself. Eventually, MGD may worsen, causing further reduction of the outflow of meibum, alteration in the normal bacterial flora, increase in inflammation, and obstruction of the glands. Thus, reduced blink rate at the computer contributes to poor tear film quality and increased evaporation, which, in turn, produces symptoms of DED, which will most likely reduce the overall efficiency and comfort of work. Furthermore, the positive correlation between lifetime computer usage and ocular surface disease index (OSDI) score shows that people who use the computer tend to have more significant ocular surface symptoms (Yee et al. 2007). Interestingly, the variable that correlates with ocular symptoms is not current computer usage, but lifetime computer usage, suggesting that prolonged computer usage has an additive negative effect on ocular surface health.

FACTORS INFLUENCING SURFACE DISEASE THROUGH COMPUTER USAGE

There are several factors that contribute to DED. They include the following.

Environmental factors

The cornea is very sensitive to drying and chemical imbalances from environmental factors. Around the office, these include dry air, ventilation fans, static buildup, airborne paper dust, laser and photocopy toner, building contaminants, and the like.

Reduced blink rate

Most individuals blink 10–15 times/min. Studies have shown that the blink rate at the computer is significantly less. A reduced blink rate at the VDT contributes to a poor-quality tear film and temporary as well as long-term stress upon the cornea and ocular surface. This results in symptoms of DED.

Increased exposure

Normally the reading of text on paper is done while looking downwards. This results in the eyelid covering a good deal of the front surface of the eye. This covering minimizes the evaporation of tears. On the other hand, computer users look at their reading material in straight ahead gaze. This results in a wider opening between the eyelids, and an increased surface area exposed to the effects of evaporation.

Gender

The prevalence of DED is twice as frequent in females (4.8%) compared to males (2.2%).

Age

Tear production normally decreases with age. Although DED can occur at any age in both men and women, postmenopausal women represent the group of individuals affected most by DED.

Menopause

Hormonal changes have been identified as contributing to DED. However, sometimes it is difficult to assess the relative contributions of menopause and aging.

Systemic diseases and disease syndromes

DED is associated with various systemic diseases. A general review of the patient's entire medical history aids in establishing a complete diagnosis. In the case of Sjögren's syndrome, dry mouth and rheumatoid arthritis can assist in making the diagnosis. Several autoimmune diseases also have association with DED. Regardless of age, an abnormal basal or Schrimer's 1 (<10 mm) warrants a referral to confirm a systemic disease associated with aqueous deficiency.

Systemic medications

There are several systemic medications contributing to ocular drying. Most prominent among them are diuretics, antihistamines, psychotomimetics, and antihypertensives.

Contact lens wear

Office workers wearing contact lenses have been found to be more likely to fall into the severe category of ocular discomfort (Wallin et al. 1994). Contact lens comfort is highly dependent on the fit of the lens and lubrication of the eye. The contact lens surfaces should skate along the eye and eyelid surfaces with minimal resistance. If the eye is dry, the lenses dry and adhere to the upper eyelid during the blink. This 'friction effect' from DED produces the discomfort described.

Cosmetics

Poorly applied eye makeup can block the openings of the oil-secreting meibomian glands and create debris and inflammation. This, in turn, contributes to a rapid evaporation of the water component of the tear film and deposition of foreign bodies from the makeup in the tear film or on the ocular surface with resultant discomfort.

Cholesterol

Patients with moderate to severe MGD may have increased levels of total cholesterol compared to control population (Dao et al. 2010). We also found a statistically significant decreased prevalence of low high-density lipoprotein (HDL) in patients with moderate to severe MGD relative to the control population. The cause of this is unknown, but the findings suggest that elevated HDL may be a risk factor for the development of meibomian gland disease, despite being known as 'good cholesterol' with its cardioprotective effects. More studies, both at the prospective and basic science levels, will be needed to examine the significance of this finding. It suggests that ophthalmologists may be instrumental in the early detection of dyslipidemia in the general population. The ability to screen for lipid abnormalities by physical examination at the slit lamp is exciting and can be telling. Prospective studies should be conducted to justify early screening of patients with moderate to severe MGD for dyslipidemia.

VISUAL EFFECTS OF DISPLAY CHARACTERISTICS

Display quality

The National Research Council Committee on Vision stated that 'poor display quality … probably contributes to the annoyance and discomfort sometimes reported by workers… Visual performance is affected by a number of display parameters, such as character size, structure, and style; and by image contrast and stability'. There appears to be little disagreement regarding the effect of monitor design and display quality on visual performance.

The images produced on a VDT consist of thousands of tiny, bright spots (pixels) or horizontal lines (rasters), which collectively form unresolved images that blur together and lack sharp edges. The more the dots or lines displayed on a monitor to produce a picture, the sharper and clearer the image will appear. It is thought that slightly blurred characters can overstimulate the ciliary muscles of the operator's eyes in a futile attempt to produce a clear image. Ziefle noted a functional characteristic of computer operators and resolution through the comparison of monitor resolutions at 62 dots per inch (dpi) and 89 dpi (Ziefle 1998). He determined that search reaction times and fixation durations when viewing documents were significantly increased with the lower resolution. In addition, the extent of visual fatigue correlated with both search reaction times and eye movement parameters. Fortunately, over the past decade the resolution of monitors has improved drastically, producing displays approaching that of typeset documents (Thomson 1998).

Several factors affect readability and legibility of characters displayed on the screen. Words containing upper case in combination with lower case are more easily interpreted than all upper case documents. The spacing between characters and lines also affects picture quality and should allow for at least one-half character space between words and one character space between lines. High levels of contrast and brightness are known to represent the most common causes of character blur. It is also recommended that screens contain dark characters against a light background display screen, rather than the opposite (Thomson 1998). When a VDT operator constantly switches from a light background hard copy to dark background display, fatigue of the iris muscle can result.

Lighting and glare

Improper lighting conditions of a workstation can also adversely affect a VDT user's ocular comfort. Constant and bright illumination from surrounding sources of light (e.g. overhead fluorescent, large windows, and desk lamps) appears to wash out screen character images, creating reflection and glare. Although these problems are not thought to produce chronic visual disorders, they can be sources of annoyance and possibly visual fatigue. One recent study compared varying amounts of background surrounding luminance with subjective evaluations of asthenopia and specific objective measurements. The results of the study showed no significance in the value of surrounding luminance on the asthenopic symptoms for either cathode ray tube or liquid crystal display monitors. However, surrounding luminance was shown to significantly reduce the accommodation amplitude (Wolska & Switula

1999). Another study revealed conflicting evidence concerning screen reflections. Glare was found to increase the amount of time required to read relatively easy passages but decrease the amount of time to read relatively difficult passages (Garcia & Wierwille 1985).

It was believed that, since screen reflections are imaged behind the computer monitor, potentially conflicting cues could be created to initiate inappropriate accommodation responses. Collins et al. (1994), however, found little evidence that reflections influence the accuracy of a user's accommodation response under binocular viewing conditions. They did, however, detect errors to a small degree (<0.25 D) under some monocular viewing conditions.

In cases where it is not practical to reduce surrounding light, reduction of reflections and increase in contrast may be obtained from antiglare filters (Sheedy 1997). While ambient light from the room passes through the glare filter twice (once on the way in and once on reflection), direct light emitted from the VDT passes through the filter only once. This increases the overall contrast of the picture because the background is attenuated more than the characters.

Recent studies demonstrate differing results in the efficacy of symptom relief with screen filters. One recent study revealed that of 60 full-time VDT workers, the 40 participants who used a screen filter reported less occurrence, shorter duration, and less intensive eye and musculoskeletal complaints after 1 month of use. The authors concluded that screen filters could improve the conditions for visual perception and thus relieve eyestrain (Hladky & Prochazka 1998). Screen filters were also found to help schoolchildren with myopia, who reported significant functional changes after 0.5 hour of computer usage, improving their overall functional indices. In contrast, a study of 25,064 participants investigated whether screen filters reduced the incidence of asthenopia with reference to weekly time spent at a VDT and duration of work at a VDT. The group shows that filters by themselves do not reduce the occurrence of asthenopia. Moreover, the ocular symptoms associated with environmental illumination may be due to keratitis from surface disease and necessitate a complete ocular examination. It is apparent that more research is needed to determine whether screen filters are effective in the relief of ocular symptoms, and if so, which specific types of filters are most supportive in symptom relief.

Refresh rates

The refresh rate of a VDT represents the number of times per minute (measured in Hz) the screen is repainted to produce an image. If the refresh rate is too slow, the characters on the screen may appear to flicker. The flicker rate is of particular importance, since the National Research Council reported that extremely low refresh rates (8–14 Hz) could induce epileptogenic seizures. Perceived flicker has resulted in subjective complaints of annoyance, fatigue, and headache. The critical fusion frequency is the refresh rate at which humans can no longer distinguish the pulsating beams of light as separate entities. In most viewing situations, this rate is 30–50 Hz. The Video Electronic Standards Association has recommended a minimum refresh rate of 75 Hz, which minimizes flicker at all brightness levels. Berman et al. (1991) supplied evidence to perhaps support this recommendation with their study on human electroretinogram (ERG) responses. They clearly identified a synchronous ERG response for a VDT stimulus, operating at 76 Hz.

Studies have shown that much higher refresh rates may decrease ocular symptoms and increase user functionality. Jaschinski et al. (1996) compared refresh rates of 300 Hz and the lowest frequency that did not produce visible flicker for each subject (50–90 Hz in this study). At the lower refresh rate, mean accommodation in monocular vision was 0.06 D weaker, median eye blink duration was 6% shorter, and mean eye blink interval was 15% longer. Another study determined that reading from a display at 500 Hz was eight words per minute (3.05%) faster than at 60 Hz (Montegut et al. 1997). Lower refresh rates (50 Hz compared to 100 Hz) increase the number of prematurely triggered, less accurate saccades and an increase in the number of disrupted saccades in flight, which land short of their intended target.

Radiation

The potential of health risk has persisted in the public eye concerning the claims that radiation emissions from VDTs could be responsible for hazardous effects to the computer user. Ionizing radiation is known to cause cellular changes and can affect living tissue through the breaking of chemical bonds and the charging neutral molecules (Scalet 1987). However, VDTs neither produce nor emit a-, b-, g-, or hard X-radiation. Small amount of soft X-rays is produced, but almost all of the radiation is contained by the monitor's glass screen. Even still, press reports continue to speculate that VDTs can potentially be responsible for skin problems, spontaneous abortions, and ocular disorders.

Numerous studies have shown that there is no evidence to support that VDT operators face health hazards or are exposed to electric, magnetic, or ionizing radiation fields significantly above ambient levels (Thomson 1998). Furthermore, Oftedal et al. (1999) determined that a reduction in the electric field surrounding a VDT, through the use of an electric-conducting screen filter, did not reveal a significant reduction of eye symptom severity. Kirsner and Federman published a review of the literature and found that the data reviewed were either inconsistent or methodically flawed. They concluded that continued research should be performed to further define and elucidate the risk of electromagnetic radiation produced by VDTs (Kirsner & Federman 1998).

TREATMENT

Without any doubt, the treatment of CVS requires a multidirectional approach due to the variety of complaints between users. When treating a patient, it is important to consider ocular therapy as well as adjustment of the user's workstation and habits in an ergo-ophthalmological approach.

A complete ocular surface examination by subspecialty corneal and ocular surface experts is imperative to rule out local and systemic events associated with DED, blepharitis, inflammation, and lid margin disease. Patients with significant aqueous deficiency basal or Schirmer's I < 5 mm should be evaluated by an internist or referred to the rheumatologist to rule out autoimmune diseases.

Local ocular surface disorders should be treated aggressively and on a chronic basis. Eye care providers and patients need to understand the chronicity of this disorder in order to maintain compliance of doctor-recommended treatment approaches. This includes restoring aqueous deficiencies with lubrication and partial or complete punctal occlusion, and short- and long-term inflammation control with varying combinations of topical steroids, omega 3s, flaxseed, and topical cyclosporin A. Isolation techniques, that is, MEGS or specialized contact lenses, are helpful if the patients are moderately to severely symptomatic or have significant findings of dry eye or lid margin disease on clinical examination.

Lighting

As mentioned earlier, proper lighting within the computer workstation area will enable the user to improve visual comfort and performance while eliminating annoyance and visual fatigue. An ideal environment would allow equalized brightness throughout the user's visual field. Intense fluorescent lights can be diminished by removing a few of the lighting tubes. Excessive window lighting should be filtered with blinds, window coverings, or window tinting. If bright spots in the visual field cannot be avoided, shifting the workstation to a more favorable position may provide relief.

The actual type of lighting also appears to be important. One study focused on the visual work capacity with different sources of illumination. After comparing natural light, filament lamps, luminescent lamps, sodium lamps, and mercury arc lamps, it was found that sodium lamps were the most adequate for high functional capacity of the visual analyzer.

Task lights, or desktop lamps, use incandescent bulbs, which are 'warmer' (contain more red), easier on the eyes, and cause less glare and eyestrain. Task lights are often too bright; thus, it is important to position the light carefully so that it does not throw bright light into the eyes.

As previously discussed, antiglare filters may not reduce symptoms of asthenopia, but have been shown to reduce glare and improve contrast from the screen. This provides an effective means to eliminate reflections and therefore improve visual comfort. Surface abnormalities are often missed; however, if detected and adequately treated, it will reduce light sensitivity-related complaints.

VDT positioning

Computer users often assume uncomfortable positions in order to properly view the screen. As previously mentioned, these postural distortions often lead to pain in the back, neck, and shoulder. It is thus important to properly distance the monitor and maintain proper monitor height.

Previously, it was recommended that the eye should be 16–30 inches from the screen. Distances outside this range usually indicate a poor screen resolution or images that are too small. Recent data suggest that further distances may be more favorable to ocular symptoms. Three studies have compared visual strain with various screen distances at lengths of 66 cm (26.0 inches) versus 98 cm (38.6 inches), 50 cm (19.6 inches) versus 100 cm (39.4 inches), and 63 cm (24.8 inches) versus 92 cm (36.2 inches). In all three cases, participants reported more eyestrain at the shorter distances from the monitor. These studies suggest that distances of 35–40 inches may produce fewer complaints of visual strain.

It is recommended that the screen should be placed 10–20° below (or the middle of the screen 5–6 inches below) the eye level. When the screen is higher than this level, VDT users often tilt back their heads, causing muscle strain on the upper trapezius and neck. Kietrys et al. (1998) also report that a raised monitor has no beneficial effect of reducing postural stress of the cervical spine. Lowering the monitor allows the VDT user to gaze downward, thus exposing less ocular surface to ambient air and reducing tear film loss. Studies have shown that high screens result in greater eyestrain than low screens, and that users actually prefer the low VDT position.

Work breaks

Research has shown that when regular breaks are implemented, work efficiency improves, usually compensating for the time lost during the break. The National Institute of Occupational Safety and Health found that short, frequent breaks demonstrated a decrease in worker discomfort and increase in productivity compared to the historical 15-minute morning and afternoon breaks. Taking a quick walk around the office provides stretching of strained and fatigued muscles, a change of scenery, and possible relaxation.

Long periods of work without breaks are thought to be detrimental to ocular symptoms. In fact, one study showed that working for >4 hours at the VDT had a significant association with asthenopia (Sanchez-Roman et al. 1996). Frequent breaks are recommended to restore and relax the accommodative system, thereby preventing eyestrain. It is commonly believed that looking away at a distant object at least twice an hour during computer usage is sufficient for prevention of visual fatigue.

Lubricating drops

One of the most simple and therapeutic modes of therapy are using lubricating eyedrops intended to relieve the symptoms of dry eyes due to decreased blink rates. Abelson states that 'an over-the-counter tear substitute can periodically rewet the ocular surface, contribute to tear volume, and maintain the proper balance of salts and acidity while viewing a terminal.' It is important, though, to find the proper lubricating eyedrop for the VDT user. One study in Japan revealed that the majority of self-medicating eyedrop users were dissatisfied with the therapeutic effects (Shimmura et al. 1999). Another study indicates that higher-viscosity eyedrops may be more beneficial than balanced salt solutions. Although the higher-viscosity eyedrops did not vary blink rates, they normalized the interblink interval and relieved ocular discomfort more efficiently than balanced salt solutions following VDT use. While artificial tears are effective, other medications such as cyclosporin A drops may need to be administered long term to effectively treat the chronic ocular surface inflammation.

Computer eyeglasses

Studies show that it is effective to reduce the evaporation rate by providing a physical barrier to air currents, evaporation, and particles by creating an increased relative humidity via an enclosed environment, with the use of glasses that isolate the ocular surface and provide a microenvironment over the eye. Isolation techniques with swim or workshop goggles or modified spectacles surrounding the eye decrease entry of particulate matter and prevent desiccation and the associated increase in cytokines (Stern et al. 2006).

HISTORICAL STUDIES

Earlier studies have evaluated signs and symptoms of DED under control conditions where the eye is open to the ambient air versus experimental conditions produced with use of side-baffled eye glasses (sometimes in combination with an added moisture pad), completely enclosed swimming goggles, or a separate steam-producing device.

Side-baffled glasses

In 10 DED patients and 10 normal controls, Tsubota et al. (1994) measured humidity near the cornea in eyes wearing (1) empty spectacle frames, (2) spectacles, (3) side-baffled glasses alone, and (4) side-baffled glasses with moisture pads. Humidity was significantly higher in the eyes wearing side-baffled glasses with moisture pads than in those wearing side-baffled glasses alone, and humidity was higher in eyes wearing side-baffled glasses with or without moisture pads than in eyes wearing spectacles or empty frames. Measurements were taken under still-air conditions and with fan-created wind directed at the face. Dry eye patients were selected based on subjective complaints and scores beyond stated cutoffs on one or more of the following tests: Rose Bengal and fluorescein staining, tear break-up time (TBUT), basal tear test, and the cotton thread test. Effectiveness was judged by subjective comfort and reduced ad libitum use of artificial tears. In a separate clinical study, 14 of 16 patients with DED reported that they were very comfortable with the use of glasses and moisture pads, and 4 of these reported complete relief of symptoms. However, of the objective tests, only the Rose Bengal and fluorescein scores showed significant improvement over the control conditions with the periocular isolation and moisture pads.

Lindstrom and Weberling reported a subjective questionnaire on commercially available (under the trade name of Panoptx) motorcycle style glasses, which use padded foam linings to isolate the eyes. They reported highly significant improvements in subjective comfort under a number of categories.

■ Completely enclosed swimming goggles

Korb et al. (1996) measured the thickness of the tear film lipid layer in 13 patients with DED, with one eye encased in swimming goggles and the other eye wearing a goggle with the lens removed. The lipid layer was monitored over a 60-minute period with goggles on, and then over an additional 60-minute period after the goggles were removed. The encased eye's lipid layer thickness (measured by color interferometry) increased significantly ($p < 0.0001$) within 5 minutes, reaching an increased thickness of 66.4 nm after 15 minutes of goggle wear, which was maintained to the end of the 60-minute postgoggle period. The control eye showed no significant changes.

■ Humidity treatment

Matsumoto et al. (2006) studied the effectiveness of raising periocular humidity in 15 patients with MGD by applying a new warm moist air steamer device for 10 minutes before measurements were taken of the temperature of eyelids and cornea. Symptoms of ocular fatigue by the visual analog scale (VAS) were measured before and after application of the device, as were the Schirmer's test, TBUT, DR-1 lipid layer interferometry, and fluorescein and Rose Bengal staining. Long-term effects were assessed in 20 additional patients with MGD, of whom 10 used the steamer device and the other 10 used warm moist pads, both applied for 10 minutes twice daily for 2 weeks. VAS scores improved significantly following use of the warm moist air device in both short-term and long-term studies, but not following the compresses. DR-1 measures of lipid layer interference showed significant thickening after 10 minutes of the steamer device and after long-term use. The warm compress increased lipid layer thickness in the long-term study, but not as much as the steamer device.

■ USE OF MICROENVIRONMENT GLASSES (MEGS)

Occasional computer viewers may be able to get away with using their general eyewear, but those who spend several hours a day, including the occupational user, can benefit from the use of computer glasses.

Presbyopes have much to consider when deciding the right format of eyewear. Conventional bifocals are designed for viewing at 16 inches at an angle of [3]20° below primary gaze. Computer screens are usually 24 inches away and only slightly below primary gaze. General-wear progressive lenses are better, providing clear vision at an intermediate distance. Although one study has shown that users have preferred progressive lenses in the past (Bachman 1992), the user must continually engage in a frustrating and fatiguing search for the perfect 'sweet spot' on the lens that gives a clear view of the screen. This results in both annoyance and head and neck strain, causing sore muscles. Occupational progressive lenses are now available, which incorporate a large area in the top half of the lens for mid-distance viewing (i.e. VDT) and a bottom half of the lens for near distance (i.e. keyboard and desktop). Some lenses even contain a small area for distance viewing, usually at the top of the lens. One study revealed that 24 symptomatic VDT users were significantly relieved from 7 of 10 symptoms reported (including neck and shoulder aches, eyestrain, and blurred intermediates) following the use of occupational lenses (Butzon & Eagels 1997).

Eyeglasses can also provide a few other benefits for the treatment of CVS. Grant has suggested that the near triad of accommodation, convergence, and miosis should be expanded to include depression of gaze and extorsion (Grant 1987). The increase in extorsion observed on elevation of gaze at near point may induce binocular disruption and strain. Lazarus has shown that base-up and base-in prism could alleviate some of the CVS complaints, since they decrease the elevation and convergence required. A double-blind study of 30 VDT users indicated a preference for prism and plus lenses over plus lenses without prism (Lazarus 1996). Color-contrast optic filters are known to improve the color-discriminating capacity when exposed to VDTs. Feigin et al. (1998) revealed that 20 of 23 subjects reported an improvement of visual fatigue after 4 weeks of using the eyeglasses with spectral filters. Micro-environment glasses (MEGS), unlike swim goggles, can be optically modified with the suggestions above and still create an increase in humidified microenvironment that successfully reduces dry eye symptoms and signs (i.e. punctate staining and improved TBUT) as well as symptoms in symptomatic computer users (Yee et al. 2007).

■ CONCLUSION

As the general public becomes more aware of CVS, it is imperative that ophthalmologists and optometrists are attentive to this rapidly evolving disorder. An important question arises whether ocular surface disease can be considered a direct consequence of long-term computer use. Researchers have found a significant correlation between cumulative lifetime computer use and OSDI scores that indicated dry eye symptoms. Unfortunately direct comparisons between computer users and non-users are not easily possible because in this day and age, the latter cannot be found in an available cohort. Even subjects who did not use computers at their workplace reported that they routinely spent several hours a day surfing the net on computers after working. It may well be that high computer usage raises the number of dry eye sufferers and/or increases the severity of symptoms, but studies have not produced any direct comparison of groups that would allow us to conclude that computer use bears a long-term causal relation to ocular surface disease. There needs to be more prospective studies to elucidate the direct relationship between ocular surface disease (i.e. MGD) and CVS.

■ REFERENCES

Abelson MB. How to fight computer vision syndrome. *Rev Ophthalmol* 1999:114–116.

Bachman WG. Computer-specific spectacle lens design preference of presbyopic operators. *J Occup Med* 1992; **34**:1023–1027.

Berman SM, Greenhouse DS, Bailey IL, et al. Human electroretinogram responses to video displays, fluorescent lighting, and other high frequency sources. *Optom Vis Sci* 1991; **68**:645–662.

Butzon SP, Eagels SR. Prescribing for the moderate-to-advanced ametropic presbyopic VDT user. A comparison of the Technica Progressive and Datalite CRT trifocal. *J Am Optom Assoc* 1997; **68**:495–502.

Collins M, Davis B, Atchison D. VDT screen reflections and accommodation response. *Ophthalmic Physiol Opt* 1994; **14**:193–198.

Costanza MA. Visual and ocular symptoms related to the use of video display terminals. *J Behav Optom* 1994; **5**:31–36.

Dao AH, Spindle JD, Harp BA, et al. Association of dyslipidemia in moderate to severe meibomian gland dysfunction. *Am J Ophthalmol* 2010; **150**:371–375.

Feigin AA, Zak PP, Korniushina TA, Rozenblium Iu Z. Prevention of visual fatigue in computer users by eyeglasses with spectral filters. *Vestn Oftalmol* 1998; **114**:34–36.

Freudenthaler N, Neuf H, Kadner G, Schlote T. Characteristics of eye blink activity during video display terminal use in healthy volunteers. *Graefes Arch Clin Exp Ophthalmol* 2003; **241**:914–920.

Garcia KD, Wierwille WW. Effect of Glare on performance of a VDT reading-comprehension task. *Hum Factors* 1985; **27**:163–173.

Grant AH. The computer user syndrome. *J Am Optom Assoc* 1987; **58**:892–901.

Hladky A, Prochazka B. Using a screen filter positively influences the physical well-being of VDU operators. *Cent Eur J Public Health* 1998; **6**:249–253.

Jaschinski W, Bonacker M, Alshuth E. Accommodation, convergence, pupil diameter and eye blinks at a CRT display flickering near fusion limit. *Ergonomics* 1996; **39**:152–164.

Kietrys DM, McClure PW, Fitzgerald GK. The relationship between head and neck posture and VDT screen height in keyboard operators. *Phys Ther* 1998; **78**:395–403.

Kirsner RS, Federman DG. Video display terminals: risk of electromagnetic radiation. *South Med J* 1998; **91**:12–16.

Korb DR, Greiner JV, Glonek T, et al. Effect of periocular humidity on the tear film lipid layer. *Cornea* 1996; **15**:129–134.

Laubli T HW, Grandjean E. Postural and visual loads at VDT workplaces II. Lighting conditions and visual impairments. *Ergonomics* 1981; **24**:933–944.

Lazarus SM. The use of yoked base-up and base-in prism for reducing eye strain at the computer. *J Am Optom Assoc* 1996; **67**:204–208 (see comments published erratum appears in J Am Optom Assoc 1996; 67:315).

Matsumoto Y, Dogru M, Goto E, et al. Efficacy of new warm moist air device on tear functions of patients with simple meibomian gland dysfunction. *Cornea* 2006; **25**:644–650.

Montegut MJ, Bridgeman B, Sykes J. High refresh rate and oculomotor adaptation facilitate reading from video displays. *Spat Vis* 1997; **10**:305–322.

Mutti DO, Zadnik K. Is computer use a risk factor for myopia? *J Am Optom Assoc* 1996; **67**:521–530.

Oftedal G, Nyvang A, Moen BE. Long-term effects on symptoms by reducing electric fields from visual display units. *Scand J Work Environ Health* 1999; **25**:415–421.

Samuelson RJ. The PC Boom—and now Bust? Newsweek 1999:52.

Sanchez-Roman FR, Perez-Lucio C, Juarez-Ruiz C, et al. Risk factors for asthenopia among computer terminal operators. *Salud Publica Mex* 1996; **38**:189–196.

Scalet EA. VDT health and safety: issues and solutions. Lawrence, Kansas: Ergosyst Associates, 1987.

Sheedy JE. How to treat computer users. *Review of Ophthalmology* 1997:181-189.

Sheedy JE. Vision problems at video display terminals: a survey of optometrists. *J Am Optom Assoc* 1992; **63**:687–692.

Shimmura S, Shimazaki J, Tsubota K. Results of a population-based questionnaire on the symptoms and lifestyles associated with dry eye. *Cornea* 1999; **18**:408–411.

Stern ME, Pflugfelder SC, Siemasko KF, et al. Desiccation stress to the ocular surface induces a transferable T-cell mediated lacrimal keratoconjunctivitis. *Invest Ophthalmol Vis Sci* 2006;47:E-abstract 3530 (www.arvo.org)

Thomson WD. Eye problems and visual display terminals—the facts and the fallacies. *Ophthalmic Physiol Opt* 1998; **18**:111–119.

Trusiewicz D, Niesluchowska M, Makszewska-Chetnik Z. Eye-strain symptoms after work with a computer screen. *Klin Oczna* 1995; **97**:343–345.

Tsubota K, Yamada M, Urayama K. Spectacle side panels and moist inserts for the treatment of dry eye patients. *Cornea* 1994; **13**:197–120.

Wallin JA ZZ, Jacobsen JL, Jacobsen SD. A preliminary study of the effects of computer glasses on reported VDT user symptoms: a field study. *J Saf Res* 1994; **25**:67–76.

Wang W, Li C, Zhan C, Long Y. Study on the psychological status of video display terminal operator. *Wei Sheng Yen Chiu* 1998; **27**:233–236.

Wolska A, Switula M. Luminance of the surround and visual fatigue of VDT operators. *Int J Occup Saf Ergon* 1999; **5**:553–581.

Yee RW, Sperling HG, Kattek A, et al. Isolation of the ocular surface to treat dysfunctional tear syndrome associated with computer use. 2007; **5**:308–315.

Ziefle M. Effects of display resolution on visual performance. *Hum Factors* 1998; **40**:554–568.

Chapter 15 Anterior blepharitis

Jose M. Benitez-del-Castillo, Pedro Arriola-Villalobos, David Diaz-Valle, Michael A. Lemp

INTRODUCTION

Anterior blepharitis is one of the most common conditions seen in the ophthalmologist's office. A prevalence of 12% in anterior blepharitis has been reported in patients with ocular discomfort (Saccà et al. 2006), with 37% of patients seen by ophthalmologists in the United States experiencing blepharitis (Lemp & Nichols 2009). However, it remains a diagnostic and therapeutic challenge, with frequent frustration both in patients and in clinicians, due to its very complex spectrum of signs and symptoms. Although rarely threatening sight, anterior blepharitis is an annoying and symptomatic disease, and patients frequently move from ophthalmologist to ophthalmologist looking for a better solution to their problem. Cornea and bulbar conjunctiva may be injured by contiguous lid inflammation, resulting in vascular congestion and infiltration of the conjunctiva and corneal damage, including new vessel growth and epithelial breakdown.

The term 'blepharitis' is a general one, describing inflammation of the lid as a whole. Anterior blepharitis describes inflammation of the lid margin anterior to the gray line and centered around the lashes (McCulley et al. 1982). Anterior blepharitis may be accompanied by squamous debris or collarettes around the base of the lashes and vascular changes of the lid skin (Nelson et al. 2011) (**Figure 15.1**).

The lid margin is a complex structure, which facilitates lid diseases. The skin is thin, and the mucocutaneous junction contains many glandular structures. Besides, the eyelid provides mechanical protection of the ocular surface, limiting exposure to the environment.

CLASSIFICATION

First of all, a fundamental distinction should be made between acute anterior blepharitis and chronic anterior blepharitis. Usually, acute blepharitis means acute infections of the lid, whereas chronic blepharitis refers to chronic low-grade inflammatory disease.

Fuchs, one century ago, made the first classification of marginal lid disease in two groups: blepharitis squamosa, with hyperemia of the lid border and dry scales; and blepharitis ulcerosa, with marginal crusting, small ulcers of the surface, and microabscesses of the follicles and sebaceous glands (Fuchs 1908). Almost 70 years ago, Thygeson described blepharitis as 'a chronic inflammation of the lid border.' He observed three main types of blepharitis: seborrheic blepharitis, staphylococcal blepharitis, and mixed seborrheic and staphylococcal blepharitis (Thygeson 1946). He theorized a main role for *Staphylococcus* and its toxic products in anterior blepharitis (Thygeson 1937), but did not give an adequate answer to penicillin-resistant blepharitis. In 1982, after previous investigations (McCulley & Sciallis 1977), McCulley and colleagues expanded the two fundamental categories of marginal lid inflammation into six groups, three of them involving anterior blepharitis, based on clinical signs of disease, including a seventh group associated with other disorders (McCulley et al. 1982) (**Table 15.1**). Nine years later, Bron et al. (1991) suggested a modification in the McCulley classification, with special emphasis on meibomian gland dysfunction (MGD) (**Table 15.2**). Despite all the efforts aimed at defining and classifying anterior blepharitis, there is not a consensus on a classification that categorizes clinical presentations

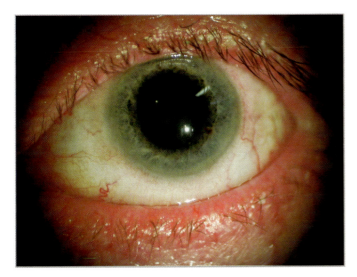

Figure 15.1 Anterior blepharitis.

Table 15.1 McCulley classification of blepharitis

Group	Clinical features
Staphylococcal blepharitis	Dry scale, collarettes, more inflammation, short story
Seborrheic blepharitis	Greasy scales, less inflammation, longer course, frequent associated seborrheic dermatitis
Seborrheic/Staphylococcal mixed	Greasy scales, more inflammation, exacerbations
Seborrheic/meibomian seborrhea	Greasy scales, meibomian secretion normal but increased
Seborrheic/secondary meibomitis	Greasy scales, meibomian inflammation patchy with clusters
Primary meibomitis	Meibomian inflammation diffuse, frequent associated rosacea
Associated with other conditions	Associated with atopy, psoriasis, fungal infection

Table 15.2 Bron's modification of the McCulley classification of blepharitis

Anterior blepharitis

Staphylococcal

Seborrheic

Alone
With staphylococci
With seborrhea
With secondary meibomitis

Posterior blepharitis

Meibomian seborrhea

Primary meibomitis
Secondary meibomitis
   Secondary to seborrheic blepharitis
   Secondary to other disorders (e.g. atopy and cicatrizing conjunctivitis)

of anterior blepharitis, unlike posterior blepharitis, now best named MGD. The MGD Workshop group has just published the new MGD definition and classification (Nelson et al. 2011).

ETIOLOGY

The cause of anterior blepharitis is unknown and probably multifactorial. Bacteria play a main role in chronic blepharitis, but the exact mechanism by which bacteria produce blepharitis is unclear. Direct infection of the lids was suggested by Thygeson (1937). Bacterial populations in patients with anterior blepharitis consist of normal skin microflora, but in greater amounts. *Staphylococcus epidermidis* and *Propionibacterium acnes* are isolated more often from patients with blepharitis, whereas *Staphylococcus aureus* is dominant in staphylococcal blepharitis (McCulley et al. 1982). Participation of staphylococcal exotoxin in the production of blepharitis has been classically suggested, but some controversy surrounds the role of toxins in blepharitis. Besides, some reports have elucidated the role of a delayed-type hypersensitivity to *S. aureus* in the development of blepharitis (Mondino et al. 1987). Finally, bacterial lipases can release some products of meibum, hydrolyzing cholesterol esters and wax esters in free fatty acids, which could contribute to the development of blepharitis. Meibum changes have been reported in patients with blepharitis. Indeed, based on individual's meibum, the clinical picture of the patient can be predicted. A complex inflammatory cascade has been involved in blepharitis development, including reactive oxygen species, lipolytic enzymes, free fatty acids, and even keratinocytes, showing the multifactorial pathogenesis of the disease (McCulley & Shine 2000). The role of *Demodex folliculorum* infestation in the development of blepharitis remains controversial because it can be found in asymptomatic subjects, although some authors report the pathogenic potential of *Demodex* mites in causing lid margin inflammation. *Demodex* blepharitis is often overlooked in differential diagnosis of corneal and external disease. Some mechanisms have been proposed to explain the pathogenic role of *Demodex* in anterior blepharitis. *Demodex* mites cause direct damage to the lid margin, with follicular distension and epithelial hyperplasia and hyperkeratinization around the base of the lashes. *Demodex* mites can also lead to anterior blepharitis because of bacteria on its surface, like streptococci and staphylococci. Recently, *Bacillus oleronius* has been implicated in rosacea and blepharitis pathogenesis. Finally, some *Demodex* components, debris, and waste can evoke host inflammatory responses, with a delayed type of hypersensitivity (Liu et al. 2010).

CLINICAL FEATURES

There are some common symptoms associated with blepharitis, such as itching, tearing, red eyes, burning and foreign body sensation, blurred vision, and photophobia. Some of these symptoms are secondary to the evaporative dry eye disease (DED) associated with some clinical categories of blepharitis, due to the abnormal polar lipid layer of the tear film, resulting in a hyperevaporative DED. Almost 50% of patients with anterior blepharitis have DED. Patients with anterior blepharitis are usually more symptomatic in the morning, after the prolonged nightly closure and contact of inflamed lids with the ocular surface.

Staphylococcal anterior blepharitis has a female preponderance, and tends to occur in younger patients, with a mean age of 42 years (Smith & Flowers 1995). Clinical signs of staphylococcal blepharitis are anterior lid inflammation, with fibrinous and hard crusting scales, surrounding individual cilia as collarettes (**Figure 15.2**). Dilated blood vessels produce hyperemia of the lid margins. Chronic disease can cause hypertrophy of the lid margin, scars, madarosis (loss of eyelashes), poliosis (white lashes), and trichiasis (misdirection of eyelashes). Acute staphylococcal infections in the lid margin produce internal hordeola (acute inflammation of the meibomian glands) or external hordeola (acute inflammation of the Zeis glands).

Seborrheic anterior blepharitis has an equal male and female preponderance, and patients tend to be older than in staphylococcal blepharitis, with a mean age of 51 years. Most of the patients have evidence of seborrheic dermatitis. They have less lid inflammation, with oily or greasy scaling (**Figure 15.3**). A small percentage of patients (~15%) develop an associated keratitis or conjunctivitis.

Some patients have a mixed condition, in which clinical signs are a combination of both groups, having more anterior lid inflammation than the seborrheic category (**Figure 15.4**). Anterior *Demodex* blepharitis refers to infestation of eyelashes and follicles by *D. folliculorum*, clustering to the root of the lashes (**Figure 15.5**). Cylindrical dandruff is seen, with lid margin inflammation associated. Chronic infestation of follicles may lead to malalignment, trichiasis, or madarosis.

Longstanding patients with anterior blepharitis can have chronic papillary conjunctivitis, thought to be secondary to staphylococcal toxins (Thygeson 1937). There are four characteristic corneal

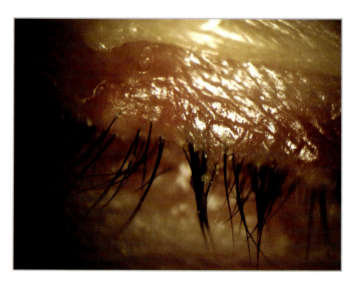

Figure 15.2 Staphylococcal blepharitis.

complications: chronic punctate epithelial keratitis, marginal corneal infiltrates, phlyctenules, and Salzmann's nodules. Superficial punctate erosions of the inferior one third of the cornea are common in chronic anterior blepharitis, with a regular pattern of small flat punctate lesions (**Figure 15.6**). Chronic superficial punctate keratitis may result in pannus formation at the inferior corneal limbus. Marginal, catarrhal infiltrates often occur at the 10 o'clock, 2 o'clock, 4 o'clock, and 8 o'clock positions on the cornea. They are secondary to a hypersensitivity reaction to staphylococcal antigens, and begin as a superficial stromal infiltrate near the limbus with a disease-free area interval between the infiltrate and the limbus. They may progress to epithelial rupture and ulceration. A wedge-shaped pannus may develop after healing. Phlyctenulosis represents another hypersensitivity reaction to staphylococcal antigens, and it usually begins with lumbar nodules that can spread to the cornea into marginal ulcers, with no lucid interval to limbus. On healing, a characteristic limbus-based triangular scar or inferior pannus can appear. Corneal involvement is recurrent, and centripetal migration of successive inflammatory lesions may develop. Occasionally, such inflammation leads to corneal

thinning and, in rare cases, perforation. Finally, Salzmann's nodules can develop in chronic anterior blepharitis due to the secondary chronic corneal inflammation.

Chronic anterior blepharitis is a significant risk factor for complications in several ocular surgeries. The most common organisms causing endophthalmitis are Gram-positive bacteria, with coagulase-negative *Staphylococcus* comprising the majority of cases. Patients with anterior blepharitis have greater amounts of normal skin microflora, leading to a higher risk of endophthalmitis. Diffuse lamellar keratitis (DLK) is an inflammation in the interface after laser-assisted in situ keratomileusis (LASIK). The causes of DLK are inflammatory cells, bacterial toxins, eyelid secretions, and other debris that get access to the area between the flap and corneal stromal bed, causing inflammation. Briefly, several causative agents, not microbial, may lead to a common inflammatory pathway, which results in the clinical picture of DLK. Anterior blepharitis, due to anterior chronic lid margin inflammation and bacterial load, has been involved as a risk factor for DLK. Because the skin and lashes are likely sources of endophthalmitis and DLK, preoperative treatment of blepharitis and proper surgical draping are

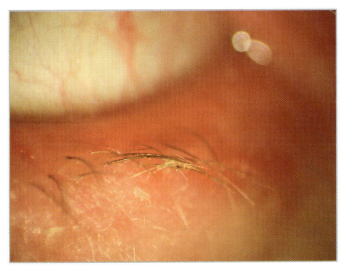

Figure 15.3 Seborrheic anterior blepharitis.

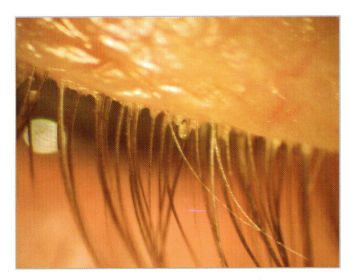

Figure 15.5 Anterior Demodex blepharitis.

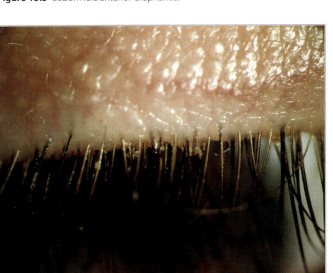

Figure 15.4 Mixed seborrheic–staphyloccocal blepharitis.

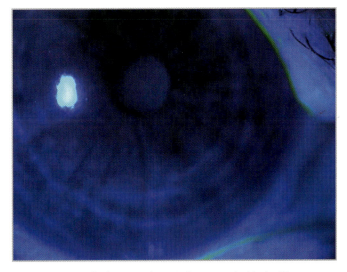

Figure 15.6 Superficial punctate keratitis due to anterior blepharitis.

important considerations. Patients with chronic anterior blepharitis may develop corneal peripheral pannus, which may increase the risk of corneal graft rejection in case corneal transplantation is needed. Current corneal transplantation guidelines recommend that ocular surface problems, including blepharitis and rosacea, must be recognized and treated prior to transplantation.

SYSTEMIC ASSOCIATIONS

Rosacea

Rosacea is a chronic inflammatory eruption of the flush areas (e.g. forehead, nose, and cheeks) of the face. It usually starts at around 30–40 years, being more common in women than in men. Rosacea is often overlooked as an important cause of ocular disease. Cutaneous lesions are characterized by the presence of telangiectasias, erythema, papules, pustules, and hypertrophic sebaceous glands. After a few months, it progresses to plaques and hypertrophic changes in the face. Rhinophyma is seen in advanced cases, especially in males. Ocular manifestations (ocular rosacea) occur in about 50% of patients with rosacea. Blepharitis is the most common associated finding. With regard to treatment, there is evidence to support the use of oral tetracyclines and topical ophthalmic steroids, although there are few well-designed studies evaluating the efficacy of therapies for ocular rosacea (Stone & Chodosh 2004).

Seborrheic dermatitis

Seborrheic dermatitis is a common chronic inflammatory disorder characterized by flaky, white-to-yellowish scales to form on oily areas (where there is a greater concentration of sebaceous glands) such as the scalp or inside the ear. It can occur with or without reddened skin. It is more likely to affect men than women. Stress, fatigue, weather extremes, oily skin, and infrequent shampooing or skin cleaning make it worse. Severe medical illnesses, including acquired immune deficiency syndrome, Parkinson's disease, head injury, and stroke, are associated with seborrheic dermatitis. These are thought to make the normal skin care that prevents seborrheic dermatitis harder to keep up with. The vast majority of people with seborrheic dermatitis have no associated conditions. Seborrheic blepharitis is often associated with seborrheic dermatitis. If both are present, the prognosis is poor, with a chronic and prolonged course.

Other diseases

Anterior blepharitis is more common in patients with Down's syndrome, atopic dermatitis, psoriasis, and 13-*cis*-retinoic acid treatment.

DIFFERENTIAL DIAGNOSIS

DED and anterior blepharitis usually occur together, and the diagnosis of DED along with blepharitis is needed to adjust the treatment. Schirmer's test, tear break-up time, and other examinations should be performed if DED is suspected.

Sebaceous gland carcinoma is a rare adnexal epithelial tumor that can mimic chronic blepharoconjunctivitis or recurrent chalazion, more often if there is no significant mass growth. Good diagnosis and recognition are crucial, due to its poor prognosis, which gets worse with the delay in diagnosis.

Other infectious and non-infectious diseases may be taken into account in the differential diagnosis, although a good patient history and examination are usually enough to obtain the correct diagnosis. Some of those diseases are herpes simplex blepharoconjunctivitis, molluscum contagiosum, phthiriasis palpebrarum, or allergic blepharitis.

Poliosis, associated with chronic anterior blepharitis, can also be caused by sympathetic ophthalmia, Vogt–Koyanagi–Harada syndrome, and Waardenburg's syndrome.

TREATMENT

The first and main step in the management of anterior blepharitis is to inform the patient that blepharitis is a chronic disease with no cure and requires a long-term treatment to keep it under control. The patient must be motivated about the goals of the treatment and about the disease prognosis. Usually, the management of anterior blepharitis consists of two phases. In the first phase, the acute phase, which lasts 2–8 weeks, intensive measures aim to bring the disease under control. In the second phase, the chronic phase, which may lasts for an unlimited period, minimal maintenance therapy is required to achieve the therapeutic goals, i.e. to control the symptoms and to prevent secondary complications.

The mainstay of treatment of anterior blepharitis is the eyelid hygiene, composed of warm compresses and eyelid scrubs (Leibowitz & Capino 1988). The warm compress partially melts the debris and crust from the base of the lids, and eyelid scrubs eliminate the debris and, due to soaps, reduce the bacterial load. The warm compress must be applied for at least 5 minutes, with washcloths or specific warm spectacles. The cloth or spectacles must be rewarmed as it cools. After the heating, the margin must be washed with baby shampoo or commercial lid scrubs or soaps, and directed to the base of the lashes and lid margins. Eyelid hygiene must be performed twice a day during the acute phase and then only in the morning during the maintenance phase. Patients should be urged to remain compliant since many are inclined to abandon the treatment during the follow-up.

Topical antibiotics are useful in staphylococcal blepharitis, by reducing the bacterial load. Several antibiotics must be used, although erythromycin and tetracycline ointments are currently the most widely used. Usually, topical antibiotics are used twice a day for 2 or 3 weeks, placing a small amount of the antibiotic ointment on the lid margins and lashes after hygienic and mechanical maneuvers. Some recent studies have emphasized the utility of azithromycin in the treatment of anterior blepharitis (Haque et al. 2010). Several studies suggest that topical azithromycin 1% may be effective as a stand-alone treatment for blepharitis as well as an adjunctive therapy with warm compresses; the studies demonstrate that topical azithromycin is more successful in treating the signs and symptoms of blepharitis than just mechanical therapy (warm compresses) alone. However, these studies are limited by their small size, open-label design, lack of a control arm, and potential bias due to the relationships of some of the investigators with the study sponsor. In addition, some concerns about high rates of resistance against azithromycin are emerging (Haas et al. 2011).

Oral antibiotics must be used in moderate or severe refractory cases. Tetracyclines are the most used drugs, due to their double mechanism of action, by killing bacteria and inhibiting lipolytic enzymes' activity (Dougherty et al. 1991). Doxycycline is the drug of choice nowadays, 100 mg/day for 2–4 weeks, followed by 50 mg/day for 6–12 weeks. Patients must be advised on the side effects of oral tetracyclines, including gastrointestinal upset, sun sensitivity, or yeast infections in women, and about the fact that response to treatment may take weeks. Other options are macrolides, such as erythromycin and azithromycin.

Topical steroids must be avoided in the management of anterior blepharitis because they do not treat the pathophysiology of the disease. If used, a short-term pulse is mandatory, preferably with 'surface steroids' such as fluorometholone, rimexolone, or loteprednol. Patients with rosacea-associated keratitis are also very sensitive to steroids; however, these drugs should be used with caution because these patients are prone to corneal thinning with chronic therapy. Marginal infiltrates and phlyctenulosis have a strong immunologic component and can thus respond to topical corticosteroid therapy.

Oral intake of omega-3 fatty acids must improve symptoms in blepharitis patients due to their anti-inflammatory effect and the improvement in the tear film stability (Macsai 2008).

If present, *Demodex* infestation-related blepharitis must be treated. Several treatments have been used to control *Demodex* mites, such as mercury oxide 1% ointment, pilocarpine gel, sulfur ointment, and camphorated oil. However, nowadays, the most used treatment is tea tree oil (TTO). Lid scrub with TTO cleanses cylindrical dandruff from the lash root and stimulates embedded mites to migrate out of the skin. Daily lid scrub with 50% TTO and lid massage with 5% TTO ointment are effective in eradicating ocular *Demodex* infestation in vivo. In addition, TTO improves patient symptoms and decreases inflammation on the ocular surface (Liu et al. 2010).

If coexistent, DED must be treated according to current recommendations (Behrens et al. 2006). DED must be suspected in patients with persistence of symptoms despite sufficient treatment of the blepharitis.

A recent meta-analysis has examined the effectiveness of interventions in the treatment of chronic blepharitis. Twenty studies focussing on anterior or mixed blepharitis were included in the review. The authors concluded that there is no strong evidence for any of the treatments in terms of curing chronic blepharitis. Topical antibiotics were shown to provide some symptomatic relief and were effective in eradicating bacteria from the eyelid margin for anterior blepharitis. Lid hygiene may provide symptomatic relief for anterior and posterior blepharitis. The effectiveness of other treatments for blepharitis, such as topical steroids and oral antibiotics, was inconclusive (Lindsley et al. 2012).

■ REFERENCES

Behrens A, Doyle JJ, Stern L, et al. Dysfunctional tear syndrome: a Delphi approach to treatment recommendations. *Cornea* 2006; **25**:900–907.

Bron AJ, Benjamin L, Snibson GR. Meibomian gland disease. Classification and grading of lid changes. *Eye* 1991; **5**:395–411.

Dougherty JM, McCulley JP, Silvany RE, Meyer DR. The role of tetracycline in chronic blepharitis. Inhibition of lipase production in staphylococci. *Invest Ophthalmol Vis Sci* 1991; **32**:2970–2975.

Fuchs HE. Textbook of ophthalmology. *Philadelphia*: JB Lippincott, 1908.

Haas W, Pillar CM, Torres M, et al. Monitoring antibiotic resistance in ocular microorganisms: results from the Antibiotic Resistance Monitoring in Ocular micRorganisms (ARMOR) 2009 surveillance study. *Am J Ophthalmol* 2011; **152**:567–574.

Haque RM, Torkildsen GL, Brubaker K, et al. Multicenter open-label study evaluating the efficacy of azithromycin ophthalmic solution 1% on the signs and symptoms of subjects with blepharitis. *Cornea* 2010; **29**:871–877.

Leibowitz HM, Capino D. Treatment of chronic blepharitis. *Arch Ophthalmol* 1988; **106**:720.

Lemp MA, Nichols KK. Blepharitis in the United States 2009: a survey-based perspective on prevalence and treatment. *Ocul Surf* 2009; **7**:S1–S14.

Lindsley K, Matsumura S, Hatef E, Akpek EK. Interventions for chronic blepharitis. Cochrane Database Syst Rev 2012; 5:CD005556.

Liu J, Sheha H, Tseng SCG. Pathogenic role of demodex mites in blepharitis. *Curr Opin Allergy Clin Immunol* 2010; **10**:505–510.

Macsai MS. The role of omega-3 dietary supplementation in blepharitis and meibomian gland dysfunction (an AOS thesis). *Trans Am Ophthalmol Soc* 2008; **106**:336–356.

McCulley JP, Sciallis GF. Meibomiankeratoconjunctivitis. *Am J Ophthalmol* 1977; **84**:788–793.

McCulley JP, Dougherty JM, Deneau DG. Classification of chronic blepharitis. *Ophthalmology* 1982; **89**:1173–1180.

McCulley JP, Shine WE. Changing concepts in the diagnosis and management of blepharitis. *Cornea* 2000; **19**:650–658.

Mondino BJ, Caster AI, Dethlefs B. A rabbit model of staphylococcal blepharitis. *Arch Ophthalmol* 1987; **105**:409–412.

Nelson JD, Shimazaki J, Benitez-del-Castillo JM, et al. The international workshop on meibomian gland dysfunction: report of the definition and classification subcommittee. *Invest Ophthalmol Vis Sci* 2011; **52**:1930–1937.

Saccà SC, Pascotto A, Venturino GM, et al. Prevalence and treatment of *Helicobacter pylori* in patients with blepharitis. *Invest Ophthalmol Vis Sci* 2006; **47**:501–508.

Smith RE, Flowers CW Jr. Chronic blepharitis: a review. *CLAO J* 1995; **21**:200–207.

Stone DU, Chodosh J. Ocular rosacea: an update on pathogenesis and therapy. *Curr Opin Ophthalmol* 2004; **15**:499–502.

Thygeson P. Bacterial factors in chronic catarrhal conjunctivitis: I. Role of toxin-forming staphylococci. *Arch Ophthalmol* 1937; **18**:373–387.

Thygeson P. Etiology and treatment of blepharitis: a study in military personnel. *Arch Ophthalmol* 1946; **36**:445–447.

Chapter 16   Episcleritis, scleritis, and peripheral ulcerative keratitis

Maite Sainz de la Maza

■ EPISCLERITIS AND SCLERITIS

■ Introduction

Scleral inflammation gives rise to a spectrum of conditions, ranging in severity from benign, superficial inflammation of the episclera to vision-threatening necrosis of the sclera. Differentiation between episcleritis and scleritis is important because there are considerable differences in clinical features, visual prognosis, ocular morbidity, therapeutic approach, and the association with potentially life-threatening underlying systemic disease.

Episcleritis is usually an acute, self-limited condition that rarely produces significant adverse ocular sequelae. It is infrequently associated with systemic disease and usually requires no more than systemic non-steroidal anti-inflammatory drugs (NSAIDs) if treatment is necessary. In contrast, scleritis is usually a chronic, painful, progressive, potentially blinding condition, involving both the episclera and the sclera. It is often associated not only with ocular complications (e.g. keratitis, uveitis, glaucoma, and cataract if anterior, or fundus abnormalities, if posterior) but also with immune-mediated systemic diseases, some of them potentially lethal. Scleritis always requires aggressive systemic therapy with NSAIDs, corticosteroids, or immunomodulatory agents, alone or in combination.

■ Classification

The classification scheme of scleral inflammatory diseases, proposed by Watson and Hayreh (Watson et al. 1976), is regarded as the most clinically useful. It is based on the anatomic site of the inflammation and on the clinical appearance of the disease at presentation. It enables one to assign most patients to a particular category and subcategory at the initial clinical examination, with almost no changes over the course of the disease. Two main groups can be differentiated: episcleritis and scleritis (**Table 16.1**). Episcleritis can be divided into simple and nodular forms, and scleritis into anterior and posterior types. Anterior scleritis may be further classified as diffuse, nodular, necrotizing with inflammation (necrotizing), and necrotizing without inflammation (scleromalacia perforans).

■ Clinical features
Episcleritis

Episcleritis occurs in young adults, usually women, with a peak incidence in the fourth decade. It is abrupt in onset, with the eye becoming red and swollen within an hour of the start of the attack. The main symptom is that of mild ocular discomfort, manifested as a burning, foreign-body sensation, or irritation. It is always localized to the eye itself and does not radiate to the forehead, jaw, temple, or sinuses. Unlike scleritis, tenderness to palpation of the globe is absent and frank pain is extremely uncommon. Mild tearing and photophobia may also

Table 16.1 Clinical classification of episcleral and scleral inflammation*

Episcleritis
Simple
Nodular
Scleritis
Anterior scleritis
Diffuse scleritis
Nodular scleritis
Necrotizing scleritis
With inflammation
Without inflammation (scleromalacia perforans)
Posterior scleritis

*Adapted from Watson et al. (1976)

be present. The main sign is redness, which may range from a mild pinkish hue to fiery red, with injection and dilation of the superficial episcleral blood vessels. Episcleritis is bilateral in approximately one third of cases, although not frequently simultaneous. Recurrences, not necessarily in the same location, are common over a period of years, decreasing in frequency after the first 3–4 years. Despite recurrent disease, vision is usually unaffected and extension of the inflammatory process to adjacent ocular structures is very uncommon. Episcleritis may be simple (sectorial or diffuse) (**Figure 16.1**) or nodular (**Figure 16.2**). In nodular episcleritis, the inflammation is confined to a round or oval mobile nodule, 2–6 mm in diameter, with little surrounding congestion. The overlying conjunctiva can be moved over the surface of the nodule, which in turn moves slightly

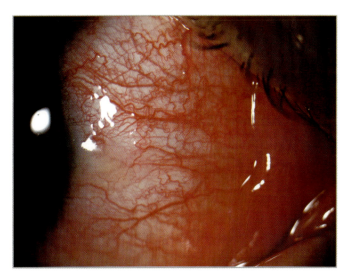

Figure 16.1 Simple episcleritis. The involved area appears diffusely congested and edematous.

on the underlying sclera. Simple episcleritis is more common than nodular episcleritis. Episcleritis rarely produces significant adverse ocular sequelae (Sainz de la Maza et al. 1994a, 2012a).

Scleritis

Scleritis is most common in the fourth to sixth decades of life, with a peak incidence in the fifth decade, and affects women more frequently than men (1.6:1.0). Scleritis is insidious in onset, with the eye becoming red, painful, and swollen within a period of 5–10 days after the start of the attack. The cardinal symptom is pain of moderate to severe intensity with exquisite tenderness to palpation of the globe, frequently radiating to the forehead, the jaw, temple, or sinuses. In some patients, such as those with necrotizing scleritis, the eye may be so painful and sensitive to touch as to be totally debilitating, even to the extent of preventing the patient from resting the head on the affected side on a soft pillow. Indeed, the pain may be unresponsive to analgesics or narcotics. Sometimes, the severity of pain may be out of proportion with the clinical signs. In these cases, the patient may be erroneously diagnosed as having migraine, temporomandibular joint arthritis, sinusitis, herpes zoster, or orbital tumor. The pain is probably caused by either distention or destruction of the sensory nerve fibers in the sclera as a result of edema, inflammatory mediators, or necrosis. Pain is, therefore, a good indicator of the presence of active scleritis; it always vanishes with adequate medical treatment of the inflammatory condition. As with episcleritis, mild tearing (never true discharge) and mild-to-moderate photophobia may be present. The main sign is redness, which has a bluish or violaceous tinge, with injection and dilation of the deep episcleral blood vessels. Recurrences, not necessarily in the same location, are common over a period of many years, and usually decrease in frequency after the first 3–6 years. Vision is sometimes affected in anterior scleritis and almost always in posterior scleritis due to extension of the inflammatory process to adjacent ocular structures, resulting in keratitis, uveitis, glaucoma, cataract, or fundus abnormalities (Benson 1988). Diffuse anterior scleritis, the most common and least severe form of disease, varies from a small, sectoral area of inflammation to involvement of the whole anterior segment (**Figure 16.3**). Nodular anterior scleritis is characterized by a deep red or violaceous scleral lesion, usually located in the interpalpebral area about 3–4 mm from the limbus, which is tender to the touch and immobile (**Figure 16.4**). Necrotizing anterior scleritis, the most destructive form of scleritis, appears as white avascular areas surrounded by scleral inflammation and diffuse congestion of the abnormal deep vascular episcleral channels. The involved tissue becomes thin, revealing the brown color of the underlying uvea (**Figure 16.5**). Scleromalacia perforans is a rare, bilateral condition that is seen most frequently among elderly women with severe rheumatoid arthritis. It is characterized by yellow to grayish patches on the sclera that gradually develop a necrotic slough and separate, leaving the uvea bare or covered by a thin layer of conjunctiva without surrounding inflammation (**Figure 16.6**). Posterior scleritis is defined as inflammation of the sclera, posterior to the ora serrata, that frequently extends to secondarily involved adjacent structures, such as the choroid, retina, optic nerve, extraocular muscles, and orbital

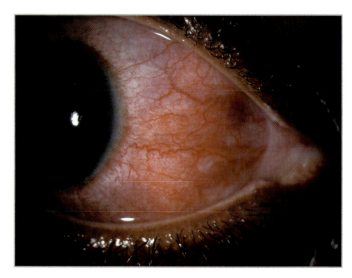

Figure 16.3 Diffuse anterior scleritis. Redness has a bluish tinge with injection and dilation of the deep episcleral blood vessels, with tortuosity, distortion, and loss of normal radial vascular architecture.

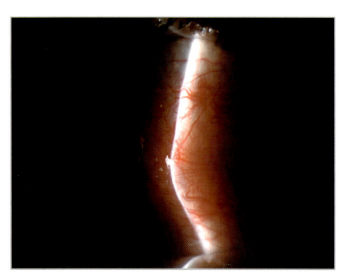

Figure 16.2 Nodular episcleritis. The inflammation is confined to a very well-defined area, forming a slightly tender, dark red nodule, usually round or oval, with little surrounding congestion.

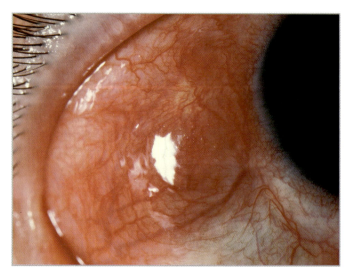

Figure 16.4 Nodular anterior scleritis. The nodule is tender and immobile, typically localized to the interpalpebral zone.

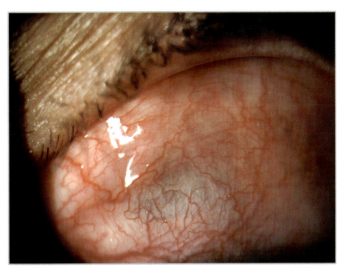

Figure 16.5 Necrotizing anterior scleritis. The damaged sclera becomes translucent and shows the brown color of the underlying choroid.

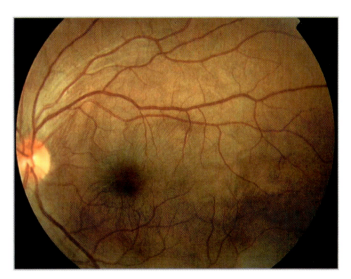

Figure 16.7 Posterior scleritis. Choroidal folds seen as series of alternating light and dark lines, confined to the posterior pole.

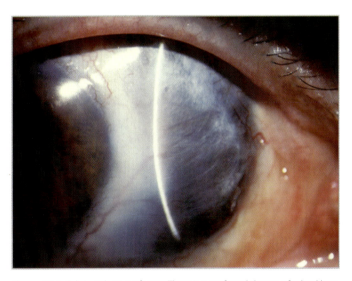

Figure 16.6 Scleromalacia perforans. There is a profound degree of scleral loss with uveal protrusion covered by a thin layer of conjunctiva without associated inflammation.

tissues. The most common presenting symptoms are decreased vision and pain. The most common posterior segment signs are choroidal folds (**Figure 16.7**), subretinal mass, disk edema, macular edema, annular ciliochoroidal detachment, and serous retinal detachment.

◼ Ocular examination

The ocular examination in scleral diseases must include an episcleral and scleral examination and a general ophthalmological examination. The episcleral and scleral examination should be performed under conditions of daylight and with the slit lamp, employing diffuse white light, the narrow slit beam, and red-free illumination.

Examination in daylight

Episcleral and scleral examination in daylight is sometimes the only way to distinguish episcleritis from scleritis because it does not distort the natural color of the sclera. In episcleritis, the eye appears pink to red, while in scleritis, the eye has a deep bluish-red or violaceous tinge. If scleral necrosis is present, blue gray to dark-brown areas corresponding to the underlying uvea may become visible through the translucent sclera. If tissue necrosis is progressive, the scleral area may become avascular, producing a central white sequestrum surrounded by a well-demarcated black or dark-brown circle. The slough may be gradually replaced by granulation tissue, leaving the underlying uvea bare or covered by a thin layer of conjunctiva.

Slit-lamp examination

Slit-lamp examination, under conditions of diffuse illumination, helps to detect congested vessels, nodules, or avascular areas with sequestra or uveal show. It also helps to differentiate the configuration of vessels; in episcleritis, congested vessels follow the usual radial pattern, while in scleritis, this pattern is altered and new, abnormal vessels are formed.

Slit-lamp examination with the narrow slit beam helps to detect the depth of inflammation, indicating which network of vessels is predominantly affected. In episcleritis, maximum congestion is in the superficial episcleral network, with no changes in the deep episcleral network. The edema is localized to the episcleral tissue. The anterior edge of the narrow slit beam is displaced forward while the posterior edge remains flat against the sclera, in its normal position. Topical application of 10% phenylephrine renders the eye white because its vasoconstrictor effect is greater on the superficial episcleral plexus with no significant effect on the deep episcleral vessels (**Figure 16.8a and b**). In scleritis, maximum congestion is in the deep episcleral plexus, although there is some in the superficial episcleral plexus. The edema is localized to the scleral and episcleral tissues. The anterior and posterior edges of the narrow slit beam are displaced forward. With the topical application of 10% phenylephrine, which only blanches the superficial episcleral plexus with no effect on the deep episcleral plexus, the eye remains congested in scleritis (**Figure 16.9a and b**).

Red free light is helpful in revealing areas of maximal vascular congestion, avascularity, and new vascular channels.

General ophthalmological examination

Evaluation of adjacent structures must always be performed at every follow-up visit of a patient with scleritis because keratitis, uveitis,

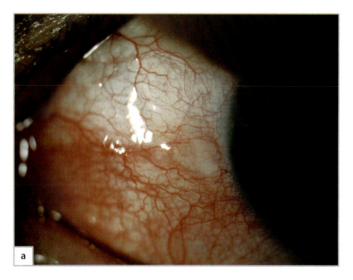
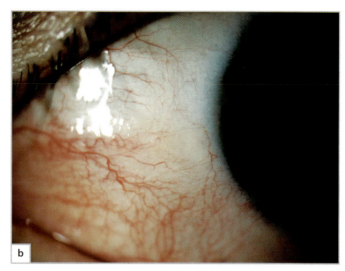

Figure 16.8 (a) Simple episcleritis. (b) The same eye after topical application of 10% phenylephrine. The eye appears white, as its vasoconstrictor effect is greater on the superficial episcleral plexus with no significant effect on the deep episcleral vessels.

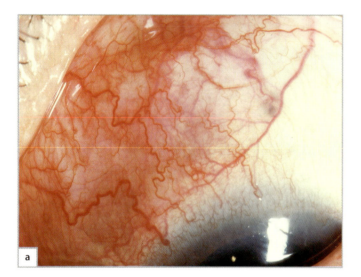
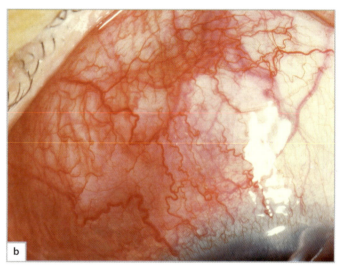

Figure 16.9 (a) Diffuse scleritis. (b) The same eye after topical application of 10% phenylephrine. The eye remains congested, as the vasoconstrictor effect only blanches the superficial episclera plexus but has no significant effect on the deep episcleral vessels.

glaucoma, cataract, or fundus abnormalities are important reasons for vision loss and, in some cases, destruction of the eye. Extension of the inflammation to the adjacent structures in episcleritis is very uncommon.

Imaging

The conjunctival, superficial episcleral and deep episcleral plexuses can be imaged with anterior-segment fluorescein angiography (FA) and indocyanine green angiography (ICGA) (Nieuwenhuizen et al. 2003). The combination of both techniques provides complementary information that may be useful in the differential diagnosis and monitoring of treatment of patients as well as in detecting subclinical pathology. Ultrasonography is the most useful test in the diagnosis of posterior scleritis (Cappaert et al. 1977), although CT and MRI may be helpful to exclude orbital inflammatory diseases or orbital tumors (Chaques et al. 1993).

Simple and nodular episcleritis

Anterior segment FA shows that the speed of circulation is very rapid in the affected area, with the whole transit of dye being complete within 3 seconds as opposed to the normal 11–15 seconds. There is also extensive leakage, mainly into the episcleral nodule in nodular episcleritis, and no changes in the normal vascular pattern. ICGA also shows extremely rapid filling and short transit time, although there is no leakage.

Diffuse and nodular scleritis

In diffuse scleritis, both anterior segment FA and ICGA show rapid filling and short transit times with a structurally normal flow pattern. There is no evidence of vascular closure. On ICGA, there is no leakage except in regions of local vascular damage, which may signify accompanying deep inflammation. The findings of anterior segment FA and ICGA in nodular scleritis are similar to those found in diffuse anterior scleritis—rapid filling and short transit times, with staining of the nodules in both techniques.

Necrotizing scleritis

Anterior-segment FA shows hypoperfusion, venular occlusion, and new vessels that leak extensively. The transit time in necrotizing scleritis is markedly increased even in the presence of ocular congestion. ICGA also shows hypoperfusion, venular occlusion, increased transit time, and late leakage from new or damaged vessels. Both FA and ICGA are useful during the early treatment phases to confirm the presence or absence of vascular occlusion and to detect active vasculitis.

Posterior scleritis

Ultrasonography is an essential investigation in the diagnosis of posterior scleritis because it demonstrates scleral and choroidal thickening and the presence of edema in Tenon space, the so-called T sign. Although CT is not as sensitive as ultrasonography, it is very helpful in excluding orbital inflammatory disease, tumors, thyroid eye disease, and sinus disease. Magnetic resonance scanning with gadolinium is able to distinguish scleral from choroidal thickening, which may be of value in patients with choroidal detachments. Likewise, FA may highlight choroidal folds, reveal neurosensory retinal and pigment epithelial detachments, disk edema, and macular edema, and serve to clarify the differential diagnosis.

■ Associated diseases and diagnostic evaluation

Investigation of the illness (e.g. major complaint and history of present illness, personal and family history), review of systems, and complete ocular and physical examination (e.g. head and extremities) are essential to the diagnosis and management of scleral inflammatory disease.

Episcleritis

Episcleritis, while most commonly idiopathic, may be associated with a wide variety of systemic and ocular conditions in up to 27% of patients (Sainz de la Maza et al. 2012b) (**Table 16.2**), including connective tissue or vasculitic diseases, spondyloarthropathies, atopy, rosacea, gout, herpes zoster, herpes simplex, and syphilis. Other entities such as drug reactions to pamidronate (Aredia) (Macarol & Fraunfelder 1994), alendronate (Fosamax) (Mbekeani et al. 1999), and risedronate (Actonel) (Barrera et al. 2005) have also been reported. Episcleritis is rare in childhood, especially in children younger than 5 years; however, in older children, it is frequently associated with rheumatic disease (Read et al. 1999).

If the episcleritis attack is the first one and is evanescent, and the medical review of systems and physical examination are unrevealing, it is unnecessary to obtain extended diagnostic studies. Selective investigations should be performed to rule out specific diseases in patients with persistent or recurrent clinical course and symptoms suggestive of an associated systemic disease.

Scleritis

An associated systemic disease is present in approximately 36–57% of patients with scleritis; 25–48% have an associated connective tissue or vasculitic disease; 5–10% have an infectious etiology; and 1–2% have atopy, rosacea, or gout (Akpek et al. 2004, Jabs et al. 2000, Sainz de la Maza et al. 1994a, 2012a, Tuft & Watson 1991, Watson et al. 1976) (**Table 16.2**). Rheumatoid arthritis is by far the most common systemic association (Sainz de la Maza et al. 1994b), followed by granulomatosis

with polyangiitis (Wegener), relapsing polychondritis, systemic lupus erythematosus, and arthritis with inflammatory bowel disease. Scleritis can be the presenting clinical manifestation of a systemic disease. Necrotizing scleritis is most frequently identified in patients with granulomatosis with polyangiitis (Wegener), rheumatoid arthritis, polyarteritis nodosa (PAN), or relapsing polychondritis, and it is less likely to be seen in those with systemic lupus erythematosus, or the seronegative spondyloarthropathies (Sainz de la Maza et al. 1995). As with anterior scleritis, rheumatoid arthritis is the most common systemic disease association in posterior scleritis, followed by other connective tissue diseases (e.g. systemic lupus erythematosus, psoriatic arthritis) and systemic vasculitides [e.g. granulomatosis with polyangiitis (Wegener), PAN, relapsing polychondritis (McCluskey et al. 1999)]; one must also consider infectious etiologies (e.g. Lyme disease, toxoplasmosis, and herpes zoster) and neoplastic masquerade syndromes.

The detection of a connective tissue or vasculitic disease in a patient with scleritis is a sign of poor general prognosis because it indicates potentially systemic complications that may be lethal unless managed with prompt and aggressive therapy. It is also a sign of poor ocular

Table 16.2 Diseases associated with episcleritis and scleritis and PUK

Non-infectious
Connective tissue diseases and other inflammatory conditions
Rheumatoid arthritis
Systemic lupus erythematosus
Ankylosing spondylitis
Reactive arthritis
Psoriatic arthritis
Arthritis and inflammatory bowel disease
Relapsing polychondritis
Vasculitic diseases
Polyarteritis nodosa
Allergic granulomatous angiitis (Churg–Strauss syndrome)
Granulomatosis with polyangiitis (Wegener)
Behçet's disease
Giant cell arteritis
Cogan's syndrome
Vasculitic diseases associated with connective tissue diseases and other inflammatory conditions
Miscellaneous
Atopy
Rosacea
Gout
Foreign body granuloma
Chemical injury
Infectious
Bacterial
Fungal
Viral
Parasitical

PUK, peripheral ulcerative keratitis.

prognosis because patients with these systemic diseases frequently have more necrotizing scleritis, peripheral ulcerative keratitis, or decrease in vision than do patients without these diseases (Sainz de la Maza et al. 1995). In addition, the ocular prognosis of scleritis with connective tissue or vasculitic disease varies depending on the specific disease: scleritis associated either with spondyloarthropathies or with systemic lupus erythematosus is usually a benign and self-limiting condition; scleritis associated with rheumatoid arthritis or relapsing polychondritis is a disease of intermediate severity; and scleritis associated with granulomatosis with polyangiitis (Wegener) is a severe disease that can lead to permanent blindness or even loss of the eye.

Miscellaneous conditions associated with scleritis include gout, atopy, rosacea, foreign body granuloma, chemical injury, and drug reactions to pamidronate, alendronate, risedronate, zoledronic acid, and ibandronate (Barrera et al. 2005, Macarol & Fraunfelder 1994, Mbekeani et al. 1999).

Infectious scleritis, either endogenous or exogenous, may be caused by the direct invasion of a microorganism or by the immune response to an infectious pathogen. Historical details that raise the index of suspicion of an infectious etiology include prior ocular trauma or surgery (especially a scleral buckling procedure, strabismus surgery, or pterygium excision), contact lens use, systemic or local immunosuppression, and local debilitating diseases (history of recurrent keratitis caused by herpes simplex virus or herpes zoster virus). All classes of microorganisms, including bacteria, viruses, fungi, and parasites, can infect the sclera and produce a clinical picture identical to that seen with immune-mediated disease. Bacterial causes of scleritis include *Pseudomonas, Streptococcus, Staphylococcus, Proteus, Haemophilus influenzae, Mycobacteria, Borrelia, Treponema,* and *Nocardia*. Bacterial scleritis may result from extension of an adjacent keratitis. An inflammatory microangiopathy in the sclera may arise by the induction of immune-mediated responses in the vessel wall, such as the formation and deposition of immune complexes containing bacterial products.

Herpes virus is probably the most common cause of infectious or late immune-related episcleral and/or scleral inflammation of viral etiology, occurring in as many as 7% of patients with scleritis and 74% of patients with infectious scleritis (Gonzalez-Gonzalez et al. 2012). Although diffuse anterior is the most common type of herpetic scleritis, nodular anterior, necrotizing anterior, and posterior can also be seen. Indeed, posterior scleritis presenting with annular choroidal detachment as a complication of herpes zoster ophthalmicus has been reported (Tranos et al. 2003) as well as that of recurrent nodular scleritis thought to be caused by reactivation of a varicella zoster virus infection (Livir-Rallatos et al. 1998). In addition, herpes zoster virus sclerokeratitis and anterior uveitis have been observed in a child following varicella vaccination (Naseri et al. 2003). Although, less often, herpes simplex virus may occasionally cause scleritis, scleral involvement may occur as a result of direct viral invasion or months after the initial viral encounter as a result of an immune-mediated reaction induced by the virus.

Fungal scleritis, such as that caused by *Aspergillus*, is typically seen after ocular trauma but has also been reported following pterygium surgery (Margo et al. 1988).

Protozoal infections with *Acanthamoeba* have also been identified as the causative agents in patients with severe sclerokeratitis (Lee et al. 2002).

The detection of scleritis, even if the attack is the first one, requires complementary studies. Based on the results obtained in the investigation of the illness (e.g. major complaint and history of present illness, past personal, and family history), review of systems, and physical examination (e.g. head, extremities, and eye), appropriate diagnostic tests can be selected to confirm or reject preliminary diagnoses. Sometimes, one series of diagnostic studies may be insufficient and regular reinvestigations may be necessary to discover the diagnosis.

Typical initial investigations might include a chest radiograph, urine analysis, serum chemistries (which may indicate renal dysfunction in systemic vasculitides), syphilis serologies (FTA-ABS and RPR), and antineutrophil cytoplasmic antibody (ANCA) testing. ANCAs are specific markers for a group of related systemic vasculitides that include PAN, granulomatosis with polyangiitis (Wegener), microscopic polyangiitis, Churg–Strauss syndrome, and pauci-immune glomerulonephritis. Specifically, ANCAs are antibodies directed against cytoplasmic azurophilic granules of neutrophils and monocytes and may be divided into two classes based on the pattern of staining seen on immunofluorescence. The cytoplasmic pattern, or c-ANCA, is both sensitive and specific for granulomatosis with polyangiitis (Wegener), whereas the perinuclear pattern, or p-ANCA, is associated with PAN, microscopic polyangiitis, relapsing polychondritis, and renal vasculitis. All positive ANCA tests should be confirmed by testing for antibodies to proteinase-3 (PR3) and/or myeloperoxidase (MPO). Between 85% and 95% of all ANCA found in granulomatosis with polyangiitis (Wegener) is c-ANCA with antigen specificity for PR3, which is highly specific for the disease, while the remainder is p-ANCA directed against MPO. In contrast, the diagnostic sensitivity of c-ANCA and p-ANCA for PAN is only 5% and 15%, respectively, while in patients with microscopic polyangiitis, p-ANCA (anti-MPO) positivity is more common (50–80%) with a smaller percentage (40%) having the c-ANCA (anti-PR3) marker (**Table 16.3**).

Further testing in the appropriate clinical context might include

- Rheumatoid factor or human leukocyte antigen-B27 in the presence of polyarthritis or spondyloarthropathy
- Lyme serology in a patient with a history of a tick bite from an endemic area
- Antinuclear antibodies in individuals where SLE is suggested on history and physical examination
- Radiographic imaging of the sinus in the presence of sinus symptomatology
- Purified protein derivative skin test or Quantiferon gold assay with a history of tuberculosis exposure
- Ultrasound examination in patients suspected of having posterior scleritis

Table 16.3 Antineutrophil cytoplasmic antibodies

Granulomatosis with polyangiitis (Wegener)
85–95% c-ANCA[*]
5–15% p-ANCA[†]
Polyarteritis nodosa
5% c-ANCA
15% p-ANCA
Microscopic polyangiitis
40% c-ANCA
50–80% p-ANCA

ANCA, antineutrophil cytoplasmic antibodies.
[*]c-ANCA: cytoplasmic pattern, antigen specificity for proteinase-3.
[†]p-ANCA: perinuclear pattern, antigen specificity for myeloperoxidase.

Therapy

Episcleritis

Since episcleritis is a benign, self-limited process, it may be left untreated except for palliative therapy with cool compresses and iced lubrication. Topical NSAIDs appear to be ineffective based on the results of a randomized double-masked placebo-controlled clinical trial (Lyons et al. 1990). Topical steroids may speed the resolution; however, there are significant side effects, such as elevated intraocular pressure and cataracts, especially with prolonged use. Recurrences frequently occur with discontinuation of the steroids (rebound effect). A small number of patients, particularly those with nodular episcleritis with persistent episodes or frequent recurrences, require oral NSAIDs (Watson et al. 1976). Patients who do not respond to one NSAID may respond to another. The selective inhibitors of COX-2 remain a viable choice in cases complicated by significant gastrointestinal adverse effects or interactions with other medications (mainly anticoagulants). Episcleritis associated with rosacea, atopy, gout, or herpes should be initially treated with specific therapy for each disease.

Scleritis

Scleritis almost always requires treatment with systemic medications. Important considerations in the formulation of a therapeutic plan include accurate classification of scleritis type and identification of concomitant local or systemic disease, the exclusion of possible infectious etiologies, and the potential for medication-related toxicity and/ or possible drug interactions (Sainz de la Maza et al. 2012b).

Non-infectious scleritis

Our suggested guidelines for appropriate therapy in patients with scleritis are the following (**Figure 16.10**):

- Patients with idiopathic diffuse and nodular scleritis, with degree of scleral inflammation <2+ (0–4+), will most often respond to NSAIDs as initial treatment, provided there are no contraindications for such therapy and the patient understands and accepts the risks and the need for monitoring; if one is not effective, another NSAID may be tried in substitution for the first one. In case of NSAID therapeutic failure, consider steroidal anti-inflammatory drugs (SAIDs) substitution with subsequent progressive tapering until discontinuing; once SAIDs have been discontinued, remission may be maintained with NSAIDs. Concomitant NSAID and SAID therapies are not appropriate given the risk of gastrointestinal ulcer. In case of SAID therapeutic failure or relapse after tapering, consider immunomodulatory therapy (IMT) addition or substitution, mainly antimetabolites such as methotrexate (MTX), azathioprine (AZA), mycophenolate mofetil (MMF), or leflunomide; MTX is the most commonly prescribed antimetabolite because of its efficacy, convenience, and safety record. In case of IMT (antimetabolites) therapeutic failure, consider biologic response modifiers (BRM) addition or substitution, mainly antitumor necrosis factor alpha (anti-TNFα) such as infliximab (INFLI), adalimumab (ADA), or certolizumab
- Patients with idiopathic diffuse or nodular scleritis, with degree of scleral inflammation >2+ (0–4+), will most often respond to SAIDs as initial treatment with subsequent progressive tapering until discontinuing; once SAIDs have been discontinued, remission may be maintained with continued NSAIDs. In case of SAID therapeutic failure or relapse after tapering, consider IMT

addition or substitution, mainly antimetabolites. In case of IMT (antimetabolites) therapeutic failure, consider BRM addition or substitution, mainly anti-TNFα

- Patients with diffuse or nodular scleritis, associated with underlying connective tissue or vasculitic disease (e.g. rheumatoid arthritis, relapsing polychondritis, inflammatory bowel disease, and systemic lupus erythematosus), will most often require IMT, mainly antimetabolites, or BRM, mainly anti-TNFα. We suggest IMT as the first choice because of BRM cost, safety, and logistical matters. In case of BRM (anti-TNFα) therapeutic failure, consider other BRM such as abatacept, rituximab (RTX), or tocilizumab. If the underlying vasculitic disease is potentially lethal, patients will most often respond to IMT, mainly alkylating agents such as cyclophosphamide (CYC)
- Patients with necrotizing scleritis will most often respond to IMT, mainly alkylating agents. However, in some specific cases, BRM such as RTX may be an alternative. For example, a 25-year-old woman with necrotizing scleritis, discovered to have Wegener's granulomatosis, may, for the sake of ovarian protection, prefer to be treated with BRM (RTX) rather than with alkylating agents (CYC) coupled with ovarian suppression or with egg harvesting. On the other hand, a 25-year-old man may conclude, after education about the data in peer-reviewed literature on the matter, that sperm banking followed by CYC therapy (intravenous CYC every 2 weeks for 6–12 months), with subsequent conversion to long-term

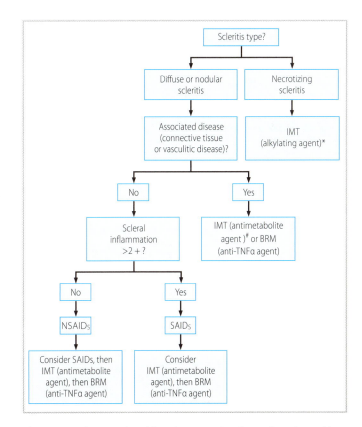

Figure 16.10 Suggested guidelines for appropriate therapy in patients with scleritis. *Consider BRM such as rituximab for ovarian protection. #Consider first IMT (antimetabolite agent). If therapeutic failure, consider BRM (anti-TNFα agent). If potentially lethal disease, the IMT should be an alkylating agent. BRM, biologic response modifiers; IMT, immunomodulatory therapy; NSAIDs, non-steroidal anti-inflammatory drugs; SAIDs, steroidal anti-inflammatory drugs; TNF, tumor necrosis factor.

maintenance therapy with an antimetabolite agent (MTX, AZA, or MMF), is his preferred path. Many risks of CYC therapy can be mitigated by employing a pulse intravenous strategy every 14 days We would caution that IMT and BRM agents should be administered by a physician, either an ophthalmologist, rheumatologist, or oncologist, specifically trained in the early recognition and management of drug-induced complications of those treatments.

Infectious scleritis

Patients with infectious scleritis should be treated with appropriate and specific antimicrobial therapy. It is important to differentiate infectious scleritis from non-infectious scleritis because corticosteroids or immunosuppressive agents are contraindicated in active infection.

PERIPHERAL ULCERATIVE KERATITIS

Introduction

The unique anatomic and physiological characteristics of the peripheral cornea explain its predilections to be involved in a variety of disorders (Mondino 1988). Blood vessels and lymphatic channels from the adjacent conjunctiva and episclera enable diffusion into the cornea of some molecules, such as immunoglobulins and complement components. IgG and IgA are found in similar concentrations in the peripheral and central corneas; however, more IgM is found in the periphery, probably because its high molecular weight restricts diffusion into the central cornea. Both classic and alternative pathway components of complement and their inhibitors have been demonstrated in healthy human corneas; however, although most of the complement components have a ratio peripheral-to-central cornea of 1.2:1.0, C1 is denser in the periphery, with a ratio peripheral-to-central cornea of 5:1. The high molecular weight of C1, the recognition unit of the classic pathway, may also restrict its diffusion into the central area.

The normal human corneal epithelium contains small numbers of Langerhans cells, with the greatest density at the limbus dropping to almost zero in the central cornea. The peripheral cornea also contains a reservoir of inflammatory cells, including neutrophils, eosinophils, lymphocytes, plasma cells, and mast cells. The presence of IgM, C1, Langerhans cells, and inflammatory cells makes the peripheral cornea more susceptible than the central cornea to ulceration in a wide variety of infectious and non-infectious local and systemic diseases, causing a specific entity named peripheral ulcerative keratitis (PUK). Whether it is the sequel of an infectious, trophic, traumatic, neurological, dermatological, anatomic, or autoimmune disease, PUK is always a local destructive process mediated by the final common pathway of collagenolytic and proteolytic enzyme release from inflammatory cells. PUK may also be the presenting manifestation of a potentially lethal systemic autoimmune vasculitic disease or may herald the onset of a potentially lethal systemic vasculitic process in a patient with an already known systemic disease (**Table 16.2**) (Tauber et al. 1990). Early diagnosis and subsequent appropriate treatment may improve the ocular and systemic prognoses.

Clinical features

The main symptoms are pain, tearing, and photophobia. If the peripheral process progresses centrally and compromises the visual axis, visual acuity decreases.

Ocular examination

PUK appears as a crescent-shaped peripheral corneal stromal ulceration with epithelial defect adjacent to the corneoscleral limbus, with an intrastromal white blood cell infiltrate visible on slit-lamp examination. Clinical disease activity can be described according to the degree of depth of corneal ulceration (0–4+) and the degree of adjacent conjunctival inflammation (0–4+). The detection of scleritis, especially the necrotizing form, is an important finding because its presence is highly associated with underlying systemic vasculitic diseases (Sainz de la Maza et al. 2002). Visual acuity, intraocular pressure, and presence or absence of anterior uveal inflammation should be recorded. Mooren ulcer presents with no scleral involvement, with the typical central corneal edge 'hanging' and with no associated systemic findings; therefore, it is a diagnosis of exclusion.

Associated diseases and diagnostic evaluation

Because PUK can be a manifestation of a systemic vasculitic disease, investigation of the illness (e.g. major complaint and history of present illness, past personal, and family history), review of systems, and complete ocular and physical examination (e.g. head and extremities) are essential to the diagnosis and management of PUK. At that point, few preliminary systemic diagnoses emerge as most likely. The next phase includes the selection of diagnostic tests for confirming the suspected possibilities. It is important to emphasize that laboratory tests will only rarely detect a systemic disorder; they will rather confirm it in the context of the clinical considerations.

Ocular tissue biopsy in suspected autoimmune PUK, such as Mooren ulcer and systemic vasculitic syndrome-associated PUK, can be very helpful in reaching a specific diagnosis and deciding a specific therapy. Ocular biopsies are taken from the bulbar conjunctiva adjacent to the ulcerating cornea. The presence of vasculitis, granulomas, eosinophils, mast cells, and neutrophil or lymphocytic infiltrate in ocular tissue can be useful in the diagnosis solving process of a systemic vasculitic disease. Vasculitis is defined as neutrophil invasion of the vessel wall, with fibrinoid necrosis seen by light microscopy, or as immunoreactant deposition in the vessel wall seen by immunofluorescence. The presence of vasculitis in ocular tissue can be very helpful in the decision making regarding therapy institution. In patients with systemic vasculitic disease and PUK, the demonstration of vasculitis in ocular tissue implies systemic involvement of the same vasculitic process. Immunosuppressive therapy can be lifesaving in this group of patients. In patients with suspected systemic vasculitic disease, but without definite diagnosis, the demonstration of a destructive vasculitic process in ocular tissue provides additional justification for the institution of immunosuppressive therapy. In patients clinically suspected of having Mooren ulcer, the absence of vasculitis is helpful in making this diagnosis of exclusion.

Therapy

Local treatment for PUK includes keratectomy, the application of cyanoacrylate (with therapeutic contact lens) or amniotic membrane in the bed of the ulcer, and adjacent conjunctival resection supplemented with topical steroids. In some cases, the conjunctival flap is necessary to maintain the integrity of the globe. In the rare cases of large areas of corneal perforation, 'hot' lamellar or penetrating keratoplasty may be required (Raizman et al. 1991), but the prognosis is poor, especially in systemic vasculitic processes due to inflammation, to the associated dryness, and to the corneal hypoesthesia. Systemic steroids may be effective as intravenous (methylprednisolone 500 mg; repeated again if no response followed by oral steroids) or oral (prednisone 80–20 mg progressively reduced) according to severity. Systemic immunosuppression with alkylating agents (e.g. cyclophosphamide) with or without oral steroids will be needed in case of PUK associated with the vasculitic process such as PAN or with granulomatosis with polyangiitis (Wegener). Systemic immunosuppression with antimetabolites (e.g. MTX, AZA, and mycophenolate mofetil) may be used in cases of allergic angeiitis, Churg–Strauss, rheumatoid arthritis, lupus erythematosus, spondyloarthropathies, relapsing polychondritis, or giant cell arteritis when steroid therapy fails to control the process or when the doses needed to control it are too high to protect the patient from side effects. Systemic immuno-

suppression may also be assessed in cases of PUK with pathological diagnosis of vasculitis in ocular tissue without specific systemic diagnosis, and in cases of bilateral PUK and/or associated progressive Mooren's ulcer in which steroid therapy fails to control the process or the doses needed are too high to protect the patient from side effects. It is important to note the patient the absolute prohibition of smoking in the ulcerative process.

Some authors have reported the efficacy of BRM for PUK, especially anti-TNFα (INFLI, ADA), when other immunosuppressive drugs are not effective (Odorcic et al. 2009, Thomas & Pflugfelder 2005). Furthermore, RTX can be effective as an alternative to alkylating agents (cyclophosphamide) in PUK, associated with granulomatosis with polyangeitis (Wegener) (Huerva et al. 2010). As in scleritis, and for the same reasons mentioned previously, BRM is not considered the first-line treatment for PUK.

REFERENCES

Akpek EK, Thorne JE, Qazi FA, et al. Evaluation of patients with scleritis for systemic disease. *Ophthalmology* 2004; **111**:501–506.

Barrera BA, Wilton L, Harris S, et al. Prescription-event monitoring study on 13,164 patients prescribed risedronate in primary care in England. *Osteoporosis Int* 2005; **16**:1989–1998.

Benson WE. Posterior scleritis. *Surv Ophthalmol* 1988; **32**:297–316.

Cappaert WE, Purnell EW, Frank KE. Use of B-sector scan ultrasound in the diagnosis of benign choroidal folds. *Am J Ophthalmol* 1977; **84**:375–379.

Chaques VJ, Lam S, Tessler HH, Mafee MF. Computed tomography and magnetic resonance imaging in the diagnosis of posterior scleritis. *Ann Ophthalmol* 1993; **25**:89–94.

Gonzalez-Gonzalez LA, Molina-Prat N, Doctor P, et al. Clinical features and presentation of infectious scleritis from herpes viruses: a report of 35 cases. Ophthalmology 2012 [Epub ahead of print].

Huerva V, Sanchez MC, Traveset A, Jurjo C, Ruiz A. Rituximab for peripheral ulcerative keratitis with Wegener granulomatosis. *Cornea* 2010; **29**:708–710.

Jabs DA, Mudun A, Dunn JP, et al. Episcleritis and scleritis: clinical features and treatment results. *Am J Ophthalmol* 2000; **130**:469–476.

Lee GA, Gray TB, Dart JK, et al. Acanthamoeba sclerokeratitis: treatment with systemic immunosuppression. *Ophthalmology* 2002; **109**:1178–1182.

Livir-Rallatos C, El-Shabrawi Y, Zatirakis P, et al. Recurrent nodular scleritis associated with varicella zoster virus. *Am J Ophthalmol* 1998; **126**:594–597.

Lyons CJ, Hakin KN. Watson PG. Topical flurbiprofen: an effective treatment for episcleritis? *Eye* 1990; **4**:521–525.

Macarol V, Fraunfelder FT. Pamidronate disodium and possible ocular adverse drug reactions. *Am J Ophthalmol* 1994; **118**:220–224.

Margo CE, Polack FM, Hood CI, et al. Aspergillus panophthalmitis complicating treatment of pterygium. *Cornea* 1988; **7**:285–289.

Mbekeani JN, Slamovits TL, Schwartz BH, Sauer HL. Ocular inflammation associated with alendronate therapy. *Arch Ophthalmol* 1999; **117**:837–838.

McCluskey PJ, Watson PG, Lightman S, et al. Posterior scleritis: clinical features, systemic associations, and outcome in a large series of patients. *Ophthalmology* 1999; **106**:2380–2386.

Mondino BJ. Inflammatory diseases of the peripheral cornea. *Ophthalmology* 1988; **95**:463–472.

Naseri A, Good WV, Cunningham ET, Jr. Herpes zoster virus sclerokeratitis and anterior uveitis in a child following varicella vaccination. *Am J Ophthalmol* 2003; **135**:415–417.

Nieuwenhuizen J, Watson PG, Jager MJ, et al. The value of combining anterior segment fluorescein angiography with indocyanine green angiography in scleral inflammation. *Ophthalmology* 2003; **110**:1653–1666.

Odorcic S, Keystone EC, Ma JJ. Infliximab for the treatment of refractory progressive sterile peripheral ulcerative keratitis associated with late corneal perforation: 3-year follow-up. *Cornea* 2009; **28**:89–92.

Raizman MB, Sainz de la Maza M, Foster CS. Tectonic keratoplasty for peripheral ulcerative keratitis. *Cornea* 1991; **10**:312–316.

Read RW, Weiss AH, Sherry DD. Episcleritis in childhood. *Ophthalmology* 1999; **106**:2377–2379.

Sainz de la Maza M, Jabbur NS, Foster CS. Severity of scleritis and episcleritis. *Ophthalmology* 1994a; **101**:389–396.

Sainz de la Maza M, Foster CS, Jabbur NS. Scleritis associated with rheumatoid arthritis and with other systemic immune-mediated diseases. *Ophthalmology* 1994b; **101**:1281–1286.

Sainz de la Maza M, Foster CS, Jabbur NS. Scleritis associated with systemic vasculitic diseases. *Ophthalmology* 1995; **102**:687–692.

Sainz de la Maza M, Foster CS, Jabbur NS, et al. Ocular characteristics and disease associations in scleritis-associated peripheral keratopathy. *Arch Ophthalmol* 2002; **120**:15–19.

Sainz de la Maza M, Molina N, Gonzalez-Gonzalez LA, et al. Clinical characteristics of a large cohort of patients with scleritis and episcleritis. 2012a; **119**:43–50.

Sainz de la Maza M, Molina N, Gonzalez-Gonzalez LA, et al. Scleritis therapy. *Ophthalmology* 2012b; **119**:51–58.

Tauber J, Sainz de la Maza M, Hoang-Xuan T, et al. An analysis of therapeutic decision making regarding immunosuppressive chemotherapy for peripheral ulcerative keratitis. *Cornea* 1990; **9**:66–73.

Thomas JW, Pflugfelder SC. Therapy of progressive rheumatoid arthritis-associated corneal ulceration with infliximab. *Cornea* 2005; **24**:742–744.

Tranos PG, Ong T, Nolan W, et al. Posterior scleritis presenting with annular choroidal detachment as a complication of herpes zoster ophthalmicus. *Retina* 2003; **23**:716–717.

Tuft SJ, Watson PG. Progression of scleral disease. *Ophthalmology* 1991; **98**:467–471.

Watson PG, Hayreh SS. Scleritis and episcleritis. *Br J Ophthalmol* 1976; **60**:163–191.

Chapter 17 — Chemical and thermal injuries of the eye

Roswell R. Pfister

INTRODUCTION

Chemical and thermal injuries of the eye continue to pose major obstacles to optimal management. Despite several decades of research, considerable controversy still exists regarding the best treatment at many stages of the disease process. Major problems might develop from seemingly small and reversible events, while relatively minor problems might continue to stymie progress and even grow into major difficulties. Continued observation over short intervals and proactive alleviation of all observed problems help ensure continued success. Given the uncertain atmosphere surrounding treatment strategies of thermal and chemical injuries of the eye, our focus is on sorting through available measures and providing sufficient data to enable subscription to a particular approach or treatment for each specific problem.

Ocular surface disease is embedded within the challenge of a chemical or thermal injury, but constitutes only one part, however significant, of a very complex process of damage and healing. As defined by the International Dry Eye Workshop (DEWS 2007) 'Dry eye is a multifactorial disease of the tears and ocular surface that results in symptoms of discomfort, visual disturbance, and tear film instability with potential damage to the ocular surface. It is accompanied by increased osmolarity of the tear film and inflammation of the ocular surface.' With these considerations in mind, a comprehensive approach to each problem enhances the possibility of finding a successful treatment.

THERMAL VERSUS CHEMICAL INJURY

Chemical injuries are far more common that thermal, with very different forms of ocular insult, postinjury problems, and treatment approaches. With thermal injury, eyelid damage is very common, leading to necrosis of tissues, eschar formation, and, finally, quantitative loss of tissue. Therefore, the eyelid and conjunctival support system of the cornea is compromised, further embarrassing any corneal or anterior segment pathology. Chronic exposure keratitis is one of the greatest threats to corneal integrity and visual rehabilitation. Direct thermal damage to the cornea produces collagen shrinkage, with prominent stress lines radiating away from the area of greatest injury, especially in case of hot metal contact to the surface. This shrinkage might be severe enough to make the cornea grossly distorted and opaque, leading to steepening of the axis of severest injury. Collagen damage can be so severe as to produce a rapidly excavating corneal ulcer originating from liquefactive necrosis. The postinjury phases of thermal injuries have not been studied as comprehensively as chemical injuries. Because thermal injuries are much less common and the data less available, most of the discussion in this chapter is focused on chemical injuries.

Tissue destruction resulting from chemical injuries is created from a wave of strongly dissociated ions flooding the eyelids and/or tear film and reservoir, penetrating the cornea and adjacent tissues, into the aqueous humor. Immediate shrinkage of the collagenous envelope of the eye results in a rapid intraocular pressure rise, followed by a second rise, lasting longer, which is a consequence of prostaglandin release. At any time, rise in pressure can occur due to the clogging of the trabecular meshwork by necrotic debris, and from organization of inflammatory components followed by cicatricial closure of the chamber angle, especially inferiorly. Inflammatory cells, most importantly, neutrophils, pour into the damaged tissue, releasing superoxide radicals and tissue degrading enzymes. Extensive data from animal models have identified incoming repair fibroblasts as scorbutic, occasioned by damage to the ascorbate concentrating mechanisms within the non-pigmented epithelium of the ciliary body. The upshot of this amalgam is the development of corneal ulcerations, perforations, and vascularization.

CLINICAL GRADING OF CHEMICAL INJURIES

Emergency treatment of the chemically injured eye must precede any attempt at classification. Once the condition has been stabilized, determine the anticipated course of the chemical injury by examining the critical features listed below. Understanding and documenting the salient features of an alkali injury of the eye permits proper classification so that appropriate treatment can be initiated and accurate prognostication adduced. Documentation of the following physical data is recommended in the form of a labeled drawing:

- **Epithelial defect:** instill 2% fluorescein and measure the size and draw the shape of the defect. It is critical to include any conjunctival epithelial defects as well, particularly concerning the palisades of Vogt (limbal stem cells). Document all epithelial defects, including those extending into the fornices
- **Corneal stromal opacity:** grade on the basis of a penlight examination: grade 0, clear cornea; grade 1, mild corneal haze; grade 2, mild to moderate opacity; grade 3, moderate opacity; grade 4, moderate to severe opacity, details of iris trabeculae can be seen but pupils are visible; grade 5, severe corneal opacity, pupils are not visible with penlight
- **Perilimbal ischemia:** document the clock hours where the conjunctiva is whitened. In these areas the conjunctiva and episclera are devoid of blood vessels. This whitening should not to be confused with less severe injury where there is chemosis and thrombosed blood vessels but some of the conjunctiva is still viable. Perilimbal whitening has proved be a useful parameter by which the extent of corneal stem cell damage and, indirectly, injury of the underlying ciliary body and trabecular meshwork, can be judged. Documentation of these findings allow for a later,

more accurate, determination of the necessity for corneal stem cell transplantation
- **Adnexa:** measure and document the blinking pattern, corneal exposure, and/or lagophthalmos

These measurements and findings can then be applied to the classification of alkali injuries as described by Hughes, and later modified by Pfister (Pfister & Koski 1982). This classification, with accompanying drawings and photographs, represents the span of damage encountered after alkali injury (**Figure 17.1a–e**). The accuracy of early assessment becomes very important in prognostication and treatment plans.

Regarding terminology, the literature is replete with allusions to alkali 'burns,' potentially confusing the alkali-injury terminology with

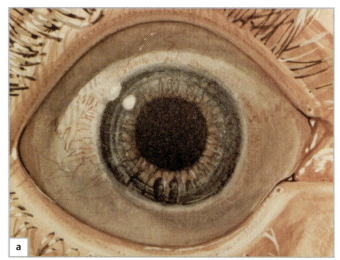

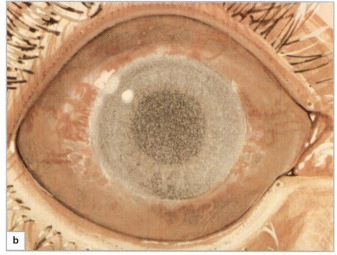

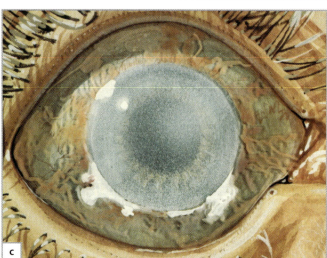

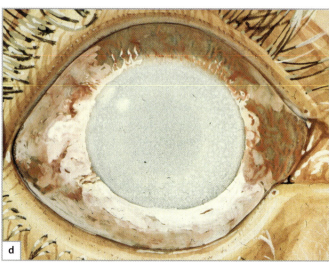

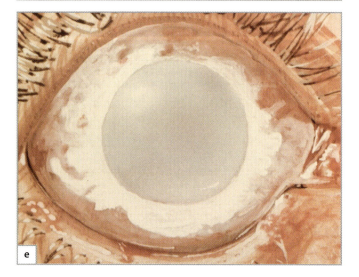

Figure 17.1 A diagrammatic representation of chemical injuries based on severity, with an accompanying prognosis. (a) Mild: corneal epithelial erosion, faint anterior stromal haziness, and no ischemic necrosis of perilimbal conjunctiva and sclera. Prognosis: healing with little or no corneal scarring, visual loss usually no greater than one to two lines. (b) Moderate: moderate corneal opacity, little or no significant ischemic necrosis of perilimbal conjunctiva. Prognosis: slow healing of epithelium with moderate scarring, peripheral corneal vascularization, and visual loss of two to seven lines. (c) Moderate to severe: corneal opacity, blurring iris details, ischemic necrosis of conjunctiva limited to less than one third of perilimbal conjunctiva. Prognosis: prolonged corneal healing with significant corneal vascularization and scarring, vision usually limited to 20/200 or less. (d) Severe: blurring of pupillary outline, ischemia of approximately one third to two thirds of perilimbal conjunctiva, cornea often marbleized. Prognosis: very prolonged corneal healing with inflammation and high incidence of corneal ulceration and perforation. In the best cases, severe corneal vascularization and scarring with counting fingers vision results. (e) Very severe: pupil not visible, greater than two-third ischemia of perilimbal conjunctiva, cornea often marbleized. Prognosis: very prolonged corneal healing with inflammation and high incidence of corneal ulceration and perforation. In the best cases, severe corneal vascularization and scarring with counting fingers vision results. Reprinted with permission from Pfister and Koski (1982).

a, usually non-existent, thermal, or even open flame component. We recommend the designation 'alkali' injury or 'acid' injury of the eye to distinguish chemical 'burns' from true thermal burns. When both chemical and thermal injuries occur simultaneously, the terms 'alkali–thermal injury' or 'thermal–alkali injury' might be used, with the most prominent injurious agent stated first. Acid injuries should be referred to in a similar way.

MAJOR CHEMICAL DIFFERENCES BETWEEN ALKALI, ACID, AND TOXIC INJURY OF THE EYE

Alkali

The pain, lacrimation, and blepharospasm following an ocular alkali injury result from direct injury of free nerve endings located in the epithelium of the cornea, conjunctiva, and eyelids. The severity of the injury is dependent on the anion concentration, the dissociation of the alkali, and the quantity of fluid. A wave of hydroxyl ions rapidly advances through ocular tissues, causing massive cell death by saponification of cellular membranes and extensive hydrolysis of glycosaminoglycans and collagen within the corneal matrix. The alkaline products in common usage have been briefly described in the following text.

Ammonia

Ammonia (NH_3) is available as a fertilizer and refrigerant and is used in the manufacture of other chemicals. It is commonly used as a household cleaning agent; and a 7% solution is capable of causing major ocular damage due to its high solubility and penetrability.

Lye

Lye [sodium hydroxide (NaOH), caustic soda, sodium hydrate] penetrates into the interior of the eye in 3–5 minutes (Grant 1974). Solid sodium hydroxide, often used as a drain cleaner, can cause pressure to develop within the drainpipe, resulting in an explosion of lye into the face and eyes of the unprepared. Warmed lye is also commonly used to straighten curly hair. Its easy availability in homes makes it a common instrument of attack among paramours. Lye injuries rank second in severity to those produced by ammonium hydroxide.

Other hydroxides

Potassium hydroxide [(KOH) caustic potash] and magnesium hydroxide [$Mg(OH)_2$] penetrate the eye slightly less rapidly than sodium hydroxide. Magnesium hydroxide is found in sparklers and flares; the combination of thermal injury and chemical injury accounts for more severe injury than that occurring as a result of heat alone.

Lime

Lime {[$Ca(OH)_2$], fresh lime, quicklime [$CaO + H_2O = Ca(OH)_2$], calcium hydrate, slaked lime, hydrated lime, plaster, mortar, cement, and whitewash} penetrates the eye less rapidly because it reacts with epithelial cell membranes, forming calcium soaps that precipitate and hinder further penetration. Despite this, these injuries can be quite severe, with the corneal opacity visible before the opacity in case of ammonium or sodium hydroxide.

Methyl ethyl ketone peroxide

Methyl ethyl ketone peroxide is a catalyst, and commonly used in various industries. Both immediate and delayed corneal injury can occur because of this. There have been reports of exacerbations and remissions of limbal and corneal disease lasting >20 years.

Acids

Weak acidic compounds contacting the outer eye precipitate proteins within the corneal and conjunctival epithelium, thus acting as a partial barrier to further ingress of the chemical. In its wake is left a grayish white epithelium, often obscuring all tissues posterior to it. Stripping off this opacified epithelial layer often reveals a relatively clear underlying corneal stroma (**Figure 17.2**). As long as the corneal stem cells ringing the cornea are not damaged, epithelial recovery is likely, with little or no stromal cloudiness.

Very strong acids, however, overcome this precipitated proteineous obstacle and progress through tissue, much as alkali. The end result of a very severe acid injury is often indistinguishable from that of an alkali injury. For this reason, this chapter deals with alkaline and acid injuries as one, unless otherwise specified.

Sulfuric acid

Sulfuric acid (H_2SO_4) is a commonly used industrial chemical as well as the acid used in batteries. The great avidity of concentrated sulfuric acid for water results in the release of heat, which causes tissue charring. Sulfuric acid produces injuries ranging from mild to very severe. Most of the injuries, especially the more severe ones, occur as a result of battery explosions. Hydrogen and oxygen are produced by electrolysis when sulfuric acid combines with water in the battery. This gaseous mixture explodes on contact with flame. Matches or cigarette lighters used as illumination sources or sparks produced by jumper cables are the most common modes of ignition. Injuries that result from battery explosions are usually combinations of acid burn and contusion from particulate matter, but might also show laceration or intraocular foreign body penetration.

Sulfurous acid

Sulfur dioxide (SO_2) forms sulfurous acid (H_2SO_3) when it combines with water in ocular tissue. It might be encountered as sulfurous

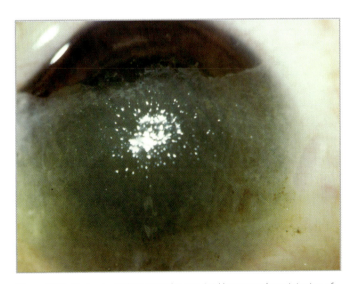

Figure 17.2 Moderate acid injury to the eye. Acid has caused precipitation of epithelial protein. Removal of epithelium discloses a clear underlying stroma. Epithelium readily recovered the cornea because deeply embedded limbal stem cells had not been injured.

anhydride or sulfurous oxide: a fruit and vegetable preservative, bleach, and refrigerant. At first, visual acuity is not severely affected, but it worsens greatly over hours to days as the ocular condition deteriorates. It is not the sulfur dioxide's freezing effect on the tissue that produces the injury but rather sulfurous acid itself, denaturing protein and inactivating numerous enzymes. Because of its high lipid and water solubility, sulfurous acid penetrates the tissues easily.

Hydrofluoric acid

Hydrofluoric acid [(HF) hydrogen fluoride] is a weak inorganic acid but a strong solvent, widely used in a variety of industries. It has been used for centuries, but currently it is found either in its pure form (in solutions ranging from 0.5 to 70.0% in strength) or mixed with other agents such as nitric acid, ammonium difluoride, and acetic acid. Hydrofluoric acid is used in etching and polishing glass and silicone, in the pickling or chemical milling of metals, and in the refining of uranium, tantalum, and beryllium. In the semiconductor industry it is essential in the manufacture of silicon chips. It is so highly toxic that as little as 7 mL of hydrofluoric acid, or 2.5% burn of the body, is sufficient to cause death from uncontrolled hypocalcemia.

Much has been written on skin burns caused by hydrofluoric acid; however, the literature is sparse regarding ocular injuries. Hydrofluoric acid produces a severe ocular injury because of its high degree of activity in dissolving cellular membranes.

Other acids

Chromic acid is a strong caustic derived from chromic oxide and chromium trioxide (Cr_2O_3). Ocular injuries caused by chromic acid are more often associated with exposure to droplets of the acid in the chrome-plating industry, resulting in chronic conjunctival inflammation and a brown discoloration of the epithelium in the interpalpebral fissure.

Hydrochloric acid (HCl) is commonly used as a 32–38% solution. Hydrogen chloride gas is irritating to the eye; thus, the profuse tearing serves to limit ocular damage. At high concentrations and with prolonged exposure, liquid hydrochloric acid produces severe ocular damage.

Injuries produced by nitric acid (HNO_3) are similar to those produced by hydrochloric acid, except that the epithelial opacity produced by nitric acid is yellowish rather than white, as it is in the other acid burns.

Acetic acid (CH_3COOH) is a relatively weak organic acid, and is also known as ethanoic acid, ethylic acid, methane carboxylic acid, vinegar acid, and glacial acetic acid. The various forms of acetic acid, especially vinegar acid (4–10% acetic acid), typically produce only minor ocular damage, unless exposure is prolonged. Exposure to a solution >10% produces a severe injury unless the time of exposure is exceedingly short. 'Essence of vinegar' (80% acetic acid) and glacial acetic acid (90%) are the most concentrated forms of acetic acid, and most likely to produce severe ocular injury.

■ Other toxic chemicals

Other types of ocular chemical injuries are usually less severe than alkali and acid injuries. The reader is referred to Grant's 'Toxicology of the Eye' for a detailed discussion of the adverse ocular effects of petroleum products and other organic chemicals (Grant 1974).

Chemical Mace and similar compounds can cause minor to severe ocular injury, depending on a number of factors. The ocular injury associated with the original Chemical Mace is caused by the lacrimator chloroacetophenone. The degree of severity of reported injuries depends on factors such as proximity of the spray can to the eye, quantity of chemical entering the eye, duration of exposure, state of normal reflex mechanisms, and the mechanism of propelling the chemical. Police recommend directing the spray away from the eyes and from a distance >2 m (6 ft). Under these conditions, only minor injury is likely to occur. Extensive exposure leads to damage including loss of ocular surface epithelium, severe persistent stromal edema, presumably secondary to endothelial damage, stromal clouding, and corneal neovascularization.

■ Preparation for vision restoration

Preparation for vision restoration must begin immediately after the injury. Successful outcomes are predicated on deliberate and timely treatment at each juncture in the rehabilitative process. In succession, these consist of emergency treatment, pressure control, suppression of inflammation, enhancing stromal repair, and establishing eyelid–globe congruity during the early days, weeks, and months after the injury. Operative procedures include amniotic membrane transplant, corneal epithelial stem cell transplants, keratoplasty, large-diameter lamellar keratoplasty, and keratoprosthesis. A brief discussion of each of these approaches is described in the following text.

■ Emergency treatment

Irrigation of the chemically injured eye with water at the scene of the injury, or with an intravenous fluid in an emergency room after the injury, can no longer be regarded as sufficient for emergency care. Several reports have shown the inability of saline or water to significantly lower the pH of the aqueous humor (Paterson et al. 1975). Newer safe and effective irrigants are now available to effectively neutralize a variety of chemicals. In the United States, only Cederroth, a borate buffer, is commercially available to neutralize alkalis (Rihawi et al. 2008). After its application, the pH profile of the aqueous humor shows rapid neutralization as compared to saline or a phosphate buffer. Diphoterine, an amphoteric, divalent, chelating irrigant, available in Europe, is effective against up to 600 different chemicals by trapping the molecules within its molecular structure (Hall et al. 2000). There are no specific irrigants available in the United States to neutralize acids or other toxic compounds.

The pultaceous character of lime used in cement compounds clings to the conjunctiva. The bulk of material can be removed with a cotton-tipped applicator but the sticky paste in contact with the conjunctiva can be loosened and removed with greater ease by irrigation with a solution of ethylene diaminetetraacetic acid (0.01 M).

■ Events controlling intraocular pressure

A multitude of causes raise the intraocular pressure to damaging levels in alkali-injured eyes. When alkali contacts the cornea and sclera, an immediate contracture of the collagen causes the intraocular pressure to rise as high as 40 mmHg above normal (Paterson & Pfister 1974). A subsequent, overlapping pressure increase, of a greater duration, reflects the release of intraocular prostaglandins. Aqueous debris from damaged anterior uveal cells accumulate on the trabecular meshwork, initially obstructing outflow but later serving as a latticework for fibrotic organization and angle closure. Fibrotic angle closure might lead to a lasting form of secondary glaucoma that might or might not be medically treatable. Filtering cicatrices are rarely successful, so shunt procedures are commonly required. Most importantly, pressure control from the inception of injury is mandatory. The major reason for failure to restore vision to a chemically injured eye is glaucomatous optic nerve damage (Cade et al. 2011).

Anterior segment inflammation

Within minutes after chemical injury, neutrophils adhere to and diapedese between vascular endothelial cells in the perilimbal arcades and uvea, bringing these inflammatory cells into damaged tissues. Powerful mediator attractants for neutrophils, N-acetyl proline-glycine-proline and N-methyl proline-glycine-proline, obtained from alkali-degraded collagen, create a gradient along which neutrophils move (Pfister et al. 1995).

Traditionally, topical steroids have been used to control the inflammatory process. If used beyond 7–10 days, however, they pose a risk of corneal ulceration from concomitant suppression of the repair process (Davis et al. 1997). A more rational approach employs research gleaned from animal models, utilizing topical buffered 10% sodium citrate, a powerful chelator of the calcium held on the plasma membrane of the neutrophil. This results in inhibition of the calcium–calmodulin molecule, a key molecular intermediary preventing locomotion, degradative enzyme release, and superoxide radical production. In a rabbit model of severe corneal alkali injury, topical citrate reduced the incidence of corneal ulceration and perforation from 78.6 to 18.8% and, in separate experiments, it encouraged healing and prevented deepening of established corneal ulcers (Pfister et al. 1981).

Enhancing stromal repair

Extensive animal research has revealed that the alkali-injured cornea is scorbutic, caused by damage to its concentrating cells, the non-pigmented epithelium of the ciliary body. Ascorbate is normally concentrated in the aqueous humor, and is 15–20 times that of the blood level. In animal eyes subjected to alkali injury, <15 mg/mL aqueous humor concentration of ascorbate often leads to corneal ulceration. When the aqueous concentration is increased by the application of topical 10% ascorbate drops, the incidence of corneal ulceration is significantly decreased (Pfister & Paterson 1977). Histology of these corneas mimics the findings of Ross and Benditt from research on the skin of scorbutic guinea pigs (Ross & Benditt 1962). Fibroblasts contained swollen, smooth endoplasmic reticulum with ribosomal disarray, while immature collagen fibrils surrounding these cells failed to assemble into the triple helical structure of collagen. The molecular events responsible for the failure of collagen to assemble properly occur because of the deficiency of the reducing agent ascorbate required to hydroxylate proline while it is held in the ribosomal cellular machinery. As a consequence, underhydroxylated collagen swells the endoplasmic reticulum and is ultimately externalized as fibrillar, immature collagen.

When topical 10% ascorbate and 10% citrate are dropped into alkali-injured rabbit eyes, alternately every hour 14 hours per day, the incidence of corneal ulceration is reduced to a transitory 4% (Pfister et al. 1991).

A single human clinical trial using ascorbate and citrate for eye treatment was conducted, showing that of 20 patients with moderately severe alkali injuries, 93% of eyes resulted in 20/40 vision. In the control group, three out of six patients had 20/40 vision (50%) (Brodovsky et al. 2000). These patients received topical 10% ascorbate and 10% citrate, as well as fluoromethalone every 2 hours, 24 hours a day. They also received oral ascorbate and citrate. This significant difference is encouraging, mirroring the findings in the animal model.

CHEMICAL AND THERMAL INJURY: A MODEL OF MULTIPLE OCULAR SURFACE DISEASES

Chemical and thermal ocular injuries invite a toxic mix of factors, all of which encourage the development of ocular surface disease. Multiple symblephara and even ankyloblepharon might develop from the apposition of raw conjunctival surfaces or from progressive subconjunctival scarring and contracture. With or without symblephara, there is often incomplete blinking and exposure keratitis resulting from conjunctival adhesions and/or periorbital and lid scarring with retraction of the lid margins, especially after thermal burns. Tear film deficiencies are common, with mucus and oil gland destruction, leading to rapid fluid evaporation.

While all of these factors are inimical to the integrity of the ocular surface, none of them is as critical as loss of the limbal epithelial stem cells. Alkalis and strongly dissociated acids rapidly penetrate the epithelial cell layers over their complete contact areas, demolishing all cellular constituents. When there is extensive damage to the limbal tissues the phenotype for corneal epithelia is destroyed; what is left are the residual conjunctival epithelial cells. Lacking the corneal cell phenotype, these conjunctival cells spread on to the corneal surface, dragging a vascular supply with its attendant scarring. If undisciplined, a pannus spreads over the cornea, curtailing useful vision. Failure of corneal epithelium to repopulate the surface also invites inflammatory cells into the void, enhancing the opportunity for enzymatic digestion of degraded collagen and the release of superoxide radicals from neutrophils. In this scenario, the ultimate fate of the cornea is the formation of a corneal ulcer, and in some cases, perforation of the globe.

Elements of surgery

Assuming that the eye has bridged the initial insult and is ready to undergo visual restoration, certain considerations must be taken. Successful visual rehabilitation after chemical injury is dependent on timing, skills, and appropriate application of tissue materials. The following is a current list of available approaches. Bear in mind that, first, the eyelids and conjunctiva must be able to support the cornea from a physiological–mechanical standpoint. Ophthalmic plastic surgery might be required initially to re-establish a semblance of normal lid–globe congruity.

Amniotic membrane

Amniotic membrane has gained an appreciable reputation in ophthalmology as a supplement to surgical procedures where coverage of raw surfaces or suppression of inflammation is required. Pterygium excision, expansion of conjunctival surfaces, and extraocular muscle surgery are but a few of the procedures benefiting from surfacing with amniotic membrane. Contained within the membrane are antiangiogenic and anti-inflammatory proteins capable of suppressing the inflammatory response (Sotozono et al. 1997, Yanxia et al. 2000). Amniotic membrane can create a new basement membrane and promote epithelial healing. Amniotic membrane might be applied very early after a chemical injury but only after emergent services have concluded, usually weeks later (Gomes et al. 2003). A combination of sutures and fibrin adhesive are used to provide a temporary covering over the cornea and adjacent conjunctiva. An alternative approach is the placement of ProKera, a preformed amniotic membrane with a ring that can be inserted into the eye in the manner of a large contact lens.

Clinical results with amniotic membrane have been favorable but not overwhelming. Tsai and coworkers treated 72 alkali, acid, or thermally injured eyes with amniotic membrane with a success rate of 87% in acute and 72.9% in chronic cases (Tsai & Tseng 1994). Despite these advantages, amniotic membrane cannot replace the need for corneal stem cells. This was demonstrated in a paper by Tandon showing that 50 patients with grade II to IV injuries, treated with amniotic membrane, healed their epithelial defects faster than controls, but these moderate injuries, along with the severe injuries in additional 50 patients, showed no long-term advantage over medical therapy (Tandon et al. 2011). Using amniotic membrane with or without cultured stem cells in acute or chronic chemical or thermal injuries gave improved results based on initial criteria indicating limbal stem cell deficiency (Tejwani et al. 2007).

Corneal stem cell transplantation

Replacement of the corneal stem cells lost due to disease or injury is an important concept in the restoration of an intact and normal corneal epithelial cell layer. These primitive, slow-cycling stem cells, located in the limbal niche, show little differentiation.

Monocular injuries allow for procurement of stem cells from the uninjured eye. The use of lenticular grafts, pioneered by Thoft, led the way to a variety of surgical approaches to replace the corneal stem cell population from related or unrelated donors (Kenyon 1989, Thoft 1982). When the injury is bilateral, research by Pfister showed that allografted limbal tissue was capable of restoring the stem cell population from an unrelated donor (Pfister 1993).

My personal technique requires removal of all pannus and epithelial cells from the recipient cornea and limbus. Conjunctiva is allowed to retract back ≥5 mm from the limbus, removing any scar under the conjunctiva down to the episclera. Limbal tissue harvested from the other eye is obtained under topical 4% xylocaine, with a subconjunctival injection of 2% xylocaine. Three pieces of tissue are obtained, about 3 mm wide and 4 or 5 mm deep, from the upper inner, upper outer, and inferior quadrants of the normal eye or a related donor. The conjunctival edge of each transplant is delineated with a wet field cautery and cut loose from its surroundings with scissors. Each piece can be moved over to the recipient eye individually or oriented on to surgical paper in a Petri dish for later transfer. Individual tissues are sutured into episclera with four 10-0 ethilon sutures or adhered with a fibrin adhesive. The procedure is completed with a covering of fresh or frozen amniotic membrane, amply cut to fit over the total corneal and conjunctival defect, suturing it to the edge of the recipient conjunctiva peripherally.

Stem cell tissue can be obtained from a related donor using the Petri dish technique. Harvesting stem cell tissue from an eye donor requires either the whole eye or an artificial anterior chamber to stabilize the tissue to harvest 360° of tissue. A small piece of cornea removed along with the stem cells makes transfer and suturing less difficult.

Allografted corneal stem cells must be protected from the recipient immune process by systemic immunosuppression, commonly azithiaprin and cyclosporin. As an adjunct, amniotic membrane stretched over the alkali-injured cornea has proved to be useful when transplanting corneal stem cells by replacing the abnormal surface of the cornea with a new surface, which tends to quiet the inflammatory process (Meller et al. 2000, Tsai & Tseng 1994). Amniotic membrane disappears over time and is not sufficient to substitute for corneal stem cells alone. Techniques to culture corneal stem cells ex vivo on amniotic membrane from unrelated, related, or fellow eyes now provide an expanded source of corneal stem cells (Gomes et al. 2003, Sharma et al. 2011).

CORNEAL TRANSPLANTATION
Penetrating keratoplasty

The prospects for restoration of vision after chemical injury have been substantially improved over the past two decades. Success in any type of restorative corneal surgery will be governed by (1) lid–globe congruity with normal blinking and the absence of corneal exposure, (2) quality and quantity of the tear film, (3) the presence of epithelial stem cells phenotypic for cornea, (4) the absence of any current ulceration, inflammation, and/or uncontrolled glaucoma, (5) flawless surgical technique, and (6) fresh corneal transplant tissue.

Preparatory procedures to lyse symblephara, expand cul-de-sacs, and eliminate lagophthalmos are often required to re-establish normal lid physiology and anatomy. Secondary glaucoma must also be controlled with medications or filtration surgery. The value of preoperative LASER of blood vessels at the limbus in high-risk patients is controversial, but at the least it would reduce bleeding at the time of surgery.

If corneal surgery is delayed 18 months to 2 years after a chemical burn, it increases the chances of success, especially without preexisting ulceration, perforation, or glaucoma. Corneal surgery is indicated for the worst eye in bilateral injuries when serviceable vision is not available. In some patients with severe monocular injuries, if a definite need for binocularity does not exist, corneal transplantation might not be contemplated, since transplantation in chemically burned eyes is fraught with numerous potential complications.

If corneal transplantation is indicated, it is important to pay meticulous attention to the rigorous protocol of fine corneal surgery. A few points of importance are mentioned here. Trephination with a vacuum cutter and vertical section of remaining attachments with scissors improves the quality of the wound architecture. If suction cannot be achieved due to surface irregularity, layering a ring of viscoelastic on the peripheral cornea usually assists vacuum adherence. Fresh blood from the wound edges is absorbed with cellulose sponges, applying pressure to active bleeders by squeezing with fine forceps until it stops or until suture placement closes the vessel. Even light application of wet field cautery causes wound retraction; hence, it should be used sparingly, if at all.

The donor cornea should be fresh, with intact epithelium, cut 0.50–0.75 mm larger than the recipient bed. Oversizing the donor corneal button by 0.5 mm or even 0.75 mm compensates for retraction of the scarred and vascularized recipient bed as well as the softness of scar tissue compared to cornea. Donor tissue is age-matched, but human leukocyte antigen (HLA) or blood typing is not usually done for the first transplant. A single continuous 10-0 nylon suture might be used if the recipient corneal tissue is firm and is of near normal thickness with mild vascularity. When the quality of the recipient bed is soft or friable, it is generally safer to use 24 interrupted sutures, eight more than that usually employed. This is especially true for more extensively vascularized or thin corneas. The knots must be buried to avoid epithelial defects and limit portals for infection. Occasionally, it is necessary to thicken the recipient bed by a lamellar graft 3–6 months in advance in preparation for penetrating keratoplasty.

When a cataract is present, it is usually wisest to remove it at the time of corneal surgery. Cataract surgery should follow modern techniques with special emphasis on the approach to the open eye. Despite the use of preoperative pressure devices to reduce vitreous volume, the crystalline lens usually tends to prolapse forward. Positive vitreous pressure usually requires a 'can-opener' technique using Vannas scissors. The lens usually self-delivers with gentle hydrodissection. Cortical cleanup, with irrigation and aspiration, followed by placement of an intraocular lens, can then be accomplished. Choice of the intraocular lens should be dictated by haptic design, namely torsional strength, slight anterior angulation (15°), easy haptic collapsibility, and null anteroposterior movement on linear collapse. The Bausch + Lomb model 122 UV fulfills these requirements and can be used in the anterior as well as the posterior chamber.

If epithelial defects are noted in the postoperative period then search for a definitive cause is important. If necessary, a soft contact lens can be fitted for continuous wear, or a one- or two-pillar tarsorrhaphy performed to reduce air exposure. It is critical to remove interrupted sutures that become loose and/or break through the epithelium as soon as it occurs.

Large-diameter penetrating keratoplasty

Replacement of the entire cornea and adjacent stem cells by large-diameter penetrating keratoplasty has been performed successfully and reported in two different series. Kukelkorn replaced the entire cornea in sterile ulcerating, alkali-injured eyes, preserving an intact epithelium and absence of ulceration over a 1-year period (Kukelkorn et al. 1993). Redbrake reported on nine eyes operated this way, preserving the epithelium but only maintaining clarity in two (Redbrake et al. 1996). Nevertheless, under the circumstances, these results should be considered a guardedly successful approach. One potential danger might be that such large transplants might interfere with the trabecular outflow channels and hence increase the likelihood of glaucoma. Proximity to the limbal blood vessels makes the specter of an immune rejection more likely.

Large-diameter lamellar keratoplasty

A very promising technique in corneal transplantation for chemical injuries includes the use of 12 or 13 mm lamellar corneal transplants, including the limbal epithelial stem cell population. Six out of nine patients showed vision improvement while epithelial integrity was re-established in an average of 5.2 days (Vajpayee et al. 2000). No systemic or topical immunosuppressive agents were given. Surgery was performed at an average of 29.5 months after injury, gaining all the advantages of replacement of the cornea and associated stem cells while reducing the chance of consequent glaucoma through less interference with the outflow channels. In the event that the deep residual corneal tissue is opaque and vision impaired, a later penetrating transplant can be performed, centered on the lamellar. Smaller lamellar transplants are useful to fill in deep corneal ulcerations, desmetocoeles, or frank corneal perforations.

Keratoprosthesis

In the most severe cases, implantation of a keratoprosthesis might afford the only means by which vision can be restored. Corneas exhibiting exuberant vascularity, repeated failures of fresh transplanted corneal tissue, chronic limbal stem cell deficiency, or the inability to restore normal lid anatomy are potential indications for this procedure. The operation is usually advised in patients with severe bilateral injuries where serviceable vision is not present in either eye. All available devices are investigational and require assembly, but are not difficult to implant. A surprising degree of success has been achieved, but this must be balanced against the sometimes serious and untreatable complications that can occur. Critical to the visual outcome of a keratoprosthesis is the control of the intraocular pressure at all times after the chemical injury.

Twenty eight eyes of 23 alkali- or acid-injured patients received Boston keratoprostheses and were followed-up over a 20-year period. While 54% achieved 20/50 vision in the short term, this dropped to 25% over the entire period of time. Eight developed retinal detachment. Glaucoma usurped significant vision in the majority of patients, 20 eyes showing glaucoma preoperatively and 3 postoperatively (Cade et al. 2011). In a separate paper, more than two thirds of 28 patients with limbal stem cell deficiency disease, followed-up for 3 years, obtained 20/50 vision after Boston keratoprosthesis implantation (Sejpal et al. 2011).

REFERENCES

Brodovsky S, McCarty C, Snibson G. Management of alkali burns: an 11-year retrospective review. Ophthalmol 2000; 107:1829–1835.
Cade F, Grosskreutz C, Tauber A, et al. Glaucoma in eyes with severe chemical burns before and after keratoprosthesis. Cornea 2011; 30:1322–1327.
Davis A, Ali Q, Aclimandos W. Topical steroid use in the treatment of ocular alkali burns. Br J Ophthalmol 1997; 81:732–734.
DEWS. Report of the International Dry Eye Workshop. Ocul Surf 2007; 5:69-202.
Gomes J, dos Santos M, Cunha C, et al. Amniotic membrane transplantation for partial and total limbal stem cell deficiency secondary to chemical burn. Ophthalmol 2003; 110:466–473.
Grant W. Toxicology of the eye, 2nd edn. Springfield, IL: Thomas, 1974.
Hall A, Blomet J, Mathieu L. Diphoterine for emergent eye/skin chemical splash decontamination: a review. Presented at Semiconductor Safety Association – Europe 2000; 3–5.
Kenyon K. Limbal autograft transplantation for chemical and thermal burns. Dev Ophthalmol 1989; 18:53–58.

Kukelkorn R, Redbrade C, Scharage N, et al. Keratoplasty with 11–12 mm diameter for management of severely chemically-burned eyes. Ophthalmologe 1993; 90:683–687.
Meller D, Pires R, Mack R, et al. Amniotic membrane transplantation for acute chemical or thermal burns. Invest Ophthalmol Vis Sci 2000; 107:980–990.
Paterson CA, Pfister R. Intraocular pressure changes after alkali burns. Arch Ophthalmol 1974; 91:211–218.
Paterson CA, Pfister R, Levinson RA. Aqueous humor pH changes after experimental alkali burns. Am J Ophthalmol 1975; 79:414–419.
Pfister R, Haddox J, Barr D. The combined effect of citrate/ascorbate treatment in alkali-injured rabbit eyes. Cornea 1991; 10:100–104.
Pfister R. Stem cell disease. CLAO J 1993; 20:64–72.
Pfister R, Koski J. The pathophysiology and treatment of the alkali burned eye. South Med J 1982; 75:417–422.
Pfister R, Haddox J, Somers C, et al. Identification and synthesis of chemotactic tripeptides from alkali-degraded whole cornea: a study of

N-acetyl-proline-glycine-proline and N-methyl-proline-glycine-proline. *Invest Ophthalmol Vis Sci* 1995; **36**:1306–1316.

Pfister R, Nicolaro ML, Paterson CA. Sodium citrate reduces the incidence of corneal ulcerations and perforations in extreme alkali-burned eyes—acetylcysteine and ascorbate have no favorable effect. *Invest Ophthalmol Vis Sci* 1981; **21**:486–490.

Pfister R, Paterson CA. Additional clinical and morphological observations on the favorable effect of ascorbate in experimental ocular burns. *Invest Ophthalmol* 1977; **16**:478–487.

Redbrake C, Buchal V, Reim M. Keratoplasty with a scleral rim after most severe eye burns. *Klin Monatsbl Augenheilkd* 1996; **208**:145–151.

Rihawi S, Grentz M, Reim M. Rinsing with isotonic saline solution for eye burns should be avoided. *Burns* 2008; **34**:1027–1032.

Ross R, Benditt E. Wound healing and collagen formation. II. Fine structure in experimental scurvy. *J Cell Biol* 1962; **12**:533.

Sejpal K, Yu F, Aldave A. The Boston keratoprosthesis in the management of corneal limbal stem cell deficiency. *Cornea* 2011; **30**:1195–1200.

Sharma S, Tandon R, Mohanty S, et al. Culture of corneal limbal epithelial stem cells: experience from benchtop to bedside in a tertiary care hospital in India. *Cornea* 2011; **30**:1223–1232.

Sotozono C, He J, Matsumoto Y, et al. Cytokine expression in the alkali-burned cornea. *Curr Eye Res* 1997; **16**:670–676.

Tandon R, Gupta N, Kalaivani M, et al. Amniotic membrane transplantation as an adjunct to medical therapy in acute ocular burns. *British J Ophthalmol* 2011; **95**:199–204.

Tejwani S, Kolari R, Sangwan V. Role of amniotic membrane graft for ocular chemical and thermal injuries. *Cornea* 2007; **26**:21–26.

Thoft R. Indications for conjunctival transplantation. *Ophthalmol* 1982; **89**:335–339.

Tsai R, Tseng S. Human allograft limbal transplantation for corneal surface reconstruction. *Cornea* 1994; **13**:389–400.

Vajpayee R, Thomas S, Sharma N, et al. Large-diameter lamellar keratoplasty in severe ocular alkali burns: a technique of stem cell transplantation. *Ophthalmol* 2000; **107**:1765–1768.

Yanxia H, Hui-Kang D, Hwang D, et al. Identification of antiangiogenic and antiinflammatory proteins in human amniotic membrane. *Cornea* 2000; **19**:348–352.

Chapter 18

Anterior corneal dystrophies and recurrent corneal erosion syndrome

Arturo E. Grau, Elío Díez-Feijóo, Juan A. Durán

GENERAL FEATURES

Corneal dystrophies are heterogeneous inherited conditions that affect the cornea. They are bilateral, slowly progressive, and not associated with prior inflammation or trauma. They are often asymmetric and preferentially affect the central cornea without vascularization. The age of onset varies, even within the same condition.

Most corneal dystrophies have no systemic manifestations and present variably shaped opacities in a clear or cloudy cornea, with varying degrees of visual dysfunction. Clinically, corneal dystrophies are classified according to the affected layer of the cornea and can be divided into three broad groups: anterior or superficial corneal dystrophies, stromal corneal dystrophies, and posterior corneal dystrophies. Recent advances in genetics have allowed the development of a new classification based on phenotypic and genotypic characteristics of these diseases.

In this chapter, we focus on the anterior corneal dystrophies. We refer to the clinical features, histological and ultrastructural changes, genetic characteristics, and treatment.

HISTORY

The word 'dystrophy' is derived from the Greek ('dys' = wrong, abnormal, difficult; 'trophe' = food, nourishment) and was introduced into medical literature by the German neurologist Wilhelm Erb in 1884. After the early studies of the French physician Guillaume Duchenne and the English physician Edward Meryon, Erb in his article 'dystrophia muscularis progressiva' suggested that muscular dystrophies were a primary degeneration of muscle. In 1890, Arthur Groenouw published his classic paper describing two patients with 'noduli corneae,' or 'nodular corneal opacities,' with one patient having macular corneal dystrophy and the other granular corneal dystrophy. In 1910, Ernst Fuchs reported 13 cases of bilateral central corneal clouding in elderly patients. Fuchs originally referred to it as 'dystrophia epithelialis corneae.'

In 1938, Max Bücklers, published the first classification of the corneal dystrophies when he described the differences between macular, granular, and lattice corneal dystrophies.

EPIDEMIOLOGY

An accurate estimate of the prevalence of the different superficial corneal dystrophies is not available, given that many individuals are asymptomatic. The presence of a corneal dystrophy may be found incidentally during routine eye examination. Determining the true frequency of these disorders in the general population is difficult; all are rare and found mainly in populations containing the responsible mutated gene. Some data are based on values derived from the histopathological diagnosis of corneas removed at keratoplasty. Musch et al. (2011) in their article 'Prevalence of corneal dystrophies in the United States: estimates from claims data' showed an overall corneal dystrophy prevalence rate of 897 per million.

The relative frequency of corneal dystrophies has relied primarily on data provided by the corneal transplantation registries:

- The Eye Bank Association of America's (EBAA 2010) Statistical Report on Eye Banking Activity for 2009 stated that Fuchs dystrophy represented 5.9% (n = 1387), keratoconus 21.7%, repeat corneal transplant 17.4%, postcataract surgery edema 15.4%, and other degenerations or dystrophies 11.8% of the 23,493 corneal transplantations
- The Australian Corneal Graft Registry Report of 2007 showed that corneal dystrophies were the fourth most frequent indication for penetrating keratoplasty (PKP) (7%) after keratoconus (32%), bullous keratopathy (26%), and failed corneal grafts (19%). Corneal dystrophies were further divided into Fuchs (83.8%), granular (4%), lattice (2.6%), posterior polymorphous (2.1%), macular (1.9%), crystalline (0.9%), juvenile (0.6%), anterior (0.4%), and unspecified (3.7%) and unspecified (3.7%) (Williams et al. 2007).
- According to the French National Waiting List, dystrophies were the third most common indication for PKP: Fuchs (65%), lattice (10%), granular (4%), macular (2%), and others (20%)

GENETICS AND ETIOLOGY

The development of genotyping has enabled more accurate characterization of the mutations responsible for different types of corneal dystrophies and has expanded our knowledge regarding their genetic and inheritance patterns. The majority of corneal dystrophies are caused by mutations in specific genes, and different phenotypes may be the result of different mutations in the same gene. Mutations in four genes (*TGFBI*, *KRT3*, *KRT12*, and *TACSTD2*) are currently known to cause inherited diseases that are probably limited to the superficial cornea (Poulaki & Colby 2008).

Additionally, molecular analysis for pathogenetic mutations can confirm the diagnosis in cases with atypical presentations of corneal dystrophies.

TGFBI DYSTROPHIES

Several clinical forms of autosomal dominant corneal dystrophies are caused by mutations in the human transforming growth factor β-induced gene (*TGFBI*), which was formerly known as the β-induced gene human cell clone number 3 (*BIGH3*). Munier et al. (1997) reported that a mutation of one gene (*TGFBI*) caused dystrophic deposits or accumulation of insoluble extracellular material noted clinically and histopathologically in different corneal layers. *TGFBI* mutations induced a heterogeneous group of dystrophies, including epithelial basement membrane corneal dystrophy, Bowman's layer dystrophies (Reis–Bücklers and Thiel–Behnke), and the stromal dystrophies: lattice corneal dystrophy type 1 and variants, and granular corneal dystrophy types 1 and 2.

The *TGFBI* gene is located in chromosome region 5q31 and encodes for transforming growth factor-b-induced protein ig-h3 (TGFBIp), known as keratoepithelin, a 68 kDa extracellular matrix protein composed of 683 amino acids. The gene contains four internal repeat domains (FAS) (Skonier et al. 1992). The majority of the mutations in *TGFBI* are located in the Fas1 domain 4.

More than 50 *TGFBI* mutations have been identified in the *TGFBI* gene and shown to affect either one of the two mutational hot spot residues Arg124 and Arg555 (Yang et al. 2010).

The gene is expressed in many tissues, including corneal epithelium, and its mutations in this tissue lead to accumulation of abnormal keratoepithelin protein or its proteolytic fragments (Kannabiran & Klintworth 2006).

GENETIC COUNSELING

While the clinical characteristics and mode of inheritance of each corneal dystrophy are well established and can be confirmed histopathologically or by appropriate genetic analysis, it is important to keep in mind that the severity of disease expression varies for each individual.

The majority of the corneal dystrophies have autosomal dominant inheritance. Patients with macular dystrophy have a poor prognosis, but are less likely to have an affected child due to its autosomal recessive inheritance. Patients with epithelial basement membrane, Fuchs, and posterior polymorphous dystrophies are rarely counseled because not all cases are known to be autosomal dominant and generally the prognosis is good. This type of information is obviously more important if the prognosis is guarded, as is the case for patients who have Reis–Bücklers, granular, and lattice dystrophies.

If the gene responsible for a corneal dystrophy can be identified, it is possible to give more accurate genetic counseling (Seitz & Lisch 2011). It is very important to provide relevant information for individuals and families about their particular corneal dystrophy—mode of inheritance, treatments, and prognosis, as well as information about relevant patient support organizations.

IMAGING

Conventionally, the clinical evaluation, diagnosis, and differentiation of corneal dystrophies have been based on slit-lamp biomicroscopy. Newer in vivo imaging modalities are able to better characterize the dystrophies and improve the clinical description of the different phenotypes. The development of confocal optics has enabled cellular morphology to be examined in detail.

There are two types of in vivo confocal microscopy: white light and laser. Both provide information at the cellular level, with high-resolution images ('non-invasive in vivo biopsy'). The axial resolution of the laser confocal microscopy is higher than the white light and allows the detection of subtle abnormalities in the cornea (Vemuganti et al. 2011). The clinical usefulness of these methods has been documented in studies of both normal human corneas and corneas affected by different pathologies including dystrophies (Niederer & McGhee 2010).

CLASSIFICATION

The dystrophies are classically classified by the level of the cornea that is involved, which separates these entities into three groups based on the anatomical location of the abnormalities: corneal epithelium and its basement membrane or Bowman's layer (anterior corneal dystrophies), the corneal stroma (stromal corneal dystrophies) and Descemet's membrane, and the corneal endothelium (posterior corneal dystrophies).

Corneal dystrophies can be classified according to their slit-lamp characteristics, the morphology and depth of the deposits, and their histopathological features.

This classification has been challenged because of the variability in phenotypic expression of the corneal dystrophies. There are dystrophies with atypical characteristics that involve multiple corneal layers that cannot be classified into a single type. Developments in corneal genetics have given more information about the pathogenesis of corneal dystrophies.

The International Committee for Classification of Corneal Dystrophies (IC3D) was founded to develop a new, internationally accepted classification of corneal dystrophies, based on modern clinical, histological, and genetic knowledge (**Tables 18.1** and **18.2**). This classification system is anatomically based, with dystrophies classified according to the layer affected. The majority of the dystrophy names are identical or similar to those in the current nomenclature. However, dystrophies with a known common genetic basis, i.e. *TGFBI* dystrophies, have been grouped together.

Each dystrophy carries a template, summarizing genetic, clinical, and pathological information. A category number from 1 through 4 is assigned that reflects the level of evidence supporting the existence of a given dystrophy. The most defined dystrophies belong to category 1, and the least defined belong to category 4 (Weiss et al. 2008).

Anterior corneal dystrophies
Meesmann's corneal dystrophy

Alternative names for this dystrophy are juvenile hereditary epithelial dystrophy and Stocker–Holt dystrophy. It is a rare, bilateral, symmetric, diffuse corneal dystrophy that affects only the epithelium and appears in the first or second year of life. It was first described clinically by Pameijer in 1935. He reported the presence of a great number of small punctate or drop-like opacities located in the very superficial layers of the cornea. The histopathological description was given by Meesmann in 1938.

Inheritance pattern

Meesmann's corneal dystrophy (MECD) has an autosomal dominant mode of inheritance with incomplete penetrance and variable expressivity. This was reported by Stocker and Holt, in 1955, in 20 individuals in a group of 200 descendants of Morovian settlers in the area of North Carolina, USA. The Moravians, a Protestant religious group, came from an area near Dresden in Saxony, East Germany, and first settled at Bethlehem, Pennsylvania, in 1741. In 1753, a group of these immigrants moved to the area of Winston-Salem, where their descendants still live.

Genetics

The molecular basis of Meesmann's dystrophy has been attributed to mutations of the cornea-specific keratin genes (Irvine et al. 1997) *KRT3* (locus 12q13) and *KRT12* (locus 17q12, Stocker–Holt

Table 18.1 The IC3D classification

Epithelial and subepithelial dystrophies

1. Epithelial basement membrane dystrophy—majority degenerative, some C1
2. Epithelial recurrent erosion dystrophy C4 (Smolandiensis variant) C3
3. Subepithelial mucinous corneal dystrophy C4
4. Mutation in keratin genes: Meesmann's corneal dystrophy C1
5. Lisch epithelial corneal dystrophy C2
6. Gelatinous drop-like corneal dystrophy C1

Bowman's layer dystrophies

1. Reis–Bücklers corneal dystrophy—granular corneal dystrophy, type 3 C1
2. Thiel–Behnke corneal dystrophy C1, potential variant C2
3. Grayson–Wilbrandt corneal dystrophy C4

Stromal dystrophies

1. *TGFBI* corneal dystrophies
    A. Lattice corneal dystrophy
        a. Lattice corneal dystrophy, *TGFBI* type (LCD): classic lattice corneal dystrophy (LCD1) C1, variants (III, IIIA, I/IIIA, and IV) are C1
        b. Lattice corneal dystrophy, gelsolin type (LCD2) C1 (This is not a true corneal dystrophy but is included here for ease of differential diagnosis)
    B. Granular corneal dystrophy C1
        a. Granular corneal dystrophy, type 1 (classic) C1
        b. Granular corneal dystrophy, type 2 (granular-lattice) C1
        c. Granular corneal dystrophy, type 3 (Reis–Bücklers corneal dystrophy) = Reis–Bücklers C1
2. Macular corneal dystrophy C1
3. Schnyder corneal dystrophy C1
4. Congenital stromal corneal dystrophy C1
5. Fleck corneal dystrophy C1
6. Posterior amorphous corneal dystrophy C3
7. Central cloudy dystrophy of François C4
8. Pre-Descemet's corneal dystrophy C4

Descemet's membrane and endothelial dystrophies

1. Fuchs endothelial corneal dystrophy C1, C2, or C3
2. Posterior polymorphous corneal dystrophy C1 or C2
3. Congenital hereditary endothelial dystrophy, type 1 C2
4. Congenital hereditary endothelial dystrophy, type 2 C1
5. X-linked endothelial corneal dystrophy C2

Corneal dystrophies categories

Category 1: A well-defined corneal dystrophy in which the gene has been mapped and identified and specific mutations are known
Category 2: A well-defined corneal dystrophy that has been mapped to one or more specific chromosomal loci, but the gene remains to be identified
Category 3: A well-defined corneal dystrophy in which the disorder has not yet been mapped to a chromosomal locus
Category 4: This category is reserved for a suspected new, or previously documented, corneal dystrophy, although the evidence for it, being a distinct entity, is not yet convincing

C, category; LCD, lattice corneal dystrophy; *TGFBI*, transforming growth factor β-induced gene.

variant). These genes encode cytoskeletal proteins keratin K3 and keratin K12, respectively. In general, these disorders are inherited as autosomal dominant traits and the mutations act in a dominant-negative manner.

Keratins

Keratins are heteropolymeric proteins that form the intermediate filament cytoskeleton in epithelial cells. Their predominant function is to impart mechanical strength to the cells. Also, keratins have a regulatory function, influencing cell size, proliferation, translation control, organelle transport, malignant transformation, and stress responses (Magin et al. 2007).

Mutations in keratin genes result in instability of intermediate filaments with tonofilament aggregation, cytoskeletal disruption, keratinocyte fragility, and cellular lysis. The abnormal fragility of epithelial cells leads to their detachment, blistering of tissues in response to even mild physical trauma, and impaired keratinization. Keratin mutations have been detected in several human diseases, e.g. epidermolysis bullosa simplex and keratoderma disorders (Smith 2003).

Onset and course

MECD is characterized by fragility of the corneal epithelium that resembles several blistering epidermal diseases. The dystrophy follows a slow, progressive course. The epithelial cysts gradually spread throughout the corneal epithelium, and the majority of patients may remain asymptomatic till the fourth or fifth decade of life, when photophobia, redness, and pain occur because of recurrent erosions due to the rupture of cysts. Subepithelial gray opacities appear at the late stage of the disease.

Signs

MECD is characterized by bilateral small cystic changes in the corneal epithelium. These cysts present in a diffuse distribution. Clusters of tiny round epithelial cysts extend to the limbus and are most numerous in the interpalpebral area, with clear surrounding epithelium and individual superficial punctate opacities.

Cysts can be visualized with slit-lamp examination like small, discrete, and grayish intraepithelial bubbles. Indirect illumination shows varying diffuse gray dots in different patterns, which may have

Table 18.2 Summary of the anterior CD: genetic characteristics IC3D classification and clinical features

	Meesmann's CD	Epithelial basement membrane dystrophy	Reis–Bücklers CD	Thiel–Behnke CD	Lisch epithelial CD	Gelatinous drop-like CD	Epithelial recurrent erosion dystrophy	Grayson–Wilbrandt CD	Subepithelial mucinous CD
IC3D abbreviation	MECD	EBMD	RBCD	TBCD	LECD	GDLD	ERED	GWCD	SMCD
MIM#*	122100	121820	608470	602082	None	104870	122400	None	None
Onset	Early childhood	Adult life	Childhood	Childhood	Childhood	First to second decade	First decade	First to second decade	First decade
Inheritance	Autosomal dominant	Not documented	Autosomal dominant	Autosomal dominant	X-chromosomal dominant	Autosomal recessive	Autosomal dominant	Autosomal dominant	Autosomal dominant
Genetic locus	Locus 12q13 (*KRT3*) Locus 17q12 (*KRT12*) Stocker–Holt variant	5q31	5q31	5q31 10q24	Xp 22.3	1p32	Unknown	Unknown	Unknown
Gene	Keratin K3 (*KRT3*) Keratin K12 (*KRT12*) Stocker–Holt variant	*TGFBI* in the minority of cases	*TGFBI*	5q31: *TGFBI* 10q24: unknown	Unknown	Tumor-associated calcium signal transducer 2	Unknown	Unknown	Unknown
IC3D category	1, including Stocker–Holt variant	Most cases are sporadic Category 1 in a minority of cases	1	1 (*TGFBI*) 2 (10q24)	2	1	4 3 (Smolandiensis variant)	4	4

CD, corneal dystrophies; *TGFBI*, transforming growth factor β-induced gene.
MIM#*, the unique six-digit number assigned to each entry listed in the catalog of human genes and genetic disorders.

a distinct border and appear as transparent vesicles or microcysts on retroillumination (**Figure 18.1**).

The cornea may be slightly thinned and corneal sensation may be reduced. Areas of the central or peripheral cornea may be unaffected. Coalescence of several cysts may result in refractile linear opacities with intervening clear cornea. The pattern changes with time because the cysts migrate to the surface and they can stain with colorants (**Figure 18.2**).

In the Stocker–Holt variant, the entire cornea demonstrates fine, grayish punctuate epithelial opacities that stain with fluorescein and fine linear opacities that may appear in a whorl pattern. Confocal microscopy shows the presence of well-delineated cystic structures with hyper-reflective material inside (**Figure 18.3a**).

Symptoms

Patients are usually asymptomatic until about middle age when intermittent, mild ocular irritation, photophobia, redness, epiphora,

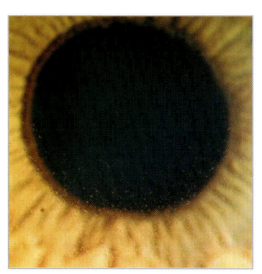

Figure 18.1 Meesmann's dystrophy: multiple epithelial microcysts. Courtesy of Stephen Tuft, Moorfield's Eye Hospital NHS Foundation Trust, London, UK.

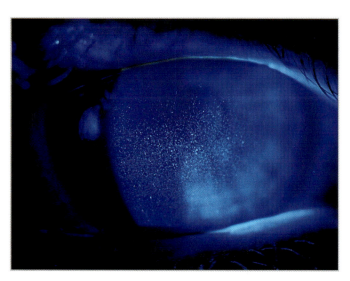

Figure 18.2 Positive fluorescein staining in a symptomatic patient with Meesmann's dystrophy. Courtesy of Alberto Arntz, Pontificia Universidad Catolica de Chile.

and pain may occur due to recurrent corneal erosions (RCE), with the rupture of mainly interpalpebral epithelial cysts. Most patients retain good functional vision; few may complain of blurred vision, fluctuating visual acuity or glare, and light sensitivity secondary to corneal irregularity and scarring. Corneal sensitivity is normal.

Patients with the Stocker–Holt variant demonstrate more severe signs and symptoms with earlier onset compared with classic MECD.

Histopathology

Under light microscopy, morphologically, the epithelium is disorganized and thickened with widespread cytoplasmic vacuolation and numerous small, round, keratin aggregate intraepithelial microcysts. Multilaminar basement membrane is thickened with projections into the basal epithelium. Cysts are filled with periodic acid-Schiff-positive cellular debris. The composition of the fibrillogranular material is unknown; it causes cell death.

Transmission electron microscopy (TEM) shows focal aggregation of electron-dense fibrillogranular keratin within the cytoplasm of the corneal epithelium—the 'peculiar substance' of Kuwabara & Ciccarelli (1964)—which is surrounded by cytoplasmic filaments and vacuoles in relation to hemidesmosomes.

In the Stocker–Holt variant, the epithelium and the basal membrane are variably thickened with vacuolated cells and evidence of degeneration.

Management

Most patients remain asymptomatic and may not require any treatment. Treatments include the following:

- Lubricants and cyclopedia reduce the severity of symptoms
- Therapeutic contact lenses decrease the number of cysts
- Epithelial debridement of the abnormal corneal epithelium has been used as a treatment modality, but this dystrophy recurs in the regenerated epithelium
- Yeung and Hodge (2009) have suggested keratectomy with mitomycin C application
- Phototherapeutic keratectomy (PTK) is an alternative treatment of recalcitrant recurrent erosions

If the visual acuity is reduced secondary to subepithelial scaring, lamellar keratoplasty can be performed but it is followed by recurrence of the epithelial cysts.

■ Epithelial basement membrane dystrophy

Alternative names for this dystrophy are map-dot-fingerprint dystrophy, Cogan's microcystic epithelial dystrophy, anterior basement membrane dystrophy, and dystrophic recurrent erosion. It is a bilateral, often asymmetrical corneal disorder. It is the most common anterior corneal dystrophy in clinical practice. The main pathological feature of the disease is the abnormal epithelial turnover, maturation, and production of basement; it manifests clinically as recurrent erosions. Onset is in adult life. It affects 76% of people older than 50 years, and 42% of people of all ages (Werblin et al. 1981).

Vogt described fingerprint lines in the corneal epithelium in his slit-lamp atlas of 1930. Cogan et al. (1964) first described the characteristic microcystic changes in the corneal epithelium in this disorder. Guerry (1965) supplemented Cogan and colleagues' description showing that dots were accompanied by map-like or 'geographic' nebulae, which lay anterior to Bowman's membrane. In 1972, Trobe and Laibson found map changes, microcysts, and fingerprints in various combinations. They coined the name map-dot-fingerprint corneal dystrophy for this condition. Bleb-like changes were described by Bron and Brown in 1971.

Inheritance pattern

Most cases have no definite hereditary pattern. Autosomal dominant inheritance has been documented with variable penetrance.

Genetics

The genetic locus is 5q31. The *TGFBI* gene can be found in the minority of cases.

Signs

The pattern of epithelial basement membrane dystrophy (EBMD) varies considerably among patients. The epithelial or anterior basement membrane includes Cogan's microcysts, Guerry's map-like changes, Vogt's fingerprint parallel lines, and Bron's bleb changes or any combination of the patterns. Combination of maps and dots is noted most frequently, followed by maps alone.

All of these tend to appear and go spontaneously and affect different areas of the cornea. On slit-lamp examination, areas of pathology are often identified best by broad-beam illumination, fluorescein with cobalt blue light to identify areas of negative staining, or retroillumination following dilation. Slit-lamp findings include the following:

- **Maps**: irregular gray geographical patches that may contain clear oval areas. Thickened, gray, hazy epithelium with scalloped circumscribed borders, particularly affecting the central or paracentral cornea. They vary greatly in size (**Figure 18.4**)
- **Dots**: irregular round, oval, or comma-shaped gray-white intraepithelial non-staining, opacities; clustered like an archipelago in the central cornea (**Figure 18.5**)
- **Fingerprints**: parallel, curvilinear branching lines with club-shaped terminations; usually paracentral (**Figure 18.6**)
- **Blebs**: small clear, round, bubble-like pebbled glass dots clustered together (**Figure 18.7**)

Confocal microscopy reveals linear hyper-reflective structures corresponding to abnormal basement membrane (**Figure 18.3b**).

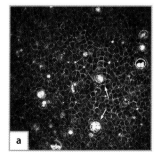
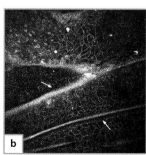
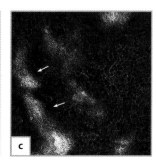

Figure 18.3 Confocal microscopy. (a) Meesmann's dystrophy: presence of well-delineated cystic structures with hyper-reflective material inside (arrows). (b) Epithelial basement membrane dystrophy: linear hyper-reflective structures corresponding to abnormal basement membrane (arrows). (c) Reis–Bücklers dystrophy: focal deposition of homogeneous hyper-reflective materials (arrows). Courtesy of Scott Hau, Moorfield's Eye Hospital NHS Foundation Trust, London, UK.

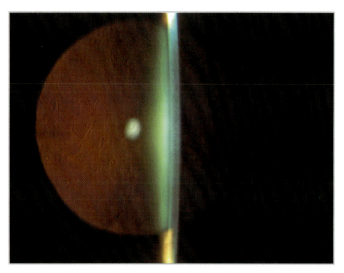

Figure 18.4 Epithelial basement membrane dystrophy. Map-like changes viewed in retroillumination.

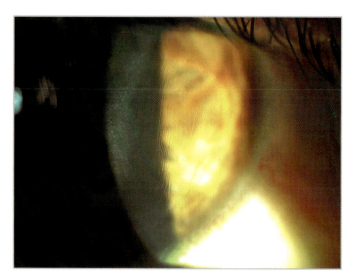

Figure 18.6 Epithelial basement membrane dystrophy. Fingerprint lines.

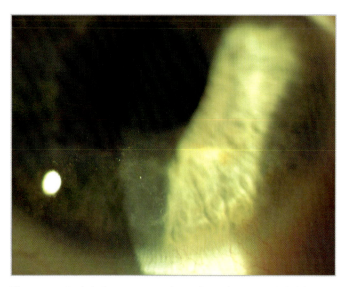

Figure 18.5 Epithelial basement membrane dystrophy. Intraepithelial dot opacities.

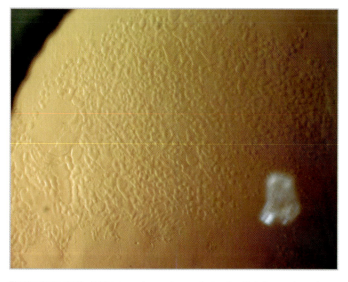

Figure 18.7 Epithelial basement membrane dystrophy. Bleb forms viewed in retroillumination. Courtesy of Stephen Tuft, Moorfield's Eye Hospital NHS Foundation Trust, London, UK.

In map-fingerprint-dot patterns, the intraepithelial basement membrane appears separated from normal basal epithelial cells. It has a droplet-shaped configuration in the epithelium, and a ring-like structure in the basal epithelium.

Bleb-like changes include areas of circular and irregular hyporeflectivity, ranging from 30 to 150 μm in diameter at the level of the basal epithelium and Bowman's layer, with apparent fragmentation of the sub-basal nerve plexus (Hau & Tuft 2011).

Symptoms

Patients with this condition may be asymptomatic, or present with moderate or sometimes severe symptomatic episodes. When the basement membrane and microcysts changes are concentrated in the visual axis, alterations in visual acuity occur. Irregular astigmatism and increase in higher order aberration may cause blurred vision, glare, ghosting, or monocular diplopia. Vision is variable and fluctuating due to migratory and intermittent corneal involvement, and refractions are often unstable.

Spontaneous RCE may be mild and transient, lasting minutes, or occasionally characterized by more severe pain. This pain can last only few minutes or persist for hours or even days. Pain may be present on awakening, or it can awaken the patient when the eyelids are opened during sleep. Symptoms in these patients with RCE vary from a foreign body sensation and photophobia to severe pain if the epithelium loosens, identifiable at slit lamp using a triangular ophthalmic surgical spear.

Patients who have recurrent erosions and no history of trauma should be examined carefully for signs of the presence of epithelial basement membrane dystrophy (EBMD).

Symptoms alone cannot distinguish the cause of RCE, whether traumatic, dystrophic, or idiopathic.

Histopathology

The major pathology in EBMD is the abnormal synthesis of the epithelial basement membrane. Maturing epithelial cells migrating from the deeper to the superficial layers of epithelium, which would eventually be discharged from the corneal surface, become entrapped beneath the sheets of basement membrane, blocking the normal maturation and forward migration, and are prevented from surfacing. These trapped cells degenerate to form intraepithelial cysts.

Light microscopy findings

Findings include:

- **Maps**: sheets of intraepithelial, multilamellar, basal laminar material
- **Fingerprint lines**: rib-like intraepithelial extensions of basal laminar material
- **Dots**: intraepithelial pseudocyst containing cytoplasmic debris
- **Bleb pattern**: irregular, subepithelial accumulation of a fibrillogranular material between the basement membrane of the epithelium and Bowman's layer

TEM findings

Findings include:

- **Maps:** thick epithelial basement membrane that extends into the epithelium as multilamellar
- **Fingerprint lines:** fine fibrillogranular substance in addition to basement membrane
- **Dots:** intraepithelial pseudocyst contains degenerating cells with pyknotic nuclei and cytoplasmic debris
- **Bleb pattern:** the anterior surface of this material forms discrete mounds, which dent the overlying basal epithelial cells. May mimic cysts clinically but no cysts present histologically

▪ Management

In mild cases, RCE may resolve spontaneously within a few hours. Most patients respond to topical lubrication therapy, topical cycloplegic agents, or eye patch to promote healing and relieve symptoms. Hypertonic sodium chloride (5%) drops and lubricant at bedtime are recommended.

Disposable extended-wear bandage contact lens removed every 2 weeks for a total of 3 months have been used (Fraunfelder & Cabezas 2011).

Treating-associated lid pathologies, such as blepharitis and meibomian gland dysfunction (MGD), facilitate corneal surface recovery.

Matrix metalloproteinase (MMP) is upregulated in the tears of patients with RCE. MMP is a generic name for a group of enzymes that can degrade part of the structure of the extracellular matrix (type IV, type VII collagen, and laminin). MMP inhibitors such as oral doxycycline (50 mg bid) and topical steroids (fluorometholone 0.1% qid) have been used (Dursun et al. 2001).

Resistant disease may require the following treatments:

- **Mechanical debridement of the epithelium:** this is performed with a diamond burr, which is used to uniformly polish the Bowman's membrane in the area of the epithelial defect
- **Alcohol delamination of the corneal epithelium:** 20% alcohol solution is placed over the defect and applied for 30–40 seconds; the treated area of the corneal epithelium is completely debrided using a surgical spear, and the corneal surface is irrigated with saline before placing a bandage contact lens (Singh et al. 2007)

- **Anterior stromal puncture:** this procedure involves making small punctures with a bent needle to minimize scarring and prevent corneal perforation. An insertion depth of 0.1 mm is sufficient to cause the production of new basement membrane attached to the anterior stroma
- **Superficial PTK:** the mechanism of action of excimer photoablation in the treatment of recurrent erosion is unknown but may lie in the strong bonds formed between the epithelial basement membrane and Bowman's layer postoperatively. Treatment for recurrent erosions due to trauma has a higher success rate than treatment for corneal dystrophies (Ewald & Hammersmith 2009, Reeves et al. 2010). For more information read Chapter 42

Other treatments

There are a few cases reported in the literature using autologous serum drops, umbilical cord serum drops, collagen punctal plug occlusion or punctal cautery, substance P-derived peptide and ILGF-I drops, botulinum toxin lid injections, and Nd:YAG laser treatment with good results.

▪ Reis–Bücklers corneal dystrophy

Alternative names for this disorder include corneal dystrophy of Bowman's layer, type 1; geographic corneal dystrophy; superficial granular corneal dystrophy; atypical granular corneal dystrophy; granular corneal dystrophy, type 3; and anterior limiting membrane dystrophy, type 1.

Reis–Bücklers corneal dystrophy (RBCD) is an inherited, bilateral corneal dystrophy characterized by superficial symmetrical reticular opacities in Bowman's layer and secondary alterations in the epithelium and stroma.

This disease was first reported by Reis in 1917 as a superficial corneal annular dystrophy with geographic opacities. Detailed description was given by Bücklers in 1949 for another family. Since then, the name Reis–Bücklers anterior membrane dystrophy has been common in the literature.

Kuchle in 1995 studied corneal dystrophy of the Bowman's layer by light and electron microscopy. He described two distinct dystrophies: type 1 (true Reis–Bücklers dystrophy or geographic) and type 2 [Thiel–Behnke corneal dystrophy (TBCD) or honeycomb-shaped previously described by Thiel and Behnke in 1967].

On the one hand, corneal dystrophy of Bowman's layer type 1 is synonymous with Reis–Bücklers original dystrophy and equivalent to what has been called the superficial variant of granular dystrophy. RCE begins in childhood, and is marked by early and fairly marked visual loss.

On the other hand, corneal dystrophy of Bowman's layer type 2 (TBCD) is often confused with RBCD, also with RCE starting in early childhood, but visual acuity is reduced later in life in comparison to RBCD.

Inheritance pattern

RBCD and TBCD have an autosomal dominant mode of inheritance, with variable expressibility.

Genetics

RBCD is caused by a specific mutation in the TGFBI gene (locus 5q31) (Small et al. 1996).

Signs

Irregular, confluent, superficial gray-white opacities with varying densities are seen in the Bowman's layer and superficial stroma.

Opacities may be linear, geographical, or ring like and are best seen with broad, oblique illumination. Peripheral cornea is usually unaffected, although a diffuse haze extends to the limbus with time. Corneal sensations are decreased, and prominent corneal nerves may be seen (**Figure 18.8**).

With confocal microscopy distinct deposits are found in the epithelium and Bowman's layer. The deposits in the basal epithelial cell layer show extremely high reflectivity from small granular material without any shadows. Bowman's layer is replaced by highly reflective irregular and granular material, even more reflective than in TBCD (**Figure 18.3c**) (Kobayashi & Sugiyama 2007).

Symptoms

RCE manifest as episodes of pain, redness, and tearing. These attacks may become less severe by the end of the second decade, with progressive deterioration of vision. The visual loss is attributable to the diffuse opaque irregular surface because Bowman's layer is progressively replaced with scar tissue. Erosions are typically more frequent and severe than in TBCD.

Histopathology

Light microscopy reveals intact epithelium or an irregular partially dehiscent epithelium. The epithelium shows edema, degeneration, and thinning, secondary to changes in the underlying Bowman's layer, which is absent in some areas. A band-shaped granular eosinophilic Masson's trichrome-positive subepithelial material, with projections into the epithelium and the anterior stroma, is widely dispersed and replaces the Bowman's layer. The material deposits do not demonstrate features of amyloid and do not stain with periodic acid-Schiff (PAS). The basement membrane of the epithelium may be normal or absent.

Subepithelial accumulations of electron-dense material, with the morphological characteristics of granular dystrophy deposits, are seen under TEM. Crescent or rod-shaped bodies are interspersed between the collagen fibrils in Bowman's layer; yet, not the curly fibers of TBCD that are observed on electron microscopy.

Electron microscopy is necessary for definitive histopathological diagnosis to distinguish from TBCD. The clinical appearance of these dystrophies is similar, and differentiation can be made only with light and, particularly, electron microscopy. Interestingly, RBCD stains positively with Masson's stain (**Figure 18.9**).

Immunohistochemistry demonstrates rod-shaped bodies immunopositive for transforming growth factor b-induced protein (keratoepithelin) (Lohse et al. 1989).

Management

Early in the course of the disease when only recurrent erosions occur, they can be managed similarly to the therapy of recurrent erosion due to EBMD. Debridement can be performed in cases with recalcitrant erosions.

PTK has been reported to be an effective modality for the treatment of this dystrophy. The procedure is performed to different depths following epithelial debridement or ablation (transepithelial). PTK is the treatment of choice when vision is disturbed sufficiently or painful erosions occur. Recurrence is common after this procedure. Dinh et al. in 1999 reported that 47% of the eyes with Reis–Bücklers dystrophy developed clinically significant recurrence an average of 21.6 months

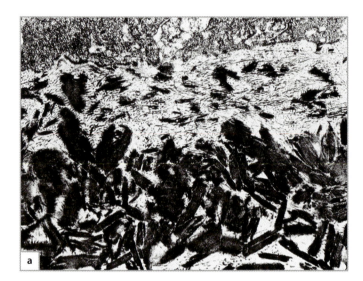

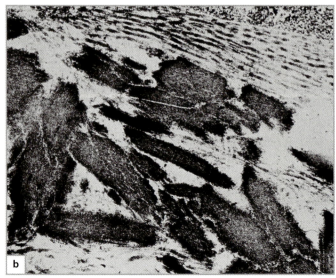

Figure 18.9 Reis–Bücklers corneal dystrophy. Rod-like bodies seen by transmission electron microscopy. Courtesy of Richard Green, Wilmer Eye Institute, Baltimore, USA.

Figure 18.8 Reis–Bücklers corneal dystrophy. Broad oblique illumination demonstrating dense, reticular, superficial opacities.

after PTK. Adjunctive application of topical mitomycin C 0.02% may be helpful in reducing the recurrence of the disease after PTK.

With significant superficial corneal scarring and opacification and a decrease in visual acuity, superficial lamellar keratoplasty can be performed but recurrence of the dystrophy in the graft is frequent (Shousha et al. 2011).

■ Thiel–Behnke corneal dystrophy

Alternative names for this dystrophy include corneal dystrophy of Bowman's layer, type 2 (CDB2); honeycomb-shaped corneal dystrophy; anterior limiting membrane dystrophy, type 2; curly fibers corneal dystrophy; and Waardenburg–Jonkers corneal dystrophy. It is a progressive dystrophy, consisting of subepithelial corneal opacities that form a honeycomb-shaped pattern in the superficial cornea, with sparing of the corneoscleral limbus. TBCD is associated to RCE and vision becomes increasingly impaired.

Thiel and Behnke in 1967 described a bilateral autosomal dominant disorder with onset in childhood.

Genetics

TBCD was mapped to chromosome 5 (5q31). It was later found to be associated with a p. Arg555Gln mutation in TGFBI. Another locus for TBCD has also been identified on chromosome 10 (10q24) (Yee et al. 1997).

Signs

Under the slit lamp, symmetrical subepithelial reticular honeycomb-like opacities are seen, sparing the peripheral cornea. In advanced cases, the opacities can progress to deep stromal layers and corneal periphery.

Confocal microscopy reveals that different deposits are found in the epithelium and Bowman's layer. The deposits in the basal epithelial cell layer show homogeneous reflectivity, with round edges accompanying dark shadows. Bowman's layer is replaced with homogeneous, relatively reflective irregular material that is less reflective than in RBCD.

Symptoms

Main symptoms are progressive RCE with episodes of pain, redness and epiphora, and alteration in visual function to different degrees.

Onset and course

Corneal erosions start in the first and second decades and cause ocular discomfort and pain, together with a slowly progressive deterioration of vision from increasing corneal opacification. RCE may resolve with time. The course is similar but frequently less aggressive than RBCD.

Histopathology

Light microscopy shows an irregular epithelium of varying thickness, with non-specific degenerative changes and destruction of Bowman's layer. Subepithelial fibrous tissue accumulates with an undulant configuration (wavy saw-toothed pattern) and absence of the epithelial basement membrane in many areas. The deposits are limited to the subepithelial region, with an abrupt transition to the anterior stroma.

In advanced stages, the anterior stroma collagen and Bowman's layer may be markedly disorganized and replaced by numerous aggregates.

There is a broad band of subepithelial material composed of irregular short, curled filaments or collagen fibers, with a diameter of 9–15 nm, which are pathognomonic of TBCD, when seen under TEM. These are interspersed among normal collagen fibrils in the Bowman's zone and the contiguous superficial corneal stroma. TEM is necessary to distinguish RBCD from the TBCD where curly fibers are present. Curly fibers are immunopositive for transforming growth factor b-induced protein (keratoepithelin) in TBCD (5q31).

■ Lisch epithelial corneal dystrophy

Alternative names for this dystrophy include band-shaped and whorled microcystic dystrophy of the corneal epithelium. It is an epithelial corneal dystrophy where diffuse gray corneal opacifications appear in different patterns. Onset occurs during childhood and the course is slowly progressive. By adulthood vision can be significantly reduced. Similar degrees of opacities are noted in both men and women.

Lisch et al. (1992) described the clinical findings of a new corneal epithelial dystrophy and established some histological features that distinguish these cases from other epithelial dystrophies. Lisch described the lesions like unilateral and bilateral, gray, band-shaped, and feathery opacities that sometimes appear in whorled patterns.

Genetics

The gene for Lisch epithelial corneal dystrophy (LECD) has been mapped to the short arm of the X chromosome (Xp22.3), and no responsible gene has been identified (Lisch et al. 2000). In spite of the X-linked inheritance pattern, both males and carrier females may have similar corneal opacities since the mutation is dominant.

Signs

LECD is characterized by feather-shaped opacities and microcysts in the corneal epithelium that often appear in a band-like or sometimes whorled pattern.

Slit-lamp examination reveals these opacities to consist of multiple, densely crowded, clear intraepithelial microcysts, which are better seen with retroillumination. The surrounding epithelium appears clinically normal (Figure 18.10).

Confocal microscopy reveals many solitary dark and well-demarcated lesions, with round and oval configuration. Some lesions demonstrate central reflective points, which probably correspond to the cell nuclei.

Symptoms

Patients are usually asymptomatic and lesions are found incidentally. The opacity is not associated with RCE. The epithelial opacities are slowly progressive and may lead to visual deterioration when the visual axis is affected, and sometimes monocular diplopia. Most individuals, however, retain relatively good visual acuity.

No concomitant alterations of palpebral conjunctiva or physical factors, suggesting a mechanical pathogenesis, have been described.

Histopathology

Under light microscopy, diffuse cytoplasmic vacuolization of the affected epithelium is seen, most evident at the wing cell layer, with a sharp delineation from non-affected areas. TEM shows intracytoplasmic vacuoles of the affected corneal epithelium. The vacuoles either are optically empty or contain weakly osmiophilic, partly homogenous, and partly lamellar material. The vacuoles tend to collapse and coalesce, resulting in a structureless transparent cytoplasm.

Management

There are only a few cases reported that discuss treatment options for this dystrophy. In his original article, Lisch performed therapeutic

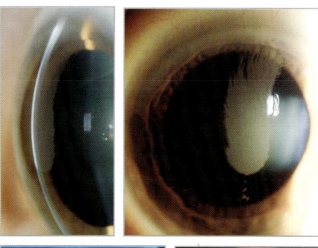

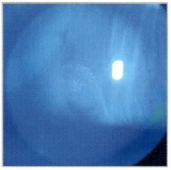
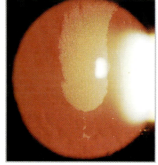

Figure 18.10 Lisch epithelial corneal dystrophy. Localized, whorl-like gray opacity on direct illumination and retroillumination. Courtesy of Rafael Barraquer, Instituto Barraquer, Barcelona, Spain.

epithelial abrasions in three patients, and despite treatment, the lesions recurred and the vision dropped to their pretreatment levels.

Lisch et al. (2010) show that wearing contact lenses for a longer duration caused a significant regression of corneal opacities; discontinued wearing of contact lenses induced again a progression of opacity in LECD. The etiology of this phenomenon was interpreted as a contact lens-induced thinning of corneal epithelium and reduction of epithelial layers.

Robin et al. (1994) treated their symptomatic patient with epithelial debridement, but this led to recurrence and progression. Subsequent treatment with a rigid gas-permeable contact lens led to partial regression.

Charles et al. (2000) reported a case of Lisch dystrophy treated with scraping of the corneal epithelium and recurrence was noted. Alvarez-Fischer et al. (2005) in another case report showed no recurrence, but the patient was only re-examined after 6 months of follow-up.

Wessel et al. (2011) treated one patient with MMC in addition to excimer laser photorefractive keratectomy (PRK); the surface ablation was successful in treating the corneal lesion.

■ Gelatinous drop-like corneal dystrophy

Alternative names for this dystrophy include subepithelial amyloidosis and primary familial amyloidosis. It is most commonly seen in ethnic Japanese people. It has an estimated prevalence of one in 300,000 in Japan but has been reported in other regions of the world

as well. First described by Nakaizumi in 1914, it is characterized by abnormal deposition of amyloid in the subepithelial and superficial cornea, leading to corneal vascularization and involvement of the underlying cornea. Onset is in the first to second decades of life with progression of protruding subepithelial deposits and stromal opacity.

Severe impairment of the corneal epithelial barrier function in gelatinous drop-like corneal dystrophy (GDLD) is also associated with lactoferrin deposition within the amyloid. The pathogenesis of amyloid deposits in the corneal stroma may be related to penetration of constituents such as lactoferrin.

Inheritance pattern

GDLD has an autosomal recessive mode of inheritance.

Genetics

GDLD has been mapped to chromosome 1 (1p32) and the gene tumor-associated calcium signal transducer 2 (*TACSTD*2). More than 20 mutations in the *TACSTD*2 (formerly *M1S1*, *TROP2*, and *GA733-1*) gene cause GDCD. Some affected individuals have been found not to have mutations in *TACSTD*2, suggesting the existence of genetic heterogeneity in this autosomal recessive disease (Tsujikawa et al. 1999).

Signs

GDLD has four distinct subtypes in the literature: band keratopathy type, stromal opacity type, kumquat-like type, and typical mulberry type (Ide et al. 2004).

Initially, the subepithelial lesions may appear similar to band-shaped keratopathy because they progress to form groups of small multiple nodules of amyloid deposits and acquire a mulberry configuration. The amyloid contains lactoferrin, but the disease is not linked to the lactoferrin gene. Fusiform deposits similar to those in lattice corneal dystrophy may also form in the deeper stroma.

These lesions show late staining with fluorescein, implying hyperpermeability of the corneal epithelium. Superficial vascularization is frequently seen. As the disease progresses, patients may develop stromal opacification or develop larger nodular kumquat-like lesions (kumquat: small golden-yellow colored fruits) (**Figure 18.11**).

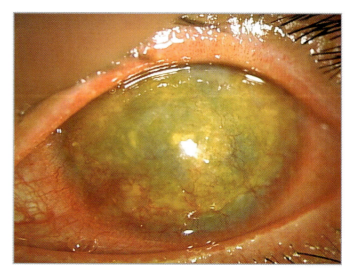

Figure 18.11 Gelatinous drop-like dystrophy. Stromal opacification with larger nodular kumquat-like lesions and superficial vascularization. Courtesy of Yukihiro Matsumoto, Keio University School of Medicine, Tokyo, Japan.

Symptoms

The main symptoms are significant decrease in vision, photophobia, irritation, redness, tearing, and corneal foreign body sensation.

Histopathology

Light microscopy demonstrates subepithelial and stromal amyloid deposits. Under TEM, disruption of epithelial tight junctions in the superficial epithelium is noted. Amyloid is noted in the basal epithelial layer.

Management

Continuous wearing of soft contact lens after a PRK is effective in preventing amyloid deposit formation.

In GDCD, corneal transplantation is required for visual rehabilitation; almost all patients develop recurrence after superficial keratectomy, lamellar keratoplasty, or PKP because amyloid recurs in the graft. Lasram et al. (1994) reported that the five cases of GDLD they treated required multiple keratoplasties at a mean interval of 5 years because of recurrence of the disease on the corneal graft.

Ito et al. (2000) have reported that PTK may be a safe and useful modality to remove corneal opacities that recur after lamellar grafts.

■ Other corneal dystrophies (category 4)

Epithelial recurrent erosion dystrophy

Alternative names for this dystrophy include corneal erosions and recurring hereditary (Franceschetti). Variants have been reported: dystrophia Smolandiensis and dystrophia Helsinglandica (Hammar et al. 2009, 2010).

Inheritance

The inheritance is autosomal dominant, but the genetic locus and gene are unknown.

Course

Onset is in the first decade of life. Attacks generally decline in frequency and intensity and cease by the age of 50 years. In the Smolandiensis variant, central subepithelial opacities will progress. In the Helsinglandica variant, the affected family members experience their first signs and symptoms of the disease between the ages of 4 and 9 years.

Symptoms

Most patients have attacks of redness, photophobia, epiphora, and ocular pain. Some experience a burning sensation and report sensitive eyes for years. Erosions are often precipitated by relatively minor trauma and are often difficult to treat.

In the Smolandiensis variant, a quarter of patients eventually need corneal grafts by a mean age of 44 years. Recurrence of opacities occurs within 15 months in the graft periphery, but the central graft can remain clear for many years. In the Helsinglandica variant, the affected individuals show subepithelial fibrosis by the mean age of 37 years. The fibrosis generally starts in the mid-periphery and is followed, in some cases, by central fibrosis and late small gelatinous formations.

Histopathology

Light microscopy does not show changes consistent with either EBMD or known dystrophy of Bowman's layer reported for the Smolandiensis variant.

■ Grayson–Wilbrandt corneal dystrophy

Grayson–Wilbrandt corneal dystrophy (GWCD) is a bilateral disorder of the central cornea characterized by accumulation of abnormal material in the basement membrane. There is only one publication describing a single family (Grayson & Wilbrandt 1966). Some authors consider GWCD a variant of EBMD or a Bowman's layer dystrophy. The corneal opacifications begin in the first to second decades of life with a progressive course. GWCD has an unknown mode of inheritance and genetics.

Signs

Bowman's layer demonstrates a variable pattern of opacification from diffuse mottling to diffuse gray-white mound-like opacities, which protrude anteriorly into the epithelium. The cornea between the deposits is clear, and the peripheral cornea is spared.

Symptoms

The onset of the disease occurs at the age of 10–12 years, which is later than in RBCD. Corneal erosions are less severe and less frequent than in RBCD and TBCD. Visual acuity is generally not affected.

Histopathology

Light microscopy demonstrates accumulation of homogeneous eosin-staining material between the epithelium and Bowman's layer, positive for periodic acid-Schiff.

■ Subepithelial mucinous corneal dystrophy

Subepithelial mucinous corneal dystrophy is a diffuse, bilateral disorder. The genetic locus and gene remain unknown. This unique condition clinically resembles Grayson–Wilbrandt dystrophy, but differs histochemically.

It was Feder et al. (1993) who described a family with an unusual autosomal dominant anterior corneal dystrophy. The onset was characterized by frequent RCE in the first decade of life. This decreased during adolescence and was followed by progressive loss of vision. The patients in this family ranged in age from 45 to 78 years.

Signs

There are bilateral, homogenous subepithelial gray-white opacities and haze, most dense centrally, involving the entire cornea.

Symptoms

Frequent, painful RCE episodes occur. In the only publication on this condition, older individuals developed subepithelial opacities and a corneal haze, causing progressive decreased vision.

Histopathology

A subepithelial band of mucinous material is seen under light microscopy: eosinophilic, periodic acid-Schiff-positive, Alcian blue-positive, and Masson's trichrome-positive, hyaluronidase-sensitive material anterior to Bowman's layer. The overlying epithelium is thinned out, and the deposits are elevated above the level of the basement membrane.

TEM shows irregular subepithelial deposits of fine fibrillar material consistent with glycosaminoglycan. Immunohistochemistry demonstrates accumulated material containing a combination of chondroitin-4-sulfate and dermatan sulfate.

RECURRENT CORNEAL EROSION SYNDROME

First described by Hansen in 1872 as a vesicular neuralgic keratitis, recurrent corneal erosion syndrome (RCES) is a common disorder, often misdiagnosed and treated only during the acute phase (Das & Seitz 2008). It is characterized clinically by repeated episodes of pain, redness, photophobia, and tearing. RCES more often presents unilaterally but can also affect both eyes.

RCES can be diagnosed at almost any age and affects men and women equally. Even though the majority of patients report trauma, an underlying factor should be suspected when there is no history of trauma or surgery. Epithelial, stromal, and endothelial corneal dystrophies have been described in association with RCES (Letko & Foster 2005). Patients with a history of trauma usually describe minor incidents commonly produced by fingernails, a leaf of a tree, or the edge of a piece of paper. The appearance of loose epithelium may occur any time, from days to several years after the initial trauma. Metallic foreign bodies and larger abrasions appear less prone to develop RCES.

Patients with RCES present with unilateral involvement, and the most commonly affected part of the cornea is central just below the pupil. When the underlying cause is a corneal dystrophy, symptoms are more often bilateral, localization of the loosely adherent epithelium more variable, and the management of symptoms often more complicated. The most frequently corneal dystrophies related to RCES are those affecting the epithelial, subepithelial basement membrane, and Bowman's layer (EBMD, Meesmann's, and Reis–Bücklers), although stromal dystrophies (e.g. lattice, granular, and macular) can also produce RCES (Hope-Ross et al. 1994). Previous refractive surgery with LASIK or PRK has also been reported as a risk factor for RCES (Jeng et al. 2004).

Clinical features

Patients with RCES develop pain, redness, photophobia, and tearing that may vary from mild to severe. Some have symptoms every day, and others have recurrences that can vary from every week or month to longer periods without symptoms. Typically pain is more severe at night or upon first waking and may be related to rapid eye movements during sleep or opening of the eyelid. Patients normally notice this situation and they try to open their eyes gently every morning, while others refer that they awake in the middle of the night because of the pain (Letko & Foster 2005). Since the pain is produced by poorly adherent epithelium, in the acute state of the disease a corneal erosion is always present, commonly within the lower half of the cornea, irrespective of the etiology. This area of the cornea is the most exposed to evaporative dry eye disease being in permanent contact with the tear film and the lower lid underlying the important contribution that dry eye disease and MGD make in RCES (Das & Seitz 2008).

Signs at the slit-lamp examination may vary. The appearance of the affected cornea ranges from loosely adherent and elevated epithelium, epithelial microcysts, or corneal epithelial defects, to stromal infiltrates and opacities. Negative fluorescein staining is a frequent finding. Tear break-up time is often diminished on the affected areas, and it is common to observe signs of MGD. Retroillumination after dilatation of the pupil may help to diagnose basement membrane dystrophies.

Epithelium adherence may be tested with a cellulose sponge: loosely adherent epithelium will fold or break when touched with the tip of the sponge under topical anesthetic (Rammamurthi et al.

2006). It is important to explore the inferior and central cornea, but other areas may be affected (**Figure 18.12**).

In some cases topography may be helpful, showing an irregular ocular surface, which may explain visual symptoms, such as a decrease in acuity or monocular diplopia.

Pathogenesis

The exact etiology and pathogenesis of RCES are not well understood, but the lack of adherence of the epithelium to the stroma sets focus on the anchoring complex of the basement membrane of the epithelium. These structures secure the basal layer of the epithelium to the anterior stroma (Letko & Foster 2005). The anchoring complex is composed of hemidesmosomes, lamina lucida, and lamina densa of the basement membrane and several molecules including integrins, laminin, and type VII collagen. Several studies have demonstrated differences in this structure when compared to normal corneas. These ultrastructural changes include abnormal basal epithelial cell layer, abnormal epithelial basement membrane, absent or abnormal hemidesmosomes, and loss of anchoring fibrils (Aitken et al. 1995). Binucleated and multinucleated cells have been found within all layers of the epithelium, and all layers are also infiltrated with neutrophils. Proteases contained on the lysozymes of these neutrophils are responsible for proteolytic degradation of the basement membrane structures. Interestingly, elevated levels of matrix metalloproteinase-9 (MMP-9) have been observed in the tear fluid and in the epithelium of patients with RCES. This collagenase is produced by neutrophils as well as by corneal epithelial cells and macrophages and is responsible for degradation of damaged matrix during re-epithelialization, and for stromal remodeling after the epithelialization is complete. Integrin α4, an integral membrane protein within the hemidesmosomes, is also cleaved by elevated levels of MMP-9, explaining the lack of hemidesmosomes in patients with RCES (Pal-Gosh et al. 2011).

In case of trauma, after the initial injury the regenerative process initiates. Since the epithelial defect is filled rapidly with epithelial cells sliding from adjacent basal layers, disassembly of hemidesmosomes must occur to allow sheet movement cell migration. The sliding of basal epithelial cells can occur over either preexisting basement mem-

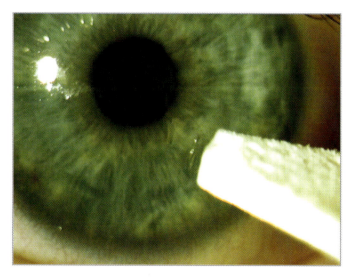

Figure 18.12 Diagnosis of loose epithelium using a triangular ophthalmic surgical spear.

brane or bare stromal collagen. If the basement membrane remains intact after trauma, the new epithelium becomes firmly adherent in a few days. However, in epithelial injuries that involve removal of basement membrane, epithelial cell migration is delayed and it takes several weeks to become adherent to the underlying stroma. Reattachment of corneal epithelium following an initial abrasion, normally a slicing-type injury, appears to be faulty in RCES (Rammamurthi et al. 2006).

Management

A wide number of treatments for RCES have been described. Palliative rather than curative options range from conservative measures to more invasive interventions, and a stepladder approach should be followed to control symptoms. During the acute phase, corneal erosions can be successfully managed with cycloplegia, therapeutic bandage contact lens, and topical antibiotic drops.

A Cochrane review of 11 trials and meta-analysis of 7 studies with dichotomous healing outcomes favored no patching on the first day of healing. These patients generally received more adjuvant treatment with antibiotics and/or cycloplegics, which is an important confounding factor (Turner & Rabiu 2006).

Treatment with lubrication measures is then started to prevent recurrences. Lubrication should be maintained and applied in the form of drops, gels, or ointments. Patients should be aware of their pathology and increase conservative treatments according to their symptoms. The bedtime application of ointments or gels is important to prevent adherence of the epithelium to the lid at night. It is also advisable to open the eyes gently upon awaking, even doing some eye movements before opening them. Most patients do well with conservative treatments, although these do not appear to reduce the recurrence rate of RCES (Reidy et al. 2000).

Ocular surface health must be evaluated and treated. Dry eye disease and MGD should be controlled as they act as important factors limiting successful re-epithelization. Lid hygiene and oral tetracyclines are useful in lowering the frequency of acute episodes. Tetracyclines have proved to be effective in reducing the free fatty acids in the tear film, the number of colony-forming units cultured from the eyelids, and the activity of MMP-9 as demonstrated in human corneal epi-

thelial cultures (Sobrin et al. 2000). Tetracyclines also act as an anti-inflammatory drug decreasing synthesis and activity of Interleukin-1 in these epithelial cultures. Successful treatment with autologous serum has been reported, since it provides substances such as vitamin A, growth factors, fibronectin, and many other cytokines involved in the healing process (Benitez del Castillo et al. 2001). Long-term bandage contact lenses have also been used as a treatment for RCES, but it may carry the risk of infection and neovascularization.

In patients with recalcitrant corneal erosions that do not respond to medical treatment, invasive steps may be implemented. These procedures include epithelial debridement, anterior stromal punctures, PTK, Nd:YAG laser keratectomy, and diamond burr superficial keratectomy. All of these techniques try to modify structures of the adherent complex at the epithelial basal membrane or at the anterior stroma, attempting to restore a strong adherence of the epithelium to the underlying stroma.

Debridement of loose epithelium is a good option during the acute phase when there is already corneal erosion or there are long areas of loose epithelium. But it is a painful procedure and there is no current evidence that this reduces recurrences of epithelial erosions (Turner & Rabiu 2006). Alcohol delamination of the epithelium has also been reported as an alternative to classical mechanical debridement (Dua et al. 2006).

Anterior stromal puncture performed under topical anesthesia, with a 25-gauge needle, is a relatively simple and inexpensive procedure that is generally performed at the slit lamp. Punctures must reach the anterior stroma and should be applied widely, avoiding the central cornea (**Figures 18.13** and **18.14**). The aim of this therapy is to enhance epithelial adhesion by scar formation on the anterior stroma. Even though it may be necessary to be repeated, success rates of up to 80% have been reported in recalcitrant RCES (Rubinfeld et al. 1990). We believe this is an effective technique, and it can be recommended as a first approach when conservative treatment fails. PTK can also be an effective treatment for RCES with high successful rates (described elsewhere in this book).

A number of prophylactic options are available for RCES; however, there is no agreement as to the best option. Randomized control trials are still needed (Watson & Barker 2007). Moreover, the physiopathology of this syndrome has not been so far elucidated.

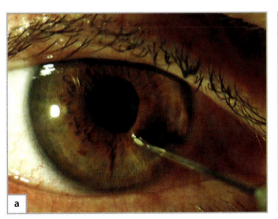 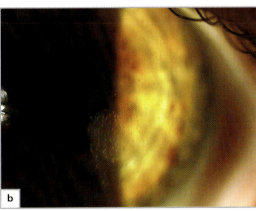

Figure 18.13 (a) Corneal micropunctures using a 20-gauge needle. (b) Corneal aspect after corneal micropunctures.

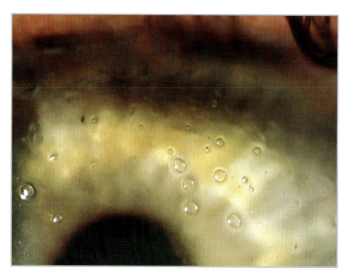

Figure 18.14 Subepithelial bubbles after corneal micropunctures due to loose or not adhered epithelium.

■ REFERENCES

Aitken DA, Beirouty ZA, Lee WR. Ultrastructural study of the corneal epithelium in the recurrent erosion syndrome. *Br J Ophthalmol* 1995; **79**:282–289.

Alvarez-Fischer M, de Toledo JA, Barraquer RI. Lisch corneal dystrophy. *Cornea* 2005; **24**:494–495.

Benitez del Castillo JM, de la Casa JM, Sardina RC, et al. Treatment of recurrent corneal erosion using autologous serum. *Cornea* 2001; **20**:807–810.

Charles NC, Young JA, Kumar A, et al. Band-shaped and whorled microcystic dystrophy of the corneal epithelium. *Ophthalmology* 2000; **107**:1761–1764.

Cogan DG, Donaldson DD, Kuwabara T, Marshall D. Microcystic dystrophy of the corneal epithelium, *Trans Am Ophthalmol Soc* 1964; **62**:213-225.

Das S, Seitz B. Recurrent corneal erosion syndrome. *Surv Ophthalmol* 2008; **53**:3–15.

Dua HS, Lagnado R, Raj D, et al. Alcohol delamination of the corneal epithelium: an alternative in the management of recurrent corneal erosions. *Ophthalmology* 2006; **113**:404–411.

Dursun D, Kim MC, Solomon A, Pflugfelder SC. Treatment of recalcitrant recurrent corneal erosions with inhibitors of matrix metalloproteinase-9, doxycycline and corticosteroids. *Am J Ophthalmol* 2001; **132**:8–13.

EBAA. 2010 Statistical Report—the EBAA statistical report is a compilation of information provided to the EBAA by 79 U.S. and nine international eye banks and reflects an essentially complete picture of eye banking activity in the United States.

Ewald M, Hammersmith KM. Review of diagnosis and management of recurrent corneal erosion syndrome. *Curr Opin Ophthalmol* 2009; **20**:287–291.

Feder RS, Jay M, Yue BY, et al. Subepithelial mucinous corneal dystrophy. Clinical and pathological correlations. *Arch Ophthalmol* 1993; **111**:1106–1114.

Fraunfelder FW, Cabezas M. Treatment of recurrent corneal erosion by extended-wear bandage contact lens. *Cornea* 2011; **30**:164–166.

Grayson M, Wilbrandt H. Dystrophy of the anterior limiting membrane of the cornea (Reis–Bücklers type). *Am J Ophthalmol* 1966; **61**:345–349.

Guerry D. Observations on Cogan's microcystic dystrophy of the corneal epithelium. *Trans Am Ophthalmol Soc* 1965; **63**:320-332.

Hammar B, Björck E, Lind H, et al. Dystrophia Helsinglandica: a new type of hereditary corneal recurrent erosions with late subepithelial fibrosis. *Acta Ophthalmol* 2009; **87**:659–665.

Hammar B, Lagali N, Ek S, et al. Dystrophia smolandiensis: a novel morphological picture of recurrent corneal erosions. *Acta Ophthalmol* 2010; **88**:394–400.

Hau SC, Tuft SJ. In vivo confocal microscopy of bleb-like disorder in epithelial basement membrane dystrophy. *Cornea* 2011; **30**:1478–1480.

Hope-Ross MW, Chell PB, Kervick GN, et al. Recurrent corneal erosion: clinical features. *Eye* 1994; **8**:373–377.

Ide T, Nishida K, Maeda N, et al. A spectrum of clinical manifestations of gelatinous drop-like corneal dystrophy in Japan. *Am J Ophthalmol* 2004; **137**:1081–1084.

Irvine AD, Corden LD, Swensson O, et al. Mutations in cornea-specific keratin K3 or K12 genes cause Meesmann's corneal dystrophy. *Nat Genet* 1997; **16**:184–187.

Ito M, Takahashi J, Sakimoto T, Sawa M. Histological study of gelatinous drop-like dystrophy following excimer laser phototherapeutic keratectomy. *Nihon Ganka Gakkai Zasshi* 2000; **104**:44–50.

Jeng BH, Stewart JM, McLeod SD, et al. Relapsing diffuse lamellar keratitis after laser insitukeratomileusis associated with recurrent erosion syndrome. *Arch Ophthalmol* 2004; **122**:396–398.

Kannabiran C, Klintworth GK. TGFBI gene mutations in corneal dystrophies. *Hum Mutat* 2006; **27**:615–625.

Kobayashi A, Sugiyama K. In vivo laser confocal microscopy findings for Bowman's layer dystrophies (Thiel-Behnke and Reis–Bücklers corneal dystrophies). *Ophthalmology* 2007; **114**:69–75.

Kuwabara T, Ciccarelli EC. Meesmann's corneal dystrophy. A pathological study. *Arch Ophthalmol* 1964; **71**:672–682.

Lasram L, Rais C, el Euch M, Ouertani A. Gelatinous dystrophy of the cornea. Apropos of 5 cases. *J Fr Ophtalmol* 1994; **17**:24–28.

Letko E, Foster CS. Recurrent erosion syndrome. In: CS Foster, Azar DT, Dohlman CH (eds), The cornea. Philadelphia: LWW, 2005:657–661.

Lisch W, Buttner A, Oeffner F, et al. Lisch corneal dystrophy is genetically distinct from Meesmann corneal dystrophy and maps to xp22.3. *Am J Ophthalmol* 2000; **130**:461–468.

Lisch W, Steuhl KP, Lisch C, et al. A new, band-shaped and whorled microcystic dystrophy of the corneal epithelium. *Am J Ophthalmol* 1992; **114**:35–44.

Lisch W, Wasielica-Poslednik J, Lisch C, et al. Contact lens-induced regression of Lisch epithelial corneal dystrophy. *Cornea* 2010; **29**:342–345.

Lohse E, Stock EL, Jones JC, et al. Reis–Bücklers corneal dystrophy. Immunofluorescent and electron microscopic studies. *Cornea* 1989; **8**:200–209.

Magin TM, Vijayaraj P, Leube RE. Structural and regulatory functions of keratins. *Exp Cell Res* 2007; **313**:2021–2032.

Munier FL, Korvatska E, Djemaï A, et al. Kerato-epithelin mutations in four 5q31- linked corneal dystrophies. *Nat Genet* 1997; **15**:247–251.

Musch DC, Niziol LM, Stein JD, Kamyar R, Sugar A. Prevalence of corneal dystrophies in the United States: estimates from claims data. *Invest Ophthalmol Vis Sci* 2011; **52**:6959–6963.

Niederer RL, McGhee CN. Clinical in vivo confocal microscopy of the human cornea in health and disease. *Prog Retin Eye Res* 2010; **29**:30–58.

Pal-Gosh S, Blanco T, Tadvalkar G, et al. MMP9 cleavage of the β4 integrin ectodomain leads to recurrent epithelial erosions in mice. *J Cell Sci* 2011; **124**:2666–2675.

Poinard C, Tuppin P, Loty B, Delbosc B. The French national waiting list for keratoplasty created in 1999: patient registration, indications, characteristics, and turnover. *J Fr Ophtalmol* 2003; **26**:911–919.

Poulaki V, Colby K. Genetics of anterior and stromal corneal dystrophies. *Semin Ophthalmol* 2008; **23**:9–17.

Rammamurthi S, Rahman MQ, Dutton GN, et al. Pathogenesis, clinical features and management of recurrent corneal erosions. *Eye* 2006; **20**:635–644.

Reeves SW, Kang PC, Zlogar DF, et al. Recurrent corneal erosion syndrome: a study of 364 episodes. *Ophthalmic Surg Lasers Imaging* 2010; **9**:1–2.

Reidy JJ, Paulus MP, Gona S. Recurrent erosion of the cornea: epidemiology and treatment. *Cornea* 2000; **19**:767–771.

Robin SB, Epstein RJ, Kornmehl EW. Band-shaped, whorled microcystic corneal dystrophy. *Am J Ophthalmol* 1994; **117**:543–544.

Rubinfeld RS, Laibson PR, Cohen EJ, et al. Anterior stromal puncture for recurrent erosion: further experience and new instrumentation. *Ophthalmic Surg* 1990; **21**:318–326.

Seitz B, Lisch W. Stage-related therapy of corneal dystrophies. *Dev Ophthalmol* 2011; **48**:116–153.

Shousha MA, Yoo SH, Kymionis GD, et al. Long-term results of femtosecond laser-assisted sutureless anterior lamellar keratoplasty. *Ophthalmology* 2011; **118**:315–323.

Singh RP, Raj D, Pherwani A, et al. Alcohol delamination of the corneal epithelium for recalcitrant recurrent corneal erosion syndrome: a prospective study of efficacy and safety. *Br J Ophthalmol* 2007; **91**:908–911.

Skonier J, Neubauer M, Madisen L, et al. cDNA cloning and sequence analysis of BIGH3, a novel gene induced in a human adenocarcinoma cell line after treatment with transforming growth factor. *DNA Cell Biol* 1992; **11**:511–522.

Small KW, Mullen L, Barletta J, et al. Mapping of Reis–Bücklers corneal dystrophy to chromosome 5q. *Am J Ophthalmol* 1996; **121**:384–390.

Smith F. The molecular genetics of keratin disorders. *Am J Clin Dermatol* 2003; **4**:347–364.

Sobrin L, Ye HQ, Azar DT. Regulation of MMP-9 activity in human tear fluid and corneal epithelial culture supernatant. *Invest Ophthalmol Vis Sci* 2000; **41**:1703–1709.

Tsujikawa M, Kurahashi H, Tanaka T, et al. Identification of the gene responsible for gelatinous drop-like corneal dystrophy. *Nat Genet* 1999; **21**:420–423.

Turner A, Rabiu M. Patching for corneal abrasion. *Cochrane Database Syst Rev* 2006.

Vemuganti GK, Rathi VM, Murthy SI. Histological landmarks in corneal dystrophy: pathology of corneal dystrophies. *Dev Ophthalmol* 2011; **48**:24–50.

Watson SL, Barker NH. Interventions for recurrent corneal erosions. *Cochrane Database Syst Rev* 2007; **17**:CD001861.

Weiss JS, Møller HU, Lisch W, et al. IC3D classification of corneal dystrophies. *Dev Ophthalmol Cornea* 2008; **27**:S1–S83.

Werblin TP, Hirst LW, Stark WJ, Maumenee IH. Prevalence of map-dot-fingerprint changes in the cornea. *Br J Ophthalmol* 1981; **65**:401–409.

Wessel MM, Sarkar JS, Jakobiec FA, et al. Treatment of lisch corneal dystrophy with photorefractive keratectomy and mitomycin C. *Cornea* 2011; **30**:481–485.

Williams KA, Lowe MT, Bartlett CM, et al. The Australian Corneal Graft Registry 2007 Report. Adelaide: Flinders University Press, 2007.

Yang J, Han X, Huang D, et al. Analysis of TGFBI gene mutations in Chinese patients with corneal dystrophies and review of the literature. *Mol Vis* 2010; **16**:1186–1193.

Yee RW, Sullivan LS, Lai HT, et al. Linkage mapping of Thiel-Behnke corneal dystrophy (CDB2) to chromosome 10q23-q24. *Genomics* 1997; **46**:152–154.

Yeung JY, Hodge WG. Recurrent Meesmann's corneal dystrophy: treatment with keratectomy and mitomycin C. *Can J Ophthalmol* 2009; **44**:103–104.

Chapter 19 Pinguecula and pterygium

David Diaz-Valle, Rosalia Mendez-Fernandez, Pedro Arriola-Villalobos,
Maria T. Iradier, Jose M. Benitez-del-Castillo

PINGUECULA

Pinguecula is a common ocular surface disorder with a broad reported range of prevalence (22.5–90%). The prevalence increases with age. It has been found in almost all people older than 80 years (Mimura et al. 2011). Pingueculae are benign, elevated, yellowish masses on the conjunctiva, found in the interpalpebral paralimbal zone. They are usually bilateral and are more common nasally than temporally. Histopathologically, they may have normal conjunctival epithelium with elastotic degeneration in the substantia propia. The etiology of pingueculae is not fully understood, but prolonged exposure to ultraviolet-B radiation seems to be the main factor involved. Pinguecula is almost always asymptomatic, but it can manifest as a foreign body sensation, pain, and tearing. Only in these symptomatic cases is topical treatment necessary, usually with lubricants, topical surface steroids, or topical non-steroidal anti-inflammatory drugs (Frucht-Pery et al. 1999). Surgical excision is rarely used, mostly for cosmetic reasons.

PTERYGIUM

Pterygium is derived from the Greek word 'pterygion,' which means 'wing.' It is a fibrovascular triangular-shaped neoformation extending from the conjunctiva to the cornea. The masses are located in the limbar interpalpebral zone, usually bilateral and asymmetric, and they are more frequently nasal than temporal.

Pterygium prevalence increases toward the equator because ultraviolet radiation is the main factor involved in its pathogenesis. Pterygium prevalence is very variable, ranging from 1.2% in a white urban community, in middle latitudes, to 31% in pigmented rural people from Peru, near to the equator. Some risk factors have been involved in pterygium pathogenesis, while other factors have been reported as protective (Table 19.1) (Arriola-Villalobos 2006).

For successful treatment of pterygium, the pathogenesis must be well understood. Nowadays, the main pathogenic factor involved is a focal limbar defect caused by ultraviolet radiation. This limbar defect is more common in the nasal area because ultraviolet light reflects in the anterior chamber, focusing on the nasal limbus. Ultraviolet radiation damages limbal stem cells through oxidative stress (Balci et al. 2011). This damage leads to the rupture of the corneoconjunctival barrier. This is the first pathogenic step in pterygion development. Matrix metalloproteinases and proinflammatory cytokines are involved in this rupture. The second step in pterygion development is mainly growth, with conjunctival fibroblasts releasing growth factors involved in cell proliferation, inflammation, connective tissue remodeling, and the angiogenesis seen in pterygium. This theory of barrier rupture and subsequent growth concurs with another reported theory that argues that pterygia have some tumor-like features, including expression of p53 gene in the epithelium of the pterygium, ultraviolet radiation as the main risk factor, frequent recurrence following resection, low levels of cellular apoptosis, and common treatment modalities such as antimetabolites. In conclusion, it seems that pterygion pathogenesis is more a of a cellular proliferation disorder than a degenerative disorder (Liang et al. 2011).

The histology of the pterygia is variable. The epithelium may be normal, but it usually shows pleomorphism with dysplastic aspects. Impression cytology of the pterygium surface is abnormal, showing increased goblet cells and dendritiform inflammatory cells, which correlate with pterygium activity (Labbé et al. 2010). Histological changes present in the connective tissue of the pterygium are extremely varied. The first alteration is probably local hyalinization followed by elastotic degeneration of the substantia propia with degenerated collagen. There is also a quantitatively reduced inflammatory infiltrate.

Clinical features
Symptoms

Pterygium symptoms are highly variable, mainly depending on the severity (Twelker et al. 2000). It is sometimes asymptomatic and the patient is usually concerned about the aesthetic appearance. Irritation, itching, photophobia, tearing, and foreign body sensation are the usual symptoms that are made worse by light, wind, and dust. Symptoms occur due to the alteration of the tear film and the epithelial surface. Eye pain is unusual, and is related to ulcerations in the line of advance of the pterygium. The following changes in vision may occur:

- Glare and reduction of contrast sensitivity. It is frequent even in early cases due to stromal opacities in the peripheral cornea and alteration of the tear film, which results in greater diffraction of light (Lin et al. 1989)
- True vision loss when growth over the cornea exceeds 2–3 mm. This effect is due to two mechanisms:
  - Static deformation of the cornea. Growth of the pterygium over the cornea causes deformation and increases corneal higher order aberrations (Zare et al. 2010). This disease also causes astigmatism with the rule related to flattening of the horizontal meridian, the degree of which is proportional to the size of the pterygium (Mohammad-Salih & Sharif 2008) (**Figure 19.1**)

Table 19.1 Risk and protective factors of pterygium

Risk factor	Protective factor	Controversy
Ultraviolet radiation	Sunglasses use	Tobacco
Outdoor work	Spectacles use	Gender
Age		Iris color
Race		Skin color
Hereditary susceptibility		Hair color
Irritant exposure (i.e. dust)		

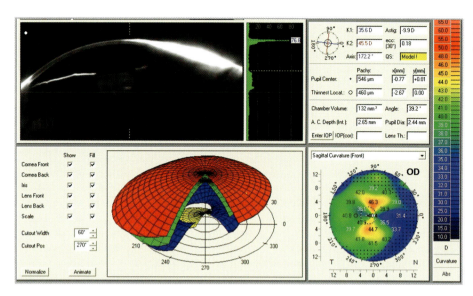

Figure 19.1 Right eye nasal pterygium topography. Note the existence of high with-the-rule astigmatism caused by the flattening of the horizontal meridian.

– Dynamic deformation of the cornea with eye movements, mainly in abduction, especially in cases with stronger adhesions

The following changes improve after surgery, but are usually not completely reversed (Yagmur et al. 2005):

- Invasion of the pupil area when highly advanced (>4 mm of corneal invasion)
- Diplopia, enophthalmos. In very advanced forms, especially in multiple recurrences, there may be a symblepharon mainly affecting the area of the medial canthus, which can lead to restriction of the gaze with diplopia, moderate enophthalmos, and sometimes ectropion or entropion of lacrimal punctum with persistent tearing (Khan 2005)

Signs

Pterygium is a triangular wing-like mass of fibrovascular tissue, extending from the conjunctiva, that encroaches a variable distance onto the cornea. The lesion is usually on the horizontal meridian, particularly on the nasal side, although either nasal or temporal (double pterygium) lesions can occur. There may be subepithelial scarring, elevated whitish opacities ('islets of Vogt') and an iron deposition line at the apex (Stocker's line), and dellen with elevated pterygia.

Slit-lamp examination can help identify various morphological and anatomical features for classification of the pterygium, and to decide whether or not it is active. This is fundamental for deciding on the treatment.

Signs of activity include rapid growth, engorged vessels with dilated capillaries and sometimes hemorrhages at the line of advancement, thick and elevated body, gray leading edge in the cornea, and punctate epitheliopathy at the head of the pterygium. Signs of stability include a visible iron line (Stocker's line) just anterior to the margin, observation of islets of Vogt, and absence of punctate epitheliopathy; the pterygium head appears flat and almost non-vascularized, and the body of the pterygium appears as a whitish band with fine and straight capillaries that allow for visualization of the episcleral vascularization.

Classification of pterygium

The pterygia are classified in a variety of ways depending on the following aspects:

- According to their morphology (T)
  - **Atrophic:** translucent, scantly vascularized, episcleral vessels under the pterygium are clearly distinguished

- **Fleshy:** thick, vascularized, episcleral vessels are completely hidden
  - **Intermediate:** episcleral vessels are partially hidden
- According to corneal invasion (C)
  - <2 mm, low visual impact
  - 2–4 mm, greater visual impact by induced astigmatism
  - >4 mm, significant visual impact by astigmatism and invasion of the optic zone
- According to limbal involvement (L)
  - <2 mm
  - 2–4 mm
  - >4 mm
- Stationary (quiescent) or active
  - Clinical features are shown in **Table 19.2**
- Primary or recurrent
- Uni- or bilateral, that is, to involve one or both eyes
- Uni-, bi-, or multipolar in the same eye

TCL classification

Different classifications have emerged in order to group together the above factors and to improve clinical usefulness when handling these patients (Anduze & Merrit 1985). In our center, we use a classification

Table 19.2 Degree of activity of the pterygium

Stationary or inactive
No apical stain
Visible Stocker's line
Visible islets of Vogt
Whitish head, scant vascularity
White body, episcleral vessels visible
Active
Apical stain
Stocker's line not visible
Visible islets of Vogt
Very vascular head
Hyperemic and thickened body, little or non-visible episcleral vessels

based on previous systems that have been adapted by us (TCL classification) (Méndez et al. 2006). We assign a value according to the morphology (T), corneal invasion (C), and limbal involvement (L), with each parameter graduated from 1 to 3 from smaller to greater aggressiveness (**Figures 19.2–19.4**). We also add to the classification according to if the pterygium is active or stationary, and if it is primary or recurrent (**Table 19.3**).

TCL classification is a quick and easy form of describing pterygia that allows for assessment of the clinical progression of the process, decide the medical or surgical therapy in each case, as well as analyze the results in terms of the rate of recurrence with the different treatment alternatives.

■ Diagnosis and differential diagnosis
Biomicroscopy

Pterygium diagnosis is clinical, according to the morphology described above. Occasionally, differential diagnosis can be performed with other limbal diseases such as pseudopterygium, limbal dermoid, nevi, and especially epithelial neoplasms.

An important differential characteristic is that pterygium is a process oriented toward the center of the cornea, while conjunctival and limbal neoplasms tend to grow in any direction. On the other hand, a pseudopterygium (after corneal injury) can develop in any quadrant and direction (sometimes oblique), and there are sometimes real bridges of tissue separating from deeper levels (Hirst 2003).

Confocal microscopy and optical coherence tomography

Optical coherence tomography can provide some data, especially about the relationship between the corneal tissue and injury (Soliman & Mohamed 2010). Confocal microscopy can be helpful in assessing the inflammatory activity of the pterygium and the differential diagnosis (Labbé et al. 2010).

Histopathology

Although pterygium has traditionally been considered a degenerative lesion, it shares some characteristics with tumors as it has a tendency to invade normal tissue and has a high rate of recurrence after removal. Pterygium can also coexist with premalignant lesions, so all pterygium removed must be studied histologically (Chui et al. 2011). Rates of up to 9.8% of unsuspected epithelial neoplasms have been published (Hirst et al. 2009), supporting the histopathological study in all removed pterygia.

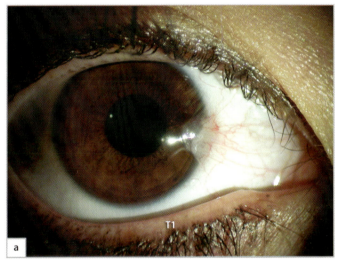

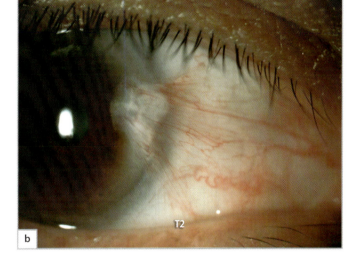

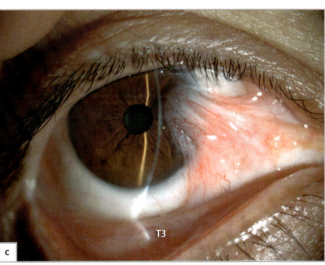

Figure 19.2 Morphology (T). (a) T1 (atrophic). (b) T2 (intermediate). (c) T3 (fleshy).

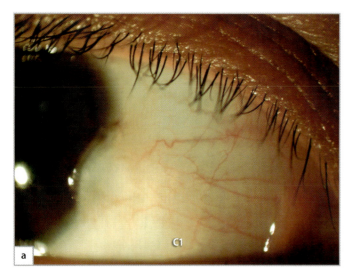

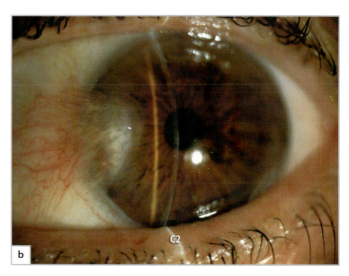

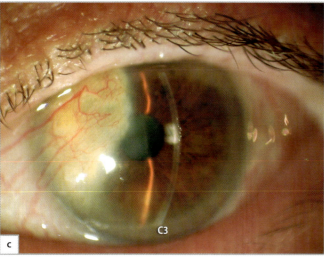

Figure 19.3 Corneal involvement (C). (a) C1 (<2 mm). (b) C2 (2–4 mm). (c) C3 (>4 mm).

Pterygium surgery

In recent decades, there have been an increased number of surgical alternatives for the treatment of pterygium. The aim of these alternatives is to eliminate the lesion and prevent recurrence. These newer treatment methods have significantly reduced the worrisome problem of recurrence. However, the field is still evolving.

The main method of pterygium treatment is surgical excision. Any conservative treatment is mainly symptomatic, and usually temporary, in the early stages of the disease. Conservative treatment involves solar protection and the use of artificial tears or preservative-free eye ointment lubricant to provide comfort and relief from foreign body sensation. Short-term anti-inflammatory eye drops may also be useful for inflamed pterygia.

Primary pterygium: indications and surgical technique

The main indications for pterygium surgery include the following:
- Decrease in or disturbance of visual function, because of proximity to the visual axis or high astigmatism, usually in favor of the rule, since the pterygium induces a flattening of the horizontal meridian (**Figure 19.1**)
- Documentation of pterygium growth
- Chronic ocular irritation and significant discomfort
- Cosmetic reasons

The classical surgical procedure involves complete excision of a pterygium from the cornea and sclera, which subsequently leaves a bare corneoscleral surface. This procedure, also known as the bare sclera technique, was first fully described by D`Ombrain (1948). The high frequency of recurrence associated with this procedure has led to the search for adjunct treatment options.

There is no standard definition of recurrence, but it is generally accepted that a recurrence occurs when a fibrovascular growth in the position of the previously excised pterygium crosses the limbus onto the cornea for any distance. At least 97% of all recurrent pterygia manifest within the first year after excision (Hirst et al. 1994).

Pterygium excision

Removal of the pterygium involves surgical excision of the head, neck, and body of the pterygium.

After adequate combination of topical and subconjunctival anesthesia, the first approach involves grasping the head of the pterygium with forceps and separating it from the cornea by avulsion or using a surgical blade. An attempt is made to identify the plane of dissection,

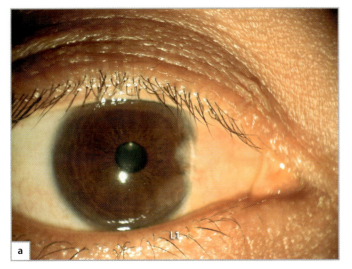

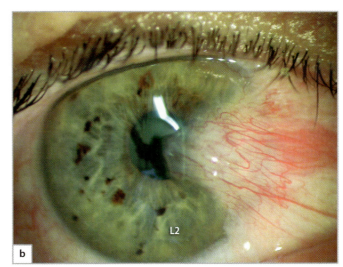

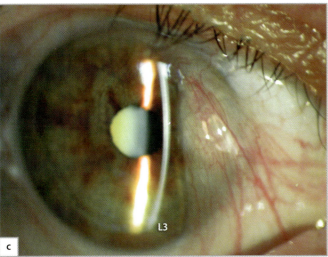

Figure 19.4 Limbal involvement (L). (a) L1 (<2 mm). (b) L2 (2–4 mm). (c) L3 (>4 mm).

which facilitates removal of the pterygium while keeping the underlying corneal surface smooth. Any pterygium tissue remnants on the cornea are gently polished with a diamond burr or scraped off with the surgical blade until a clear corneal bed is obtained. Care should be taken to scrape superficially, and not to cut deeply into the cornea, creating a permanent thinning. Any bleeding points found are gently cauterized. Diathermy should be avoided or minimally applied in order to reduce the risk of scleral necrosis, especially after the use of mitomycin C (Singh 1989).

In case of a difficult dissection of the head of the pterygium, or in recurrent cases, it has been recently suggested that alcohol should be used on the cornea prior to surgical excision of the pterygium to split the basal membrane and destroy hemidesmosome junctions between corneal epithelial cells. It has been in use for a long time in corneal refractive surgery. Unlike blunt dissection, prior alcohol application seems to create a smoother and clearer separation plane (Chen & Hsu 2006). Despite the various methods for pterygium surgical excision, there is to date no definitive evidence to show that outcome is influenced by the excision technique.

Blunt and sharp dissections are usually performed to separate the pterygium from the underlying sclera and surrounding conjunctiva. The neck and body of the pterygium are then dissected with Westcott scissors posteriorly up to about 4 mm from the limbus and then excised. As the body of the pterygium has no clearly defined margin,

Table 19.3 TCL classification of the pterygium

Pterygium morphology (T)
T1: atrophic pterygium
T2: intermediate pterygium
T3: fleshy pterygium
Corneal invasion (C)
C1: <2 mm
C2: 2–4 mm
C3: >4 mm
Limbar involvement (L)
L1: <4 mm
L2: 4–6 mm
L3: >6 mm
Degree of activity
Active
Inactive
Primary or recurrent
Primary
Recurrent

the extent of surgical excision of the pterygium and subconjunctival fibrovascular tissue varies between reports. Our preferred method is to excise the base of the pterygium approximately no more than 4 mm from the limbus, as retraction of the surrounding conjunctiva results in enlargement of the surgical defect. Thereafter, a wide tenonectomy should be performed and the subconjunctival fibrous tissue under the pterygium should be excised much wider than the area covered by the pterygium in order to ensure that the edges of the resection remain free of fibrous tissue.

If no additional measures are performed, pterygium excision alone is commonly referred to as bare sclera excision. The recurrence rates for bare sclera excision alone are unacceptably high (ranging from 30 to 80%) when compared with other treatment modalities (Frucht-Pery et al. 1996). As such, bare sclera excision alone is no longer recommended for the treatment of pterygium.

■ Prevention of pterygium recurrence

Pterygium excision is often combined with various adjunct measures to prevent recurrence of the disease. These include further surgical or grafting procedures, chemotherapy, and the use of radiation therapy. The availability of a variety of modalities makes it possible to use another method when one fails. It also allows for a combination of methods such as chemotherapy and grafting in cases of pterygium that are difficult or have been recurrent multiple times (Ang et al. 2007).

Surgical methods

Surgery could be the sole adjunct or could be combined with radiation therapy or chemotherapy, especially for multiple recurrent pterygia. Applicable surgical procedures include lamellar keratoplasty, amniotic membrane transplantation (AMT), and conjunctival grafting including all its variants (conjunctival or limbal-conjunctival grafts). These various surgical options could be applied alone or in combination.

For conjunctival grafting and AMT, attachment of the graft could be by either sutures or fibrin tissue glue (Koranyi et al. 2004); however, the fibrin glue (Tisseel, Baxter Corporation, Canada) is now generally preferred over sutures. Use of fibrin glue reduces both the operation time and postoperative discomfort experienced by the patient. In a prospective comparative study by Karalezli et al. (2008), the average duration of surgery using fibrin glue was 15.7 minutes compared to 32.5 minutes for sutures. Recent studies (Ratnalingam et al. 2010, Srinivasan et al. 2009) have also shown that it reduces postoperative inflammation and the pterygium recurrence rate as compared to sutures. It has also been shown by histological examination to be safer on ocular tissues (Ozdamar et al. 2008) causing no complications, and in the rare event of graft dehiscence, fibrin glue can be reapplied or the graft can be sutured. There is, however, the potential but yet undocumented risk of cross-infection with its use and issues related to added costs can become significant.

Conjunctival autograft

Since its introduction by Kenyon et al. (1985), conjunctival autograft has gradually become the gold standard for the treatment of primary pterygia. Although different types of grafts can be used, the preferred technique to cover the bare sclera is to use a free conjunctival autograft. The graft is typically harvested free of tenon tissue from the superior bulbar conjunctiva and sutured or, more preferably, glued to the bare sclera defect after pterygium excision. Although more time-consuming and technically demanding, conjunctival autografting is safer and probably more effective than radiation therapy or chemotherapy, since it is free of any serious side effects. Graft success is enhanced by, among other things, the use of minimal cautery; tenon-free grafts; removal of excess fibrin glue; and countering postoperative graft retraction by using a slightly oversized (by 1 mm) graft (Ang et al. 2007).

The advantages of this technique highlight the excellent restoration of the anatomy of the ocular surface because of the placement of a fragment of healthy conjunctiva over the area of the lesion. It provides good cosmetic and functional results (**Figure 19.5a–b**). Also, it can be performed in most cases, unless there is compromise of the donor conjunctiva in the affected or the contralateral eye, or if there is a risk of performing glaucoma surgery in the future (Marticorena et al. 2006).

A variant of this technique is the use of sliding grafts or a limbal-conjunctival graft, which includes about 2 mm of limbal tissue in the graft. The limbal-conjunctival graft aims to replenish damaged limbal stem cells with fresh tissue in order to reduce the tendency towards

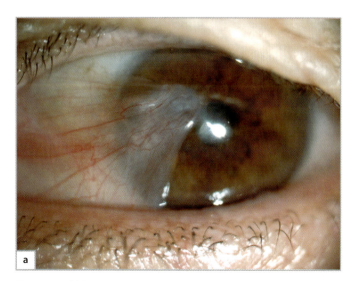
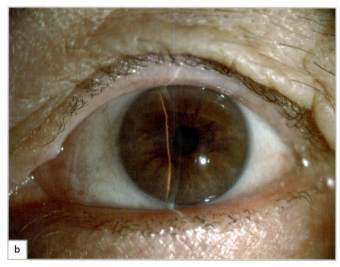

Figure 19.5 (a) Preoperative aspect. Primary pterygium stage T1 C3 L3 in the left eye. (b) One-month postoperation (surgical excision and conjunctival autograft fixated with fibrin glue).

recurrence. In terms of preventing recurrence, there is no conclusive additional advantage over the free or sliding conjunctival autograft (Abdallah 2009). However, limbal-conjunctival autograft is technically demanding and increases surgical time, in addition to the possibility of limbal tissue damage to the donor site.

Amniotic membrane transplantation

AMT has been proposed as a treatment option because of its antiscarring, antiangiogenic, and anti-inflammatory properties, which may be useful for treating pterygium. An additional advantage is that it removes the need for harvesting large autografts, thereby minimizing iatrogenic injury to the rest of the conjunctival surface. AMT is our preferred technique in cases where it is not possible to obtain a conjunctival autograft.

However, in a randomized prospective study by Tananuvat and Martin (2004), AMT was associated with an unacceptably high recurrence rate when compared with conjunctival autograft. This result is also supported by Luanratanakorn et al. (2006) in a prospective randomized controlled study. **Table 19.4** shows the published recurrence rate encountered by different authors in primary pterygium with conjunctival autograft and AMT.

Recurrent pterygium: surgical technique

The main problem of primary pterygium surgery is the possibility of recurrence. Recurrence seems to be related to the method of removal of the pterygium and the morphologic type according to TCL classification. Ocular surface inflammation also plays an important role; therefore, control of inflammation before and after surgery is important for minimizing recurrences.

Recurrence is defined as any new growth that exceeds 1.5 or 2 mm onto the cornea (Hirst 2009). It is recommended to wait for at least 6 months before reoperation to avoid more inflammation.

When recurrent pterygium is removed, a different and more aggressive technique than performed for primary pterygium should be used to prevent a new recurrence. Extended removal with extended conjunctival autograft (Arenas 2006), lamellar corneal keratoplasty, AMT, adjunctive treatments with mitomycin C (Donnenfeld et al. 2003) or cyclosporine A (Aydin et al. 2008), or a combination of such techniques are the most common methods of this type of surgery

depending on the severity of the recurrence. Subconjunctival bevacizumab has also been investigated resulting in a short-term decrease in vascularization and irritation, which regresses to its preinjection state in 6–7 weeks (Teng et al. 2009).

Reconstruction of the ocular surface should be the purpose of the procedure. The first key step in recurrent pterygium is to dissect and recess the conjunctiva back to the fornix to avoid symblepharon.

In case of severe recurrences, lamellar corneal keratoplasty has been proposed to be a good surgical option (Mc Clellan et al. 2006).

Lamellar corneal keratoplasty

The goal of this method is to remove the damaged cornea and pterygium followed by substitution of a lamellar graft of fresh cornea of the same thickness and diameter, creating a smooth ocular surface. The donor tissue is a preserved corneoscleral button with intact epithelium.

Subtenon or peribulbar anesthesia is applied. The first step of the procedure is to perform a partial-thickness trephination of the lesion followed by a lamellar dissection of the fibrovascular tissue and the injured cornea, limbus, and sclera. The donor lamella is then obtained with the Moria automated lamellar therapeutic keratoplasty (ALTK) microkeratome system (Moria/Microtek Inc., Doylestown, Pennsylvania, USA) from a donor cornea with a scleral rim of at least 3 mm in diameter to guarantee proper vacuum during the lamellar cut.

Table 19.4 Recurrence rate observed by different authors in primary pterygium with conjunctival autograft and amniotic membrane transplantation (AMT)

Author (year)	Surgical technique	Number of eyes	Recurrence rate (%)
Prabhasawat (1997)	Conjunctival autograft	78	2.6
Tan (1997)	Conjunctival autograft	61	2
Tananuvat (2004)	Conjunctival autograft	44	4.76
	AMT	42	40.9
Luanratanokorn (2006)	Conjunctival autograft	106	12
	AMT	148	25
Mejía (2005)	Conjunctival autograft	111	1.8

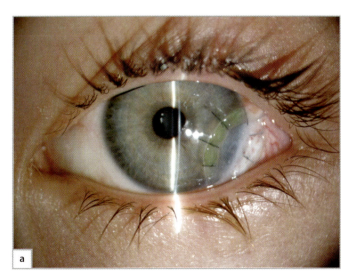
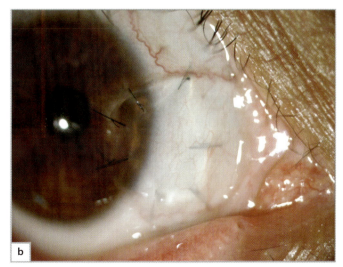

Figure 19.6 (a) Lamellar keratoplasty in recurrent pterygium. (b) Lamellar keratoplasty and conjunctival autograft in recurrent pterygium. Two-month follow-up visit.

Overlying or radial 10/0 nylon sutures can be used to hold the implant in place on the recipient's cornea, sclera, and conjunctiva. While radial sutures penetrate recipient cornea, overlying sutures do not go through and would induce less astigmatism (**Figure 19.6a**). A conjunctival autograft can also be performed in order to restore the conjunctival surface (**Figure 19.6b**).

It is essential that this lamellar grafting procedure establish a smooth ocular surface and that the graft epithelium heal as soon as possible. To facilitate this, the eye is kept patched to accomplish re-epithelization.

Postoperative treatment comprises antibiotic and steroid eye drops tapered for 6 months with intraocular pressure monitoring. Drops without preservative are preferred. Artificial tears are prescribed at least for 6 months. Although surgical technique is essential for a good result, postoperative management remains crucial for outcome. Conjunctival sutures are removed within a month when the tissues have healed completely. Lamellar graft sutures are removed any time they become loose, or routinely within the first 6 months.

Excellent cosmetic results, low rate of recurrences, and improved best corrected visual acuity are the main advantages of this technique.

■ REFERENCES

Abdallah WM. Efficacy of limbal-conjunctival autograft surgery with stem cells in pterygium treatment. *Mid E Afr J Ophthalmol* 2009; **16**:260–262.

Anduze AL, Merrit JC. Pterygium: clinical classification and management in Virgin Islands. *Ann Ophthalmol* 1985; **17**:92–95.

Ang LP, Chua JL, Tan DTH. Current concepts and techniques in pterygium treatment. *Current Opin Ophthalmol* 2007; **18**:308–313.

Arenas E. Manejo del Pterigión recidivante. In: Iradier Urrutia MT (ed.), Cirugía del Pterigión. *Madrid: Sociedad Española de Oftalmología*, 2006:103–114.

Arriola-Villalobos P. Pterygium epidemiology. In: Iradier-Urrutia MT (ed.), Pterygium Surgery. *Madrid: Sociedad Española de Oftalmología*, 2006; 45–49.

Aydin A, Karadayi K, Aykan U, Colakuglu K, Bilge AH. Effectiveness of topical ciclosporine A treatment after excision of primary pterygium and limbal conjunctival autograft. *Journal Francais d'Ophtalmologie* 2008; **31**:699–704.

Balci M, Sahin S, Mutlu FM, et al. Investigation of oxidative stress in pterygium tissue. *Mol Vis* 2011; **17**:443–447.

Chen KH, Hsu WM. Intra operative ethanol treatment as an adjuvant therapy of pterygium excision. *Int J Biomed Sci* 2006; **2**:413–420.

Chui J, Coroneo MT, Tat LT, et al. Ophthalmic pterygium: a stem cell disorder with premalignant features. *Am J Pathol* 2011; **178**:817–827.

D'Ombrain A. The surgical treatment of pterygium. *Br J Ophthalmol* 1948; **32**:65–71.

Donnenfeld ED, Perry HD, Fromer S. Subconjunctival mitomycin C as adjunctive therapy before pterygium excision. *Ophthalmology* 2003; **110**:1012–1026.

Frucht-Pery J, Charalambos SS, Ilsar M. Intraoperative application of topical mitomycin C for pterygium surgery. *Ophthalmology* 1996; **103**:674–677.

Frucht-Pery J, Siganos CS, Solomon A, et al. Topical indomethacin solution versus dexamethasone solution for treatment of inflamed pterygium and pinguecula: a prospective randomised clinical study. *Am J Ophthalmol* 1999; **127**:148–152.

Hirst LW. The treatment of pterygium. *Surv Ophthalmol* 2003; **48**:145–180.

Hirst LW. Recurrent pterygium surgery using pterygium extended removal followed by extended conjunctival transplant: recurrence rate and cosmesis. *Ophthalmol* 2009; **16**:1278–1286.

Hirst LW, Axelsen RA, Schwab I. Pterygium and associated ocular surface squamous neoplasia. *Arch Ophthalmol* 2009; **127**:31–32.

Hirst LW, Sebban A, Chant D. Pterygium recurrence time. *Ophthalmology* 1994; **101**:755–758.

Karalezli A, Kucukerdonmez C, Akova YA, Yaycioglu RA, Borazan M. Fibrin glue versus sutures for conjunctival autografting in pterygium surgery: a prospective comparative study. *Br J Ophthalmol* 2008; **92**:1206–1210.

Kenyon KR, Wagoner MD, Hettinger ME. Conjunctival autograft transplantation for advanced and recurrent pterygium. *Ophthalmology* 1985; **92**:1461–1470.

Khan AO. Inverse globe retraction syndrome complicating recurrent pterygium. *Br J Ophthalmol* 2005; **89**:640–641.

Koranyi G, Seregard S, Kopp ED. Cut and paste: a no suture small incision approach to pterygium surgery. *Br J Ophthalmol* 2004; **88**:911–914.

Labbé A, Gheck L, Iordanidou V, et al. An in vivo confocal microscopy and impression cytology evaluation of pterygium activity. *Cornea* 2010; **29**:392–399.

Liang K, Jiang Z, Ding BQ, et al. Expression of cell proliferation and apoptosis biomarkers in pterygia and normal conjunctiva. *Mol Vis* 2011; **17**:1687–1693.

Lin BS, Reiter MS, Dreher AW, Frucht-Pery J, Feldman ST. The effects of pterygia on contrast sensivity and glare disability. *Am J Ophthalmol* 1989; **107**:407–410.

Luanratanakorn P, Ratanapakorn T, Suwan-Apichon O, Chuck RS. Randomised controlled study of conjunctival autograft versus amniotic membrane graft in pterygium excision. *Br J Ophthalmol* 2006; **90**:1476–1480.

Marticorena J, Rodríguez-Ares MT, Touriño R, et al. Pterygium surgery: conjunctival autograft using a fibrin adhesive. *Cornea* 2006; **25**:34–36.

Mc Clellan K, Butler TKH, Wechsler AW, et al. Lamellar keratoplasty in recurrent pterygium. In: Thomas John (ed.), Step by step anterior and posterior lamellar keratoplasty. *New Delhi: Jaypee Brothers Medical Publishers*, 2006; 197–216.

Mejía LF, Sánchez JG, Escobar H. Management of primary pterygia using free conjunctival and limbal-conjunctival autografts without antimetabolites. *Cornea* 2005; **24**:972–975.

Méndez Fernández R, López Abad C, Díaz Valle D. Clínica y clasificación del pterigium. In: Iradier Urrutia MT (ed), Cirugía del pterigión. *Madrid: Sociedad Española de Oftalmología*, 2006: 19–29.

Mimura T, Usui T, Obata H, et al. Severity and determinants of pinguecula in a hospital-based population. *Eye Contact Lens* 2011; **37**:31–35.

Mohammad-Salih PA, Sharif AF. Analysis of pterygium size and induced corneal astigmatism. *Cornea* 2008; **2**:434–438.

Ozdamar Y, Mutevelli S, Han U, et al. A comparative study of tissue glue and vicryl suture for closing limbal-conjunctival autografts and histologic evaluation after pterygium excision. *Cornea* 2008; **27**:552–558.

Prabhasawat P, Barton K, Burkett G, Tseng SC. Comparison of conjunctival autografts, amniotic membrane grafts, and primary closure for pterygium excision. *Ophthalmology* 1997; **104**:974–985.

Ratnalingam V, Keat Eu AL, Ng GL, Taharin R, John E. Fibrin adhesive is better than sutures in pterygium surgery. *Cornea* 2010; **29**:4859.

Soliman W, Mohamed TA. Spectral domain anterior segment optical coherence tomography assessment of pterygium and pinguecula. *Acta Ophthalmol* 2012; **90**:461–465.

Singh G. Postoperative instillation of low-dose mitomycin C in the treatment of primary pterygium [letter]. *Am J Ophthalmol* 1989; **107**:570–571.

Srinivasan S, Dollin M, McAllum P, et al. Fibrin glue versus sutures for attaching the conjunctival autograft in pterygium surgery: a prospective observer masked clinical trial. *Br J Ophthalmol* 2009; **93**:215–218.

Tan DT, Chee SP, Dear KB, Lim AS.Effect of pterygium morphology on pterygium recurrence in a controlled trial comparing conjunctival autografting with bare sclera excision. *Arch Ophthalmol* 1997; **115**:1235–1240.

Tananuvat N, Martin T. The results of amniotic membrane transplantation for primary pterygium compared with conjunctival autograft. *Cornea* 2004; **23**:458–463.

Teng CC, Patel NN, Jacobson L. Effect of subconjunctival bevacizumab on primary pterygium. *Cornea* 2009; **28**:468–470.

Twelker JD, Bailey IL, Mannis MJ, Satariano WA. Evaluating pterygium severity: a survey of corneal specialists. *Cornea* 2000; **19**: 292–296.

Yagmur M, Ozcan AA, Sari S, Ersoz TR. Visual acuity and corneal topographic changes related with pterygium surgery. *J Refract Surg* 2005; **21**:166–170.

Zare M, Zarei-Ghanavati S, Ansari-Astaneh MR, Baradaran-Rafiee A, Einolahi B. Effects of pterygium on ocular aberrations. *Cornea* 2010; **29**:1232–1235.

Chapter 20   Ocular surface tumors

Rosario Touriño, Maria Lopez-Valladares, Teresa Rodríguez-Ares

■ INTRODUCTION

The ocular surface is a sensitive structure that includes two major territories—the cornea and the conjunctiva—bordered by the upper and lower lids and covered by a thin layer of tear film. The plica semilunaris and caruncula are special regions of the conjunctiva. All parts of this surface are directly exposed to the external environment and are thus vulnerable to potential environmental insults. For this reason, the ocular surface can be affected by a wide variety of lesions, including neoplastic lesions, which range from benign to highly malignant.

The tumors of the conjunctiva and the cornea can be classified into tumors of the surface epithelium (benign and malignant), melanocytic tumors, congenital lesions, vascular tumors, fibrous tumors, neural tumors, histiocytic tumors, myxoid tumors, myogenic tumors, lipomatous tumors, lymphoid tumors, leukemia, metastatic lesions, caruncular cysts, and secondary and miscellaneous lesions.

This chapter describes the most frequent tumors, and those that could deserve special attention for their malignancy.

■ TUMORS OF THE SURFACE EPITHELIUM

■ Benign lesions of the surface epithelium

Squamous papilloma

Squamous papilloma is reported to be associated with human papillomavirus (HPV). There is a strong association between HPV types 6/11 and 16/18, and the development of conjunctival papillomas (Di Girolamo 2012, Nagaiah et al. 2010); however, other studies have not found a relationship between HPV infection and this lesion (Guthoff et al. 2009).

In appearance, squamous papilloma is a strawberry red sessile or pedunculated lesion, with multiple, fine, vascular channels ramifying through the stroma beneath the epithelial surface. This lesion may be asymptomatic or associated with ocular surface-related symptoms, such as foreign body sensation, itching, irritation, mucoid discharge, tearing, and visual disturbances. In adults, these lesions are usually solitary, and when they become large enough, they may extend to cover the corneal surface, simulating a malignant tumor. Multiple pedunculated papillomas are most commonly found in children, and sometimes, they may regress spontaneously over time.

Microscopic examination shows acanthotic squamous epithelium, covering fibrovascular fronds. There may be associated koilocytosis and inflammation.

There are several treatment options. Topical interferon α-2b (IFNα2b) has been shown to be an effective adjunct therapy for small-to-medium-size lesions but not for larger lesions, where it is necessary to remove the bulk of the lesion, with double freeze-thaw cryotherapy, to prevent possible recurrences. Several authors suggest that topical IFNα2b and mitomycin C (MMC) can be utilized as adjunctive therapy for recurring conjunctival papilloma and for those lesions refractory to conventional treatment (Chen et al. 2004, Galor et al. 2010, Nemet et al. 2006). In cases of recalcitrant and diffuse conjunctival papillomas, oral cimetidine has been demonstrated to be effective by stimulating the patient's immune system and consequently causing tumor regression (Shields et al. 1999).

Epithelial inclusion cyst

Epithelial inclusion cyst is a translucent subconjunctival mass (with mucinous material and/or proteinaceous fluid) originated when conjunctival epithelial cells are buried beneath the conjunctival surface during surgery, trauma, or inflammation. Congenital cysts have also been described. Epithelial inclusion cysts are usually small and asymptomatic, and therefore do not require treatment. Occasionally, they have to be removed, in which case it is better to perform a complete excision and marsupialization to prevent recurrences, particularly with large cysts.

Keratotic plaque and actinic keratosis

Both lesions may be considered as precancerous, with proliferative activity and few possibilities to transform into conjunctival intraepithelial neoplasia or squamous cell carcinoma. Keratotic plaque is a white conjunctival mass usually localized in the interpalpebral region. Actinic keratosis appears as a frothy white lesion often located over a pingueculae or pterygium. Although they are clinically similar, they have different pathology. The former has acanthosis and parakeratosis with keratinization of the epithelium, and the latter has proliferation of the surface epithelium with keratosis (Shields & Shields 2004).

Keratoacanthoma

Keratoacanthoma generally occurs on the skin; it is rarely found in the conjunctiva. It is a benign epidermal tumor usually detected in the elderly, characterized by fast and painless nodular growth. Differential diagnosis between conventional squamous cell carcinoma and keratoacanthoma can be difficult. Histopathologically, this lesion is characterized by a central keratin deposit surrounded by acanthosis and parakeratosis, similar to a volcano crater. Treatment involves complete resection. Some authors have recently suggested the use of topical 0.04% MMC in the postoperative period.

■ Malignant lesions of the surface epithelium

Ocular surface squamous neoplasia

Ocular surface squamous neoplasia (OSSN) includes a wide spectrum of dysplastic alterations of the squamous epithelium of the ocular surface, cornea, and conjunctiva, ranging from precancerous lesions to bona fide invasive carcinoma. It can be classified into two groups: cornea and conjunctiva intraepithelial neoplasia (CCIN), when they are restricted to the epithelium; and invasive squamous cell carcinoma (ISCC), when it breaks the basal membrane, invading the underlying stroma.

This type of neoplasia has received different denominations: epithelioma, Bowen's disease, carcinoma in situ, conjunctival squamous dysplasia, and dyskeratosis. Pizzarello and Jakobiec were the first to use the term 'intraepithelial neoplasia,' which subsequently classified into mild, moderate, and severe dysplasia, according to the extent of disease (Pizzarello & Jakobiec 1978). Other terms such as 'ocular surface squamous neoplasia,' which covers both dysplasia and carcinoma in situ, have also been used by other authors such as Lee and Hirst (1995).

Cornea–conjunctival intraepithelial neoplasia

Cornea–conjunctival intraepithelial neoplasia (CCIN) presents as a unilateral progressive slow-growing lesion on the conjunctiva or cornea with low malignant potential. Epidemiologically, intraepithelial neoplasias of the conjunctiva and cornea are among the most common ocular surface tumors, with an estimated incidence of 1.9/100,000 new patients per year. Although this is a rare tumor compared with other ocular–orbital tumors, CCIN is the third most common ocular tumor after melanoma and lymphoma. This tumor is usually found in advanced age. However, patients with acquired immunodeficiency syndrome (AIDS) and patients with xeroderma pigmentosum have a higher risk of developing these tumors at earlier ages (Gupta et al. 2011, Nagaiah et al. 2010). These disorders also predispose to more severe disease.

CCIN´s etiology is multifactorial. There are several factors and different theories that could be involved in the development of this lesion:

- Alteration of the regulatory mechanism of the limbal stem cells located in the interpalpebral area
- Excessive exposure to ultraviolet light, which could cause irreversible damage to the DNA and mutations in the p53 tumor suppressor gene
- Different authors have demonstrated the presence of HPV (subtypes 16 and 18) in the conjunctival epithelium of patients with CCIN, using polymerase chain reaction techniques. This was even more obvious in bilateral tumors and immunosuppressed patients
- Other reported factors included dust, wind, abnormalities in the palpebral closure, chemical exposure to trifluridine, arsphenamine or beryllium, chronic inflammation of the ocular surface, vitamin A deficiency, or exposure to petroleum products, smoking cigarettes, and viruses such as herpes simplex type 1

Clinically, these tumors are slightly elevated lesions, with pearl-gray to red-gray color (depending on the tumor vascularization). They are often asymptomatic, but some patients may have foreign body sensation and eye redness. There are two clinicopathological variants:

1. Actinic variant, a well-delimited nodule, with keratinized surface, localized in the exposed interpalpebral zone. It is more common in elderly men and can be associated with pingueculae and pterygium
2. Diffuse variant, less frequent than the former. It usually affects palpebral and bulbar conjunctiva. It does not have well-demarcated margins and, consequently, recurrences are frequent after surgery. Sometimes, this type is difficult to diagnose, especially in nascent stages, and it may be confused with a chronic conjunctivitis. In several occasions, they may extend onto the adjacent cornea, especially limbal lesions (**Figure 20.1**)

It may show three macroscopic slit-lamp appearances: gelatinous (as bouquet vessels), leukoplakic (white plaque-associated secondary hyperkeratosis), and papilliform.

CCIN grows slowly and has a low malignancy potential (progression to ISCC), and spontaneous regression has been described in some cases (Char 2001).

Many lesions are difficult to diagnose and the pathological evaluation is necessary. Excisional biopsy is the usual technique for smaller tumors (≤15 mm basal dimension or ≤4 clock limbal hours), but other techniques such as exfoliative cytology or impression cytology are also currently used. Cytological analysis shows dysplastic ocular surface cells, which in itself cannot differentiate between CIN and squamous cell carcinoma. The use of 1% toluidine blue eye drops has recently been described for the diagnosis of OSSN and premalignant lesions, yet the intensity of the staining does not correlate with the degree of malignancy of these tumors (Romero et al. 2012). Incisional biopsy should be performed in extensive lesions, suspected to be malignant, because the treatment can be planned based on the pathological results. Pathological examination of squamous conjunctival lesions has been described by many authors (Koreishi & Karp 2007, Lee & Hirst 1995; Shields & Shields 2004) and can be classified as follows:

- Mild dysplasia or CIN 1: atypical cells (epidermoid and spindle cells) in less than one third of the thickness of the epithelium
- Moderate dysplasia or CIN 2: when atypia is found in the middle third
- Severe dysplasia, CIN 3, or carcinoma in situ: atypia extends throughout the full thickness of the epithelium. The basement membrane is always intact

Differential diagnosis must be made with inflamed pterygium and pingueculae, phlyctenulosis, episcleritis, keratoacanthoma, and less often with dermoid cysts, pyogenic granuloma, and malignant melanoma. Some lesions may also have histopathological similarities with pseudoepitheliomatous hyperplasia, melanocytic lesions, or sebaceous carcinoma.

Invasive squamous cell carcinoma

Invasive squamous cell carcinoma is the most common malignant tumor of the conjunctiva. This type of lesion is less frequent than CCIN; however, CCIN may be a precursor of carcinoma when the abnormal cells break through the basal membrane into conjunctival stroma. ISCC is considered a tumor with low-grade malignancy.

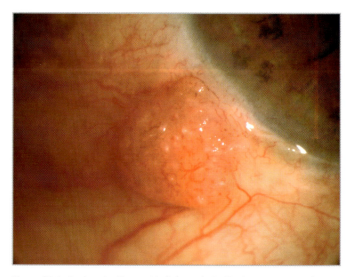

Figure 20.1 Conjunctival intraepithelial neoplasia. Carcinoma in situ in the interpalpebral zone.

ISCC usually appears in patients of advanced age, but young persons can also be affected (i.e. xeroderma pigmentosum and HIV patients). Clinically ISCC is more elevated and aggressive than CCIN, although both lesions have similar clinical appearances (**Figure 20.2**). ISCC develops on the interpalpebral conjunctiva area, but can also be detected in the tarsal conjunctiva, can spread onto the cornea, and can invade the orbit and the globe. ISCC cells can occasionally access to blood vessels and lymphatic channels causing metastasis, but this is not common.

Microscopic examination reveals epithelial layer basement membrane ruptures and atypical cells in the conjunctival stroma. Anatomopathological studies show hypercellularity, pleomorphism and weak intercellular adhesion, especially in the deeper layers. Ultrastructurally, there is a decrease in desmosomes adhesions, an increase in intracytoplasmic keratin filaments, and gaps in the basal membrane as well as loss of hemidesmosomes.

Two variants, mucoepidermoid carcinoma (with mucous-secreting cells within the cyst) and spindle cell carcinoma, are both very aggressive.

MELANOCYTIC TUMORS

Nevi

The conjunctival nevus is the most common melanocytic tumor. It is congenital and usually presents in the first or second decade of life. It is small and slightly elevated with variable pigmentation, and tends to contain fine and clear cysts that may be seen on the slit-lamp examination (**Figure 20.3**). Over time, a nevus can increase its pigment and a portion not pigmented previously can acquire it, simulating neoplastic growth (especially during puberty, coinciding with hormonal changes). Between 20% and 30% of the nevi are non-pigmented.

Nevi are located most often in the interpalpebral area near the limbus and remain stable throughout life, although in some cases, they might eventually become malignant. A retrospective study (Shields et al. 2011) on outcomes based on conjunctival tumor origin in 382 consecutive patients showed that 7% of the conjunctival melanomas were reported to arise from preexisting nevi.

This lesion usually shows a typical clinical appearance, but some amelanotic or diffuse and irregular growing nevi may be difficult to diagnose and sometimes may be confused with other disorders such as primary acquired melanosis or melanoma. For this reason, these lesions must be photographed for future comparisons of the degree of pigmentation. If surgery is to be performed, total elimination of the mass using the 'no touch technique' is recommended (Shields & Shields 2004).

Histopathologically, nevi are stromal nests of benign melanocytes adjacent to the basal layers of the epithelium. They may be, depending on the location of melanocytes and as cutaneous nevi, junctional (at the epithelial–substantia propria junction), compound (involving both junctional and subepithelial areas), or deep (subepithelial).

Primary acquired melanosis

Clinically, the primary acquired melanosis (PAM) is a diffuse or patchy lesion, flat and not cystic. This benign pigmented conjunctival lesion can occasionally transform into a conjunctival melanoma when it contains atypical cells (up to 74%, according to a recent study by Shields et al. 2011). It is a melanocytic proliferation, which takes place in the conjunctival epithelium. This lesion, which tends to be unilateral, is characterized by the presence of brown patches of conjunctival pigmentation (**Figure 20.4**). This lesion can regress, remain unchanged, or progress to malignant melanoma.

The differential diagnosis must be made based on different pigmented lesions of the conjunctiva. The presence of cysts within the lesion supports a diagnosis of conjunctival nevus rather than PAM. Unlike racial melanosis (bilateral pigmentation of the bulbar conjunctiva found in dark-skinned individuals), PAM is usually unilateral and found in fair-skinned individuals. Unlike ocular melanocytosis (congenital pigmentation of sclera with or without associated pigmentation of the skin, 'nevus of Ota'), PAM can grow or diminish over time, is acquired, located into the conjunctiva, and brown. PAM may occasionally be difficult to distinguish from melanoma.

Histopathological examination shows the presence of abnormal melanocytes near the basal layer of the epithelium. Classifying

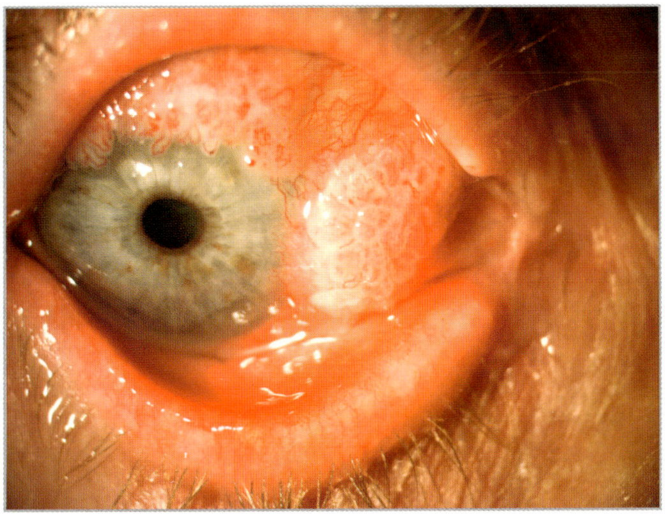

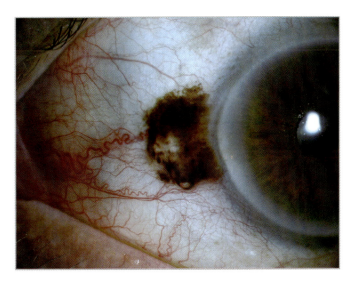

Figure 20.2 Invasive squamous cell carcinoma. Nodular and extensive invasive squamous carcinoma.

Figure 20.3 Conjunctival nevus. A typical nevus with cystic elements in a young patient.

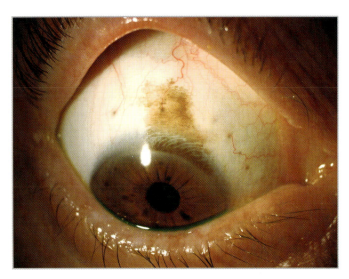

Figure 20.4 PAM with atypia. Localized PAM in the upper bulbar conjunctiva, adjacent to the limbus. PAM, primary acquired melanosis.

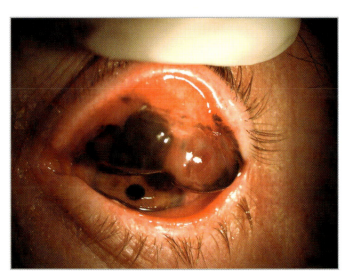

Figure 20.5 Conjunctival melanoma. Nodular tumor localized in the upper palpebral conjunctiva of the left eye.

melanocytes according to atypia (based on nuclear features and growth pattern of the cell) is important because PAM without atypia (benign) and PAM with atypia (several severity levels) have different prognoses. PAM with atypia has a high risk of turning into malignant, whereas in PAM without atypia, this risk is very low. Shields et al. found the risk for progression to melanoma in 311 eyes, with 0% in PAM without atypia, 0% in PAM with mild atypia, and 13% in PAM with severe atypia. In this study, the most significant factor for PAM recurrence and progression to melanoma was the extension of the lesion in clock hours (Shields et al. 2008).

Conjunctival melanoma

Conjunctival melanoma is a rare ocular neoplasia. It represents 2% of all ocular malignant tumors, and its annual incidence is estimated at 0.02–0.05%. In a study of 4836 cases of melanoma of the entire body, 5.2% of them involved structures of the eye, the uvea being the most common location (85%) followed by the conjunctiva (4.8%) (Chang et al. 1998). According to a recent study, 74% of conjunctival melanoma arose from PAM, 7% from preexisting nevi, and 19% were primary tumors (Shields et al. 2011).

The role of environmental factors in the etiology of conjunctival melanomas is not clear; however, patients affected by atypical nevus syndrome have a particular tendency to develop conjunctival malignant melanoma.

This tumor usually occurs in middle-aged patients, although there are rare cases reported in children.

Its clinical manifestation is variable. The most frequent presentation is a pigmented and elevated lesion that can be located on limbus, fornix, tarsal or bulbar conjunctiva, and cornea (**Figure 20.5**). However, primary melanoma of the cornea is very rare, and many of them represent a corneal invasion from a limbal melanoma. Sometimes, in this tumor we can see prominent feeder vessels associated with PAM. Few cases of conjunctival amelanotic melanoma have been described.

Several studies have reported different rates of metastasis for this type of tumor (16% of patients at 5 years, 26% at 10 years, and 32% at 15 years) (Missotten et al. 2007, Shields et al. 2000). Recently, a retrospective study of 382 patients with conjunctival melanoma has established several predictive factors for metastasis: tumor origin de

novo, fornix location, nodular tumor, tumor margin pathology (lateral margin involved), and orbital invasion (Shields et al. 2011). Metastasis can be localized in the regional lymph nodes and in brain, liver, lung, or disseminated. This study estimated a local tumor recurrence of 26% at 5 years, 51% at 10 years, and 65% at 15 years; and the factors related with this recurrence were extralimbal location (not touching the limbus) and positive surgical margins.

Nowadays, we know that about 30% of patients die of metastasis. Shields et al. found a tumor-related mortality rate of 7% at 5 years and 18% at 8 years, and the risk factors for death included the number of local recurrence and the presence of symptoms and pathological findings (as de novo melanoma). These authors have found that the surgical technique may affect ultimate tumor recurrence, need for orbital exenteration, tumor metastasis, and patient death; thus surgery must be meticulously planned and performed by experienced surgeons (Shields et al. 2000).

Other signs of poor prognosis are diffuse forms, multifocality, cell type, and pigmentation of the margins. Conjunctival melanomas away from limbo and tumor infiltration in the surgical margins should be deemed poor prognosis.

Melanoma is composed, histopathologically, of variably pigmented malignant melanocytes (small polyhedral, spindle, balloon, and round epithelioid) located in the epithelium and invading substantia propria. Immunohistochemical staining (S-100, MART-1, and HMB-45) can help in identifying abnormal melanocytes in amelanotic melanoma.

Malignant conjunctival melanoma must be differentiated from other pigmented lesions, such as racial melanosis, ocular melanocytosis, PAM, or nevus. There are other benign lesions, which must also be included (above all if they are pigmented): pingueculae, pterygium, conjunctival cysts, and gunpowder- or epinephrine-related adrenochrome deposits.

TREATMENTS OF EPITHELIAL AND PIGMENTED TUMORS

There are several treatment options for epithelial and pigmented tumors of the ocular surface (e.g. surgery, cryotherapy, radiotherapy, enucleation, exenteration and topical chemotherapy, and immunotherapy), which can be used alone or in combination.

Surgery

Simple resection of the lesion is the traditional method of treating these tumors, but presents a high rate of recurrence (25–53%) due to the difficulty in obtaining non-infiltrated margins. The conjunctival incision should be 2–3 mm outside the tumor margin to ensure clear surgical margins. Staining with Rose Bengal or lissamine green can help to define the extent of the abnormal tissue (Shields & Shields 2004).

Sometimes, if the cornea is involved, lamellar keratoplasty and scleroplasty may be necessary. In these cases, it is recommended that absolute alcohol is applied for 20–40 seconds (followed by copious irrigation with balanced salt solution) to facilitate the removal of the epithelium (Shields et al. 1997). If the lesion affects >50% of the limbal area, they have a worse prognosis and a limbal transplantation is needed (from the contralateral eye), associated with partial lamellar scleroconjunctivectomy. When it is necessary to sacrifice extensive areas of conjunctiva, reconstruction can be made with a transpositional conjunctival flap, a free conjunctival flap from the other eye, buccal mucous membrane graft, or amniotic membrane transplantation. The recurrences usually occur in the first 2 years after surgical removal and, for this reason, the full conjunctival component along with the underlying Tenon´s fascia should be excised using the 'no touch technique.'

More radical surgeries as enucleation must be taken into account in those tumors that involve the globe. If the tumor extends widely and involves the orbit, exenteration will probably be required.

Cryotherapy

This treatment is used combined with surgery and applied in the affected areas and conjunctival margins, in a double freeze-slow-thaw technique. Cryotherapy acts by destroying cells by a thermal effect and obliterates the microcirculation causing an ischemic stroke. To obtain a suitable cell destruction, a fast freezing and a slow thawing are recommended, repeating this process two or three times. When we use this treatment in the limbal region, we should not spend >3 seconds of application to avoid a limbal deficiency. Cryotherapy can be used as a first treatment, but it is most commonly used as an adjunctive therapy to surgery (to eliminate any residual tumor cells) or alone for treating recurrences. A too aggressive cryotherapy can cause iritis, alteration of intraocular pressure (both increase and decrease), and conjunctival inflammatory edema; and, apart from this, it could cause further complications such as corneal scarring, sectoral iris atrophy, peripheral retinal ablation, ectropion, and, occasionally, hemorrhage and superficial corneal vascularization. With the combination of surgery and cryotherapy, the rate of recurrence of the ocular surface epithelial tumor is considerably lower (7%) than that using both techniques separately (22%).

Radiotherapy

Radiotherapy has been used since 1930. There are several sources of radiation employed: strontium 90 and β-γ-radiation. Complications that can occur after radiation therapy range from moderate to severe postradiation conjunctivitis, dry eye disease, cataracts, telangiectasias, scleral thinning, symblepharon, and ulceration to even corneal perforation. Radiotherapy is not recommended as a unique treatment, but it may be necessary in conjunction with other procedures such as the exenteration, especially in extensive tumors.

Topical treatment
Chemotherapy

Chemotherapeutic agents have been proposed as a primary treatment for epithelial and pigmented ocular surface tumors and to treat their recurrences. Chemotherapy presents certain advantages over the classic treatment (surgery and cryotherapy): (1) it is not dependent on the surgical margins; (2) it reduces the risk of limbal deficiency secondary to extensive surgical resections or adjuvant therapies, such as cryotherapy; and (3) it simplifies the treatments and avoids repeated surgeries or cryotherapy applications in patients with tumor recurrences. The main drawback of topical chemotherapy is its limited penetration, which could lead to failures in the eradication of the lesion if it is used as a single treatment, especially in squamous cell carcinomas.

It is advisable to perform the occlusion of the lacrimal points to prevent exposure of nasopharyngeal tissue and toxicity.

The drugs used include 5-fluorouracil and MMC.

5-Fluorouracil

Topical 5-fluorouracil (5-FU) 1% has also been used in the treatment of OSSN (Parrozzani et al. 2011, Yamamoto et al. 2002). This drug is a pyrimidine analogue that inhibits DNA and RNA synthesis in the S phase of the cell cycle, causing cell death.

In this type of tumors, 5-FU is used four times a day but there is no consensus regarding the duration of each cycle (2–4 days up to 4 weeks) as well as the time between cycles. Different side effects have been described: conjunctival inflammation, epithelial defects, and cutaneous erythema. Topical corticosteroid administration improves the tolerance of this drug and MMC.

Mitomycin C

MMC is an alkylating antibiotic agent isolated from the *Streptomyces caespitosus*, which interrupts cell growth by cross-linking of DNA, inhibiting DNA synthesis and cell proliferation. MMC is cell-cycle non-specific, but it is more effective in the G1 and S phases. Alkylating agents resemble the radiation in its mechanism of action, being more sensitive to those cells with the highest rate of mitosis.

MMC is the topical chemotherapy most used in the treatment of OSSN and can be applied as a primary treatment or as surgical adjuvant (e.g. preoperative, intraoperative, and postoperative) (Kemp et al. 2002). Different publications have confirmed the efficacy of this drug in the treatment of primary and recurrent OSSN. MMC may be used in different concentrations (0.002, 0.015, 0.02, or 0.04%), and it must be prescribed four times a day for 7–14 to 21 days. These cycles can be repeated after 4–6 weeks (Chen et al. 2004, Frucht-Pery & Rozenman 1994, Prabhasawat et al. 2005, Russell et al. 2010). Several side effects have been described after topical MMC instillation: keratoconjunctivitis, photophobia, pain, and corneal epithelial defects, and less frequently blepharospasm, contact dermatitis, palpebral and corneal edema, corneal and scleral melting, limbal deficiency, and cataract (Lichtinger et al. 2010).

Immunotherapy

Immunotherapy with interferon represents a recent alternative in the treatment of OSSN (Galor et al. 2010, Karp et al. 2010, Kim et al. 2012, Nemet et al. 2006, Shields et al. 2012). Interferons are a family of glycoprotein molecules that bind to cellular membrane receptors and stimulate an intracellular cascade of events that result in antiviral and antitumor effects. IFNα2b can be used either topically or intralesionally (Vann & Karp 1999). The intralesional dose is 3 million IU/0.5 mL, and it is injected subconjuctivally or perilesionally every week (up to three times a week); topical dose is 1 million IU/mL four times a day. Both of them should be administered until clinical resolution.

Recently, one study has demonstrated the effectiveness of two different doses of topical INFα2b (1 million IU vs. 3 million IU) in the treatment of OSSN (Galor et al. 2010).

Other authors used topical INFα2b in seven eyes with CCIN, with a frequency of four to six times a day, until complete resolution of the tumor. They observed that the eradication time ranged from 28 to 188 days (Schechter et al. 2002).

Adverse effects of INFα2b topical application are mild (e.g. conjunctival hyperemia and follicular conjunctivitis), but the local injections can be associated with fever, myalgia, and pseudoinfluenza syndrome.

Combined therapy

The combination of different topical treatments may be an alternative in patients who have intolerances, poor response to other treatments, or recurrences. Several studies have shown that the combination of topical chemotherapeutic agents can remove CCIN. Yamamoto et al. (2002) described the eradication of CCIN refractory to MMC after topical 5-FU administration.

Other authors obtained good results using topical MMC in patients who had a poor response to topical 5-FU (Yeatts et al. 1995). Another study reported the elimination of CCIN after the combined administration of topical MMC and INFα2b in cycles (Di Pascuale et al. 2004); and Zaki and Farid used topical MMC and cyclosporine as an adjunct to surgery for CCIN and ISCC (Zaki & Farid 2009).

SELECTIVE TREATMENTS ACCORDING TO THE TYPE OF EPITHELIAL OR MELANOCYTIC TUMOR

Corneal–conjunctival intraepithelial neoplasia

Total surgical excision with at least 3–4 mm of healthy margins is the traditional procedure in this type of tumor; however, as mentioned earlier, the recurrence rate is high. When the CCIN affects the cornea, limbus, conjunctiva, or sclera, the excision will include these structures, using surgical techniques described previously ('no touch technique'). In these cases, it is important to perform reconstructive surgeries to prevent later complications. Several authors have reported a reduction of these recurrences with the association of cryotherapy. Adjunctive cryotherapy, in a double freeze-slow-thaw technique, is regularly applied to the affected limbus and the conjunctival margins, and sometimes in the scleral bed, if the tumor was fixed to it. Topical chemotherapy (with MMC and 5-FU, fundamentally) or INFα2b can be used, either as primary or as adjunctive therapy, because they offer important advantages in tumors with high recurrence rates (such as, to repeat the treatment if it was necessary and to reach the entire surface of the lesion). If the tumor does not seem to be responding to the initial agent used, a different one may be tried.

Recently, Shields et al. (2012) have demonstrated the efficacy of IFNα2b in the management of OSSN. This retrospective case series

study of 80 patients with 81 tumors reports complete control in 95% of cases overall.

Invasive squamous cell carcinoma

The treatment will depend on the degree of aggressiveness of the tumor, the fixation to underlying ocular structures, and intraocular and/or orbital extension. Basically, the invasive squamous carcinoma is handled similarly to the CCIN; however, when the carcinoma involves the eyeball, it must be treated with enucleation, and in those cases where the extension is very important or there is orbital invasion, an exenteration will be needed.

Nevi

The complete local excision should be considered if size changes are detected or for cosmetic reasons. When the excision is made, the entire mass is removed using the 'no touch technique' and standard double freeze-thaw cryotherapy is applied to the remaining conjunctival margins. These precautions are intended to prevent the recurrence that could degenerate into melanoma.

Primary acquired melanosis

The treatment of these lesions will depend on the degree of cell atypia. In cases with low-grade atypia, a regular observation is the management of choice. On the other hand, when the degree of atypia is high or there are changes or progression of the pigmented lesion, it must be treated by surgical excision, cryotherapy, topical chemotherapy, or a combination of these treatments.

An accepted treatment modality, when there are several regions of PAM, is to make additional small incisional map biopsies of the lesions, followed by cryotherapy in all the pigmented lesions. There are studies that demonstrate a good response to the treatment with topical MMC, which was well tolerated and considerably promising, particularly in the treatment of diffuse PAM with atypia (Anandajeya et al. 2009, Chalasani et al. 2006, Chen et al. 2007, Rodríguez-Ares et al. 2003).

Conjunctival melanoma

Conjunctival melanoma is a tumor difficult to treat because it has frequent relapses and may cause distant metastasis. All patients with conjunctival melanoma should be subjected to a complete medical examination and followed by an oncologist.

Treatment varies depending on size, location, and distribution of the lesion, as well as the patient's wishes to preserve vision and/or the anatomy of the eye. In recent years, there is a trend towards a more conservative treatment since radical resection and exenteration have failed to reduce the number of metastasis (Shields et al. 2012).

There is a correlation between the prognosis and the thickness of the lesion in the conjunctival melanoma, as in skin melanoma. Tumors of ≤1.5 mm in thickness usually do not produce metastasis, and tend to have an excellent prognosis. Tumors of >2.5 mm present a grim prognosis, even applying radical treatments. In general, melanomas of ≤1.5 mm in thickness are treated with surgery and cryotherapy. There is a therapeutic dilemma in lesions of 2.5–3.0 mm in thickness, since early exenteration does not improve the vital prognosis. Nowadays, the ophthalmologists tend to be more conservative.

Shields et al. (2000) have reported, in a retrospective study of 150 melanomas, that a complete resection of the pigmented lesion with the 'no touch technique,' combined with cryotherapy and absolute alcohol corneal epitheliectomy (when there is limbal or cornea involvement), could be an important factor in preventing eventual tumor recurrences. We know that the majority of recurrences occur in patients if surgery has been practiced without cryotherapy. On the other hand, surgical resection with free margins of 3–4 mm can be difficult to carry out, especially in diffuse tumors, so it is necessary to associate complementary treatments such as cryotherapy or/and topical chemotherapy with MMC. But even so, sometimes it is necessary to practice the exenteration when the tumor extends to intraocular structures or the orbit.

Radiotherapy may be relatively effective to control local disease, but its effect on metastasis is not clear (Seregard 1998). It can cause significant ocular complications (in 12% patients), including the loss of the eyeball.

OTHER TUMORS OF OCULAR SURFACE (CONJUNCTIVAL STROMAL TUMORS)

The conjunctival stroma contains different structures (vascular, fibrous and neural tissues, lymphatic channels, and others); and benign and malignant lesions may originate from any of them (**Table 20.1**). We describe only the most frequent tumors.

Table 20.1 Other tumors of the ocular surface

Conjunctival stromal elements	Benign tumors	Malignant tumors
Vascular	Pyogenic granuloma Hemangiomas (capillary, cavernous, and racemose) Benign lymphangioma Varix Hemangiopericytoma	Malignant lymphangioma Kaposi´s sarcoma
Fibrous	Fibroma Benign fibrous histiocytoma Nodular fasciitis	Malignant fibrous histiocytoma
Histiocytic cells	Xanthoma Reticulohistiocytoma Juvenile xanthogranuloma	
Myxoid tissue	Myxoma	
Myogenic tissue	Infantile myofibromatosis	Rhabdomyosarcoma Leiomyosarcoma
Adipose tissue	Herniated orbital fat Lipoma	Liposarcoma
Lymphoid tissue	Reactive lymphoid hyperplasia Atypical lymphoid hyperplasia	Lymphoma
Normal tissue in an abnormal location (choristoma)	Dermoid Dermolipoma Osseous choristoma Lacrimal gland choristoma Complex choristoma	
Metastatic tumors		Metastatic carcinoma from breast carcinoma or cutaneous melanoma

Vascular tumors
Pyogenic granuloma

Pyogenic granuloma is a fleshy mass with blood supply and circumscribed to the conjunctiva. It is an exaggerated inflammatory response to surgical or non-surgical trauma. 'Pyogenic granuloma' is a wrong term since there is no purulent exudate or granulomatous inflammation. This vascular tumor (a polypoid form of acquired capillary hemangioma) may respond to topical corticosteroids, but in many cases it requires surgical excision.

Hemangiomas
Capillary hemangioma

Capillary hemangioma of the conjunctiva is a reddish stromal mass that appears in childhood, usually after birth. Sometimes it is associated with a capillary hemangioma of the skin or orbit, and it may also appear in Sturge–Weber syndrome. Similar to the skin, the conjunctival hemangioma can grow for months and then regress spontaneously. It is not necessary to treat them except on certain occasions, where a surgical resection can be performed or intralesional or systemic prednisone can be administered.

Cavernous and racemose hemangiomas

These conjunctival tumors—cavernous and racemose hemangiomas—are rare and benign. The first one appears as a red or blue lesion in the deep stroma in young patients, and can be treated with local resection. The second is a dilated arteriovenous communication without an intervening capillary bed. It usually requires only observation, insofar as it remains stable, which usually occurs for years. It is also important to rule out Wyburn–Mason syndrome in these patients.

Lymphangioma

Lymphangioma is an uncommon venolymphatic lesion. It is characterized by dilation of lymphatic vessels, and it appears as a multiloculated cyst-like lesion. Dilated cystic channels have different sizes and are clear-colored, but occasionally they are filled with blood ('chocolate cysts'). It can present as a solitary or multifocal lesion that usually represents the surface component of a deeper, diffuse orbital lymphangioma. The treatment of superficial lymphangioma by surgical excision can be curative; however, alternative treatments such as carbon dioxide laser, beta irradiation or cryotherapy have been described.

Kaposi´s sarcoma

Kaposi's sarcoma is an uncommon endothelial malignant tumor that can affect the conjunctiva and eyelids. It is typically found in patients with AIDS, but it can also occur in the elderly and other immunocompromised patients (transplanted patients). Classic Kaposi's sarcoma occurs in the elderly and is slowly progressive.

Kaposi's sarcoma is a nodular or diffuse reddish conjunctival lesion that sometimes may be confused with a hemorrhagic conjunctivitis. It has a good response to low doses of radiotherapy, but moderate response to chemotherapy.

Fibrous and histiocytic tumors
Fibroma

Fibroma is very rare in the conjunctiva. It is composed of closely compact fibroblasts and collagen. It can be nodular or diffuse and generally develops in adulthood. The treatment is surgical excision.

Fibrous histiocytoma

Fibrous histiocytoma is a rare mass of the conjunctiva composed of histiocytes and fibroblasts. Clinically and histologically, it can remind of other amelanotic stromal tumors. In the conjunctiva it can have a benign, locally invasive, or malignant behavior. The treatment is a wide excision with free surgical margins.

Juvenile xanthogranuloma

Juvenile xanthogranuloma is a benign histiocytic disease of uncertain pathogenesis that usually appears as a cutaneous lesion in the head and neck region of young children (<2 years). This tumor is rarely located in the conjunctiva, orbit, or intraocular structures. In the conjunctiva it appears as an orange-pink stromal mass. The histopathological diagnosis is based on the presence of histiocytes mixed with Touton's giant cells. The treatment consists of observation or application of topical steroids.

■ Myxoid tumors
Myxoma

Myxoma is a rare and solitary conjunctival tumor whose clinical aspect is an orange-pink mass located in the temporal bulbar conjunctiva. This mesenchymal tumor is composed of stellate and spindle-shaped cells interspersed in a loose stroma (Koreishi & Karp 2007). All patients with ocular (e.g. eyelid, conjunctiva, and orbit) myxoma should be referred for medical evaluation to rule out potentially life-threatening cardiac myxoma.

■ Neural tumors
Neurofibroma

It presents as a well-circumscribed solitary mass or a diffuse or plexiform lesion. The well-circumscribed solitary form is not usually associated with a systemic disease, whereas the diffuse form is generally a part of von Recklinghausen´s neurofibromatosis. It appears as a sessile or dome-shaped yellow-gray mass. The plexiform variant is an ill-defined, firm, and irregular mass, which is often in continuity with the same lesion in the eyelid and orbit. The plexiform type is more difficult to remove and often needs complementary therapies.

Schwannoma

Schwannoma is a benign peripheral nerve sheath tumor. In the conjunctiva, it is a light pink-yellow elevated stromal mass. It is more frequently located in the orbit than in the conjunctiva. The best management of this conjunctival tumor is a complete surgical resection.

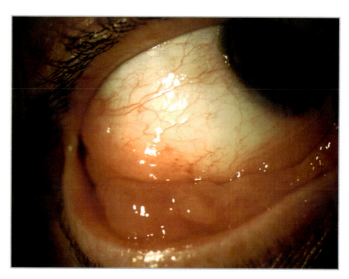

Figure 20.6 Conjunctival lymphoma. Lymphoma located in the lower bulbar and palpebral conjunctiva.

■ Lymphoid tumors

Lymphoid tumors can appear in the conjunctiva as a single lesion or can be a manifestation of a systemic lymphoma. Clinically, this tumor is a diffuse and slightly elevated fleshy pink mass located in the forniceal or bulbar conjunctiva (**Figure 20.6**). It usually presents in adulthood, either as irritation or as painless swelling. Sometimes, lymphoid infiltrate is bilateral, and in this case the chance for systemic lymphoma is 47% (Shields & Shields 2004).

It is not usually possible to differentiate clinically between benign (reactive lymphoid hyperplasia or atypical lymphoid hyperplasia) and malignant lymphoid tumors. Consequently, it is necessary to perform a biopsy for the diagnosis and carry out a medical examination to rule out systemic involvement. Malignant lymphoma may be further subdivided into: mucosa-associated lymphoid tissue (MALT) lymphoma and non-MALT lymphoma. Most of conjunctival lymphomas are B-cell lymphomas (non-Hodgkin´s type-MALT lymphomas).

If it is a systemic lymphoma, it requires treatment with chemotherapy. There are several alternatives for the conjunctival lesion: external radiotherapy or excisional biopsy and cryotherapy. Recently, subconjunctival interferon-α, in repeated injections, has been used with goods results (Blasi et al. 2012).

■ REFERENCES

Anandajeya WV, Corrêa ZM, Augsburger JJ. Primary acquired melanosis with atypia treated with mitomycin C. *Int Ophthalmol* 2009; **29**:285–288.

Blasi MA, Tiberti AC, Valente P, et al. Intralesional interferon-α for conjunctival mucosa-associated lymphoid tissue lymphoma: long-term results. *Ophthalmology* 2012; **119**:494–500.

Chalasani R, Giblin M, Conway RM. Role of topical chemotherapy for primary acquired melanosis and malignant melanoma of the conjunctiva and cornea: review of the evidence and recommendations for treatment. *Clin Experiment Ophthalmol* 2006; **34**:708–714.

Chang AE, Karnell LH, Menck HR. The national cancer date base report on cutaneous and noncutaneous melanoma: a summary of 84,836 cases from the past decade. *Cancer* 1998; **83**:1664–1678.

Char DH. Conjunctival malignancies. In: Char DH (ed.), Tumors of the eye and ocular adnexa. Hamilton, London: BC Decker Inc., 2001:57–91.

Chen C, Louis D, Dodd T, et al. Mitomycin C as an adjunct in the treatment of localised ocular surface squamous neoplasia. *Br J Ophthalmol* 2004; **88**:17–18.

Chen JY, Chappell AJ, Klebe S, et al. Resolution of primary acquired melanosis with atypia after minimal mitomycin C treatment. *Clin Experiment Ophthalmol* 2007; **35**:865–867.

Di Girolamo N. Association of human papilloma virus with pterygia and ocular-surface squamous neoplasia. *Eye* 2012; **26**:202–211.

Di Pascuale MA, Espana EM, Tseng SC. A case of conjunctiva-cornea intraepithelial neoplasia successfully treated with topical Mitomycin C and Interferon alfa-2b in cycles. *Cornea* 2004; **23**:89–92.

Frucht-Pery J, Rozenman Y. Mitomycin C therapy for corneal intraepithelial neoplasia. *Am J Ophthalmol* 1994; **117**:164–168.

Galor A, Karp CL, Chhabra S, et al. Topical interferon alpha 2b eye-drops for treatment of ocular surface squamous neoplasia: a dose comparison study. *Br J Ophthalmol* 2010; **94**:551–554.

Gupta N, Sachdev R, Tandon R. Ocular surface squamous neoplasia in xeroderma pigmentosum: clinical spectrum and outcome. *Graefes Arch Clin Exp Ophthalmol* 2011; **249**:1217–1221.

Guthoff R, Marx A, Stroebel P. No evidence for a pathogenic role of human papillomavirus infection in ocular surface squamous neoplasia in Germany. *Curr Eye Res* 2009; **34**:666–671.

Karp CL, Galor A, Chhabra S, et al. Subconjunctival/perilesional recombinant interferon α2b for ocular surface squamous neoplasia: a 10-years review. *Ophthalmology* 2010; **117**:2241–2246.

Kemp EG, Harnett AN, Chatterjee S. Preoperative topical and intraoperative local mitomycin C adjuvant therapy in the management of ocular surface neoplasias. *Br J Ophthalmol* 2002; **86**:31–34.

Kim HJ, Shields CL, Shah SU, et al. Giant ocular surface squamous neoplasia managed with interferon alpha-2b as immunotherapy or immunoreduction. *Ophthalmology* 2012; **119**:938–944.

Koreishi AF, Karp CL. Ocular surface neoplasia. Focal points. Clinical modules for ophthalmologist. *Am Acad Ophthalmol* 2007; **25**:1–213.

Lee GA, Hirst LW. Ocular surface squamous neoplasia. *Surv Ophthalmol* 1995; **39**:429–450.

Lichtinger A, Pe'er J, Frucht-Pery J, et al. Limbal stem cell deficiency after topical mitomycin C therapy for primary acquired melanosis with atypia. *Ophthalmology* 2010; **117**:431–437.

Missotten GS, de Wolff-Rouendaal D, de Keizer RJ. Screening for conjunctival melanoma metastasis: literature review. *Bull Soc Belge Ophtalmol* 2007; **306**:23–30.

Nagaiah G, Stotler C, Orem J, et al. Ocular surface squamous neoplasia in patients with HIV infection in sub-Saharan Africa. *Curr Opin Oncol* 2010; **22**:437–442.

Nemet AY, Sharma V, Benger R. Interferon alpha 2b treatment for residual ocular surface squamous neoplasia unresponsive to excision, cryotherapy and mitomycin-C. *Clin Experiment Ophthalmol* 2006; **34**:375–377.

Parrozzani R, Lazzarini D, Alemany-Rubio E, et al. Topical 1% 5-fluorouracil in ocular surface squamous neoplasia: a long-term safety study. *Br J Ophthalmol* 2011; **95**:355–359.

Pizzarello LD, Jakobiec FA. Bowen´s disease of the conjunctiva: a misnomer. In: Jakobiec FA (ed.), Ocular adnexal tumors. Birmingham, AL: Aesculapius, 1978:553–571.

Prabhasawat P, Tarinvorakup P, Tesavibul N, et al. Topical 0.002% mitomycin C for the treatment of conjunctival-corneal intraepithelial neoplasia and squamous cell carcinoma. *Cornea* 2005; **24**:443–448.

Rodríguez-Ares T, Tourino R, De Rojas V, et al. Topical mitomycin C in the treatment of pigmented conjunctival lesions. *Cornea* 2003; **22**:114–117.

Romero IL, Barros JD, Martins MC, et al. The Use of 1% Toluidine blue eye drops in the diagnosis of ocular surface squamous neoplasia. *Cornea* 2012; 19. [Epub ahead of print].

Russell HC, Chadha V, Lockington D, et al. Topical mitomycin C chemotherapy in the management of ocular surface neoplasia: a 10-year review of treatment outcomes and complications. *Br J Ophthalmol* 2010; **94**:1316–1321.

Schechter BA, Schrier A, Nagler RS, et al. Regression of presumed primary conjunctival and corneal intraepithelial neoplasia with topical interferon alpha-2b. *Cornea* 2002; **21**:6–11.

Seregard S. Conjunctival melanoma. *Surv Ophthalmol* 1998; **42**:321–350.

Shields CL, Shields JA. Tumors of the conjunctiva and cornea. *Surv Ophthalmol* 2004; **49**:3–24.

Shields CL, Kaliki S, Kim HJ, et al. Interferon for ocular surface squamous neoplasia in 81 cases: outcomes based on the American Joint Committee on Cancer Classification. *Cornea* 2012; 10. [Epub ahead of print].

Shields CL, Lally MR, Singh AD, et al. Oral cimetidine (Tagamet) for recalcitrant, diffuse conjunctival papillomatosis. *Am J Ophthalmol* 1999; **128**:362–364.

Shields CL, Markowitz JS, Belinsky I, et al. Conjunctival melanoma: outcomes based on tumor origin in 382 consecutive cases. *Ophthalmology* 2011; **118**:389–395.

Shields CL, Shields JA, Gunduz K, et al. Conjunctival melanoma: risk factors for recurrence, exenteration, metastasis and death in 150 consecutive patients. *Arch Ophthalmol* 2000; **118**:1497–1507.

Shields JA, Shields CL, De Potter P. Surgical management of conjunctival tumors. *Arch Ophthalmol* 1997; **115**:808–815.

Shields JA, Shields CL, Mashayekhi A, et al. Primary acquired melanosis of the conjunctiva: risks for progression to melanoma in 311 eyes. The 2006 Lorenz E. Zimmerman lecture. *Ophthalmology* 2008; **115**:511–519.

Vann RR, Karp CL. Perilesional and topical interferon alfa 2b for conjunctival and corneal neoplasia. *Ophthalmology* 1999; **106**:91–97.

Yamamoto N, Ohmura T, Suzuki H, et al. Successful treatment with 5-fluorouracil of conjunctival intraepithelial neoplasia refractive to mitomycin C. *Ophthalmology* 2002; **109**:249–252.

Yeatts RP, Ford JG, Stanton CA, et al. Topical 5-fluorouracil in treating epithelial neoplasia of the conjunctival and cornea. *Ophthalmology* 1995; **102**:1338–1344.

Zaki AA. Farid SF. Management of intraepithelial and invasive neoplasia of the cornea and conjunctival: a long-term follow-up. *Cornea* 2009; **28**:986–988.

Chapter 21
Conjunctivochalasis, lymphangiectasia, and conjunctival concretions

Stefano Barabino, Cristiana Valente, Eszter Fodor, Carlo Enrico Traverso

CONJUNCTIVOCHALASIS

Introduction

Conjunctivochalasis (CCh) is described as a redundant, loose, non-edematous inferior bulbar conjunctiva interposed between the globe and the lower eyelid. The condition tends to be bilateral and can be localized in the medial, central, or lateral part of the lower eyelid. The term 'conjunctivochalasis' comes from conjunctivus (Latin), and chálasis (Greek), which means relaxation, redundancy, and looseness. Meller et al.'s (1998) historical review demonstrates the importance of CCh in the last century. In the first few decades, severe CCh was found worthy of attention. In those early reports, pain, marginal corneal ulcers, and subconjunctival hemorrhage were associated with CCh. In the 1980s moderate CCh was described as a reason for disorder of tear clearance with intermittent but frequent tearing, and occlusion of the inferior lacrimal punctum. Nowadays, mild CCh is also taken into consideration as a possible reason for an unstable tear film and dry eye disease.

The prevalence and incidence of CCh have been only partially studied. Mimura et al. (2009) reported that in the first two decades of life, the prevalence of CCh is very low and increases steadily after the third decade, becoming a common condition in elderly people. Temporal conjunctiva is more involved than the nasal part. The disease is seen more frequently in females than in males.

Pathogenesis

Several hypotheses have been suggested about the etiology and pathogenesis of CCh in the last few decades, but the two most reported etiological theories are breakdown of elastic fibers in the redundant conjunctiva with negligible inflammatory cell infiltrates (Yokoi et al. 2005), and inflammation of the conjunctiva (Meller et al. 2000). The first theory is supported by histopathological studies showing that elastotic degeneration is an important pathogenetic mechanism responsible for the development of CCh, and that inflammation markers in the conjunctiva show low expression levels. Collagenolysis due to accumulation of degrading enzymes in tears because of delayed tear clearance (more frequent in old age, female sex, and decreased ocular sensitivity) might independently contribute to the formation of CCh (Meller et al. 1998). In vitro cultures of conjunctival fibroblast showed a significant overexpression of matrix metalloprotease (MMP)-1 and MMP-3 mRNA with a correlation of increased protein levels and proteolytic activities (Li et al. 2000).

Several researches have described an important role of inflammation in CCh pathogenesis. Elevated levels of inflammatory mediators [interleukin (IL)-1β, tumor necrosis factor (TNF)-α, IL-6, and IL-8] have been reported in in vitro cultures (Meller et al. 2000), and in tears collected from patients with CCh (Erdogan-Poyraz et al. 2009, Wang et al. 2007). Increased expression of HLA-DR – a proinflammatory factor in ocular surface disorders – in conjunctival epithelial cells was found in patients with severe cases of CCh than compared with moderate and mild cases, but the authors' hypothesis is that inflammation is the consequence and not the cause of the presence of conjunctival folds (Fodor et al. 2010).

Further pathogenetic mechanisms are friction of the eyelids movements on the ocular surface and consecutive elongation of the conjunctiva, extended exposure and consequent damage of the ocular surface by hypotonic eyelids, lymphatic flow obstruction, and actinic radiation.

Clinical characteristics

Different symptoms are reported by patients according to the severity of the clinical stage. At the mild stage, CCh may be asymptomatic or may induce significant changes of the tear film and therefore irritation, foreign body sensation, and transient blurring of vision (especially during reading). All symptoms are exacerbated by the exposure to dry environment, wind, and air conditioning. In more severe cases, the presence of the folds may occlude the lower lacrimal puncta and induce lacrimation, dellen formation, and, in some cases, corneal ulcers. Because of the poor affixation of the conjunctiva to the sclera, subconjunctival vessels are prone to rupture by blinking or rubbing, and subconjunctival hemorrhage becomes the most important sign complained by patients.

Slit-lamp examination shows conjunctival folds as redundant, excessive tissue (**Figure 21.1**), which can be moved over the sclera by digital pressure of the lower eyelid. In most cases, CCh occurs in both eyes, increases with downgaze (**Figure 21.2**), and decreases with upgaze. A thorough examination of the ocular surface should be performed, including blink rate, lid margin, tear meniscus height, tear film break-up time (BUT), and lissamine green staining. The tear film stability is altered in most forms of CCh with possible alteration of the quality of vision (**Figure 21.3**); the evaluation of fluorescein distribution and BUT are important indicators that should be considered. The use of lissamine green staining may demonstrate a discrete punctate or linear staining on the mucosal aspect of the lid margin adjacent to the redundant conjunctiva, the redundant bulbar conjunctiva and the adjacent lid margin, and tarsal conjunctiva.

The differential diagnosis of CCh includes dry eye disease, meibomian gland dysfunction, allergy, and all the conditions inducing tearing such as trichiasis, entropion, ectropion, lacrimal punctual stenosis, nasolacrimal obstruction, and thyroid eye disease.

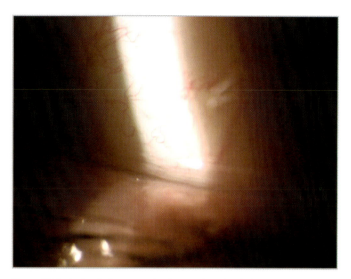

Figure 21.1 At the slit-lamp examination, conjunctivochalasis appears as redundant, loose, non-edematous inferior bulbar conjunctiva interposed between the globe and the lower eyelid.

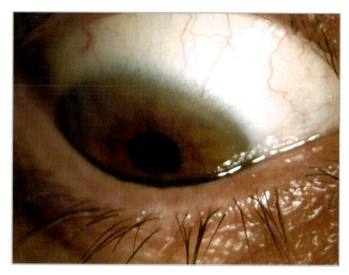

Figure 21.2 A characteristic sign of conjunctivochalasis is the increase in downgaze.

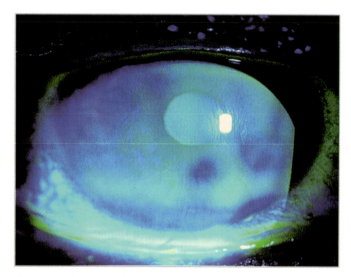

Figure 21.3 Conjunctivochalasis (CCh) alters the stability of the tear film on the ocular surface. In this 65-year-old female patient CCh determines an irregular tear film, which significantly decreases the quality of vision.

Classification

In 1995, Höh et al. reported the 'Lidkantenparallele conjunctivale Falten' (LIPCOF) classification based on the number of folds and the height of the redundant conjunctiva with respect to that of the tear meniscus. They found that the four grades of LIPCOF also had a high predictive value for the diagnosis of dry eye disease, ranging from grade 0 (no permanently present fold) and absence of dry eye disease, to grade 3 where multiple folds higher than the normal tear meniscus were indicative of severe dry eye disease.

The location of the redundant conjunctiva on the lower lid is variable, and the size of the conjunctival fold can be increased by downgaze or digital compression onto the globe; in the advanced forms of CCh, the folds may overlap the cornea and occlude the inferior lacrimal puncta. Therefore, Meller et al. (1998) developed the classification of folds with five parameters: location, relation to the lower

tear meniscus height, presence of punctal occlusion, changes in gaze, and changes when pressing the lower lid backward. The new grading system defines the extension of redundant conjunctiva as grade 1 = one location, 2 = two locations, and 3 = whole lid. Grades 1 and 2 are further specified as T, M, or N, according to if CCh is found in the temporal, middle (or inferior to the limbus), or nasal aspects of the lower lid, respectively. Each location (T, M, and N) is further given a notation to indicate if the height of folds is less than (A), equal to (B), or greater than (C) the tear meniscus height, and if it changes with digital pressure. If CCh is found in the nasal (N) location, the extent of chalasis is further determined as to whether it occludes the inferior lacrimal puncta or not.

Yokoi et al. (2003) described the conjunctival folds of the upper bulbar conjunctiva in three grades as mild, moderate, and severe in patients with superior limbic keratoconjunctivitis.

Therapy

For asymptomatic patients, no treatment is needed. Patients with ocular irritation, foreign body sensation, and blurred vision due to tear film instability should be treated with unpreserved tear substitutes. To date, in the literature, there are no clinical studies reporting the effect of different artificial tears on symptoms and signs in CCh patients. Topical drops with preservatives should be avoided because of ocular irritation and increased aggressive effect caused by their accumulation on the surface of the folds. Treatment with topical non-steroid anti-inflammatory drops or topical corticosteroids may be used to decrease the level of inflammation of the ocular surface in order to relieve symptoms and improve tear film conditions. The use of substitute tears containing omega-3 fatty acids may increase tear film stability and decrease the level of ocular surface inflammation (Rashid et al. 2008). However, so far, there have been no studies demonstrating possible changes in inflammatory markers on conjunctival cells in cases of CCh.

In patients with mild or moderate grade of CCh, surgical procedures have limitations such as postoperative inflammation and suture-related complication. For this reason, some authors used electrosurgery technique with high-frequency radio waves, which induces the fibroelastic shrinkage of the conjunctiva via intracellular water boiling

(Youm et al. 2010), or bipolar cauterization of the excess conjunctiva (Kashima et al. 2011). Another possible procedure to avoid excision of the conjunctival tissue and goblet cells, and mucosa associated lymphoid tissue (MALT) zones' damage is scleral fixation of the lower bulbar conjunctiva by single sutures. The attachment of the bulbar conjunctiva to the sclera occurs by focal inflammation around the sutures (Otaka & Kyu 2000).

In the more severe forms of CCh, a conventional surgical procedure consists of simple, fornix-based, crescent excision of the redundancy, with or without tenonectomy. Elliptical resection, trapezoidal excision, and circumferential resection are more recent techniques to remove conjunctival folds. After removal of the redundant tissue in severe CCh, transplantation of amniotic membrane is an important technique. The graft can be placed by interrupted sutures or fibrin glue. The anti-inflammatory, antiscarring, antiangiogenesis, and wound healing effects are well known for the amniotic membrane. Furthermore, it has been demonstrated that amniotic membrane is effective in ocular surface reconstruction after tenonectomy.

LYMPHANGIECTASIA OF THE CONJUNCTIVA

Lymphangiectasia is an uncommon condition of the bulbar conjunctiva in which lymphatic vessels are dilated and prominent. Despite congenital cases being reported as a component of Turner and Klippel–Trénaunay–Weber syndrome, the disruption or obstruction of lymphatic pathways that determines lymphedema, and therefore lymphangiectasia, may be determined by head or neck mass, radiotherapy, blepharoplasty, pterygium, and vascular tumors of the conjunctiva (Welch et al. 2012).

Clinically, patients may complain of visual disturbances, ocular discomfort, and tearing. Slit-lamp examination shows lymphangiectasia as a diffuse conjunctival chemosis, a localized cyst, or a series of cysts. Sometimes the lymphatic channels of lymphangiectasia are filled with blood and the conjunctival swelling is associated with hemorrhage. This condition is termed 'hemorrhagic lymphangiectasia,' as first described by Leber in 1880. It may develop spontaneously or it can follow a chronic inflammation or a trauma that cause a failure in the valvular mechanism of the lymphatic vessels and alterations in the connections with blood vessels, resulting in the intermittent rapid filling of conjunctival lymphatics with blood (Lochhead & Benjamin 1998). In the literature, lymphangiectasia hemorrhagica has also been reported as a possible complication of phacoemulsification with peribulbar injection (Kyprianous et al. 2004).

Histopathologically, lymphangiectasia is characterized by clear lymphatic channels lined by thin endothelial cells, and surrounded by a lamina propria that is often edematous. Specific markers for lymphatic vessels, such as vascular endothelial growth factor receptor 3, the monoclonal antibody D2-40, and the lymphatic vessel endothelial hyaluronate receptor 1, may be used to differentiate lymphatic vessels from capillaries (Chen et al. 2005).

The differential diagnosis of lymphangiectasia includes allergy, vasomotor instability, systemic hypoproteinemia, thyroid eye disease, and carotid-cavernous fistula, all being conditions that could induce accumulation of fluid in the conjunctiva without dilation of lymphatic vessels. Also, CCh and lymphangioma should be taken into consideration in the differential diagnosis. CCh is characterized by redundant conjunctiva without involvement of lymphatic vessels, while lymphangioma is a neoplasm of lymphatic origin that differs from lymphangiectasia because it is characterized by a prominent accumulation of vessels infiltrating the surrounding normal tissue.

Lymphangiectasia is often managed by observation because it is usually asymptomatic, and rarely shows progression. A therapy is required if the diagnosis is uncertain or if persistent and severe bleeding occurs from the dilated vascular channels. In these cases, techniques such as localized conjunctival resection, direct treatment with diathermy, argon laser photocoagulation, or liquid nitrogen cryotherapy have been used (Fraunfelder 2009). The administration of substitute tears may be helpful in improving tear film stability altered by ocular surface irregularity and, therefore, ameliorating symptoms of ocular discomfort often reported by patients affected by lymphangiectasia.

CONJUNCTIVAL CONCRETIONS

Conjunctival concretions are small avascular, granular, yellow-white deposits found in the palpebral conjunctiva in the elderly or in patients with chronic inflammatory conditions (**Figure 21.4**). They are usually idiopathic, but they have been also associated with chronic atopic keratoconjunctivitis, Herbert's pits, following post-trachomatous degeneration and sulfadiazine eye drop administration (Kulshrestha & Thaller 1995). They are frequently discrete, but confluent concretions are not uncommon. Haicl and Janková (2005) studied the prevalence of conjunctival concretions in a cohort of 500 consecutive patients and found a prevalence of almost 40%; although, only 6% of patients were symptomatic. In this study, no significant difference was found between the localization on the upper and lower eyelids, and most of the deposits were superficial and hard, and mainly single. Interestingly, in this study, 30% of patients with conjunctival concretions showed dysfunction of meibomian glands.

Concretions are almost always asymptomatic because they usually remain hidden into the palpebral conjunctiva, unnoticed by patients, until they become larger and protrude through the palpebral tissues. They may cause foreign body sensation, but only if the concretions erode the overlying conjunctival epithelium and come in contact with the cornea. A recent article has emphasized how patients with conjunctival concretions are potentially affected with the dry eye disease. Decreased values of the Schirmer's test and tear film BUT were demonstrated in 50 asymptomatic patients with accidentally detected

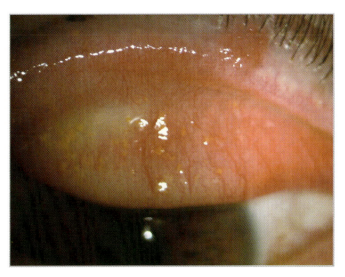

Figure 21.4 Conjunctival concretions appear as small avascular, granular, yellow-white deposits in the palpebral conjunctiva.

conjunctival concretions (Haicl et al. 2006). These results, together with the previous demonstration of an alteration of meibomian glands, are strongly suggestive of a relationship between tear film dysfunction and conjunctival concretion formation; further studies are necessary to demonstrate this hypothesis.

Histopathologically, concretions appear to be epithelial inclusion cysts filled with epithelial and keratin debris. Chang et al. (1990) confirmed that deposits are composed mainly of mucinous secretions of transformed conjunctival glands admixed with degenerated epithelial cells. Histochemically, concretions have been found to stain strongly for phospholipid and elastin, weakly for polysaccharides, and negatively for amyloid, iron, and glycogen. Very little calcium is integrated within the accumulated material, as previously thought. Secondary calcification occurs occasionally, in which case the lesion are sometimes referred to as conjunctival lithiasis.

The use of artificial tears and/or ointments is recommended for those patients who have signs of dry eye disease or are mildly symptomatic. In more severe cases with corneal erosion or persistent symptoms, concretions can be easily removed under topical anesthesia using small gauge needle.

REFERENCES

Chang SW, Hou PK, Chen MS. Conjunctival concretions. Polarized microscopic, histopathological, and ultrastructural studies. *Arch Ophthalmol* 1990; **108**:405–407.

Chen L, Cursiefen C, Barabino S, Zhang Q, Dana MR. Novel expression and characterization of lymphatic vessel endothelial hyaluronate receptor 1 (LYVE-1) by conjunctival cells. *Invest Ophthalmol Vis Sci* 2005; **46**:4536–4540.

Erdogan-Poyraz C, Mocan MC, Bozkurt B, et al. Elevated tear Interleukin-6 and Interleukin-8 levels in patients with conjunctivochalasis. *Cornea* 2009; **28**:189–193.

Fodor E, Barabino S, Montaldo E, Mingari MC, Rolando M. Quantitative evaluation of ocular surface inflammation in patients with different grade of conjunctivochalasis. *Curr Eye Res* 2010; **35**:665–669.

Fraunfelder FW. Liquid nitrogen cryotherapy for conjunctival lymphangiectasia: a case series. *Trans Am Ophthalmol Soc* 2009; **107**:229–233.

Haicl P, Janková H. Prevalance of conjunctival concretions. *Cesk Slov Oftalmol* 2005; **61**:260–264.

Haicl P, Janková H, Jirsová K. Dry eye syndrome in patients with conjunctival concretions. *Cesk Slov Oftalmol* 2006; **62**:415–422.

Höh H, Schirra F, Kienecker C, Ruprecht KW. Lidparallele konjunctivale falten (LIPCOF) sind ein sicheres diagnostisches zeichen des trockenen Auges. *Ophthalmologe* 1995; **17**:104–117.

Kashima T, Akiyama H, Miura F, Kishi S. Improved subject symptoms of conjunctivochalasis using bipolar diathermy method for conjunctival shrinkage. *Clin Ophthalmol* 2011; **5**:1391–1396.

Kulshrestha MK, Thaller VT. Prevalence of conjunctival concretions. *Eye* 1995; **9**:797–798.

Kyprianous I, Nessim M, Kumar V, Chew C. A case of lymphangiectasia haemorrhagica conjunctivae following phacoemulsification. *Acta Ophthalmologica Scandinavia* 2004; **82**:627–628.

Li D, Meller D, Liu Y, Tseng SCG. Overexpression of MMP-1 and MMP-3 by cultured conjunctivochalasis fibroblasts. *Invest Ophthalmol Vis Sci* 2000; **41**:404–410.

Lochhead J, Benjamin L. Lymphangiectasia haemorrhagica conjunctivae. *Eye* 1998; **12**:627–629.

Meller D, Li D, Tseng SCG. Regulation of collagenase, stromelysin, and gelatinase B in human conjunctival and conjunctivochalasis fibroblasts by interleukin-1b and tumor necrosis factor-alpha. *Invest Ophthalmol Vis Sci* 2000; **41**:2922–2929.

Meller D, Scheffer C, Tseng G. Conjunctivochalasis: literature review and possible pathophysiology. *Surv Ophthalmol* 1998; **43**:225–232.

Mimura T, Yamagami S, Usui T, et al. Changes of conjunctivochalasis with age in a hospital-based study. *Am J Ophthalmol* 2009; **147**:171–177.

Otaka I, Kyu N. A new surgical technique for management of conjunctivochalasis. *Am J Ophthalmol* 2000; **129**:385–387.

Rashid S, Jin Y, Ecoiffier T, et al. Topical omega-3 and omega-6 fatty acids for treatment of dry eye. *Arch Ophthalmol* 2008; **126**:219–225.

Wang Y, Dogru M, Matsumoto Y, et al. The impact of nasal conjunctivochalasis on tear functions and ocular surface findings. *Am J Ophthalmol* 2007; **144**:930–937.

Welch J, Srinivasan S, Lyall D, Roberts F. Conjunctival lymphangiectasia: a report of 11 cases and review of the literature. *Surv Ophthalmol* 2012; **57**:136–148.

Yokoi N, Komuro A, Maruyama K, et al. New surgical treatment for superior limbic keratoconjunctivitis and its association with conjunctivochalasis. *Am J Ophthalmol* 2003; **135**:303–308.

Yokoi N, Komuro A, Nishii M, et al. Clinical impact of conjunctivochalasis on the ocular surface. *Cornea* 2005; **24**:S24–S31.

Youm DJ, Kim JM, Choi CY. Simple surgical approach with high-frequency radio-wave electrosurgery for conjunctivochalasis. *Ophthalmology* 2010; **117**:2129–2133.

Chapter 22 Infectious conjunctivitis and keratitis

Eric Gabison, Serge Doan, Thanh Hoang-Xuan

■ INFECTIOUS CONJUNCTIVITIS

Acute infectious conjunctivitis is a frequent disorder, more often caused by viruses (especially adenoviruses) than by bacteria. Indeed, a predisposing factor is often present in bacterial conjunctivitis. The ocular symptoms of acute infectious conjunctivitis include tearing, burning, stinging, and ocular redness. Blurred vision and pain point to keratitis. The occurrence of similar symptoms in the circle of acquaintances also provides an indication. The systemic infectious syndrome or specific infections of the nose, throat, or ears suggest an infectious cause. Ocular signs of infectious conjunctivitis include conjunctival hyperemia, chemosis or lid edema, and discharge. Purulent discharge is more frequent in bacterial conjunctivitis. Whereas papillar hypertrophy may evoke a bacterial infection, follicles are usually the sign of viral or chlamydial infection, or of Parinaud oculoglandular syndrome (**Figure 22.1**). Conjunctival pseudomembranes and membranes (**Figure 22.2**) are a sign of severe inflammation and can induce corneal erosions and lead to symblephara and foreshortening of the fornix.

The main differential diagnosis is allergic conjunctivitis. A personal or family history of atopy, seasonal recurrences, especially in the spring, and pruritus are main indicators of allergy.

■ Bacterial conjunctivitis
Clinical aspect

Bacterial conjunctivitis is not frequent, representing <5% of all conjunctivitis, with a seasonal peak during winter and a higher frequency in children. There are predisposing factors, either systemic (e.g. systemic immunodeficiency, alcohol abuse, atopy, and diabetes) or local (e.g. tear drainage obstruction, medication with topical steroids, use of contact lenses, dry eye disease, and eye burns). Infection can be hyperacute, acute, or chronic. Bacterial conjunctivitis is suspected in patients with unilateral conjunctival inflammation and purulent discharge.

Hyperacute conjunctivitis (incubation <24 hours)

Hyperacute conjunctivitis is caused by *Neisseria gonorrhoeae* or, occasionally, by *N. meningitidis* and requires microbiological diagnosis. *N. gonorrhoeae* is directly transmitted from the infected genital organ to the eye. Gonococcal conjunctivitis is characterized by marked inflammation associated with a purulent discharge, the formation of conjunctival pseudomembranes, and preauricular lymphadenopathy. Corneal involvement is frequent (15–40%) and consists of epithelial haze or defects, marginal infiltrates, or ulcers that may progress to perforation. Treatment is urgent and is based on systemic ceftriaxone or fluoroquinolones. *N. meningitidis* conjunctivitis may also be associated

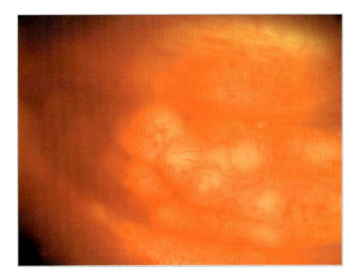

Figure 22.1 Chlamydial follicular conjunctivitis.

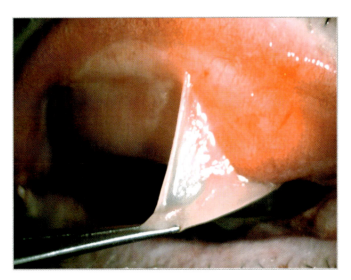

Figure 22.2 Pseudomembranous conjunctivitis

with keratitis. The treatment consists of systemic penicillin G aimed at preventing meningeal involvement.

Acute or subacute conjunctivitis

Acute or subacute conjunctivitis is caused by *Staphylococcus aureus*, *S. epidermidis*, and *Streptococcus pneumoniae* in adults and by *Haemophilus influenzae*, *S. pneumoniae*, and *S. aureus* in children.

H. influenzae and *S. pneumoniae* are often associated with otitis media. *S. pneumoniae* and streptococci can cause conjunctival pseudomembranes. Haemophilus aegyptius is responsible for Brazilian purpuric fever. *Moraxella lacunata* causes acute recurrent or chronic follicular and angular blepharoconjunctivitis in alcoholic or malnourished subjects.

Chronic bacterial conjunctivitis

Chronic colonization of the lid margin by *S. aureus* can cause acute recurrent or chronic conjunctivitis, associated with anterior blepharitis, inferior punctate keratopathy, marginal infiltrates, and phlyctenular keratoconjunctivitis.

Parinaud oculoglandular syndrome

Parinaud syndrome is characterized by chronic unilateral follicular conjunctivitis, with conjunctival granulomas and preauricular, retromandibular, or cervical adenopathies, which may evolve toward suppuration. The most frequent cause is cat scratch disease (*Bartonella henselae*), but other bacteria may be responsible, such as *Francisella tularensis* (tularemia), *Mycobacterium tuberculosis*, *Treponema pallidum* (syphilis), or *Chlamydia trachomatis* (lymphogranuloma venereum).

Laboratory investigations

Diagnosis is usually clinical. Conjunctival swabs with smears and culture may be indicated in particular cases such as in newborns, immunocompromised subjects, cases of hyperacute purulent conjunctivitis, or resistance to first-line treatment (a treatment-free period of 36 hours is required). Several culture media can be used, e.g. blood agar, chocolate agar, or thioglycolate-enriched medium. The antibiogram should be adapted to the antibiotics used in ophthalmology.

Treatment

Acute bacterial conjunctivitis is a self-limiting disease. In a randomized double-blind study, the rate of clinical cure was the same after 8 days of treatment with either saline or topical polymyxin–bacitracin (Gigliotti et al. 1984). However, topical antibiotic therapy shortened the healing time and enhanced bacterial eradication. Antibiotic eye drops (**Table 22.1**) are usually chosen empirically, and prescribed four to six times daily for 7 days, except for azithromycin, which may be administered bid for 3 days (Cochereau et al. 2007a). Fluoroquinolones should be reserved for severe conjunctivitis. In some countries, chloramphenicol is not recommended because of potentially adverse hematological effects. In case of bacterial identification, antibiotics should be chosen according to the antibiogram, although ocular concentrations of topically administered antibiotics are usually far beyond minimal inhibitory concentrations.

■ Chlamydial conjunctivitis

C. trachomatis is responsible for several conjunctival infections, including inclusion conjunctivitis in adults or neonates (serovars D–K), trachoma (serovars A–C), and lymphogranuloma venereum (serovars L1, L2, and L3).

Although clinical examination is sufficient to diagnose trachoma, chronic inclusion conjunctivitis often needs to be confirmed by conjunctival swabs. Because *Chlamydia* is an intracellular bacterium, conjunctival scraping is required to obtain epithelial cells. Direct examination of smears after May–Grünwald–Giemsa staining may show epithelial cells with basophilic intracellular inclusions, but the technique lacks sensitivity because the bacterial load may be low in cases of conjunctival infection. Rapid techniques for detecting the chlamydial antigen are based on direct immunofluorescence examination and enzyme-linked-immunosorbent serologic assay (ELISA), but these tests lack adequate sensitivity. The highly sensitive polymerase chain reaction (PCR) technique now widely used allows the detection of even a single chlamydial genome. Cultures on Hela 229 or McCoy cells represent the gold standard techniques but remain expensive. Serologic evaluation is not of much interest in chlamydial conjunctivitis since antibody levels are usually low.

Adult inclusion conjunctivitis

C. trachomatis is often transmitted by infected genital secretions (sexually transmitted urethritis or cervicitis) but less frequently by other sources such as contaminated swimming pool water. The disease is characterized by chronic unilateral follicular conjunctivitis, affecting mainly the inferior tarsal conjunctiva (**Figure 22.2**), or papillary conjunctivitis, affecting the superior tarsal conjunctiva, with various symptoms including pink/red eye, mucous discharge, tearing, photophobia, foreign body eye sensation, and decreased vision. The disease is also associated with mucopurulent discharge, chemosis, lid edema, preauricular adenopathy, and, more rarely, fine punctate epithelial keratitis, limbal subepithelial infiltrates, and micropannus. If untreated, the disease can last for weeks to months. Treatment combines topical antibiotics (azithromycin, tetracycline, or fluoroquinolone for 3 weeks) and oral azithromycin (1 g single dose), doxycycline (100 mg bid for 10 days), or erythromycin (500 mg qid for 10 days). Sexual partners should also be examined and treated.

Neonatal chlamydial conjunctivitis

Neonatal chlamydial conjunctivitis is due to infection of the neonate during the passage through the birth canal. Signs appearing 5–15 days after birth include congestive hyperemic conjunctivitis with a mucopurulent discharge and the formation of conjunctival pseudomembranes. Whereas there are no follicles or adenopathies, cultures are more frequently positive, unlike the case in adults. Pneumonitis and otitis may be associated. Conjunctival swabs should be performed to rule out other differential diagnoses. Treatment consists of oral erythromycin (50 mg/kg/day for 2 weeks), associated with topical antibiotics according to some authors. Prophylactic tetracycline or erythromycin ophthalmic ointment for 1 week is indicated in the newborn if the mother has chlamydial genital infection.

Trachoma

Trachoma is still a leading cause of blindness in developing countries, affecting about 84 million people, of whom about 8 million are visually impaired (World Health Organization 2011). It is transmitted by flies and contact with infected secretions in communities with poor hygiene.

Chronic follicular conjunctivitis with a mucopurulent discharge is characteristic of the disease. The follicles are more frequently situated in the superior tarsal conjunctiva and at the limbus. They may be associated with a papillary reaction in the acute form. Corneal punctate epitheliopathy or infiltrates may occur. Evolution toward corneoconjunctival fibrosis is typical, consisting of linear scarring of the superior tarsal conjunctiva (Arlt line), oval depressions of the superior limbus (Herbert's pits), superior corneal pannus, tear drainage obstruction, tear deficiency, entropion, and trichiasis. Corneal

Table 22.1 Main clinical and therapeutic characteristics of the infectious agents affecting the cornea

	Bacteria	Mycobacteria	Fungus	Acanthamoeba	Herpesvirus
Pathogens	*Staphylococcus coagulase* ±	**M. Chelonae**	Yeast: *Candida*		
	Streptococcus pneumoniae	*M. abscessus, fortuitum*	Filamentous *Fusarium, Aspergillus*		
	Pseudomonas spp.				
	Neisseria gonorrhoea				
	Haemophilus spp.				
Medical history	Lid abnormality–trauma	Refractive surgery (e.g. LASIK and RK)	Ocular surface disorder	Contact lenses	HSV recurrent keratitis
	Trauma—dacryocystitis	Trauma	Contact lens—vegetal trauma	Vegetal trauma	Treatment by steroid, immunosuppressive, atopic dermatitis, UV light irradiation, stress
	Contact lenses—reanimation		Topical steroid treatment	Chronic keratitis not responding to conventional therapy	
	Neonate—sexually active adult				
	ENT infection in child				
Symptoms	Pain, foreign body sensation, redness, photophobia, tearing, purulent discharge	Late-onset infiltrate, slowly progressive lesion	Variable onset (slow/rapid progression)	Extremely severe pain	
Clinical signs	Small infiltrates, healthy epithelium outside the infected area	Cracked windshield appearance of corneal infiltrate	Feathery, hyphate edges, satellite lesions, 'collar button' configuration, epithelial defect may be absent	Superficial keratitis, epithelial irregularities, dendritiform epithelial lesions, radial keratoneuritis, nummular anterior stroma infiltrates, ring infiltrate with intact central epithelium	Epithelial lesions (dendritis, geographic)
	Serpiginous edges, deep stromal involvement, hypopyon				Marginal lesion, archipelago keratitis
	Sapid evolution, epithelial edema, 'ground-glass' stromal appearance, ring infiltrate, hypopyon				Stromal infiltrate ± epithelial lesion
	Purulent conjunctivitis, chemosis, deep corneal ulcer				Endotheliitis, disciform lesions
Laboratory investigation	Corneal scrapes (margin and base ulcer)	Ziehl–Nielsen stain	Periodic acid-Schiff/Gomori stain, acridine orange, calcofluor	May–Grünwald–Giemsa stain, acridine orange, calcofluor	PCR
	Gram stains (± additional stains)	Lowenstein–Jensen special medium	Special culture medium (Sabouraud)	PCR	Viral culture if resistance to antiviral therapy is suspected
	Cultures on blood, chocolate agar		In vivo confocal microscopy (filament)	Special culture medium (*Escherichia coli* enriched)	
				In vivo confocal microscopy	
Local treatment	Commercially available topical antibiotics: moxifloxacin/gatifloxacin/ciprofloxacin/chloramphenicol/aminosides	Ciprofloxacin	Amphotericin B	Propamidine 0.1%	Trifluridine

Contd...

Contd...

	Fortified topical antibiotics: cephalosporins/aminosides/vancomycin	Azithromycin	Natamycin	Chlorhexidine 0.02%	Ganciclovir
		Amikacin	Voriconazole, fluconazole, itraconazole	Polyhexamethylene biguanide 0.02%	Topical steroids ± (except for dendritic and geographic keratitis)
Systemic treatment	In case of corneal perforation		Deep corneal involvement	Ketoconazole, miconazole, itraconazole	Acyclovir
			Oral: ketoconazole, fluconazole	Voriconazole	Valacyclovir

HSV, herpes simplex virus; PCR, polymerase chain reaction; UV, ultraviolet.

opacification is a frequent sequella. The World Health Organization (WHO) recommends a simplified grading system defined by grades TF (trachomatous inflammation, follicular), TI (trachomatous inflammation, intense), TS (trachomatous scarring), TT (trachomatous trichiasis), or CO (corneal opacity).

The treatment is based on topical tetracycline 1% or erythromycin ointment bid for 2 months, oral doxycyclin (100 mg/day for 3 weeks) or azithromycin (20 mg/kg in children, 1 g in adults, single dose). Topical azithromycin, 1.5% bid for 3 days, has recently been used with results comparable to those obtained with systemic azithromycin (Cochereau et al. 2007b). Surgical treatment of trichiasis may prevent corneal sequellae. Prevention through education imposing hand and facial hygiene is indispensable. The WHO has developed the SAFE (surgery for trichiasis, antibiotics, facial cleanliness, and environmental improvement) strategy for eliminating trachoma (World Health Organization 2006).

Lymphogranuloma venereum

Lymphogranuloma venereum is a sexually transmitted disease. It is characterized by follicular conjunctivitis, conjunctival granuloma, and homolateral adenopathy. The treatment includes antibiotics and drainage of the buboes or abscesses.

■ Viral conjunctivitis

Viral conjunctivitis is usually follicular, and frequently associated with preauricular adenopathy and corneal involvement.

Adenoviral keratoconjunctivitis

Adenovirus is the most frequent cause of viral conjunctivitis. Adenoviruses can cause two distinct syndromes according to their serotype, i.e. epidemic keratoconjunctivitis (mainly serotype 8 but also serotypes 11, 19, and 37) and pharyngoconjunctival fever (serotypes 3, 4, and 7).

Epidemic keratoconjunctivitis

Viral transmission occurs by contact with infected individuals, or with contaminated media such as hands, medical instruments, and swimming pools. The virus can survive for 5 weeks on an inert surface and 9 weeks in eye drop bottles (Uchio et al. 2002). Incubation varies from 2 to 21 days. Red, watery stinging eyes with acute bilateral papillary/follicular conjunctivitis, clear serous discharge, and preauricular adenopathy are typically found during the early phase of the disease. Chemosis, eyelid edema, and conjunctival hemorrhage are frequent.

In severe forms, pseudomembranes and membranes develop on the tarsal conjunctiva (**Figure 22.2**) and may cause corneal ulceration. Anterior uveitis is rare. Conjunctival inflammation is maximal 5–7 days after the onset of the symptoms and lasts for 1–3 weeks. Diffuse punctate epithelial erosions are frequently noted in the acute phase. Nummular fluorescein-negative subepithelial infiltrates may develop between the second and third weeks (**Figure 22.3**). Subepithelial nummular corneal scars often replace the infiltrates, which can cause glare, photophobia, irregular astigmatism, and decreased visual acuity. The scars slowly disappear with time. Severe forms may cause sequellar conjunctival fibrosis and tear drainage obstruction. Chronic viral infection is rare.

The diagnosis is clinical. However, quick diagnostic methods are available at the office, based on immunochromatography antigen detection in tears. PCR and immunofluorescence methods may also be used on conjunctival swabs in specialized laboratories.

Pharyngoconjunctival fever

Pharyngoconjunctival fever is similar to epidemic keratoconjunctivitis. It is associated with an upper respiratory tract infection, but corneal involvement is less frequent.

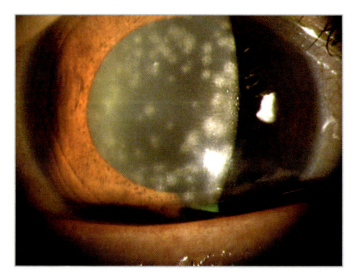

Figure 22.3 Nummular subepithelial corneal infiltrates postadenoviral conjunctivitis.

Treatment of adenoviral conjunctivitis

Strict hygiene is mandatory in order to avoid viral dissemination, and patients should stay at home for at least 7 days from the onset of symptoms. Hand hygiene and the use of personal linen are recommended. Contagiosity persists for 14 days after the onset of ocular signs. Cold compresses and ocular lubrication are the mainstay treatment, whereas antibiotics are not recommended. There are no antiviral treatments with proven efficacy. Topical steroids are indicated in cases of severe conjunctival pseudomembranes but should be used with caution during the acute phase because they may prolong viral replication (Romanowski et al. 1996). In case of nummular epithelial keratitis, topical steroids may be prescribed especially if the vision is altered, but they should be tapered off slowly because of the risk of recurrence. In steroid-dependent cases, topical cyclosporine A 1% eye drops may be prescribed (Jeng & Holsclaw 2011). Rigid contact lenses can correct sequellar irregular corneal astigmatism. If vision is impaired after several months or years, sequellar superficial subepithelial central corneal scars may be treated by laser phototherapeutic keratectomy with or without topical mitomycin C (Yamazaki et al. 2011). Induced hyperopic shift is frequent. Ophthalmologists should apply preventive measures such as hand hygiene, the use of gloves, cleansing of equipment with quaternary ammoniums or peracetic acid, and the use of single-dose eye drops.

◼ Molluscum contagiosum

Molluscum contagiosum is caused by a poxvirus and transmitted by direct contact or autoinoculation. The condition is more frequent in children, and may be florid in atopic and immunocompromised subjects, particularly in HIV-infected patients. The diagnosis is clinical, based on the presence of small pearly umbilicated nodules on the eyelids (molluscums), associated with chronic follicular conjunctivitis and sometimes a conjunctival pannus. The disease is often unilateral. The diagnosis may be difficult if the molluscums are not detected. The evolution of the disorder is chronic over several months, with possible spontaneous resolution. The histopathological examination of molluscums shows characteristic eosinophilic inclusions. Eyelid molluscums may be treated by photodestruction with an argon laser or by excision. Extraocular lesions should also be treated.

Papillomavirus conjunctivitis

Human papillomavirus (especially types 6 and 11) is responsible for conjunctival papilloma. The lesion is sessile or, more frequently, pedunculated, with a typical hypervascularized raspberry appearance. Evolution toward epithelial dysplasia and carcinoma is more frequent with some viral serotypes (16 and 18).

Laboratory investigations

Histopathological examination of the lesion is often useful in order to rule out carcinoma. The PCR, in situ hybridization, and electronic microscopy can be used to detect papillomavirus.

Treatment

Papilloma may regress spontaneously. Treatment is based on surgical resection, with additional cauterization or cryotherapy to reduce the rate of recurrence, and/or administration of topical interferon α2b eye drops, 1 million units/cc qid, until clinical resolution (Schechter et al. 2002).

Other viral conjunctivitis

Herpes simplex virus

Herpes simplex virus conjunctivitis is frequent but often misdiagnosed. It is usually unilateral (except in case of primo-infection), follicular, and may be associated with conjunctival ulcers. Laboratory investigations and treatment are detailed in section 'Infectious Keratitis.'

Chickenpox

Chickenpox may be associated with conjunctival papillar conjunctivitis and, in rare cases, with conjunctival vesicles. Zoster ophthalmicus-related conjunctivitis is rarely associated with conjunctival vesicles, pseudomembranes, conjunctival scarring, and lacrimal punctal stenosis.

Epstein–Barr virus

Epstein–Barr virus systemic infection is also frequently accompanied by unilateral follicular or nodular conjunctivitis and, in rare cases, by Parinaud oculoglandular syndrome.

Enterovirus 70 and Coxsackie A24 virus

Enterovirus 70 and Coxsackie A24 virus are responsible for outbreaks of acute hemorrhagic conjunctivitis. Signs appear 24 hours after contact with contaminated media. Evolution is usually favorable within 7 days.

Many other viruses may be associated with conjunctivitis during systemic infection, such as those of measles, rubella, influenza, mumps, Newcastle virus, chikungunya, dengue, and yellow fever.

Fungal conjunctivitis

Fungal infections are rare and occur mainly in subjects who are on long-term topical steroid therapy or have a history of vegetal ocular trauma.

◼ INFECTIOUS KERATITIS

Infections of the cornea are due to a wide variety of pathogens. In the majority of the cases, bacteria, fungi, or parasites, such as *Acanthamoeba*, contaminate the cornea through an epithelial defect. More rarely, infectious agents such as *N. gonorrhoeae* may penetrate the healthy corneal epithelium directly or be delivered in situ through the corneal nerves as in the case of herpesviruses. Hence, special care should be taken to identify the risk factors associated with corneal ulcer. The management of this sight-threatening condition calls for a precise diagnostic and therapeutic approach regarding the three main pathogenic components of the disorder, namely infection, inflammation, and ulceration. **Table 22.2** summarizes the main clinical and therapeutic characteristics of the infectious agents affecting the cornea.

◼ Defense mechanisms of the ocular surface

While the impermeability of the corneal epithelium, ensured by molecular structures, such as the tight junctions, is essential to the prevention of corneal infection, other factors may contribute to the protection of a damaged epithelium. The prevention of the adhesion and infiltration of pathogens involves several elements of defense, such as the apical glycocalyx, soluble mucin glycoproteins, secretory IgA, and surfactant proteins. The antimicrobial activity of tears under

Table 22.2 Risk factors of infectious keratitis

Lid abnormalities
Entropion
Trichiasis
Lagophthalmia
Corneal injury
Surgery
Trauma
Contact lenses
Corneal disorders
Fuchs dystrophy
Recurrent erosion
Neurotrophic keratitis
Ocular surface disorders
Chronic inflammation
Topical corticosteroids
Patient characteristics
Diabetes mellitus
Immunosuppression
Rheumatoid arthritis

inflammatory and homeostatic conditions is another protective stratagem of the ocular surface. Lysozyme, lactoferrin, and b-lysin have long been known to contribute to this activity, and recently, antimicrobial peptides such as defensins and cathelicidin have been added to the list. Since the pathogenesis of corneal infection involves the disruption of these protective barriers, it is essential to identify the specific cause in planning the management of corneal infection (Argueso & Gipson 2001, Thomas & Geraldine 2007).

Diagnosis
Clinical features

The history of corneal infection with the presenting signs and symptoms of the disorder should be methodically recorded together with the associated risk factors (**Table 22.3**). All past history of herpetic

keratitis, ocular surgery, ocular trauma, or the use of contact lenses should be assessed together with the effects of potentially iatrogenic topical medication, e.g. steroids, non-steroidal anti-inflammatory drugs, and antibiotics. Whereas acute pain is typically reported in cases of corneal infection, a foreign body eye sensation alone may be the main symptom, especially in herpetic or fungal infections. Patients usually experience tearing, photophobia, and ocular injection associated with circumlimbal redness. Ocular discharge may be absent, particularly in herpetic, acanthamoebic, or fungal infection (van Bijsterveld & Jager 1996).

Slit-lamp examination shows an epithelial defect (**Figure 22.4**) associated with an epithelial or a stromal infiltrate. In rare cases, a persistent epithelial defect may be the only presenting sign of corneal infection, but the presence of a stromal infiltrate with an intact overlying epithelium should evoke a fungal infection. The number and the size of the lesions, and their distance from the visual axis should be carefully recorded. The aspect and topographical pattern of the infiltrates may indicate the pathogen involved. Thus, smooth, regular edges would suggest bacterial or yeast infections, whereas irregular, indistinct margins with satellite lesions would evoke filamentous fungal infections. The loss of transparency of the corneal epithelium, giving the cornea a 'ground glass' aspect at a distance from the ulcer, may indicate a *Pseudomonas aeruginosa* infection (**Figure 22.5**). The clinical presentation of *Acanthamoeba* keratitis in its early phase often mimics herpetic keratitis with a dendritic pattern, but all types of superficial keratitis can be seen, resulting in delayed diagnosis and treatment. Later, deep stromal infiltrates occur and coalesce to form the typical diskiform necrotic stromal keratitis (**Figure 22.6**). A very characteristic pattern is also the radial keratoneuritis with stromal infiltrates following the corneal nerves. The diagnosis of *Acanthamoeba* keratitis should be suspected when these signs occur in patients with a history of misusage of contact lenses. Signs of local gravity include proximity of the visual axis, intense endocular inflammation (hypopyon), and involvement of the sclera.

Repeated slit-lamp examination is mandatory in order to assess the efficacy of the treatment. The first signs of clinical response to treatment include decreased pain, reduction in size and density of the stromal infiltrates, and the initiation of epithelial healing. Signs of toxicity due to the topical treatments and any exacerbation of the infectious or inflammatory corneal condition should be closely monitored with respect to the density of the superficial keratitis, the size of the persistent epithelial defect, and the stromal thinning or infiltrate.

Table 22.3 Bacterial spectrum of commercially available topical antibiotics

	Gram + cocci	Gram – bacilli		Intracellular		
	Staph Meti S	Staph Meti R	Streptococci	Haemophilus	Pseudomonas	Chlamydiae
Aminoglycosides	+	+	R	+	+	R
Azithromycin	+	±	+	+	R	+
Bacitracin	+	+	+	R	R	R
Chloramphenicol	+	+	+	+	R	+
Cyclins	+	±	+	+	R	+
Erythromycin	+	R	R	+	R	+
Fluoroquinolones	+	±	R (except for the 3rd and 4th generations)	+	+	+
Polymyxin	R	R	R	+	+	R
R, resistance.						

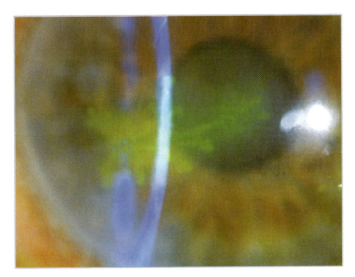

Figure 22.4 Herpes simplex virus dendritic superficial keratitis.

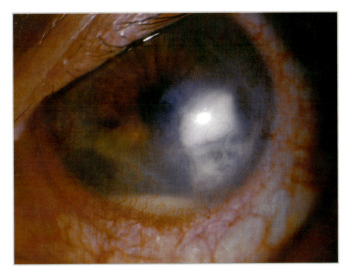

Figure 22.5 *Pseudomonas aeruginosa* keratitis in a contact lens wearer.

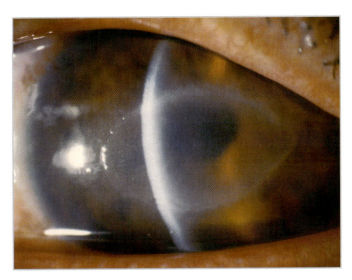

Figure 22.6 Acanthamoebic keratitis.

Differential diagnosis

Non-infectious peripheral ulcerative keratitis, catarrhal marginal infiltrates, and contact lens-related corneal infiltrates seen in the peripheral cornea rarely induce a loss of best-corrected visual acuity. In these cases, conjunctival injection is mild, usually sectorial, without discharge, and endocular inflammation is rare. In some cases, corneal scraping can be indicated to rule out superinfection.

Aseptic paracentral keratolysis linked with Sjögren's syndrome is usually not associated with stromal inflammatory infiltrates and may be misdiagnosed as herpetic keratitis.

■ Laboratory investigations

Although not systematically requested by ophthalmologists in non-sight-threatening cases of infectious keratitis, microbiological examination of corneal scrapes from the margin and the base of the ulcer, and eventually from contact lenses, should allow isolation of the pathogen involved and determine its susceptibility to anti-infectious therapies. Gram stains and cultures on blood, chocolate, and Sabouraud agar

plates should be routinely examined. When *Acanthamoeba* or atypical mycobacteria are suspected, non-nutrient *Escherichia coli*-enriched agar or Loewenstein–Jensen media may be required for culture. PCR analysis should be carried out on corneal scrapes, particularly when *Acanthamoeba* or herpesviruses are suspected. Collaboration between the biologist and the ophthalmologist is essential to optimize the chances of isolating the pathogen. In the absence of positive results, rescraping or corneal biopsy may be performed, particularly if antibiotics were empirically prescribed.

■ Treatment

The therapeutic management of corneal infectious keratitis should target the three main pathogenetic aspects of the disease, namely the infection, the inflammation, and the ulceration.

Infection

Corneal ulcer is a sight-threatening condition generally considered as an ophthalmologic emergency, requiring antibiotic therapy based on clinical signs and symptoms and on the aspect and severity of the lesion. Because an antibiotic treatment has often been initiated before the microbiologic tests are performed, the cultures may prove negative. Hence, clinical examination remains essential in the management of infectious keratitis.

Topical anti-infectious therapy represents a first-line treatment for corneal ulcer with medications, ranging from monotherapy based on commercially available antibiotics to combinations of fortified antibiotics. While combinations of fortified antibiotics are generally used in severe cases of corneal ulcer, several studies have reported the efficacy of wide-spectrum, commercially available topical antibiotics, such as the latest generation of quinolones. However, it should be noted that the use of quinolones as monotherapy carries the potential risk of developing resistance. Thus, the choice between commercially available antibiotics compared with fortified combinations will depend on their relative safety ratios weighted according to the severity of the corneal ulcer. The bacterial spectrum of commercially available topical antibiotics is shown in **Table 22.1**.

Recently, intrastromal injections of anti-infective agents, such as cefuroxime, amphotericin B, and voriconazole, have been proposed for the treatment of severe bacterial and fungal corneal ulcers.

Whereas additional studies are required to confirm tolerance and efficacy of this technique, this mode of treatment may enhance the corneal concentration of the anti-infective agents and the healing rate (Garcia-Valenzuela & Song 2005, Prakash et al. 2008).

Inflammation

Herpetic keratitis involving the corneal stroma or endothelium has been shown to benefit from topical steroid therapy in association with antiviral agents. This therapeutic approach is also advocated by several corneal specialists for bacterial ulcers, with the objective of reducing immune-mediated tissue damage and scarring. Steroids should be avoided when fungal infection cannot be excluded or before the first clinical signs of improvement are observed (Araki-Sasaki et al. 2009, Gabison et al. 2007, O'Brien et al. 1996).

Ulceration

Several factors contribute to the progression of stromal thinning. They include the presence of a persistent epithelial defect with abnormal corneal epithelial–stromal interactions, the infiltration of inflammatory cells, and the toxicity of topical antibiotics or anti-inflammatory agents (Gabison et al. 2009). Proteases, such as matrix metalloproteinases, are overexpressed in corneal ulcers so that corneal epithelial and stromal cells, inflammatory cells, and infectious agents may all contribute to proteolysis of the corneal stroma. The modulation of the rate of instillation of the topical treatment and the use of appropriate therapeutic windows may help in the healing process.

The amniotic membrane (AM) inlay graft has been proposed in cases of severe infectious corneal ulcers. An AM graft may ameliorate healing and offer antalgic benefits. Moreover, in perforated ulcers, an AM graft could replace 'à chaud' keratoplasty. In such cases, penetrating keratoplasty would be performed secondarily with a lower risk of graft rejection (Gicquel et al. 2007, Nubile et al. 2007, Yildiz et al. 2008).

An AM graft may also be used in the management of a persistent epithelial defect or sterile corneal ulceration following intense topical antibiotherapy. Therapeutic keratoplasty is usually performed in the case of large corneal perforations or in uncontrolled fungal keratitis with a centrifugal extension (Parthasarathy & Tan 2007, Sony et al. 2002, Xie et al. 2007, Yildiz et al. 2008).

◼ REFERENCES

Araki-Sasaki K, Sonoyama H, Kawasaki T, et al. Candida albicans keratitis modified by steroid application. *Clin Ophthalmol* 2009; **3**:231–234.

Argueso P, Gipson IK. Epithelial mucins of the ocular surface: structure, biosynthesis and function. *Exp Eye Res* 2001; **73**:281–289.

Cochereau I, Goldschmidt P, Goepogui A, et al. Efficacy and safety of short duration azithromycin eye drops versus azithromycin single oral dose for the treatment of trachoma in children—a randomised, controlled, double-masked clinical trial. *Br J Ophthalmol* 2007a; **91**:667–672.

Cochereau I, Meddeb-Ouertani A, Khairallah M, et al. 3-Day treatment with azithromycin 1.5% eye drops versus 7-day treatment with tobramycin 0.3% for purulent bacterial conjunctivitis: multicentre, randomised and controlled trial in adults and children. *Br J Ophthalmol* 2007b; **91**:465–469.

Gabison EE, Alfonsi N, Doan S, et al. Archipelago keratitis: a clinical variant of recurrent herpetic keratitis? *Ophthalmology* 2007; **114**:2000–2005.

Garcia-Valenzuela E, Song CD. Intracorneal injection of amphotericin B for recurrent fungal keratitis and endophthalmitis. *Arch Ophthalmol* 2005; **123**:1721–1723.

Gicquel JJ, Bejjani RA, Ellies P, Mercie M, Dighiero P. Amniotic membrane transplantation in severe bacterial keratitis. *Cornea* 2007; **26**:27–33.

Gigliotti F, Hendley JO, Morgan J, et al. Efficacy of topical antibiotic therapy in acute conjunctivitis in children. *J Pediatr* 1984; **104**:623–626.

Jeng BH, Holsclaw DS. Cyclosporine A 1% eye drops for the treatment of subepithelial infiltrates after adenoviral keratoconjunctivitis. *Cornea* 2011; **30**:958–961.

Nubile M, Carpineto P, Lanzini M, et al. Multilayer amniotic membrane transplantation for bacterial keratitis with corneal perforation after hyperopic photorefractive keratectomy: case report and literature review. *J Cataract Refract Surg* 2007; **33**:1636–1640.

O'Brien WJ, Segundo AP, Guy J, Dorn EM, Taylor JL. Herpetic stromal disease: response to acyclovir/steroid therapy. *Acta Ophthalmol Scand* 1996; **74**:265–270.

Parthasarathy A, Tan DT. Deep lamellar keratoplasty for acanthamoeba keratitis. *Cornea* 2007; **26**:1021–1023.

Prakash G, Sharma N, Goel M, Titiyal JS, Vajpayee RB. Evaluation of intrastromal injection of voriconazole as a therapeutic adjunctive for the management of deep recalcitrant fungal keratitis. *Am J Ophthalmol* 2008; **146**:56–59.

Romanowski EG, Roba LA, Wiley L, et al. The effects of corticosteroids of adenoviral replication. *Arch Ophthalmol* 1996; **114**:581–585.

Schechter BA, Rand WJ, Velazquez GE, et al. Treatment of conjunctival papillomata with topical interferon Alfa-2b. *Am J Ophthalmol* 2002; **134**:268–270.

Sony P, Sharma N, Vajpayee RB, Ray M. Therapeutic keratoplasty for infectious keratitis: a review of the literature. *Clao J* 2002; **28**:111–118.

Thomas PA, Geraldine P. Infectious keratitis. *Curr Opin Infect Dis* 2007; **20**:129–141.

Uchio E, Ishiko H, Aoki K, et al. Adenovirus detected by polymerase chain reaction in multidose eyedrop bottles used by patients with adenoviral keratoconjunctivitis. *Am J Ophthalmol* 2002; **134**:618–619.

van Bijsterveld OP, Jager GV. Infectious diseases of the conjunctiva and cornea. *Curr Opin Ophthalmol* 1996; **7**:65–70.

World Health Organization. Trachoma control. A guide for program managers. 2006.

World Health Organization. *Global Health Observatory*. 2011.

Xie L, Zhai H, Shi W. Penetrating keratoplasty for corneal perforations in fungal keratitis. *Cornea* 2007; **26**:158–162.

Yamazaki ES, Ferraz CA, Hazarbassanov RM, et al. Phototherapeutic keratectomy for the treatment of corneal opacities after epidemic keratoconjunctivitis. *Am J Ophthalmol* 2011; **151**:35–43.

Yildiz EH, Nurozler AB, Ozkan Aksoy N, et al. Amniotic membrane transplantation: indications and results. *Eur J Ophthalmol* 2008; **18**:685–690.

Chapter 23 Ocular allergy

Stefano Bonini, Flavio Mantelli

INTRODUCTION

Allergic diseases have dramatically increased in the last decades, and ocular allergy has become one of the most common clinical conditions encountered in the general and ophthalmologic clinical practice (Canonica et al. 2007). Specifically, in a recent survey it has been reported that this condition accounts for up to 25% of all the ocular surface diseases (Lambiase et al. 2009b). The worldwide increase in ocular allergy prevalence has been attributed to an increased use of contact lenses, an increased exposure to environmental factors such as smoke and pollution, and an increase in related atopic disorders (Mantelli et al. 2011a).

The clinical features of ocular allergic disease are characterized by their wide variety and include several different clinical entities: the most common forms are the seasonal allergic conjunctivitis (SAC)—often named 'hay fever'—and perennial allergic conjunctivitis (PAC); other forms include the atopic keratoconjunctivitis (AKC), vernal keratoconjunctivitis (VKC), and giant papillary conjunctivitis (GPC). Allergic reactions to topical ophthalmic drugs are also common, although the recent advent of preservative-free compounds has largely reduced their frequency. These clinical entities include a wide variety of clinical conditions with different clinical features, different immunopathology, different evolution, and different response to therapy (Friedlaender 2011). The differential diagnosis between these different forms of ocular allergy may be difficult, but the presence of conjunctival papillae or follicles, the type of conjunctival secretion, the involvement of the cornea, and the prevalence of specific symptoms, such as itching, redness, burning, photophobia, tearing, or dryness, usually allow a proper identification of most cases (Belfort et al. 2000). Moreover, in spite of the substantial differences in clinical presentation, all the allergic manifestations of the ocular surface generally show a favorable response to topical steroids, and the use of antiallergic eye drops (such as mast cells stabilizers or the new generation of multiple action agents) seems to control the ocular manifestations of the disease (Bielory 2008). In line with these characteristics, it is not uncommon that ocular allergies are grouped together, since they all share common anamnestic, immune, clinical, and therapeutic features: the presence of personal and/or family history for other atopic-associated diseases; the detection of high serum and tear levels of total IgE and the presence of specific allergen sensitization detectable by radioallergosorbent test (RAST); inflammatory cells such as mast cells, eosinophils, lymphocytes, as well as Th2-derived cytokines and chemical mediators infiltrating the conjunctival epithelium and substantia propria, probably responsible for the common clinical signs (e.g. hyperemia and papillae) and symptoms (e.g. itching) observed in all the ocular allergic patients (Mantelli et al. 2009).

Nevertheless, once the initial diagnosis of ocular allergy is made, there are several well-accepted parameters available that can be used to identify different ocular allergy subgroups. For instance, SAC and PAC are generally benign and self-limited conditions, with mild to moderate symptoms and no corneal involvement or long-term complications caused by the allergic inflammatory process. On the other hand, VKC and AKC frequently involve the cornea in the inflammatory process and have a wide spectrum of clinical presentations, ranging from mild to severe sight-threatening conditions. In fact, during the course of these diseases, the intense allergic inflammation does not spare the cornea, and at a later stage, the signs of tissue remodeling may appear with fibrosis, scarring, and reduction of the corneal transparency, which ultimately lead to permanent visual impairment.

The following is an overview of the main forms of ocular allergic disease, with a brief presentation of their specific diagnostic, therapeutic, and prognostic characteristics.

SEASONAL ALLERGIC CONJUNCTIVITIS

SAC, also known as hay fever, is the most common form of ocular allergy. Several studies have highlighted that grass and ragweed pollens are the most important seasonal triggers for this condition (Halken 2004). SAC usually affects young adults, 20–40 years old, with similar prevalence in males and females. Patients usually complain the onset of their allergic symptoms during spring and fall. Ocular symptoms are usually bilateral and include red, itchy eyes, with associated burning and watering. In more severe cases, patients also refer to photophobia and blurred vision, and swollen eyelids and conjunctival chemosis are observed at the physical examination. Allergic rhinitis symptoms are often associated to the ocular clinical picture, with watery nasal discharge and sneezing (Canonica et al. 2007).

Diagnosis is usually confirmed by a personal or family history of atopic diseases, positive allergy testing for seasonal or perennial allergies, and symptoms suggestive of ocular allergic diseases. Among all the available laboratory tests, the following may help making a proper diagnosis: elevated serum IgE levels are found in 78% SAC patients; increased mast cell infiltration of the conjunctiva in 61%; and elevated mast cell tryptase in tears following conjunctival allergen challenge in almost all patients. Eosinophil infiltration in conjunctival scraping may also be helpful but is not highly specific of SAC, being observed in only 25% of all confirmed cases. Among all the symptoms of SAC, ocular allergy specialists have clearly and unanimously stated that itching is the hallmark of ocular allergy. While this is certainly not specific for diagnosing SAC, it could be safely assumed that there is no ocular allergy without itching and in the absence of this important symptom a different diagnosis should be taken into account. Lastly, the response to antiallergic therapy may also help in the differential diagnosis. Specifically, a positive response to topical antihistamine medications is helpful in confirming the diagnosis of SAC, while failure to respond to such medications should move to a search for a different form of ocular allergy or for a different cause of conjunctivitis (Bielory et al. 2005). Further effective therapeutic options for SAC patients include mast cell stabilizers and novel multiple-action antiallergic compounds, such as azelastine, epinastine, ketotifen, and olopatadine (Lambiase et al. 2009a). Corticosteroids and other immunomodulatory agents are usually not required in the management of patients with SAC.

Since the allergic inflammatory process does not affect the cornea, the prognosis of SAC is benign even in the more severe and long-lasting cases.

PERENNIAL ALLERGIC CONJUNCTIVITIS

PAC is another very common form of ocular allergy, considered a less severe variant of SAC but characterized by year-round symptoms with seasonal exacerbations in up to 79% of cases. Patients with PAC and SAC do not have substantial differences in age and gender, and share the same prevalence of associated symptoms of asthma or eczema. However, patients with PAC have a significantly higher prevalence of associated perennial rhinitis or other allergic manifestations (up to 95% of patients). Some reports indicate a higher prevalence of eosinophils in PAC conjunctival scraping as compared to SAC (up to 43% as compared to 25%, respectively), but this finding has yet to be confirmed by large population studies and remains non-specific and of relative diagnostic value. Another difference with SAC is that dust mites and animal dander/feathers are thought to be the most important triggers for PAC (Dart et al. 1986).

Taken into account the above-mentioned differences, the diagnosis of PAC is usually made following the same clinical and laboratory evaluations described for SAC, with allergen testing directed primarily toward dust mites. Positive response to topical antiallergic treatment is typical of PAC and the prognosis is also benign.

ATOPIC KERATOCONJUNCTIVITIS

AKC is a severe chronic inflammatory disease of the conjunctiva, possibly leading to visual impairment due to the associated corneal involvement. The disease occurs more frequently in males and is observed in both young children and adults (20–50 years old), being more common and usually more severe in the latter. Symptoms referred by patients with AKC are often non-specific and include intense itching, photophobia, burning, and foreign body sensation. Therefore, diagnosis is better addressed through the observation of typical ocular signs associated with eczema of the lids and/or of other parts of the body. In fact, the presence or history of atopic dermatitis is recorded in 95% of patients with AKC, often associated with asthma (87%) and allergic rhinitis. The classical clinical signs of AKC are represented by hyperemia of the conjunctiva and episcleral vessels, papillae on the upper tarsal conjunctiva, mucous filaments in the morning urine, maceration of the eyelids' skin, and the presence of concomitant blepharitis. Conjunctival scarring with subepithelial fibrosis, fornix foreshortening, symblepharon and corneal ulceration,

and neovascularization may also be observed in more severe cases (Bonini 2004). Conjunctival scarring and loss of corneal transparency are also seen as long-term complications and are common to all the severe forms of chronic allergic keratoconjunctivitis (**Figure 23.1**). Although the diagnosis should be straightforward in most cases presenting the above characteristics, specific laboratory parameters may help identify uncertain cases: increased levels of total serum IgE, conjunctival eosinophil infiltration, and eosinophils in tears are typical but non-specific; squamous metaplasia of the conjunctival epithelium and goblet cell loss with decreased levels of the goblet cell-specific secretory gel-forming mucin MUC5AC are more characteristic of this form of ocular allergy. These cytologic alterations trigger a detrimental loop in which the reduced lubrication increases the allergen exposure, induces a progressive loss of the ocular surface wet-surfaced phenotype, and ultimately leads to epithelial damage (Mantelli & Argüeso 2008). Concomitant to the decrease in MUC5AC documented in tear and impression cytology samples from patients with AKC, there is an increase in the expression of membrane-bound mucins MUC1, MUC2, and MUC4, which may represent a defense mechanism to compensate for the loss of protection provided by the goblet cell mucin MUC5AC (Dogru et al. 2005).

The management of AKC is often a therapeutic challenge because of the chronicity of the disease and the possible complications secondary to corneal ulceration, such as infection and scarring. Moreover, therapy for AKC needs to be aimed solely not only at the corneal and conjunctival involvement but also at all the other components of the disease, especially the eyelids. Lid margin and periorbital eczema are treated with emollients and steroid ointment, while topical antibiotics or systemic tetracyclines and macrolides are useful for managing ulcerative blepharitis.

Assuming that the marginal lid disease is controlled by the above measures, AKC therapy may be divided into conservative measures and higher risk second-line therapeutic agents. Conservative measures include cold compresses, lubrication with preservative-free eye drops, and the use of topical multiple-action antiallergic compounds. Patients with more severe disease often require the use of second-line therapeutic agents, starting with prolonged courses of topical or oral steroids. To reduce the risk of secondary cataract and glaucoma in these patients, topical steroid-sparing immunosuppressive agents, including cyclosporin A and tacrolimus, can be used.

The prognosis of AKC is variable, but it is often poor in terms of patients' comfort and vision in the most severe cases, aggravated by long-term complications of both the disease and its treatments.

VERNAL KERATOCONJUNCTIVITIS

VKC is a recurrent bilateral chronic allergic inflammatory disease of the ocular surface affecting mainly young men in the first decade of life. Diagnosis is based on signs and symptoms, including intense itching, intense photophobia, sticky mucus discharge, giant papillae ('cobblestone papillae') on the upper tarsal conjunctiva or at the

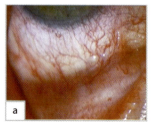
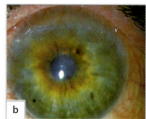
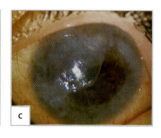

Figure 23.1 Scarring sequelae including fornix foreshortening, symblepharon (a), and neovascularization of the cornea in chronic keratoconjunctivitis (b) AKC and (c) VKC. A long-term control of the allergic inflammation is crucial to avoid permanent visual damage in patients affected by severe ocular allergies. AKC, atopic keratoconjunctivitis; VKC, vernal keratoconjunctivitis.

limbus, conjunctival hyperemia, superficial keratopathy, and corneal shield ulcer in up to 10% of patients (Leonardi 2002). Punctiform limbal concretions, known as 'Trantas dots,' may also be observed. As compared to the other forms of allergic conjunctivitis, photophobia is a major symptom in VKC and the typical patient is a young boy presenting to the ophthalmologist with dark sunglasses and a baseball hat to protect his eyes from light. Moreover, patients with VKC have a greater increase in the number of conjunctival goblet cells and MU-C5AC, which contribute to the abundant mucus discharge observed in these patients but might represent a protective mechanism aimed at clearing allergens from the ocular surface (Mantelli & Argüeso 2008). Patients with VKC frequently have a personal or family history of atopic diseases (such as asthma, rhinitis, and eczema), increased serum levels of total and specific IgE, and a positive response to antiallergic therapy. However, VKC is not associated with a positive skin test or RAST in approximately 45% of patients, suggesting that it is not solely an IgE-mediated disease. On the basis of challenge studies as well as immunohistochemical and mediator studies, a Th2-driven pathogenetic mechanism, with the involvement of mast cells, eosinophils, and lymphocytes at the conjunctiva, has been suggested. However, the exact pathogenic mechanism has yet to be fully elucidated. To date, VKC has largely been considered a type I hypersensitivity reaction.

Generally considered to be self-limited, the disease tends to subside spontaneously at puberty; however, some therapeutic measures may be required to control the disease in its active years. In fact, VKC is of widely varying severity, and complications secondary to severe and long-standing inflammation may lead to fibrovascular reaction, new collagen deposition, tissue remodeling, corneal opacification, and permanent visual impairment. Therefore, an early correct diagnostic and therapeutic approach is needed to avoid long-standing permanent inflammatory sequelae that make the visual prognosis poor (Mantelli et al. 2007).

As previously mentioned, the exact pathogenetic mechanism of VKC is still unknown and there is no specific therapy to treat this disease. Therapeutic management generally requires a combination of environmental control to avoid allergen exposure and pharmacotherapy or sometimes specific immunotherapy.

Pharmacotherapy may include the same agents used in the treatment of the other forms of allergic conjunctivitis such as topical antihistamine (H1 blockers), mast cell stabilizers, multiple-action antiallergic compounds, non-steroidal anti-inflammatory drugs (NSAIDs), corticosteroids, and cyclosporin A. These different agents need to be used depending on disease activity and severity, and based on the clinical characteristics of each patient, making it difficult to identify a gold standard treatment that may be suitable for all cases. To help ophthalmologists manage this challenging disease, a standardized grading system has recently been developed that allows to identify the more severe forms of VKC that are at higher risk of long-term complications and, therefore, need a more aggressive therapeutic approach (Sacchetti et al. 2010). Following a disease grading scheme to identify the best therapeutic regimen may be useful in all forms of ocular allergy. A therapeutic scheme for ocular allergy based on severity is proposed in **Figure 23.2**. It must be remembered, however, that all the available topical drugs do not completely control disease activity in VKC. In fact, they have been demonstrated to be effective only in reducing signs and symptoms during active phases, and cyclosporin A has also been shown effective in reducing the number of recurrences (Lambiase et al. 2011). Moreover, our recent meta-analysis has demonstrated that while currently available topical therapies (e.g. mast cell stabilizers, immunomodulators, NSAIDs, and antimitotic agents) are significantly more effective than placebo for treating most signs and symptoms of VKC, there is a lack of evidence to recommend the use of a specific type of medication for treating this disorder (Mantelli et al. 2007).

Interestingly, it has been proven that following topical antiallergic and anti-inflammatory treatments in VKC, there are reductions in conjunctival goblet cell number and MUC5AC expression. This, in turn, may reduce the sticky mucus discharge that represents one of the major symptomatic burdens for the young patients. Cold compresses may also provide symptomatic relief.

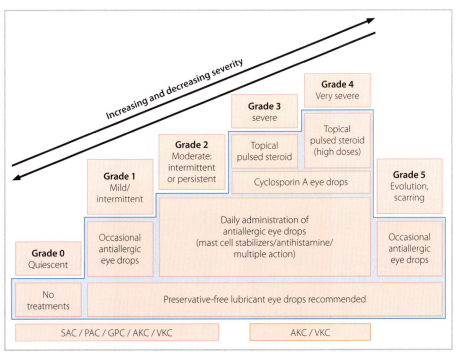

Figure 23.2 A therapeutic scheme for the different forms of allergic conjunctivitis based on disease activity and severity level is proposed. Antiallergic eye drops, from older antihistamine to newer multiple-action compounds, are useful to control disease activity in most forms of ocular allergy. In more severe cases, pulsed corticosteroid treatment may be needed and steroid-sparing agents such as cyclosporin A should always be considered to avoid long-term complications. Preservative-free lubricant eye drops should always be recommended because they act both to relieve symptoms, to reduce shear stress of follicles/papillae during blinking, and to dilute the allergen tear concentration. AKC, atopic keratoconjunctivitis; GPC, giant papillary conjunctivitis; PAC, perennial allergic conjunctivitis; SAC, seasonal allergic conjunctivitis; VKC, vernal keratoconjunctivitis

Corticosteroids must be used with extreme caution only in selected cases with severe inflammation and corneal involvement, to avoid the risk of long-term steroid use in these young patients. Cyclosporin A is an excellent steroid-sparing drug for VKC.

Due to its self-limited course, if disease activity is properly controlled without an excessive use of corticosteroids, the final prognosis of VKC is usually benign.

GIANT PAPILLARY CONJUNCTIVITIS

GPC is a condition observed in contact lens wearers, where contact lens deposits act as allergens. Contact lens wearers with a medical history of atopic diseases are at greater risk. Other people at risk of developing GPC include patients with exposed corneal and/or conjunctival sutures, and patients with ocular prostheses. The allergic response is considered to be an over-reaction of the immune system to immunogens/allergens that are deposited on foreign bodies at prolonged contact with the conjunctiva (Donshik et al. 2008). In fact, GPC incidence has drastically reduced with the advent of disposable contact lenses.

Initial presentation of GPC may occur even after years of prolonged contact lens wear, with intense itching after lens removal, mucus discharge, photophobia, and intolerance to contact lenses. The giant (measuring ^{3}1 mm) papillae at the upper tarsus may also cause mechanical corneal abrasion, resulting in intense pain and sudden decrease in vision.

This clinical giant papillary presentation, associated with the clinical history, should allow a proper and timely diagnosis. However, in somewhat doubtful cases laboratory testing may support the diagnosis: the histamine level in tears of patients with GPC remains in the normal range, while it is usually increased in all other forms of ocular allergy; cytologic scrapings from the conjunctiva of patients with GPC show the presence of T lymphocytes, mast cells, eosinophils, and basophils, suggesting an antigen–antibody mechanism (Ehlers & Donshik 2008).

Treatment of GPC requires the discontinuation of contact lens wear. However, while with this simple approach the prognosis is benign and long-term sight-threatening complications are rare, removing the contact lenses may result in an unbearable reduction in the quality of life for patients with severe ametropia who depend on contact lenses for their everyday activities. Similar is the case of patients with ocular prosthesis. Therefore, a variety of treatment strategies have been developed that enable patients with this condition to keep using contact lenses. Therapy can either be directed at decreasing the coating on the contact lens (which decreases the antigen load and trauma to the conjunctival surface) or can involve modulation of the immune reaction to these foreign bodies. In order to decrease the coating of contact lenses, it is necessary to instruct the patients on improving the cleaning and decreasing wearing time, or sometimes it is necessary to change the contact lens material or design. Topical corticosteroids, topical non-steroidal anti-inflammatory agents, and mast cell stabilizers help modulate the immune response.

ALLERGIC REACTIONS TO TOPICAL OPHTHALMIC COMPOUNDS

An allergic reaction is the most frequent clinical picture of ocular surface damage, induced by preservatives, additives, and/or drugs contained in topical ophthalmic preparations (Mantelli et al. 2011b). These reactions may take minutes to hours to manifest and generally require a sensitization time to develop, ranging from days to weeks after the exposure to a sensitizing agent.

The allergic reaction to ophthalmic compounds is characterized by conjunctival hyperemia and chemosis, lid swelling, eczema of the periorbital skin, tearing, photophobia, and intense itching caused by an IgE-mediated (type I) or by a delayed (type IV) hypersensitivity reaction (Baudouin 2005). As previously mentioned, these signs and symptoms are common to all the forms of ocular allergy, making it difficult for the ophthalmologist to diagnose the allergic reaction to a previous treatment. Therefore, a careful medical anamnesis is mandatory. Moreover, in chronic ocular allergy sufferers, vasodilation appears superficial and conjunctival hyperemia tends to appear pink rather than a deep red, as it appears in the case of an acute allergic reaction to a topical treatment (**Figure 23.3**).

An allergic reaction to a topical ophthalmic compound could affect any patient, but ocular allergy sufferers are at greatest risk, which is probably due to a higher frequency of conjunctival hyper-reactivity to non-specific stimuli among allergic patients. Therefore, especially for these patients, it is important to discriminate whether an ocular surface reaction is caused by allergic conjunctivitis or it is a consequence of a topical eye drop therapy.

The therapeutic approach to this disorder is straightforward because it requires the elimination of the sensitizing agent. In most cases the choice of preservative-free analogues resolves the clinical picture. Although there is plenty of literature showing an increased risk of developing an allergic reaction to preservatives in eye drops, a similar response may also be elicited by hypersensitivity to the medical compound itself.

The prognosis is excellent, although if it becomes necessary to eliminate a topical treatment that the patient was using for a preexisting condition, there could be difficulties in managing the underlying disease.

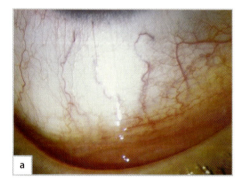

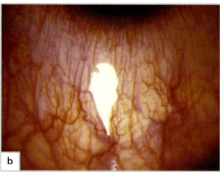

Figure 23.3 A red eye is a common sign of ocular surface disease and is not specific for the different forms of ocular allergy. However, some characteristics of the red eye may help the ophthalmologist identify the correct diagnosis. In chronic ocular allergy sufferers (a), vasodilation appears superficial and conjunctival hyperemia tends to appear pink rather than deep red, as it appears in the case of an acute allergic reaction to a topical treatment (b).

■ DIFFERENTIAL DIAGNOSIS

As previously mentioned, ocular allergic disorders include a wide variety of clinical conditions with different clinical features, which may be common to other forms of ocular surface disease. In this chapter, we focus on the most common disorders that share clinical characteristics with ocular allergic reactions and go often misdiagnosed in the clinical practice.

Probably the most frequent ocular surface disorder, primarily affecting the conjunctiva and resembling ocular allergy, is chlamydia infection, which is the most common treatable sexually transmitted infection, with up to 10% prevalence in young adults (Baguley & Greenhouse 2003). The typical presentation of this disease is with a chronic follicular conjunctivitis lasting >16 days (often several months, especially if misdiagnosed), in which a corneal involvement with punctate keratitis, subepithelial infiltrates, and limbal edema may manifest as early as in the second week. Not only the clinical sign but also the chronic course characterized by several remission and exacerbation phases may be overlooked as an allergic conjunctivitis or keratoconjunctivitis (Bielory 2007). However, the absence of a personal or family history of atopy, the lack of association with other allergic diseases, and the lack of response to common antiallergic therapies should help in the differential diagnosis. Laboratory testing may also be helpful, with a conjunctival scraping, providing certain diagnosis through the identification of chlamydial intracytoplasmic inclusion bodies.

Another clinical condition sharing many aspects of the classical ocular allergies has recently been described in a group of young women with bilateral, persistent ocular surface discomfort characterized by itching, excessive mucus production, dryness, and contact lens intolerance (Bonini et al. 2007). All these women were affected by polycystic ovary syndrome (PCOS), the most common endocrine abnormality in women of reproductive age. With a prevalence of PCOS estimated between 6.5% and 8%, 4 million reproductive-age women in the United States and approximately 105 million women affected worldwide, we believe it is important to include this condition in the differential diagnosis of ocular allergy.

In our prospective study, we described the presence of conjunctival hyperemia, follicular reaction, mucus hypersecretion, and occasional superficial punctate keratopathy, associated with itching, dryness, and contact lens intolerance in 94% of the consecutive patients with PCOS enrolled. The affected patients had signs and symptoms resembling those of two major ocular surface disorders: dryness and punctate keratopathy as usually seen in dry eye disease; and mucus discharge, itching, follicular reaction, and contact lens intolerance as usually seen in ocular allergy (**Figure 23.4**). Therefore, we have proposed that these ocular surface symptoms represent a distinct clinical entity associated with hormonal imbalance in PCOS and named the condition 'IDEA' for the acronym of 'itchy-dry eye associated' with PCOS.

It is interesting that, although most symptoms of IDEA syndrome are common to ocular allergy, there was evidence of systemic sensitization in only 20% of the symptomatic patients, and there was no history or evidence of previous ocular allergy, no association with other allergic diseases, and no response to common antiallergic treatments to support the diagnosis of allergic conjunctivitis.

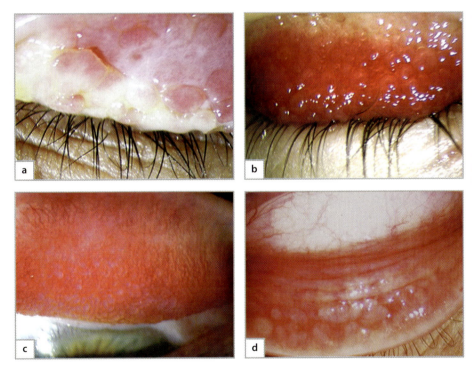

Figure 23.4 Mucus secretion and conjunctival follicular or papillar reaction may be observed in both ocular allergy—(a) VKC, (b) GPC, (c) chlamydia infection, and (d) IDEA syndrome—and other ocular surface diseases. Although a careful ophthalmic evaluation including upper eyelid eversion is mandatory for a correct diagnosis of ocular allergy, several diseases may mimic its characteristic clinical features. Therefore, a careful investigation of associated allergic disorders and family history of atopy, and additional laboratory tests, are often necessary. GPC, giant papillary conjunctivitis; IDEA, itchy-dry eye associated; VKC, vernal keratoconjunctivitis.

REFERENCES

Baguley S, Greenhouse P. Non-genital manifestations of *Chlamydia trachomatis*. *C Clin Med* 2003; **3**:206–208.

Baudouin C. Allergic reaction to topical eyedrops. *Curr Opin Allergy Clin Immunol* 2005; **5**:459–463.

Belfort R, Marbeck P, Hsu CC, Freitas D. Epidemiological study of 134 subjects with allergic conjunctivitis. *Acta Ophthalmol Scand Suppl* 2000; **230**:38–40.

Bielory L. Differential diagnoses of conjunctivitis for clinical allergist-immunologists. *Ann Allergy Asthma Immunol* 2007; **98**:105–114.

Bielory L. Ocular allergy treatment. *Immunol Allergy Clin North Am* 2008; **28**:189–224.

Bielory L, Lien KW, Bigelsen S. Efficacy and tolerability of newer antihistamines in the treatment of allergic conjunctivitis. *Drugs* 2005; **65**:215–228.

Bonini S. Atopic keratoconjunctivitis. *Allergy* 2004; **59**:71–73.

Bonini S, Mantelli F, Moretti C, et al. Itchy-dry eye associated with polycystic ovary syndrome. *Am J Ophthalmol* 2007; **143**:763–771.

Canonica GW, Bousquet J, Mullol J, Scadding GK, Virchow JC. A survey of the burden of allergic rhinitis in Europe. *Allergy* 2007; **62**:17–25.

Dart JK, Buckley RJ, Monnickendan M, Prasad J. Perennial allergic conjunctivitis: definition, clinical characteristics and prevalence. A comparison with seasonal allergic conjunctivitis. *Trans Ophthalmol Soc U K* 1986; **105**:513–520.

Dogru M, Okada N, Asano-Kato N, et al. Atopic ocular surface disease: implications on tear function and ocular surface mucins. *Cornea* 2005; **24**:S18–S23.

Donshik PC, Ehlers WH, Ballow M. Giant papillary conjunctivitis. *Immunol Allergy Clin North Am* 2008; **28**:83–103.

Ehlers WH, Donshik PC. Giant papillary conjunctivitis. *Curr Opin Allergy Clin Immunol* 2008; **8**:445–449.

Friedlaender MH. Ocular allergy. *Curr Opin Allergy Clin Immunol* 2011; **11**:477–482.

Halken S. Prevention of allergic disease in childhood: clinical and epidemiological aspects of primary and secondary allergy prevention. *Pediatr Allergy Immunol* 2004; **15**:4–5; 9–32.

Lambiase A, Leonardi A, Sacchetti M, et al. Topical cyclosporine prevents seasonal recurrences of vernal keratoconjunctivitis in a randomized, double-masked, controlled 2-year study. *J Allergy Clin Immunol* 2011; **128**:896–897.

Lambiase A, Micera A, Bonini S. Multiple action agents and the eye: do they really stabilize mast cells? *Curr Opin Allergy Clin Immunol* 2009a; **9**:454–465.

Lambiase A, Minchiotti S, Leonardi A, et al. Prospective, multicentre demographic and epidemiological study on vernal keratoconjunctivitis: a glimpse of ocular surface in Italian population. *Ophthalmic Epidemiol* 2009b; **16**:38–41.

Leonardi A. Vernal keratoconjunctivitis: pathogenesis and treatment. *Prog Retin Eye Res* 2002; **21**:319–339.

Mantelli F, Argüeso P. Functions of ocular surface mucins in health and disease. *Curr Opin Allergy Clin Immunol* 2008; **8**:477–483.

Mantelli F, Lambiase A, Bonini S. A simple and rapid diagnostic algorithm for the detection of ocular allergic diseases. *Curr Opin Allergy Clin Immunol* 2009; **9**:471–476.

Mantelli F, Lambiase A, Bonini S, Bonini S. Clinical trials in allergic conjunctivitis: a systematic review. *Allergy* 2011a; **66**:919–924.

Mantelli F, Santos MS, Petitti T, et al. Systematic review and meta-analysis of randomised clinical trials on topical treatments for vernal keratoconjunctivitis. *Br J Ophthalmol* 2007; **91**:1656–1661.

Mantelli F, Tranchina L, Lambiase A, Bonini S. Ocular surface damage by ophthalmic compounds. *Curr Opin Allergy Clin Immunol* 2011b; **11**:464–470.

Sacchetti M, Lambiase A, Mantelli F, et al. Tailored approach to the treatment of vernal keratoconjunctivitis. *Ophthalmology* 2010; **117**:1294–1299.

Chapter 24 — Limbal stem cell deficiency

Takashi Kojima, Murat Dogru

INTRODUCTION

Corneal stem cells lie in the corneal limbus, the junctional area between the cornea and the conjunctiva. They contribute to a healthy smooth corneal surface, which is essential for achieving a perfect optical surface. Stem cells are defined as undifferentiated cells that can divide indefinitely and generate differentiated cells. Under stable conditions, they divide in an asymmetric manner. The daughter cells move toward the central cornea and become transient amplifying cells (TACs) (**Figure 24.1**). TACs correspond to the corneal basal epithelial cells and divide more frequently than stem cells, but have a limited proliferative potential (Lehrer et al. 1998). The basal epithelial cells divide, differentiate, and finally slough off from the surface. Stem cells are believed to lie in a protected microenvironment called the niche. This area contains heavily pigmented cells to avoid the adverse effects of ultraviolet light. The area surrounding stem cells is also highly innervated and vascularized (Goldberg & Bron 1982, Lawrenson & Ruskell 1991), which provides the limbal epithelium with nutrition and greater exposure to blood-borne factors that may play a role in stem cell function (Zieske 1994).

Lack of limbal stem cells is referred to as limbal stem cell deficiency (LSCD). There are various disorders that cause LSCD, such as burns (thermal or chemical), congenital aniridia, Stevens–Johnson syndrome (SJS), ocular mucous membrane pemphigoid (OcMMP), ocular surface tumors, and infections. The corneal epithelium has a homeostasis to maintain a smooth epithelial surface. The balance of homeostasis in corneal epithelium is often explained by the XYZ theory of Thoft and Friend (**Figure 24.2**) (Thoft & Friend 1983). The corneal epithelium is maintained by three factors: healthy function of stem cells, centripetal movement of TACs, and sloughing of epithelium. Imbalances of this system may cause superficial punctate keratopathy and epithelial defects. Patients complain of various symptoms such as foreign body sensation, pain, photophobia, and decreased vision.

DIAGNOSIS OF LSCD

There is no direct methodology to confirm the existence of limbal stem cells. Clinically, the existence of palisades of Vogt (POV) is believed to be the marker of healthy corneal limbal cell function (Townsend 1991). POV are fold-like structures at the limbus (**Figure 24.3a**). There are racial and age-related variations in the observability of POV (Goldberg & Bron 1982). Additionally, it is getting hard to confirm POV by aging (Goldberg & Bron 1982, Zheng & Zu 2008). Generally, POV at the 12 o'clock and 6 o'clock positions are easy to confirm, but hard to confirm at the 3 o'clock and 9 o'clock positions (Goldberg & Bron 1982). Recently laser scanning confocal microscopy has been used for examining a variety of ocular surface diseases such as dry eye disease (Kojima et al. 2010), meibomian gland dysfunction (Ibrahim et al. 2010), corneal dystrophies (Kobayashi et al. 2007), and ocular surface tumors. Four characteristic structures in the limbal area have been observed with the laser scanning confocal microscopy (Kobayashi & Sugiyama 2005, Patel et al. 2006, Shortt et al. 2007, Zheng & Zu 2008): (i) hyper-reflective parallel trabecular extensions with an internal acellular region, (ii) border of bright cell groups and dark cell groups, (iii) hyper-reflective cells, and (iv) bright corpuscular particles with a dendritic cell-like morphology. Takahashi et al. (2009) reported that hyper-reflective parallel trabecular extensions with an internal acellular region were correlated with the existence of POV among these four features.

In partial LSCD, remaining stem cells can maintain a healthy corneal epithelium. However, if the area of LSCD enlarges, the remaining stem cells may not maintain the regenerative process related to the

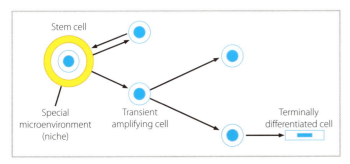

Figure 24.1 Differentiation of corneal limbal stem cell. Corneal limbal stem cell lies in a special microenvironment called the niche. The corneal epithelial stem cell divides into daughter cells. One daughter cell becomes the transient amplifying cell and the other replenishes the stem cell. Transient amplifying cells further divide and differentiate, and finally become terminally differentiated cells.

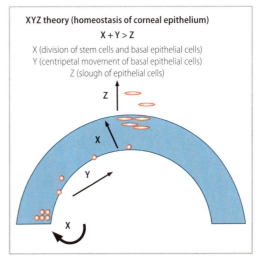

XYZ theory (homeostasis of corneal epithelium)

$$X + Y > Z$$

X (division of stem cells and basal epithelial cells)
Y (centripetal movement of basal epithelial cells)
Z (slough of epithelial cells)

Figure 24.2 XYZ theory to explain the homeostasis of corneal epithelium. In the stable condition, X (division of stem cells and basal epithelial cells) plus Y (centripetal movement of basal epithelial cells) exceeds Z (slough of epithelial cells).

corneal epithelium, which will lead to the invasion of conjunctiva. In these conditions, the cornea is partially covered with conjunctiva, resulting in an irregular optical surface. Fluorescein staining can reveal the conjunctival invasion in terms of hyperpermeability to fluorescence staining and observability of an irregular surface at slit-lamp microscopy (**Figure 24.3b** and **24.3c**). When total limbal deficiency occurs, the conjunctiva invades the cornea from a 360° perimeter (**Figure 24.3d**). Under such conditions, conjunctival invasion is accompanied by new vessel invasion. The presence of neovascularization depends on the existence of corneal epithelium that harbors antiangiogenic factors (Lim et al. 2009).

◼ Ocular surface diseases associated with LSCD

Causes of LSCD may be congenital and acquired. Causes of congenital LSCD include aniridia, whereas etiologies of acquired LSCD include thermal burns, chemical burns, SJS, OcMMP, graft-versus-host disease, drug toxicity, radiation, and trachoma.

Thermal or chemical burn

Burns on the ocular surface by radiant energy or chemicals damage the limbal stem cells. Alkali chemicals are lipophilic and penetrate the eyes more rapidly than acids, causing more severe ocular damage. According to the Kinoshita grading system after chemical burns, grade 3b (total corneal epithelial defect and total loss of POV) and grade 4 (>50% of area in limbal conjunctiva showing necrosis, total corneal epithelial defect, and total loss of POV) end up with a poor prognosis regarding visual function (Kinoshita & Manabe 1993).

Stevens–Johnson syndrome

In SJS, high fever, malaise, and upper respiratory infection symptoms, such as sore throat and cough, are usually followed by a vesicular eruption of the mucous membranes. In some patients, the acute immune response may damage the limbal stem cell functions. Inflammation of the conjunctiva may result in scar formation and obstruct the secretion of tear fluid. Even if the acute phase of SJS is resolved, chronic dryness, inflammation, and ulceration of the conjunctiva or cornea may destroy corneal epithelial stem cells at the limbus. Additionally, acute and chronic inflammation of the conjunctival tissues can cause keratinization of the eyelid margin and obstruction of the lacrimal gland duct, which can result in friction between the eyelid and ocular surface and worsen the LSCD (Wall et al. 2003).

Ocular mucous membrane pemphigoid

OcMMP is an autoimmune disease that causes deposition of immunoreactants (e.g. IgG, IgA, IgM, and/or complement) along the epithelial basement membrane zone (Kirzhner & Jakobiec 2011). Chronic inflammation may result in the loss of conjunctival/corneal stem cells and scarring. Subsequently, keratinization of the eyelid margin, meibomian gland dysfunction, and decreased tear volume may cause corneal epithelium damage (Foster & Sainz De La Maza 2004, Saw & Dart 2008). Obstruction of the lacrimal glands by inflammatory adhesions is thought to be the cause of decreased tear secretion volume (Dart 2005, Foster & Sainz De La Maza 2004).

Many OcMMP patients complain of severe dry eyes. For the differential diagnosis of dry eye disease, OcMMP should always be kept in mind.

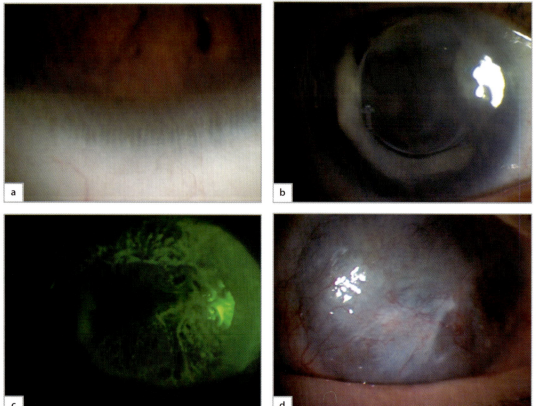

Figure 24.3 (a) Palisades of Vogt showing the presence of healthy limbal stem cells. (b) A case of aniridia (35 years old woman) showing partial LSCD. Partial LSCD generally accompanies non-vascularized conjunctiva. (c) Corneal fluorescein staining of the same patient. Fluorescein staining revealed conjunctival invasion, showing irregular and hyperfluorescence area on the cornea. (d) Total LSCD showing invasion of vascularized conjunctiva with subconjunctival fibrovascular tissue in the entire cornea. LSCD, limbal stem cell deficiency.

Aniridia

Aniridia is a congenital, bilateral, panocular disorder that occurs with an incidence of 1:64,000–1:96,000 (Kokotas & Petersen 2010, Shaw et al. 1960). This disorder is characterized by complete or partial absence of the iris and iris hypoplasia. Aniridia is commonly associated with other ocular anomalies, including cataracts, glaucoma, optic nerve hypoplasia, foveal hypoplasia, and LSCD. Based on the research using transgenic animals, involvement of *PAX6* gene mutation has been identified as a cause of aniridia. The incidence of LSCD in aniridia has been reported to be 20% (Tseng & Li 1996).

■ Treatment of limbal stem cell dysfunction

Drug treatment

There is currently no effective treatment to improve total LSCD by pharmaceutical means. For partial LSCD, artificial tear eye drops can maintain the corneal smooth epithelium, especially in patients with dry eye disease. However, none of the commercially available artificial tear preparations include essential tear components such as epidermal growth factor, hepatocyte growth factor, fibronectin, neurotrophic growth factor, and vitamin A—all of which have been shown to play an important role in the maintenance of ocular surface epithelial milieu. As reported previously, autologous serum eye drops contain these essential factors, and autologous serum eye drops have been beneficial in the treatment of ocular surface diseases such as persistent epithelial defects, superior limbic keratoconjunctivitis, keratoconjunctivitis sicca, and neurotrophic keratopathy (Goto et al. 2001, Kojima et al. 2005, Matsumoto et al. 2004, Ogawa et al. 2003, Tsubota et al. 1999a and 1999b). Furthermore, serum contains lysozyme, IgG, and complement, which may reduce the risk of infection (Schrader et al. 2006). These characteristics of autologous serum eye drops may explain the beneficial effects related to the treatment of epithelial damage due to partial LSCD.

Bandage contact lenses have been shown to decrease the desquamation of the corneal epithelium by prevention of blink-associated mechanical stress and subsequent acceleration of wound healing (van Klink et al. 1993). Combination of therapeutic contact lens and serum eye drops has been reported to be effective in the treatment of severe persistent epithelial defect due to partial LSCD (Schrader et al. 2006).

Surgical treatment

For patients with partial LSCD, mechanical debridement of the conjunctivalized epithelium can be performed. This procedure can prevent conjunctival epithelial invasion and allow the corneal epithelium to heal efficiently (Dua et al. 1994). The success of this procedure depends on the remaining limbal stem cell function. Amniotic membrane transplantation has also been used as a biological contact lens after debridement in cases of partial LSCD (Anderson et al. 2001).

Limbal stem cell transplantation (LSCT) can be carried out for patients with total LSCD. During the corneal limbal transplantation procedure, the healthy corneal limbal and subepithelial tissues are sutured at the limbal area of the patients. Amniotic membrane transplantation can be performed with corneal limbal transplantation to accelerate the corneal epithelial wound healing (Dogru & Tsubota 2005). If the LSCD is limited to one eye, the patient can undergo an autologous LSCT. In autologous LSCT, the donor limbal tissue is harvested from the unaffected fellow eye. The advantage of this procedure is that no systemic immunosuppression is required. However, there is a risk of affecting the limbal stem cell function in the fellow eye. If the fellow eye also has weak limbal stem cell functions, this procedure cannot be chosen. Bilateral LSCD needs an allogenic LSCT. In this procedure, the donor tissue is obtained from a living related or cadaveric donor. Patients who undergo limbal allografts require systemic immunosuppression to prevent rejection of the grafts. Several studies have reported good short-term results of LSCT, but long-term results have been disappointing (Solomon et al. 2002, Tsubota et al. 1999). Since the cornea before LSCT is highly vascularized, rejection tends to occur and subsequent corneal limbal transplants cannot survive for a long time. The limbal graft survival rate is about 50% at 5 years despite the use of systemic immunosuppression, and it is even less if penetrating keratoplasty (PKP) is performed with LSCT to improve the visual function. Solomon et al. (2002) reported that LSCT performed alone resulted in higher survival of ambulatory vision at 2 years (86.1 ± 9.1%) compared with LSCT with PKP (46.9 ± 10.6%).

When the graft is created from central to paracentral part of the allogeneic cornea, it is called keratoepithelioplasty. Since the graft tissue does not include the limbal tissue, lower risk of immunological rejection compared to limbal transplantation is an advantage (Kinoshita 2002).

Recently, cultivated limbal epithelial stem cell transplantation has been performed to treat total LSCD. Pellegrini et al. (1997) reported the first successful results of autologous cultivated transplantation of the corneal epithelium from contralateral eyes. Corneal limbal tissue is taken by a small biopsy; the limbal stem cells are expanded ex vivo and then transplanted to the diseased eye. Stem cells can be cultivated on human amniotic membrane or other substrates, such as temperature-responsive cell culture surfaces. Typically, a 3T3 fibroblast feeder layer is used to facilitate cell growth and development of stem cell characteristics. A major advantage of using the patient's own cells is that systemic immunosuppression is not required.

Most of the previous reports on cultivated epithelial transplantation used animal-derived materials such as fetal bovine serum (FBS) and murine fibroblast cells as feeder cells (3T3 cells). However, the use of animal-derived materials may be associated with the risk of transmission of zoonotic infection or aggravated immunological responses. Ang et al. (2006) reported successful clinical results of using autologous serum instead of FBS for cultivation of oral epithelial sheets. Human dermal fibroblasts and human mesenchymal stem cells were reported as promising candidates of feeder cells (Omoto et al. 2009, Sharma et al. 2012).

Unfortunately, the majority of LSCD cases suffered from bilateral ocular surface damage where autologous transplantation was not indicated. However, immunological rejection and failure are still significant risks especially in inflammatory diseases such as OcMMP. Such inflammatory diseases need systemic immunosuppression for a long time to keep the transplanted limbal tissues in a healthy status. Shimazaki et al. (2002) reported a successful outcome of the cultivated limbal epithelium transplantation for severe ocular surface disorders such as SJS and OcMMP. Corneal epithelialization was achieved in 46.2% of cases, suggesting that cultivated limbal allografts on amniotic membranes have similar surgical prognosis for severe limbal stem cell dysfunction, compared to conventional limbal and amniotic membrane transplants (Shimazaki et al. 2002).

A new treatment for bilateral total LSCD is autologous cultivated oral mucosal epithelial transplantation (COMET). The successful use of autologous buccal epithelium was first reported in rabbits (Kinoshita et al. 2004, Nakamura et al. 2003) and later in humans with promising results (Inatomi et al. 2005, Nakamura et al. 2004,

Nishida et al. 2004, Satake et al. 2011). The main concept is to use the smooth surface of the oral mucosa instead of using corneal limbal stem cells, along with its stem cell properties, to reconstruct the ocular surface. After fibroblasts and vascular components are carefully removed, the cellular suspension is cultivated on human amniotic membrane with an inactivated 3T3 feeder layer or temperature-sensitive culture dishes. Short-term results of COMET are promising. Inatomi et al. (2006) reported the clinical results of 15 eyes treated with cultivated autologous oral mucosa. A stable ocular surface without any major complication was achieved in 10 of the eyes (67%), showing an increase in visual acuity after a mean follow-up period of 20 months. Satake et al. (2011) reported the outcomes of 36 eyes after cultivated oral mucosal epithelial sheet with a mean follow-up of 25.5 months. The Kaplan–Meier analysis revealed an early decline in transplanted oral mucosal epithelial stability within the first 6 months, which stayed stable (59% at 2 years) afterwards. Long-term results of this procedure, however, need to be investigated. Additionally, transplanted oral epithelium has shown a different phenotype from the corneal epithelium including superficial peripheral neovascularizaion (Inatomi et al. 2006, Nakamura et al. 2004, Nishida et al. 2004). Further studies assessing the proangiogenic factors in the oral mucosal epithelium are needed to prevent the neovascularization and achieve highly stable ocular surfaces. The main advantage of cultivated autologous oral mucosal epithelium is the absence of tissue rejection and avoidance of immunosuppression, ease of obtaining the mucosal tissues, inconspicuous location of the remained small scars, and the repeatability of the methods.

Osteo-odontokeratoprothesis has been performed to restore the vision in patients with total limbal deficiency, with keratinized ocular surface and severe tear deficiency. However, meticulous management of ocular complications, such as glaucoma and infections, is essential to achieve successful results (Hille et al. 2005).

From the viewpoint of evidence-based medicine, there are no studies with solid evidence that prove the superiority of one type of LSCD treatment over another (Cauchi et al. 2008). Further studies with prospective randomized protocols should be needed to establish the treatment guidelines for LSCD.

■ REFERENCES

Anderson DF, Ellies P, Pires RT, Tseng SC. Amniotic membrane transplantation for partial limbal stem cell deficiency. Br J Ophthalmol 2001; **85**:567–575.

Ang LP, Nakamura T, Inatomi T, et al. Autologous serum-derived cultivated oral epithelial transplants for severe ocular surface disease. Arch Ophthalmol 2006; **124**:1543–1551.

Cauchi PA, Ang GS, Azuara-Blanco A, Burr JM. A systematic literature review of surgical interventions for limbal stem cell deficiency in humans. Am J Ophthalmol 2008; **146**:251–259.

Dart J. Cicatricial pemphigoid and dry eye. Semin Ophthalmol 2005; **20**:95–100.

Dogru M, Tsubota K. Survival analysis of conjunctival limbal grafts and amniotic membrane transplantation in eyes with total limbal stem cell deficiency. Am J Ophthalmol 2005; **140**:305–306.

Dua HS, Gomes JA, Singh A. Corneal epithelial wound healing. Br J Ophthalmol 1994; **78**:401–408.

Foster CS, Sainz De La Maza M. Ocular cicatricial pemphigoid review. Curr Opin Allergy Clin Immunol 2004; **4**:435–439.

Goldberg MF, Bron AJ. Limbal palisades of Vogt. Trans Am Ophthalmol Soc 1982; **80**:155–171.

Goto E, Shimmura S, Shimazaki J, Tsubota K. Treatment of superior limbic keratoconjunctivitis by application of autologous serum. Cornea 2001; **20**:807–810.

Hille K, Grabner G, Liu C, Colliardo P, Falcinelli G, Taloni M. Standards for modified osteoodontokeratoprosthesis (OOKP) surgery according to Strampelli and Falcinelli: the Rome-Vienna Protocol. Cornea 2005; **24**:895–908.

Ibrahim OM, Matsumoto Y, Dogru M, et al. The efficacy, sensitivity, and specificity of in vivo laser confocal microscopy in the diagnosis of meibomian gland dysfunction. Ophthalmology 2010; **117**:665–672.

Inatomi T, Nakamura T, Koizumi N, Sotozono C, Kinoshita S. Current concepts and challenges in ocular surface reconstruction using cultivated mucosal epithelial transplantation. Cornea 2005; **24**:S32–S38.

Inatomi T, Nakamura T, Koizumi N, et al. Midterm results on ocular surface reconstruction using cultivated autologous oral mucosal epithelial transplantation. Am J Ophthalmol 2006; **141**:267–275.

Kinoshita S. Ocular surface reconstruction by tissue engineering. Nihon Ganka Gakkai Zasshi 2002; **106**:837–868; discussion 869.

Kinoshita S, Koizumi N, Nakamura T. Transplantable cultivated mucosal epithelial sheet for ocular surface reconstruction. Exp Eye Res 2004; **78**:483–491.

Kinoshita S, Manabe S. Chemical burns. St Louis: Mosby, 1993.

Kirzhner M, Jakobiec FA. Ocular cicatricial pemphigoid: a review of clinical features, immunopathology, differential diagnosis, and current management. Semin Ophthalmol 2011; **26**:270–277.

Kobayashi A, Fujiki K, Fujimaki T, Murakami A, Sugiyama K. In vivo laser confocal microscopic findings of corneal stromal dystrophies. Arch Ophthalmol 2007; **125**:1168–1173.

Kobayashi A, Sugiyama K. In vivo corneal confocal microscopic findings of palisades of Vogt and its underlying limbal stroma. Cornea 2005; **24**:435–437.

Kojima T, Ishida R, Dogru M, et al. The effect of autologous serum eyedrops in the treatment of severe dry eye disease: a prospective randomized case-control study. Am J Ophthalmol 2005; **139**:242–246.

Kojima T, Matsumoto Y, Dogru M, Tsubota K. The application of in vivo laser scanning confocal microscopy as a tool of conjunctival in vivo cytology in the diagnosis of dry eye ocular surface disease. Mol Vis 2010; **16**:2457–2464.

Kokotas H, Petersen MB. Clinical and molecular aspects of aniridia. Clin Genet 2010; **77**:409–420.

Lawrenson JG, Ruskell GL. The structure of corpuscular nerve endings in the limbal conjunctiva of the human eye. J Anat 1991; **177**:75–84.

Lehrer MS, Sun TT, Lavker RM. Strategies of epithelial repair: modulation of stem cell and transit amplifying cell proliferation. J Cell Sci 1998; **111**:2867–2875.

Lim P, Fuchsluger TA, Jurkunas UV. Limbal stem cell deficiency and corneal neovascularization. Semin Ophthalmol 2009; **24**:139–148.

Matsumoto Y, Dogru M, Goto E, et al. Autologous serum application in the treatment of neurotrophic keratopathy. Ophthalmology 2004; **111**:1115–1120.

Nakamura T, Endo K, Cooper LJ, et al. The successful culture and autologous transplantation of rabbit oral mucosal epithelial cells on amniotic membrane. Invest Ophthalmol Vis Sci 2003; **44**:106–116.

Nakamura T, Inatomi T, Sotozono C, et al. Transplantation of cultivated autologous oral mucosal epithelial cells in patients with severe ocular surface disorders. Br J Ophthalmol 2004; **88**:1280–1284.

Nishida K, Yamato M, Hayashida Y, et al. Corneal reconstruction with tissue-engineered cell sheets composed of autologous oral mucosal epithelium. N Engl J Med 2004; **351**:1187–1196.

Ogawa Y, Okamoto S, Mori T, et al. Autologous serum eye drops for the treatment of severe dry eye in patients with chronic graft-versus-host disease. Bone Marrow Transplant 2003; **31**:579–583.

Omoto M, Miyashita H, Shimmura S, et al. The use of human mesenchymal stem cell-derived feeder cells for the cultivation of transplantable epithelial sheets. Invest Ophthalmol Vis Sci 2009; **50**:2109–2115.

Patel DV, Sherwin T, McGhee CN. Laser scanning in vivo confocal microscopy of the normal human corneoscleral limbus. Invest Ophthalmol Vis Sci 2006; **47**:2823–2827.

Pellegrini G, Traverso CE, Franzi AT, et al. Long-term restoration of damaged corneal surfaces with autologous cultivated corneal epithelium. Lancet 1997; **349**:990–993.

Satake Y, Higa K, Tsubota K, Shimazaki J. Long-term outcome of cultivated oral mucosal epithelial sheet transplantation in treatment of total limbal stem cell deficiency. *Ophthalmology* 2011; **118**:1524–1530.

Saw VP, Dart JK. Ocular mucous membrane pemphigoid: diagnosis and management strategies. *Ocul Surf* 2008; **6**:128–142.

Shaw MW, Falls HF, Neel JV. Congenital Aniridia. *Am J Hum Genet* 1960; **12**:389–415.

Schrader S, Wedel T, Moll R, Geerling G. Combination of serum eye drops with hydrogel bandage contact lenses in the treatment of persistent epithelial defects. *Graefes Arch Clin Exp Ophthalmol* 2006; **244**:1345–1349.

Sharma SM, Fuchsluger T, Ahmad S, et al. Comparative analysis of human-derived feeder layers with 3t3 fibroblasts for the ex vivo expansion of human limbal and oral Epithelium. *Stem Cell Rev* 2012; **8**:696–705.

Shimazaki J, Aiba M, Goto E, et al. Transplantation of human limbal epithelium cultivated on amniotic membrane for the treatment of severe ocular surface disorders. *Ophthalmology* 2002; **109**:1285–1290.

Shortt AJ, Secker GA, Munro PM, et al. Characterization of the limbal epithelial stem cell niche: novel imaging techniques permit in vivo observation and targeted biopsy of limbal epithelial stem cells. *Stem Cells* 2007; **25**:1402–1409.

Solomon A, Ellies P, Anderson DF, et al. Long-term outcome of keratolimbal allograft with or without penetrating keratoplasty for total limbal stem cell deficiency. *Ophthalmology* 2002; **109**:1159–1166.

Takahashi N, Chikama T, Yanai R, Nishida T. Structures of the corneal limbus detected by laser-scanning confocal biomicroscopy as related to the palisades of Vogt detected by slit-lamp microscopy. *Jpn J Ophthalmol* 2009; **53**:199–203.

Thoft RA, Friend J. The X, Y, Z hypothesis of corneal epithelial maintenance. *Invest Ophthalmol Vis Sci* 1983; **24**:1442–1443.

Townsend WM. The limbal palisades of Vogt. *Trans Am Ophthalmol Soc* 1991; **89**:721–756.

Tseng SC, Li DQ. Comparison of protein kinase C subtype expression between normal and aniridic human ocular surfaces: implications for limbal stem cell dysfunction in aniridia. *Cornea* 1996; **15**:168–178.

Tsubota K, Goto E, Fujita H, et al. Treatment of dry eye by autologous serum application in Sjögren's syndrome. *Br J Ophthalmol* 1999a; **83**:390–395.

Tsubota K, Goto E, Shimmura S, Shimazaki J. Treatment of persistent corneal epithelial defect by autologous serum application. *Ophthalmology* 1999b; **106**:1984–1989.

Tsubota K, Satake Y, Kaido M, et al. Treatment of severe ocular-surface disorders with corneal epithelial stem-cell transplantation. *N Engl J Med* 1999c; **340**:1697–1703.

van Klink F, Alizadeh H, He Y, et al. The role of contact lenses, trauma, and Langerhans cells in a Chinese hamster model of Acanthamoeba keratitis. *Invest Ophthalmol Vis Sci* 1993; **34**:1937–1944.

Wall V, Yen MT, Yang MC, Huang AJ, Pflugfelder SC. Management of the late ocular sequelae of Stevens-Johnson syndrome. *Ocul Surf* 2003; **1**:192–201.

Zheng T, Xu J. Age-related changes of human limbus on in vivo confocal microscopy. *Cornea* 2008; **27**:782–786.

Zieske JD. Perpetuation of stem cells in the eye. *Eye (Lond)* 1994; **8**:163–169.

Chapter 25

Superior limbic keratoconjunctivitis

Javier Celis Sánchez, Diana Mesa, Eva Avendaño, Fernando Gonzalez del Valle

INTRODUCTION

Superior limbic keratoconjunctivitis (SLK) is an ocular surface disease of unclear etiology, characterized by marked inflammation of the upper bulbar conjunctiva. It was first described in detail as a clinical entity by Theodore (1963), though Thygeson and Kimura had already commented on some of its manifestations (Thygeson 1961, Thygeson & Kimura 1963). They found that it is associated with tear hyposecretion in 20% of patients and with thyroid dysfunction in 65%. Theodore extended these findings later and published data from a number of patients with SLK and thyroid disorders (Theodore 1968).

SLK is a poor prognostic factor for patients with thyroid disease: in one study 90% of the patients with thyroid dysfunction and SLK had thyroid ophthalmopathy and 49% of them required orbital decompression (Kadrmas & Bartley 1995).

SLK is a rare disorder without racial predilection. It is usually bilateral and asymmetric. Patients are typically 30–60 years of age. The average age of onset is 50 years. It is found more commonly in women than in men (3:1). Although it is not a hereditary disease, it has been described in one pair of identical twins (Darrell 1992).

CLINICAL MANIFESTATIONS

SLK is clinically characterized by unilateral or bilateral redundant superior bulbar conjunctiva and inflammation of the superior tarsal and bulbar conjunctiva, with dilatation of the superior bulbar conjunctival blood vessels, fine papillary reaction, punctate staining, and filaments on the superior cornea (**Figures 25.1** and **25.2**). Vision is usually unaffected. Rose Bengal or lissamine green staining typically reveals punctate uptake of the stain over the region of involved conjunctiva.

In Theodore's study (Theodore 1963) the patients showed:
- Marked inflammation of the superior bulbar conjunctiva and tarsal conjunctiva of the upper lid
- Fine punctate staining of the cornea and the adjacent conjunctiva above the limbus
- Superior limbic proliferation
- Filaments on the superior cornea or limbus

Typical complaints include foreign body sensation, burning, photophobia, and pain. Patients who have filaments may have blepharospasm. The superior bulbar and limbal conjunctiva shows sectoral injection and appears thickened and redundant. In general, the prognosis for SLK is excellent, characterized by episodes of recurrent autolimited inflammation, although symptoms may last for years.

DIAGNOSIS

Diagnosis is mainly based on clinical symptoms and slit-lamp examination, by lifting the upper eyelid while the patient looks down and then everting the eyelid. It is very useful to stain with Rose Bengal or lissamine green to observe the typical pattern of conjunctival staining in the rubbing area (**Figure 25.3**).

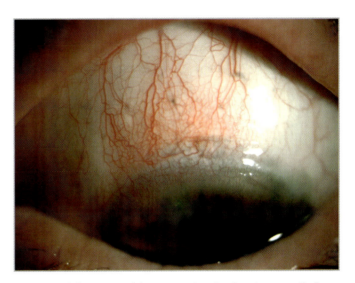

Figure 25.1 Inflammation of the upper conjunctiva. Superior sectoral bulbar conjunctiva showing a hyperemic, thickened, and superior epithelial corneal defect associated with filamentary keratitis in a patient with superior limbic keratoconjunctivitis.

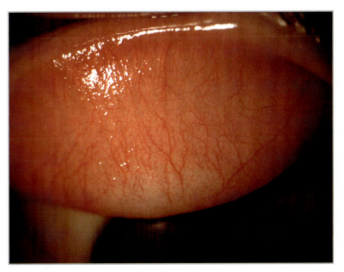

Figure 25.2 Inflammation of the tarsal conjunctiva of the upper lid. The everted eyelid shows dilatation of conjunctival blood vessels and fine papillary reaction on palpebral conjunctiva.

Checking the conjunctiva with a cotton-tipped applicator may also be helpful to demonstrate a loose and mobile superior bulbar conjunctiva (**Figure 25.4**). One study showed that the most common signs associated with SLK were dry eyes and conjunctival corrugation, occurring in 100% of patients, and lid wiper epitheliopathy with positive vital dye staining, occurring in 75% (Kim & Chun 2009).

Impression cytology and laser scanning confocal microscopy are useful tools in the diagnosis of SLK, (they are also especially useful for checking the effectiveness of a treatment). Both methods are efficient in the evaluation of phenotypic alterations of the conjunctival epithelium. Impression cytology examines the ocular surface epithelium with an application of cellulose acetate filter material to remove the superficial layers of the epithelium. The technique is easy to perform and can be used to observe ocular surface epithelial cell changes over time.

Confocal microscopy is a technology that evaluates tissue structure and cell phenotype in vivo. SLK findings on both tests have different degrees of conjunctival squamous metaplasia, marked enlargement of cell size with pyknotic nuclei, and sloughing of superficial epithelium in some areas. Furthermore, the nucleocytoplasmic ratio and the inflammatory cell density appear to be promising new parameters in the assessment of ocular surface disease in SLK (Kojima et al. 2010).

This condition not only is associated with thyroid dysfunction but also involves other potential risk factors: dry eye disease, exophthalmos, floppy eyelid syndrome, scarring of the palpebral conjunctiva, prolonged eyelid closure with associated hypoxia, and morphological or functional changes in superior conjunctival apposition to the globe following upper eyelid procedures (Sheu et al. 2007).

In our experience, SLK presents more often in patients with dry eye disease and floppy syndromes than in patients with thyroid dysfunction.

DIFFERENTIAL DIAGNOSIS

There is a syndrome associated with the use of soft contact lenses that resembles SLK. It was initially related to thimerosal-preserved solution (Sendele et al. 1983). Subsequently, several reports showed a similar syndrome in soft contact lens wearers who were not using thimerosal.

One theory postulates that a superior-riding soft contact lens may cause a mechanical effect on the bulbar conjunctival tissue and superior cornea. It would be another clinical entity. This syndrome, which is associated with contact lenses, presents some clinical signs that differ from those seen in SLK. It is more heterogeneous, not always bilateral, has no relationship with thyroid disease, no sex predilection, appears in younger patients, less commonly involves filaments, and produces more loss of visual acuity because the corneal involvement is greater. Symptoms improve with discontinuation of contact lenses (Fuerst et al. 1983).

Another entity that may mimic SLK is an ocular surface squamous neoplasia because clinical features of conjunctival lesions (e.g. location of the lesion and classic slit-lamp appearance) and clinical symptoms may show similarities (Moshirfar et al. 2011).

Some features of limbal insufficiency can resemble SLK if they affect the upper half of the limb (e.g. conjunctival epithelial ingrowth, vascularization, and chronic keratitis). In this case, the presence of goblet cells in corneal impression cytology or specific detection of mucin MUC5AC transcript in cornea by real-time polymerase chain reaction (Limbotest, Bioftalmik Applied Research) may help confirm the diagnosis.

HISTOPATHOLOGY

Theodore and Ferry (1970) described the histopathological findings in SLK. The superior bulbar conjunctiva show keratinization, acanthosis, and dyskeratosis with the presence of polymorphonuclear leukocytes and balloon degeneration of nuclei in some areas. The superior palpebral conjunctiva reveals infiltration with polymorphs, lymphocytes, plasma cells, and normal epithelium.

There is also a difference in goblet cell concentration in affected tissues. The superior palpebral conjunctiva shows goblet cell hypertrophy, while the bulbar conjunctiva, which is thickened and keratinized, shows very few goblet cells.

Electron microscopic examination shows abnormal distribution and aggregation of nuclear chromatin filaments within nuclei, as well as in the cytoplasm surrounding nuclei, resulting in a description of 'nuclear strangulation.' These findings are considered specific to SLK (Collin et al. 1978).

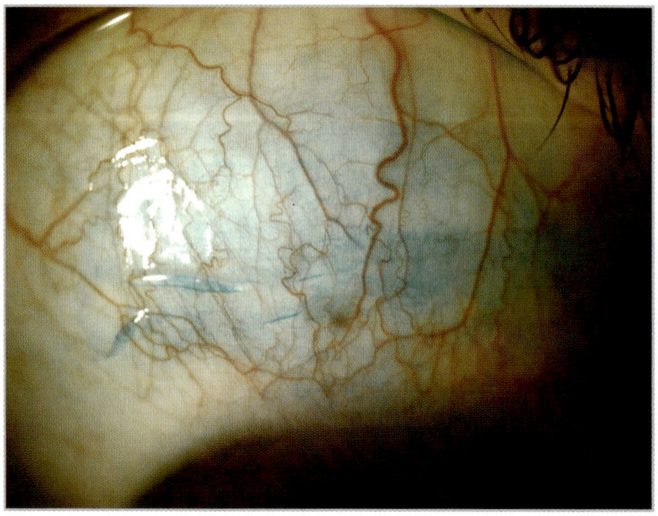

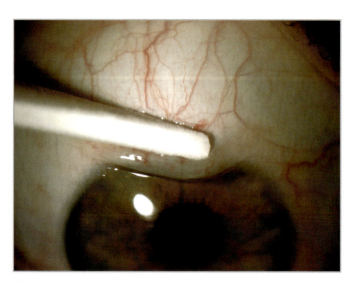

Figure 25.3 Vital dye staining. Lissamine green staining of the superior bulbar conjunctiva with horizontal corrugation parallel to the lid margin in the lax conjunctiva.

Figure 25.4 Diagnostic maneuvers. Checking the conjunctiva with a cotton-tipped applicator to show the conjunctival laxity.

Matsuda found an altered expression of cytokeratins in SLK and suggested that upregulated proliferation of conjunctival epithelial cells might be another feature of the disease (Matsuda et al. 1996).

PATHOGENESIS

Both the etiology and the pathogenesis of SLK are poorly understood, but inflammatory changes as a result of mechanical soft tissue microtrauma are the final common pathway. During a blink, the upper lid has vertical movement, so it exerts enough force to squeeze the globe, resulting in elevation of the eyeball according to Bell's phenomenon (Doane 1980). Protection from friction is derived from the membranous mucin of the corneal and conjunctival epithelium, and from goblet cells in the conjunctival and lacrimal glands (Gipson & Argüeso 2003).

Under certain conditions, such as dry eye disease, eyelid inflammation due to thyroid dysfunction, and exophthalmos, vertical lid pressure induces more friction on the ocular surface and leads to more damage to the conjunctival epithelium and goblet cells. As a result of the deficiency of mucin production, more irritation and friction will occur and the ocular surface will be caught in a vicious cycle.

The mechanical theory suggests that the superior bulbar conjunctiva is continually rubbed by the upper tarsus during blinking (because of the increased pressure of the upper eyelid against the globe or increased motility of the upper bulbar conjunctiva), resulting in chronic inflammation. Increased upper eyelid tightness may be the result of thyroid eye disease or chronic inflammation and, in addition, may impair the normal turnover of bulbar conjunctival epithelial cells (Cher 2000).

Superior bulbar conjunctivochalasis plays an important role in the pathogenesis of SLK, which is associated with laxity of the conjunctiva. However, we still do not know if conjunctival redundancy is the origin of the disease or a result of mechanical interaction between the conjunctiva and the eyelid (Yokoi et al. 2003).

Overexpression of matrix metalloproteinase-1 and -3 has been found in surgical specimens and cultured conjunctival fibroblasts from SLK patients. This imbalance may contribute to SLK pathogenesis (Sun et al. 2011).

Another study has also shown that, in SLK, there is abnormal T-cell function and upregulation of transforming growth factor b-2, tenascin, and integrin b-1. They are induced by mechanical stress in the conjunctiva of these patients (Matsuda et al. 1999).

Topical mast cell stabilizer is an efficient medication in the management of SLK. The increasing numbers of mast cells in one study seem to suggest that these cells play a role in the pathogenesis of SLK (Sun et al. 2008).

TREATMENT

Reviewing the large number of proposed treatments for this disease confirms the lack of a fully effective protocol. The options advocated for SLK management include the following.

Medical treatment

Various therapeutic approaches have been used in response to the various pathogenetic mechanisms. Sun et al. (2008) reported that 79% of SLK responded to medical treatment. However, the effect of medical treatment is limited, and in recurrent cases, or when the treatments fail, surgical management becomes necessary.

Redundancy of superior bulbar conjunctiva

Chemical cautery (silver nitrate 0.5–1.0%) is applied topically to the superior bulbar and tarsal conjunctiva. This treatment chemically cauterizes the irregular tissue, promoting regrowth of new and healthy epithelium.

Dry eye disease

Artificial tears, punctual occlusion, topical vitamin A, autologous serum 20%, and topical cyclosporine 0.5 or 0.005% can be used:
- **Cyclosporin A** acts in several ways. It improves the keratoconjunctivitis sicca, it has an immunomodulatory effect through inhibiting T-cell proliferation and activity, and it has an inhibitory effect on eosinophil and mast cell activation and on release of granule proteins, inflammatory mediators, and cytokines
- **Vitamin A (retinyl palmitate 0.05%) therapy** could reverse keratinization of conjunctival epithelium and eliminate the mechanical stimulation between the rough surface and the oppositional palpebral conjunctiva of SLK patients

A theory regarding the etiology of SLK implicates a local deficiency to the superior conjunctiva. Some researchers have proposed that this deficiency results in significantly reduced levels of vital tear-based nutrients to the affected regions as well as increased mechanical friction from the superior lid.

Mast cell infiltration

Mast cell-stabilizing agents such as cromolyn sodium 4% and lodoxamide tromethamine 1% have shown efficacy against SLK in the short term.

Filamentary keratitis

Treatment for filamentary keratitis involves eliminating the mucus filaments as thoroughly as possible. N-Acetylcysteine (10% topical) is a mucolytic agent used for dissolving corneal filaments.

Excess friction

Therapeutic lenses ('bandage' contact lenses), pressure patching, and botulinum toxin A can be used:
- **Therapeutic lenses (14–20 mm in diameter):** these can produce rapid symptom relief in SLK. They relieve pain and facilitate healing of punctate epithelial erosions by protecting the ocular surface from the eyelids, reducing upper lid pressure on the globe, and increasing tear production. Bilateral symptoms are relieved by unilateral lens use. This suggests that contact lenses reduce the tactile corneal sensation, which would decrease the bilateral reflex blinking rate and blinking power (Watson et al. 2002)
- **Pressure patching:** this eliminates the mechanical effect of the lid on the globe
- **Botulinum toxin A:** this is used to weaken the pretarsal orbicularis muscle (the muscle of Riolan), which maintains lid tone and adjusts normal apposition of lid margin to ocular surface. The injections are given subcutaneously at the lateral and medial fifth aspects of the upper eyelid as near as possible to the gray line (Kim & Chun 2009)

Inflammation

Topical anti-inflammatory agents such as ketotifen fumarate and topical corticosteroids (dexamethasone, methylprednisolone) can be used.

Others

Topical antibiotics can be given. (Infectious agents such as bacteria, viruses, fungi, and other intracellular parasites appear to be unrelated to this condition.)

▉ Surgical treatment

Surgical options for the treatment of SLK can be divided into three categories based on the mechanism of action:
* Reinforcing the adhesion of the conjunctiva to sclera
* Correcting the redundancy of the superior bulbar conjunctiva
* Reducing the inflammation

Reinforcing the adhesion of the conjunctiva to sclera

Procedures include thermal cautery and liquid nitrogen cryotherapy. Liquid nitrogen acts on the redundant superior conjunctiva by causing a scar similar to that produced by thermal cautery to form a greater adhesion between the superior bulbar conjunctiva and the underlying Tenon capsule and sclera. The disease can recur after a single application, but there are no recurrences after repeated cryotherapy (Fraunfelder 2009).

Correcting the redundancy of the superior bulbar conjunctiva

The procedure comprises conjunctival resection with or without amniotic membrane transplantation, resection of a 'crescent' of superior conjunctiva, and conjunctival fixation sutures. Redundant superior bulbar conjunctiva is a constant finding in SLK and contributes to the mechanical hypothesis of SLK. The areas of involved conjunctiva and underlying Tenon tissue are both excised. To identify the pathological area, conjunctival staining with Rose Bengal or lissamine green is used. Superior bulbar conjunctival resection combined with Tenon layer excision provides several beneficial effects:

* The involved conjunctiva, with the keratinized epithelium, is removed to eliminate the mechanical stimulation. This surgery may also eliminate the problem of redundant superior conjunctiva and redistribute the unstable tear film
* The excision of the underlying Tenon layer provides more space for redistribution of originally redundant conjunctiva in SLK patients and also supplies a free space to reduce the attrition from the oppositional superior palpebral conjunctiva. This surgical technique appears to be more effective than simple resection of superior bulbar conjunctiva without Tenon excision, and it is associated with fewer recurrences (Sun et al. 2008)

Another surgical technique (Yokoi et al. 2003) consists of four steps:
1. Rose Bengal staining is used to localize the abnormal conjunctival area
2. An arc-like conjunctival incision is placed from the 2 o'clock to the 10 o'clock position adjacent and distal to the Rose Bengal-stained area
3. The conjunctiva is removed to form a crescent using the arc-like incision at the base. The size of the resection is determined by conjunctival redundancy after removal of the subconjunctival connective tissue
4. The crescent conjunctival opening is closed with interrupted sutures

The use of amniotic membrane graft with conjunctival resection did not provide any additional advantage according to the report of Gris et al. (2010).

Reducing the inflammation—supratarsal triamcinolone injection

One hypothesis proposes that the SLK could be associated with upper tarsal inflammation that is immune based, and this could be exacerbated in the dry eye disease. According to this hypothesis, corticosteroids may improve the SLK. The technique is as follows: after topical application of anesthesia, triamcinolone acetonide 3 mg/0.3 mL is injected with a 27-gauge needle into the subconjunctiva via the temporal supratarsal conjunctiva and allowed to diffuse through the entire upper palpebral conjunctiva (Shen et al. 2007).

▉ REFERENCES

Cher I. Superior limbic keratoconjunctivitis: multifactorial mechanical pathogenesis. *Clin Exp Ophthalmol* 2000; **28**:181–184.

Collin HB, Donshik PC, Boruchoff SA, Foster CS, Cavanagh HD. The fine structure of nuclear changes in superior limbic keratoconjunctivitis. *Invest Ophthalmol Vis Sci* 1978; **17**:79–84.

Darrell RW. Superior limbic keratoconjunctivitis in identical twins. *Cornea* 1992; **11**:262–263.

Doane MG. Interactions of the eyelids and tears in corneal wetting and the dynamics of the normal human eyeblink. *Am J Ophthalmol* 1980; **89**:507–516.

Fraunfelder FW. Liquid nitrogen cryotherapy of superior limbic keratoconjunctivitis. *Am J Ophthalmol* 2009; **147**:234–238.

Fuerst DJ, Sugar J, Worobec S. Superior limbic keratoconjunctivitis associated with cosmetic soft contact lens wear. *Arch Ophthalmol* 1983; **101**:1214–1216.

Gipson IK, Argüeso P. Role of mucins in the function of the corneal and conjunctival epithelia. *Int Rev Cytol* 2003; **231**:1–49.

Gris O, Plazas A, Lerma E, et al. Conjunctival resection with and without amniotic membrane graft for the treatment of superior limbic keratoconjunctivitis. *Cornea* 2010; **29**:1025–1030.

Kadrmas EF, Bartley GB. Superior limbic keratoconjunctivitis. A prognostic sign for severe Graves ophthalmopathy. *Ophthalmology* 1995; **102**:1472–1475.

Kim JC, Chun YS. Treatment of superior limbic keratoconjunctivitis with a large-diameter contact lens and botulium toxin A. *Cornea* 2009; **28**:752–758.

Kojima T, Matsumoto Y, Ibrahim OM, et al. In vivo evaluation of superior limbic keratoconjunctivitis using laser scanning confocal microscopy and conjunctival impression cytology. *Invest Ophthalmol Vis Sci* 2010; **51**:3986–3992.

Matsuda A, Tagawa Y, Matsuda H. Cytokeratin and proliferative cell nuclear antigen expression in superior limbic keratoconjunctivitis. *Curr Eye Res* 1996; **15**:1033–1038.

Matsuda A, Tagawa Y, Matsuda H. TGF-beta2, tenascin, and integrin beta1 expression in superior limbic keratoconjunctivitis. *Jpn J Ophthalmol* 1999; **43**:251–256.

Moshirfar M, Khalifa YM, Kuo A, Davis D, Mamalis N. Ocular surface squamous neoplasia masquerading as superior limbic keratoconjunctivitis. *Middle East Afr J Ophthalmol* 2011; **18**:74–76.

Sendele DD, Kenyon KR, Mobilia EF, et al. Superior limbic keratoconjunctivitis in contact lens wearers. *Ophthalmology* 1983; **90**:616–622.

Shen YC, Wang CY, Tsai HY, Lee YF. Supratarsal triamcinolone injection in the treatment of superior limbic keratoconjunctivitis. *Cornea* 2007; **26**:423–426.

Sheu MC, Schoenfield L, Jeng BH. Development of superior limbic keratoconjunctivitis after upper eyelid blepharoplasty surgery: support for the mechanical theory of its pathogenesis. *Cornea* 2007; **26**:490–492.

Sun YC, Hsiao CH, Chen WL, et al. Conjunctival resection combined with tenon layer excision and the involvement of mast cells in superior limbic keratoconjunctivitis. *Am J Ophthalmol* 2008; **145**:445–452.

Sun YC, Hsiao CH, Chen WL, Hu FR. Overexpression of matrix metalloproteinase-1 (MMP-1) and MMP-3 in superior limbic keratoconjunctivitis. *Invest Ophthalmol Vis Sci* 2011; **52**:3701–3705.

Theodore FH. Comments on findings of elevated protein-bound iodine in superior limbic keratoconjunctivitis: Part I. *Arch Ophthalmol* 1968; **79**:508.

Theodore FH. Superior limbic keratoconjunctivitis. *Eye Ear Nose Throat Monthly* 1963; **42**:25–28.

Theodore FH, Ferry AP. Superior limbic keratoconjunctivitis. Clinical and pathological correlations. *Arch Ophthalmol* 1970; **84**:481–484.

Thygeson P. Further observations on superficial punctate keratitis. *Arch Ophthalmol* 1961; **66**:158–162.

Thygeson P, Kimura SJ. Chronic conjunctivitis. *Trans Am Acad Ophthalmol Otolaryngol* 1963; **67**:494–517.

Watson S, Tullo AB, Carley F. Treatment of superior limbic keratoconjunctivitis with a unilateral bandage contact lens. *Br J Ophthalmol* 2002; **86**:485–486.

Yokoi N, Komuro A, Maruyama A, et al. New surgical treatment for superior limbic keratoconjunctivitis and its association with conjunctivochalasis. *Am J Ophthalmol* 2003; **135**:303–308.

Chapter 26 — Neurotrophic keratoconjunctivitis

Alessandro Lambiase, Marta Sacchetti

DEFINITION AND CAUSES

Neurotrophic keratitis (NK) is a rare degenerative corneal disease first described in 1824 by Magendie. It is characterized by the impairment of corneal sensitivity, corneal epithelial breakdown, and impaired healing, leading to corneal ulceration, melting, and perforation. A decrease or absence of corneal sensation is the hallmark of this condition (Groos 1997).

Corneal sensitivity is controlled by trigeminal nerve endings. Corneal nerves also supply trophic support, playing a key role in maintaining the anatomical integrity and function of the cornea, particularly of the epithelium (Müller et al. 2003).

Many ocular and systemic diseases can produce lesions at various levels of the fifth cranial nerve, from the trigeminal nucleus to the corneal nerve endings. The most common causes of corneal anesthesia are herpetic viral keratitis, followed by trigeminal ophthalmic branch damage from intracranial space-occupying lesions and/or neurosurgical procedures.

Other local causes of trigeminal nerve damage include chemical burns, physical injuries, corneal dystrophy, and chronic topical medications. A decrease in corneal sensitivity is also observed after corneal transplantation or anterior segment surgery involving nerve transection. Systemic diseases, such as diabetes, multiple sclerosis, congenital syndromes, and leprosy, can also decrease corneal sensitivity, leading to corneal anesthesia (**Figure 26.1**) (Bonini et al. 2003).

Although the history and the clinical findings associated with a decrease in corneal sensation may aid in the diagnosis of NK, the management of this condition is one of the most difficult and challenging tasks in dealing with corneal diseases. Prompt and aggressive treatment is important in NK to prevent serious complications, such as corneal ulceration, perforation, and infection.

EPIDEMIOLOGY

NK is a rare disease (ORPHA137596) with an estimated prevalence of <5 per 10,000 individuals. No data are available in the literature on the epidemiology of NK. However, the prevalence and incidence of NK may be extrapolated from its causes. Specifically, NK complicated herpetic keratitis in 4.4–8.0% of cases (Labetoulle et al. 2005). Based on an average NK prevalence of 6% of all cases of herpetic keratitis (the prevalence of herpetic keratitis is 149/100,000), the NK prevalence can be estimated as 0.89/10,000. Similarly, the prevalence of NK from herpes zoster keratitis (HZO) may be calculated as 0.33/10,000 by applying an average NK prevalence of 12.8% to the estimated prevalence

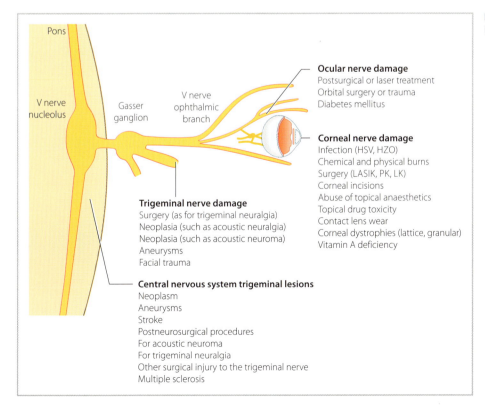

Figure 26.1 Causes of trigeminal nerve damage leading to neurotrophic keratitis development.

of HZO (26/100,000) (Dworkin et al. 2007). NK has been reported to be a complication of various surgical procedures for trigeminal neuralgia, at a percentage ranging from 0.6 to 5% (mean value 2.8%), depending on the procedure (Bhatti & Patel 2005). As the prevalence of trigeminal neuralgia has been reported at 1.5/10,000, the NK prevalence can be estimated as 0.02/10,000.

The prevalence of NK caused by other conditions, such as diabetes, multiple sclerosis, acoustic neuroma, and congenital diseases, cannot be estimated because no data are available in the literature. Therefore, the final prevalence of NK within the population of Europe can be estimated at <1.6/10,000.

PATHOPHYSIOLOGY

The cornea is the most richly innervated tissue in the body and is supplied by both sensory and autonomic nerve fibers. The sensory nerves, which are derived from the ophthalmic branch of the trigeminal nerve, are sensitive to touch, temperature, and chemical stimulation.

The loss of corneal sensory innervation leads to morphological and metabolic epithelial disturbances. In animal models, ocular nerve injury causes the swelling of squamous epithelial cells, the loss of cell surface microvilli, and acceleration of the sloughing off into the tear film, with consequent epithelial breakdown. Mitosis is decreased in basal epithelial cells, and epithelial thickness gradually diminishes. Abnormal epithelial permeability and metabolism have also been described. As a consequence of these effects, corneal epithelial healing is significantly impaired after corneal denervation, leading to recurrent corneal erosions and ulcerations.

The mechanisms by which corneal innervation exerts trophic effects in maintaining a healthy cornea and promoting wound healing are not completely understood. However, it has been clearly demonstrated that ocular surface epithelia and sensory and autonomic nerve fibers interact through the mutual release of cytokines, neuropeptides, and neuromediators, influencing the structures and functions of each other. The tear gland also helps to maintain a healthy ocular surface epithelium by providing growth factors and other nutrients and is, in turn, influenced by the neurosecretory reflex.

Several studies have focused on the role of sensory neuromediators in corneal epithelium pathophysiology. These studies have indicated that corneal sensory nerves express substance P (SP), calcitonin gene-related peptide (CGRP), galanin, and/or pituitary adenylate cyclase-activating peptide, a neuropeptide with high homology to vasoactive intestinal polypeptide, and opioid growth factor (Bonini et al. 2003).

In vitro studies have demonstrated that SP, CGRP, and acetylcholine may induce epithelial cell proliferation, migration, and adhesion, and that trigeminal neurons influence the production of type VII collagen by rabbit corneal epithelium in vitro. In vivo and in vitro studies have revealed that SP associated with insulin-like growth factor-1 (IGF-1) synergistically facilitates corneal epithelial wound healing. In response, corneal epithelium and stromal keratocytes release neuropeptides, neurotrophins, and growth factors that may influence nerve fiber extension and survival. More specifically, nerve growth factor (NGF), ciliary neurotrophic factor, epidermal growth factor, brain-derived neurotrophic factor, and glial cell-derived neurotrophic factor represent the main participants of nerve–epithelium cross-talk, modulating corneal tropism and healing (Müller et al. 2003).

Consequently, corneal sensory nerve damage impairs the neuromediator–epithelium interactions, leading to an impairment of epithelial maintenance and physiological renewal and the development of recurrent or persistent epithelial defects.

CLINICAL PRESENTATION

Impairment of corneal sensation due to damage of trigeminal nerve fibers leads to NK, which is clinically characterized by ocular surface disorders, such as a dry and cloudy corneal epithelium, superficial punctate keratopathy (SPK), and corneal edema, recurrent and/or persistent epithelial defects and ulcers with stromal melting and perforation. The damage to trigeminal sensory fibers also affects tear film production due to the diminished stimulation of the tear gland by sensory afferent input mediated by trigeminal sensory fibers. A decrease in the blink rate and in tear film stability, with decreased break-up time, is also associated with NK. Using the Mackie classification, NK can be classified based on the severity of corneal damage (**Table 26.1**) (Mackie 1995).

Stage 1 is characterized by Rose Bengal staining of the inferior conjunctiva, a decrease in the break-up time, and SPK. In chronic cases, epithelial hyperplasia and irregularity, superficial neovascularization, and stromal scarring may also be observed (**Figure 26.2**).

Stage 2 is characterized by a persistent epithelial defect, with an oval or circular shape, most frequently localized to the superior half of the cornea. There is usually an area of poorly adherent opaque and edematous epithelium around the epithelial defect that can spontaneously detach to produce an enlargement of the defect. Epithelial healing is inadequate, and the edges of the defect become smooth and rolled. Descemet's membrane folds and stromal swelling may be observed with an inflammatory reaction in the anterior chamber, which is rarely associated with sterile hypopyon.

Stage 3 is characterized by stromal involvement, with a corneal ulcer that may progress to perforation and/or stromal melting. The inappropriate use of topical steroids and/or secondary infections may worsen corneal melting and lead to perforation.

Patients with NK rarely complain of symptoms, as they are hypoanesthetic; however, they may describe ocular surface discomfort symptoms and/or blurred vision as a result of corneal scarring (Bonini et al. 2003).

DIAGNOSIS

The diagnosis of NK is mainly based on the patient's history, the clinical findings, and a corneal sensitivity evaluation. Testing of corneal

Table 26.1 Clinical staging of neurotrophic keratitis—neurotrophic keratitis classification*

Stage 1	Rose Bengal staining of the palpebral conjunctiva Increased viscosity of tear mucus Decreased tear break-up time Scattered small facets of dried epithelium (Gaule spots) Superficial punctate keratopathy Dellen Corneal superficial vascularization Stromal scarring Epithelial hyperplasia and irregularity Hyperplastic precorneal membrane
Stage 2	Epithelial defects, usually in the superior half cornea Surrounding rim of loose epithelium Stromal edema Anterior chamber inflammatory reaction (rare) Edges of the defect becoming smooth and rolled with time
Stage 3	Corneal ulcer Stromal melting Perforation

*Modified from Groos E. Cornea 2004; 94:1189–1196.

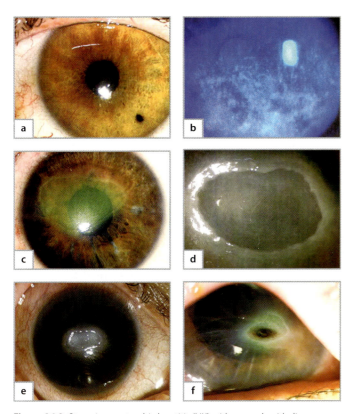

Figure 26.2 Stage 1 neurotrophic keratitis (NK) with corneal epithelium dystrophy (a) and superficial punctuate keratitis (b). Stage 2 NK with persistent epithelial defect and (c) oval epithelial defect with rolled edges (d). Stage 3 neurotrophic ulcer with stromal melting and (e) corneal perforation (f).

sensitivity and imaging of corneal nerves may aid in the management of NK patients who are poor candidates for corneal transplantation.

Clinical history

The patient's clinical history should be accurately investigated and should include systemic diseases (such as diabetes), therapies (neuroleptic, antipsychotic, and antihistamine drugs) that can cause impairment of trigeminal innervation, and local causes (previous corneal surgery or traumas, topical anesthetic abuse, chronic topical drug use, chemical burns, or contact lens abuse) that can cause local injury to corneal sensory nerves. Brain neoplasms and vascular accidents may damage the fifth cranial nerve or its nucleus. Congenital diseases, such as familial dysautonomia, Goldenhar–Gorlin syndrome, Moebius syndrome, familial corneal hypesthesia, and congenital insensitivity to pain with anhydrosis, have also been associated with the development of NK.

Cranial nerve examination

Cranial nerve examination can help localize the cause of the decreased corneal sensation. Dysfunction of the seventh and eighth cranial nerves may indicate damage from acoustic neuroma or from its surgical resection. Paresis of the third, fourth, and sixth cranial nerves may indicate an aneurysm or cavernous sinus that also affects the trigeminal nerve. Assessing the presence of associated neurological signs requires strict collaboration with a neurologist and cranial imaging evaluation (Bonini et al. 2003).

Eyelid examination

The eyelids should be examined carefully for both diagnostic and prognostic symptoms. In fact, the presence of lagophthalmos may indicate an association with seventh cranial nerve palsy and may lead to epithelial exposure, accelerating the clinical progression of NK. The blink rate is markedly decreased if bilateral NK occurs. However, the disease is frequently unilateral, and blinks can be normal because the unaffected eye elicits a normal, symmetrical blink.

Ocular examination

Accurate ocular examination must be performed. Corneal and conjunctival epithelial changes should also be evaluated and graded using vital staining, such as fluorescein, Rose Bengal, or lissamine green. Corneal stromal scarring may indicate prior infection, and iris atrophy may be a sign of a previous herpetic infection.

Tear film evaluation

Tear film evaluation should be performed during the evaluation of NK patients, as tear film may be qualitatively and quantitatively affected by the reduction of corneal sensitivity. Specifically, Schirmer's test to evaluate tear production and the break-up time test to evaluate tear film stability are recommended in the evaluation of patients with NK. Tear film function changes severely worsen the prognosis of NK.

Ocular fundus examination

Ocular fundus examination should be performed to reveal diabetic retinopathy, optic nerve pallor, or swelling due to an intracranial tumor.

Corneal sensitivity

Corneal sensitivity is a vital piece of information to confirm the diagnosis of NK. It can be measured qualitatively by touching the central and peripheral cornea with the tip of a cotton swab or quantitatively by a corneal esthesiometer (Faulkner & Varley 1997). Because the severity of NK is generally related to the severity of the corneal sensory impairment, a corneal sensitivity assessment may be useful to assess the severity of corneal nerve impairment. Different devices are available to measure corneal sensitivity. One of the most common devices is the Cochet–Bonnet esthesiometer; it quantifies corneal sensitivity by the length of a nylon filament required to initiate a blink or a patient response. The nylon filament may be extended from 0 to 6 cm. Each quadrant of the cornea may be tested separately (Norn 1974). Recently, new, non-contact esthesiometers have been developed, allowing the evaluation of the mechanical, chemical, and thermal sensitivity on the ocular surface. The Belmonte non-contact esthesiometer is based on corneal stimulation, with a series of pulses of warmed air (constant temperature of 42°C at the tip of the probe) at multiple pressures between 20 and 160 mL/min applied to the surface of the central cornea. The lowest airflow that is able to elicit a response from the patient is identified as the mechanical threshold. The chemical detection threshold is assessed by stimulating the central cornea with a mixture of air and various concentrations of CO_2. To prevent mechanical stimulation, the flow of the air and CO_2 mixture is restricted to 10 mL/min below the previously established mechanical detection threshold. Changes in the temperature of the airflow allow for the identification of the thermal sensitivity threshold (Belmonte et al. 1999). In contrast to the Cochet–Bonnet esthesiometer, the non-contact instruments allow for the evaluation of all three types of neuroreceptors on the ocular surface and improve control of the stimulus characteristics. The administration of hypertonic (3%) saline solution in the conjunctival sac for testing ocular surface sensitivity was proposed by Mandahl. The hypertonic (3%) saline test showed higher sensitivity than the use of the cotton wool thread, but it was not significantly more sensitive than the Cochet–Bonnet esthesiometer. To date, Cochet–Bonnet and non-contact esthesiometers have been the most frequently used methods to assess corneal sensitivity, and cotton thread test represents an easy and rapid method to test corneal sensitivity in clinical practice (Mandahl 1993).

In vivo corneal confocal microscopy

The exponential increase in the use of in vivo corneal confocal microscopy (IVCM) over the past years has increased understanding of corneal nerve morphology in health and in ocular and systemic diseases. IVCM is a rapid and non-invasive imaging method, with good interobserver variability.

Several studies demonstrated the role of corneal nerves and the correlation with corneal sensation in patients with NK. Specifically, in both HZO and herpes simplex keratitis eyes, ICVM studies showed a significant decrease in the number of sub-basal nerve fibers, and in nerve density significantly correlated with the decrease in corneal sensation. Similarly, a strong correlation between corneal sensation and sub-basal nerve morphology and density was described after refractive surgery. ICVM analysis in diabetic patients showed a decrease in corneal sub-basal nerve density and an increase in nerve fiber tortuosity, which correlated with the stage of peripheral neuropathy. A correlation has also been shown between reduced corneal nerve bundles, loss of corneal sensation, and severity of somatic neuropathy in patients with type 1 diabetes (Rosenberg et al. 2000). It has also been reported that in patients with diabetes the decrease of nerve density precedes the impairment of corneal sensitivity, allowing early detection of peripheral neuropathy (Cruzat et al. 2010).

DIFFERENTIAL DIAGNOSIS

In all cases, the diagnosis of NK may be made without difficulty based on the history and examination findings associated with a decrease in corneal sensation. However, some clinical findings of NK can be caused by different ocular surface diseases. Symptoms of stage 1 NK, such as SPK and tear film abnormalities, may also be observed in other conditions, including dry eye disease, blepharitis, exposure keratopathy, topical drug toxicity, mild chemical injury, contact lens-related disorders, and corneal limbal stem cell deficiency. Clinical history, systemic signs and symptoms, and laboratory tests help identify the correct diagnosis, although all of these conditions may be associated with the impairment of corneal sensation due to local sensory nerve damage, as observed in patients with NK (**Figure 26.3**).

The presence of corneal ulcers warrants the investigation of other possible causes, including infectious and immune etiologies, which always present with important ocular inflammation and stromal infiltrates. A microbiological examination should be performed to exclude bacterial, fungal, or viral infections, and an immune analysis should be considered. Any local treatment should be discontinued to exclude toxic corneal ulcers (Bonini et al. 2003).

TREATMENT

Once the diagnosis of neurotrophic keratopathy has been established, treatment must begin immediately to prevent the progression of cor-

neal damage and promote epithelial healing. The therapy must be prompt and based on the clinical stage of the disease (**Figure 26.4**) (Nishida & Yanai 2009).

Stage 1 disease requires the discontinuation of all topical medications. The topical administration of preservative-free artificial tears may help improve the corneal surface. Therapy at this stage should aim to improve epithelial quality and transparency and avoid epithelial breakdown. Ocular surface-associated diseases, such as exposure keratitis, dry eye disease, and limbal deficiency, may worsen the prognosis of the disease and require specific treatment. In these cases, it is mandatory to correct the eyelid dysfunction, consider punctal occlusion, and/or perform limbal cell transplantation (Lambiase et al. 1999).

Stage 2 epithelial defects must be treated to prevent the development of corneal ulcers, promote healing, and prevent the recurrence of the epithelial breakdown. The withdrawal of all topical drugs is always required, and preservative-free artificial tears may be used to improve the corneal surface. Corneal or scleral therapeutic contact lenses have been proposed, but their use may increase the risk of secondary infections and cause sterile hypopyon.

In unresponsive cases, tarsorrhaphy is the most simple and diffuse procedure. If healing occurs, the tarsorrhaphy opening may be enlarged after a few weeks, but opening the tarsorrhaphy prematurely may result in the recurrence of corneal epithelial breakdown. Alternatively, it is possible to cover the epithelial defect using an amniotic membrane transplantation (AMT) or utilizing a palpebral spring or botulinum A toxin injection of the eyelid elevator. Specifically, AMT is a surgical technique for ocular surface reconstruction that should be considered in the management of refractory neurotrophic corneal ulcers. AMT is relatively easy to perform and is effective in promoting corneal epithelial healing and reducing vascularization and ocular surface inflammation. It has been shown showed that multilayer AMT was also useful in treating deep neurotrophic corneal ulcers (Kruse et al. 1999). A randomized controlled trial compared AMT with the conventional treatments in eyes with refractory neurotrophic corneal ulcers and showed that both AMT and conventional management (tarsorrhaphy and bandage contact lens) were effective in treatment of NK, with a median time of 21 days for complete epithelialization in both groups (Khokhar et al. 2005).

Topical steroids have been recommended because prostaglandins inhibit epithelial growth, and the use of steroids may reduce the activity of these inflammatory mediators, particularly in patients with chemical burns. However, steroids may increase the risk of corneal stromal melting and perforation by inhibiting stromal healing; their use should therefore be considered with caution. Topical non-steroidal anti-inflammatory drug treatment does not improve the healing process. The patients should be carefully monitored because the disease can frequently progress without symptoms.

Stage 3 disease requires immediate attention to stop the stromal lysis and prevent the perforation. As in stages 1 and 2, it is important to avoid the toxic effects of topical treatment; therefore, only prophylactic topical antibiotic and preservative-free artificial tears are suggested. In the case of stromal melting, topical collagenase inhibitors, such as *N*-acetylcysteine, tetracycline, or medroxyprogesterone, may be administered.

Tarsorrhaphy and conjunctival flap are effective surgical procedures for promoting corneal healing, but they provide a poor cosmetic outcome and visual function is sacrificed. Conjunctival flap is a standard surgical procedure that could restore ocular surface integrity and provide metabolic and mechanical support for corneal healing. This surgery is effective for the treatment of chronic corneal ulceration with or without corneal perforation. Specifically, the area of

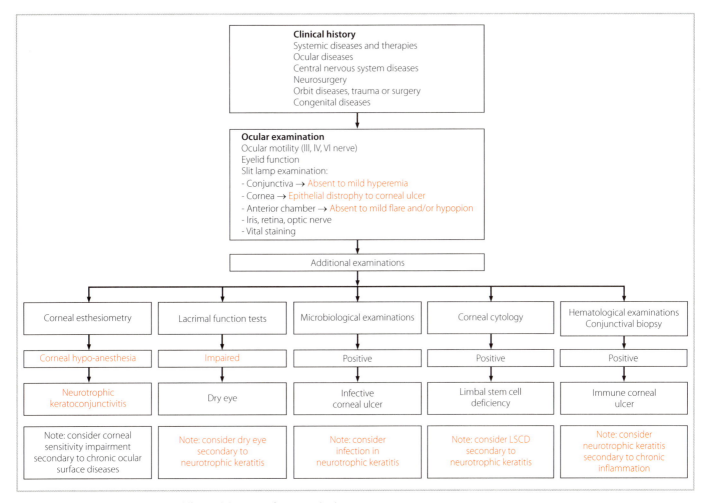

Figure 26.3 Diagnostic algorithm and differential diagnosis of neurotrophic keratoconjunctivitis.

the diseased cornea may be covered by a pedunculated conjunctival flap tailored and secured in place by fine sutures. This technique may be performed in a minor surgical procedure room under a microscope, and postoperative recovery is rapid (Khodadoust & Quinter 2003). The main goal of this procedure is to preserve the anatomical integrity of the eye, but it does not restore visual function.

Small perforations can be treated with the application of cyanoacrylate glue followed by a soft bandage contact lens, whereas larger defects require lamellar or penetrating keratoplasty. The success rate of corneal transplants is low because of poor wound healing and the persistent risk of epithelial defects from corneal anesthesia.

PROGNOSIS

NK represents one of the most difficult and challenging ocular diseases that lack a recommended course of treatment. The prognosis of NK depends on several factors, such as the cause of the impairment of corneal sensitivity, the degree of corneal hypoanesthesia, and the association with other ocular surface diseases (such as dry eye disease, exposure keratitis, and limbal deficiency). It is generally accepted that the more severe the corneal sensory impairment, the higher the probability of disease progression.

It is important to frequently assess patients with NK because the disease often lacks clinical signs and symptoms. At present, the treatment of NK is conservative, and any surgical procedure aimed at restoring corneal transparency should be avoided because of the

high risk of epithelial defects, ulcers, corneal melting, and perforation after surgery.

FUTURE DEVELOPMENTS

Several experimental and clinical studies have focused on new medical and surgical treatments for NK (Bonini et al. 2003).

Experimental sympathectomy in the rabbit may reduce corneal changes after sensory nerve damage. However, no practical application of surgical cervical sympathectomy exists in humans, and these findings have not been confirmed by sympathectomy induced by chemical substances.

Surgical procedures in which the contralateral, supraorbital, and supratrochlear nerves were inserted at the contralateral anesthetic corneal limbus for sensory neurotization have been reported to improve NK outcome in six patients with unilateral facial palsy and corneal anesthesia (Terzis et al. 2009).

Diabetic patients treated with topical aldose reductase inhibitor have shown improvement of corneal sensitivity and morphological characteristics of corneal epithelial cells. The preliminary data from an open study of nine patients with NK have indicated that treatment with thymosin β-4 eye drops is effective in promoting corneal ulcer healing (Dunn et al. 2010).

Open studies have proposed the use of autologous serum eye drops, topical non-gelified platelet-rich plasma, and umbilical cord serum eye drops in patients with NK. These studies have reported

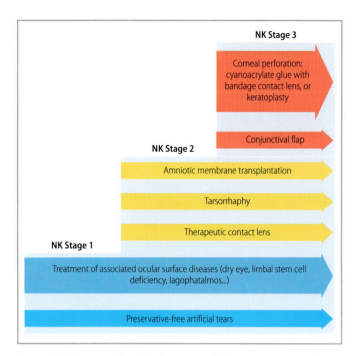

Figure 26.4 Treatment algorithm for neurotrophic keratoconjunctivitis. The therapy is based on the clinical stage of the disease. At stage 1, preservative-free artificial tears and specific treatment for ocular surface-associated diseases are required. At stage 2, preservative-free artificial tear treatment may be associated with therapeutic contact lenses. In unresponsive cases, tarsorrhaphy or amniotic membrane transplantation may be performed. Stage 3 disease often requires an additional surgical approach such as tarsorrhaphy or conjunctival flap.

a high corneal healing success rate in patients with NK, probably by providing neurotrophic factors to the damaged cornea (Jeng & Dupps 2005).

Several studies have proposed the use of neuropeptides and growth factors for the treatment of NK. The preliminary data on the use of epidermal growth factor eye drops in patients with NK were not confirmed in larger studies.

Topical treatment with SP and IGF-1 has been described in 25 patients with NK in an open uncontrolled study, and complete resurfacing of the epithelial defects has been observed in 73% of the patients within 4 weeks (Yamada et al. 2008).

Topical NGF treatment was also effective in patients with moderate to severe NK (stages 2 and 3). An open, uncontrolled study reported complete corneal healing in 100% of patients after 12 days to 6 weeks of NGF treatment. Corneal scarring was also decreased, and an improvement of visual acuity was observed. The restoration of corneal integrity was associated with a recovery of corneal sensitivity in most of the patients. The therapeutic action of NGF in NK patients is related to the multiple effects of the neurotrophin on the ocular surface (Bonini et al. 2000, Lambiase et al. 1998). In fact, NGF modulates the function, regeneration, and survival of sensory nerves; it supports epithelial proliferation and differentiation, influences the production and release of neuropeptides, and modulates tear function.

In conclusion, the management of NK poses a real challenge for ophthalmologists. Several medical and surgical treatments have been proposed to stop the progression of the disease and to avoid corneal perforation. Although surgical procedures preserve ocular integrity, they often sacrifice cosmetic appearance and visual function. Neuropeptides and growth factors may represent a future therapeutic approach for the treatment and prevention of NK.

■ REFERENCES

Belmonte C, Acosta MC, Schmelz M, Gallar J. Measurement of corneal sensitivity to mechanical and chemical stimulation with a CO_2 esthesiometer. *Invest Ophthalmol Vis Sci* 1999; **40**:513–519.

Bhatti MT, Patel R. Neuro-ophthalmic considerations in trigeminal neuralgia and its surgical treatment. *Curr Opin Ophthalmol* 2005; **16**:334–340.

Bonini S, Lambiase A, Rama P, Caprioglio G, Aloe L. Topical treatment with nerve growth factor for neurotrophic keratitis. *Ophthalmology* 2000; **107**:1347–1351.

Bonini S, Rama P, Olzi D, Lambiase A. Neurotrophic keratitis. *Eye (Lond)* 2003; **17**:989–995.

Cruzat A, Pavan-Langston D, Hamrah P. In vivo confocal microscopy of corneal nerves: analysis and clinical correlation. *Semin Ophthalmol* 2010; **25**:171–177.

Dunn SP, Heidemann DG, Chow CY, et al. Treatment of chronic nonhealing neurotrophic corneal epithelial defects with thymosin beta4. *Ann N Y Acad Sci* 2010; **1194**:199–206.

Dworkin RH, Johnson RW, Breuer J, et al. Recommendations for the management of herpes zoster. *Clin Infect Dis* 2007; 44(suppl 1):S1–S26.

Faulkner WJ, Varley GA. Corneal diagnostic tecnique. In: Krachmer JH, Mannis MJ, Holland EJ (eds), Cornea: fundamentals of cornea and external disease. St Louis, MO: Mosby, 1997:275–281.

Groos Jr EB. Neurotrophic keratitis. In: Krachmer JH, Mannis MJ, Holland EJ (eds), Cornea: clinical diagnosis and management. St Louis, MO: Mosby, 1997:340.

Jeng BH, Dupps WJ Jr. Autologous serum 50% eyedrops in the treatment of persistent corneal epithelial defects. *Cornea* 2009; **28**:1104–1108.

Khodadoust A, Quinter AP. Microsurgical approach to the conjunctival flap. *Arch Ophthalmol* 2003; **121**:1189–1193.

Khokhar S, Natung T, Sony P, et al. Amniotic membrane transplantation in refractory neurotrophic corneal ulcers: a randomized, controlled clinical trial. *Cornea* 2005; **24**:654–660.

Kruse FE, Rohrschneider K, Völcker HE. Multilayer amniotic membrane transplantation for reconstruction of deep corneal ulcers. *Ophthalmology* 1999; **106**:1504–1510.

Labetoulle M, Auquier P, Conrad H, et al. Incidence of herpes simplex virus keratitis in France. *Ophthalmology* 2005; **112**:888–895.

Lambiase A, Rama P, Aloe L, Bonini S. Management of neurotrophic keratopathy. *Curr Opin Ophthalmol* 1999; **10**:270–276.

Lambiase A, Rama P, Bonini S, Caprioglio G, Aloe L. Topical treatment with nerve growth factor for corneal neurotrophic ulcers. *N Engl J Med* 1998; **338**:1174–1180.

Mackie IA. Neuroparalytic keratitis. In: Fraunfelder F, Roy FH, Meyer SM (eds), Current ocular therapy. Philadelphia, PA: WB Saunders, 1995:452–454.

Mandahl A. Hypertonic saline test for ophthalmic nerve impairment. *Acta Ophthalmol (Copenh)* 1993; **71**:556–559.

Müller LJ, Marfurt CF, Kruse F, Tervo TM. Corneal nerves: structure, contents and function. *Exp Eye Res* 2003; **76**:521–542.

Nishida T, Yanai R. Advances in treatment for neurotrophic keratopathy. *Curr Opin Ophthalmol* 2009; **20**:276–281.

Norn MS. Measurement of sensitivity. In: Norn MS (ed.), External eye diseases. Methods of examination. Copenhagen: Munksgaard International Publisher Ltd, 1974.

Rosenberg ME, Tervo TM, Immonen IJ, et al. Corneal structure and sensitivity in type 1 diabetes mellitus. *Invest Ophthalmol Vis Sci* 2000; **41**:2915–2921.

Terzis JK, Dryer MM, Bodner BI. Corneal neurotization: a novel solution to neurotrophic keratopathy. *Plast Reconstr Surg* 2009; **123**:112–120.

Yamada N, Matsuda R, Morishige N, et al. Open clinical study of eye-drops containing tetrapeptides derived from substance P and insulin-like growth factor-1 for treatment of persistent corneal epithelial defects associated with neurotrophic keratopathy. *Br J Ophthalmol* 2008; **92**:896–900.

Chapter 27

Mechanical causes of ocular surface disease

David H. Verity, J. Richard O. Collin

The health of the ocular surface is dependent on diverse factors that can individually or collectively promote or impair ocular surface function (**Table 27.1**). Because the purpose of the lids is to protect and nourish the ocular surface, it follows that both mechanical and physiological changes within their tissues jeopardize the integrity of the corneal surface, and therefore vision (**Table 27.2**). This chapter reviews both congenital and acquired mechanical causes of ocular surface disease, with an emphasis on etiology and pathophysiology. These include lid diseases per se, and other mechanical processes that can indirectly cause corneal surface disease. Comprehensive description of the management of these conditions is beyond the scope of this review, and for this the reader is referred to the wider literature.

CONGENITAL AND HEREDITARY CAUSES

Epiblepharon and congenital entropion of the lower eyelid

Epiblepharon is most commonly encountered among children of Asian descent, and describes a fold of excess skin and orbicularis muscle in the lower eyelid (**Figure 27.1a**). Rarely this fold can progress to inversion of the lid margin resulting in a true lower lid entropion, which can cause ocular irritation and corneal abrasion, with significant astigmatism as a further reported complication (Kim et al. 2010, Noda et al. 1989). Epiblepharon typically improves spontaneously; treatment is usually reserved for patients with entropion and marked signs of

Table 27.1 Requisite eyelid anatomy and function for a healthy ocular surface

1.	Structural integrity of the eyelid, including healthy anterior, middle and of anterior, middle, and posterior lamellae
2.	Adequate volume and surface area of lid lamellae, and without excess
3.	Correct position of the eyelids relative to the globe
4.	Full innervation of all parts of the orbicularis muscle, including preseptal, pretarsal, and 'lacrimal pump' components
5.	Freedom of movement of the eyelids over the ocular surface (i.e. sufficiency of blink sweep)
6.	Normal movements of the globe relative to the eyelids (i.e. adequate Bell's phenomenon)
7.	Sufficient production, and even surface distribution, of the aqueous component of tears from the major and accessory lacrimal glands
8.	Adequate secretion of meibomian gland secretions onto the tear film surface (these stabilizing the precorneal tear film)
9.	Effective drainage of the precorneal tear film away from the eye (i.e. normal lacrimal outflow)
10.	Normal corneal sensation

Table 27.2 Pathophysiology of ocular surface disease - structural causes

Abnormalities of the tear film
• Irregular distribution
– Eyelid notches and peaks
– Eyelid malposition: entropion and ectropion
– Floppy eyelid syndrome
• Deficiency in lacrimal gland tear production (true dry eye disease)
– Lacrimal gland surgery or radiotherapy
– Cicatricial or traumatic obliteration of the lacrimal gland ductules
– Injury to ocular surface goblet cells with reduced mucus production
• Toxic tear lake and/or mucus trapping
– Lacrimal outflow impedance
– Lower eyelid ectropion
– Giant fornix syndrome
– Floppy eyelid syndrome
Abrasion of the ocular surface
• Entropion
– Involutional
– Cicatricial disease of the posterior lamella
• Trichiasis and Distichiasis
• Distichiasis
• Keratinization of the ocular surface
• Eyelid tumors
Lagophthalmos and exposure keratopathy
• Full-thickness eyelid defects
• Reduced compliance of the anterior lamella after surgery
• Neuropraxia, or palsy, of the facial nerve or its branches
• Impaired globe movement relative to the eyelids
– Direct injury to the superior rectus muscle
– Adhesions (synechiae) between the ocular surface and the eyelid
• Thyroid eye disease (TED)
– Upper lid retraction
– Inferior rectus tethering and reduced elevation of the globe
– Exophthalmos
• All causes of proptosis
Exposure of implanted material
• Retinal bands
• Posterior lamella suture exposure (i.e. after eyelid reconstruction)
• Exposed brow suspensory material within the conjunctival fornix
• Globe abrasion by orbital plates or screws

corneal irritation. It involves the excision of a horizontal crescent of excess eyelid skin and muscle. The defect is closed with skin sutures, which include a pass through the deep inferior tarsal border and lower lid retractors to prevent recurrence of entropion.

Congenital entropion of the lower eyelid is rare, and is due to an excess of skin and orbicularis oculi muscle with a relatively loose attachment of the eyelid retractors. This causes a posterior rotation of the lid margin and eyelashes toward the ocular surface, with ocular irritation further exacerbating the effect. Corneal epithelial defects can occur soon after birth, and are corrected with transverse lid sutures and horizontal stabilization of the lateral canthal tendon.

Congenital upper lid retraction and entropion

Congenital retraction of the upper eyelid levator muscle is rare, and can be associated with shortage of skin (**Figure 27.1b**). Treatment involves releasing or lengthening the retractor complex, and addressing any shortage of the anterior lamella with a full-thickness skin graft (Morax & Hurbli 1988).

Congenital horizontal tarsal kink is an unusual form of upper lid entropion, which presents in infancy with trichiasis and secondary blepharospasm and corneal ulceration. Horizontal kinking of the tarsal plate permits a rotation of the lid margin toward the globe; treatment with a simple anterior lamella reposition is generally effective (Price & Collin 1987).

Eyelid coloboma

Eyelid colobomas vary in size from small, localized notches compatible with normal corneal protection, to large defects with subtotal loss of lid tissues and corneal exposure in severe cases (**Figure 27.1c**) (Collin 1986). They may be idiopathic, occur as part of a first-arch syndrome, such as Goldenhar's syndrome, or be associated with facial clefts or amniotic bands. Large colobomas require urgent repair to prevent corneal opacification, but frequently carry a poor prognosis for visual development despite surgical reconstruction. Ocular surface abnormalities may also be present; these include limbal dermoids and conjunctival forniceal choristomatous lesions and traction bands; the latter restricts ocular vertical ductions and is a further risk for the development of amblyopia. This spectrum of disease, from small local notches, which are of aesthetic concern but carry no risk to vision, to major lid defects with derangement of the conjunctival fornices probably reflects embryological abnormalities occurring at different stages of development. The more profound defects are likely to occur early in development—before fusion of the lid folds—whereas smaller defects probably result from a failure of separation of these folds at a later stage.

Management principles include addressing conjunctival shortage and bands, and either a direct closure of the defect or other reconstruction of the eyelid. The latter can involve mucous membrane grafting to create new conjunctival fornices, and rotational skin and muscle flaps from the adjacent tissues to complete the anterior lamella. In severe cases a two-stage switch flap from the lower eyelid into the upper lid defect can be considered, which effectively replaces the defect with healthy lower eyelid tissues (Collin 1986).

Distichiasis

True congenital distichiasis is defined by an abnormal additional line of eyelashes emanating from the meibomian gland orifices, with all

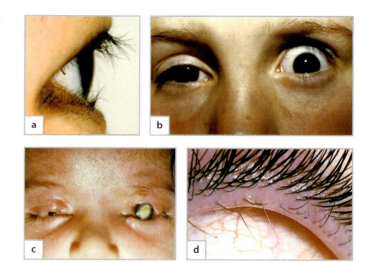

Figure 27.1 Congenital eyelid disease. (a) Epiblepharon showing proximity of the eyelashes to the globe (note the absence of true entropion in this case). (b) Congenital left upper lid retraction. (c) Bilateral upper eyelid colobomas with severe left corneal exposure and scarring. (d) True congenital distichiasis.

four eyelids frequently involved (**Figure 27.1d**). Inheritance is autosomal dominant (with incomplete penetrance), and associations with diverse systemic abnormalities have also been reported (including epicanthus, telecanthus, blepharophimosis, ptosis, color blindness, lymphedema, eyelid edema, and the Pierre Robin syndrome) (O'Donnell & Collin 1993). Various treatments have been proposed, including cryotherapy to the posterior lamella after performing a lid-split examination, although this carries a risk of secondary tissue instability, entropion, and ectropion. The best approach, but also the most time-consuming, is direct surgical exposure of the individual lash follicles and electrolysis.

ACQUIRED STRUCTURAL CAUSES

Involutional causes

Eyelid structure and function are largely dependent on horizontal and vertical collagen support. With age, or recurrent periocular inflammation or irritation, collagen strength and density are reduced, and the stabilizing effect of the medial and lateral canthal tendons is impaired. This destabilizing effect, in terms of position of the eyelid relative to the cornea, is further exacerbated by similar collagen changes within the insertions of the eyelid retractor muscles and the tarsi themselves; where there is also dissociation between the anterior and posterior lamellae, eyelid ectropion or entropion can result, with the etiologies for these two conditions being very similar.

Involutional ectropion

The etiological factors in acquired ectropion are similar to those for entropion. However, tissue laxity in the absence of orbicularis hypertrophy tends to cause ectropion, and, in the case of the lower eyelid, where there is also a dissociation of the retractors from the tarsus, complete eversion of the tarsus along its horizontal axis axis can occur (**Figure 27.2a**). Although ectropion has a less deleterious effect on the ocular surface than entropion, where there is preexisting ocular surface disease or exophthalmos (either constitutional or pathological), the effect of ectropion on the ocular surface can be more severe.

Involutional entropion

In addition to the tissue laxity described previously, vertical dissociation of the orbicularis oculis muscle and skin from the underlying tarsal plate plays an important role in involutional entropion. Clinically, this can be seen as tissue crowding along the palpebral aperture during forced lid closure, with dermatochalasis often contributing to upper lid entropion. Indeed, overriding of the preseptal orbicularis muscle on the pretarsal muscle can result in total inversion of the lower eyelid (**Figure 27.2b**). This causes chronic ocular surface irritation, with secondary blepharospasm often exacerbating the entropion.

The symptoms of entropion include ocular irritation, lid spasm, pain, redness, and watering, and are worse where there is a keratinized lid margin (more commonly seen in cicatricial disease) or where the ocular surface is already compromised.

Complications of entropion include conjunctival migration over the eyelid margin, sometimes extending beyond the meibomian gland orifices, misdirected or absent eyelashes, metaplastic lashes arising from meibomian glands, marginal telangiectases, and the formation of keratin near the eyelid margin. All of these changes can lead to further compromise of the ocular surface, and the clinician should always examine the tear film and corneal epithelium in a patient with an eyelid malposition.

■ Primary collagen failure: floppy eyelid syndrome

The hallmark of floppy eyelid syndrome (FES) is hyperelasticity of the eyelid tarsus and loss of tissue rigidity (**Figure 27.2c**). This is associated (though not exclusively) with major obesity and sleep apnea, the latter being due to recurrent complete or partial upper airways obstruction. Ocular complications, including spontaneous eyelid eversion, imbrication of the upper eyelid over the lower eyelid, mucus trapping under the lax eyelids, a chronic papillary conjunctivitis, keratinization of the posterior lamella, and even corneal perforation, have been reported (Rossiter et al. 2002). The cause of FES remains uncertain, although a reduction in mature elastin and upregulation of elastase activity have been identified. Whether these findings reflect the underlying etiology, repeated eyelid rubbing, or trauma sustained during spontaneous nocturnal eversion remains unknown.

Treatment of FES is aimed at addressing the excess laxity, and this is best performed by plicating the medial or lateral canthal tendon, depending on the position of maximum laxity (Ezra et al. 2010). However, due to the etiology of FES, repeat surgery is often required, this carrying a risk of secondary upper lid ptosis, and reduction of the horizontal palpebral aperture.

■ Trichiasis

Trichiasis describes eyelashes whose follicles arise at an abnormal site (e.g. metaplastic lashes and distichiasis), or which are normal in origin, being in the lash line, but are misdirected. Causes include trauma, chronic lid inflammation, and scarring (see later). Not infrequently, trichiasis is diagnosed in the presence of lid malposition, and injudicious electrolysis without correction of the underlying lid malposition can cause unnecessary scarring and is, at best, ineffective.

For localized trichiasis, splitting of the gray line and full-thickness excision of the abnormal anterior lamella (or a full-thickness pentagon excision of the central eyelid) is very effective. Although cryotherapy is frequently performed for more extensive areas, this can occasionally cause skin depigmentation and further scarring. Electrolysis alone is associated with recurrence in up to half of cases (Khandekar et

al. 2001), but if a cutdown to the lash follicle is first performed, the follicle can be electrolyzed directly, which is considerably more effective. Targeted ablation of the lash follicle can also be achieved using the argon laser, with success rates ranging from 28 to 89% (Oshry et al. 1994). The complications of this approach are minimal, although repeat treatments may be required.

■ Giant fornix syndrome

First reported in 2004, giant fornix syndrome describes a chronic purulent conjunctivitis associated with an unusually deep upper conjunctival fornix in an elderly patient (**Figure 27.2d**) (Rose 2004). Trapping of bacteria (exclusively *Staphylococcus aureus*) and protein coagulum within such a capacious conjunctival fornix can lead to a relapsing bacterial conjunctivitis, with a diagnostic delay of up to 4 years, and a high risk of secondary corneal scarring, thinning, and even perforation. Management is with systemic antibiotics (ciprofloxacin or ofloxacin), intensive topical antibiotics, and frequent application of steroids; patients may also require continued once-daily topical application of a combined steroid antibiotic to prevent relapse.

■ Neurological: facial nerve paresis

The ocular complications of facial nerve paresis or palsy are well described and require little further explanation (Lee et al. 2004a). Broadly, ocular surface disease results from four chief mechanisms: (i) upper lid retraction, (ii) lower lid atony with secondary ectropion, (iii) reduced lacrimal 'pump' function with stagnation of the precorneal tear film and secondary ocular surface toxicity, and, finally, (iv) reduced eyelid blink excursion and lagophthalmos (this typically persisting despite apparent clinical recovery). The great majority of patients with idiopathic facial nerve palsy (Bell's palsy) require supportive measures only with topical lubricants and lid taping until orbicularis power has improved. Patients with a structural cause

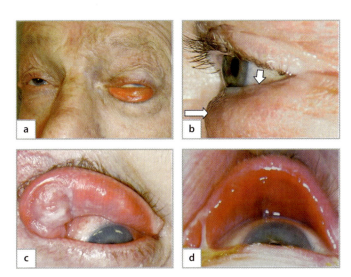

Figure 27.2 Lid malposition: age-related tissue atrophy, and collagen failure. (a) Left lower eyelid 'shelf' ectropion. (b) Total lower lid entropion (short arrow showing 180° inversion of lid margin) due to horizontal laxity and overriding of the preseptal on the pretarsal orbicularis oculis muscle (long arrow). (c) Floppy eyelid syndrome: tarsal conjunctival keratinization with irritation of the ocular surface. (d) Giant fornix syndrome: tarsal conjunctival inflammation and mucus trapping.

frequently have reduced corneal sensation, and are thus more likely to require intervention to prevent corneal exposure, including upper lid weighting or retractor recession, lower lid support or tightening, or tarsorrhaphies.

Eyelid tumors

Neoplastic disease of the eyelids can lead to corneal pathology either as a result of direct extension and involvement of the ocular surface, or through a mechanical effect with secondary failure of adequate eyelid closure. Commonly misdiagnosed as 'unilateral blepharitis,' sebaceous cell carcinoma of the eyelid can present with chronic ocular irritation and a remarkably bland clinical picture; in some there may be localized lash loss, significant ocular injection, and ulceration of the lid margin, but in others the clinical signs are less evident. A history of chronic unilateral symptoms and signs should, however, always prompt the clinician to consider a biopsy. Management depends on the extent of disease. All patients require a full head and neck oncology review to exclude metastatic disease. Younger patients should also be screened for Muir–Torre syndrome, a rare autosomal genodermatosis characterized by sebaceous neoplasms and visceral carcinomas (Ponti & de Leon 2005). Where disease is limited to the eyelid (defined by widespread conjunctival mapping biopsies), local resection and reconstruction can be considered. However, where there is more widespread intraepithelial (pagetoid) spread onto the ocular surface, exenteration (with or without sentinel lymph node biopsy) offers the best chance of survival (Savar et al. 2011, Shields et al. 2004).

CICATRIZING CONJUNCTIVAL DISEASE

The primary causes of cicatricial conjunctival disease include trachoma, chronic topical medication, ocular mucous membrane pemphigoid (OcMMP), and other autoimmune reactions such as Stevens–Johnson syndrome (SJS), toxic epidermal necrolysis (TEN), and graft-versus-host disease. Management is directed at limiting the early inflammatory reaction with topical and systemic immunosuppressants and antibacterial agents, providing supportive corneal lubrication, and correcting secondary eyelid and eyelash malposition to prevent corneal opacification.

Upper and lower eyelid cicatricial entropion is due to vertical scarring and shortening of the tarsoconjunctiva. Abrasion of the ocular surface by the posteriorly orientated lid margin is typically further aggravated by eyelid retraction, secondary lagophthalmos, and impaired blink excursion. Although lower eyelid entropion causes mild-to-moderate irritation of the inferior cornea, upper lid entropion tends to cause more severe corneal changes, and this is further exacerbated by secondary keratin formation and metaplastic or misdirected eyelashes. Conjunctival keratinization often resolves with correction of eyelid malposition, but persistent keratinization may require eversion of the terminal tarsus. Although persistently aberrant eyelashes can be treated with electrolysis or cryotherapy, this can lead to further posterior lamellar scarring and hence increase the tendency to cicatricial entropion. Direct excision of the anterior lamella that bears the aberrant lash follicles is frequently a better option, with re-epithelialization of the bare tarsus occurring rapidly and with a very acceptable aesthetic result.

Trachoma

Trachoma, caused by *Chlamydia trachomatis*, is one of the earliest recorded diseases in ancient medical literature, and remains the leading infectious cause of blindness worldwide. It is estimated to account for the loss of approximately 1.3 million disability-adjusted life years, and occurs chiefly in sub-Saharan Africa (World Health Organization 2008). In 2009, the WHO estimated that 40 million people suffered from active trachoma, that over 8 million had untreated trachomatous trichiasis, and that it was endemic in many parts of Africa and Asia, and prevalent in Latin America and the Middle East.

With repeated infection of the ocular surface, chronic inflammation within the tarsal conjunctiva leads to trachomatous trichiasis, this leading to moderate-to-severe entropion in about half of all patients. Visually significant ocular surface opacification is recorded in about one third of patients, of which over a half have bilateral disease.

Treatment includes antibiotics with a single dose of oral azithromycin, repeated every 6–12 months, improving hand and face hygiene, and surgery to correct eyelid entropion. (The extent of surgery depends on severity of entropion, but typically involves upper eyelid retractor recession, splitting the gray line, and anterior lamellar repositioning sutures, with or without tarsal incision to aid external rotation of the eyelid. More severe cases require complete anterior–posterior lamella dissociation—lamellar slide—and where there is keratinization of the eyelid margin, terminal marginal rotation may be required.) *C. trachomatis* is active chiefly among children younger than 10 years, and single-dose community-based antibiotic treatment is also effective in reducing the prevalence of active trachoma in affected communities. Whether oral or topical antibiotic is more effective is less certain, although controlled azithromycin treatment seems more effective than unsupervised topical tetracycline use (Evans & Solomon 2011).

Ocular mucous membrane pemphigoid

With a rapid onset, and unpredictable and severe relapses, OcMMP can cause bilateral blindness despite optimum medical and surgical management (Chan et al. 2002, Miserocchi et al. 2002). The onset of OcMMP typically occurs after the second decade of life, but has a peak onset age after 70 years, and a diagnostic delay of months to years is not uncommon. Three quarters of patients require immunosuppression to control the disease at some point in their life, and a half also experience extraocular disease, be it oral or cutaneous. Repeated and unpredictable episodes of inflammation directed against the conjunctival basement membrane lead to progressive cicatricial conjunctival changes, with, variably, secondary shortening of the conjunctival fornices, entropion and lid retraction (**Figure 27.3a**), destruction of conjunctival and corneal limbal stem cells, and obliteration of the lacrimal ductile orifices (Elder et al. 1996). Collectively, these changes threaten the cornea due to direct eyelid and lash irritation, impaired regenerative ability of the conjunctival and corneal stem stems, and reduced ocular lubrication. In severe cases, lagophthalmos and microbial keratitis can occur, with chronic surface inflammation eventually leading to a scarred, vascularized, or keratinized ocular surface (**Figure 27.3b** and **c**).

Treatment of OcMMP should be directed by experienced clinicians; early diagnosis and recognition of the potential severity of ocular surface inflammation with prompt treatment are essential, as ocular complications can ensue rapidly and without warning. Medical treatment should be overseen by a clinician experienced in the use of immunosuppressants and biological agents. Early intervention is required, using either a 'stepladder' approach based on the severity of disease activity, or the primary use of oral cyclophosphamide; both can affect a long-lasting remission. Drugs used in the stepladder approach include dapsone, azathioprine, mycophenolate mofetil, and cyclophosphamide (Saw et al. 2008), and surgery may be required to correct entropion, trichiasis, and lid retraction. Where there is lagophthalmos and reduced globe movement due to major conjunctival shrinkage, conjunctival fornix reconstruction may also be required. However, the active inflammatory process should be controlled first, and the patient should be monitored closely for evidence of reactivation where surgery has involved the posterior lamella.

Stevens–Johnson syndrome (SJS)

SJS is an acute life-threatening mucocutaneous disease characterized by cutaneous erythema, hemorrhagic erosions of mucous membranes, and severe blepharoconjunctivitis. Characteristic histological features include keratinocyte necrosis, which can involve the entire thickness of the epidermis, and vacuolization in the basal membrane zone, which leads to subepidermal blistering. Previously considered similar to erythema multiforme, SJS is now thought to be be related to toxic epidermal necrolysis (TEN), sharing similar histological features, etiology, and genetic susceptibility. Typically drug-induced, SJS is caused by a cell-mediated cytotoxic reaction and has a high mortality (10%) despite supportive measures [over 100 drugs have been implicated, in addition to mycoplasma pneumonia, viral infections, and varicella vaccination (Auquier-Dunant et al. 2002)]. Complications of SJS include mucous membrane strictures and non-progressive nonprogressive conjunctival cicatricial changes; the latter can cause entropion, recurrent metaplastic eye lashes, and dry eye disease due to obliteration of accessory lacrimal glands, corneal limbal goblet cells, and the lacrimal gland ductules.

Linear IgA disease

Linear IgA dermatosis is a very rare autoimmune subepidermal blistering disorder of the skin and mucous membranes. The majority of cases are idiopathic, but associations with vancomycin and other drugs have infrequently been reported. Ophthalmic complications, such as ocular surface inflammation (**Figure 27.3d**), subconjunctival fibrosis, symblepharon formation, and entropion, are virtually identical to those seen in OcMMP, with the diagnosis depending on the identification of IgA autoantibodies in a linear distribution at the dermal–epidermal junction (Ramos-Castellón et al. 2010).

Burns and chemical injuries

Severe chemical and thermal burns to the eyelids and ocular surface—due to acidic, caustic, or thermal injuries—can cause catastrophic destruction of corneal limbal stem cells, goblet cells, and, frequently, the lacrimal ductule orifices. The effect on the ocular surface is often compounded by anterior segment ischemia, eyelid entropion, and trichiasis. This picture is similar to that seen in other devastating ocular surface disorders such as SJS and TEN, and the prognosis of these patients is largely dependent on the immediate management. Early measures include correcting the pH of the ocular surface, treating any associated extra- and intraocular inflammation, providing adequate

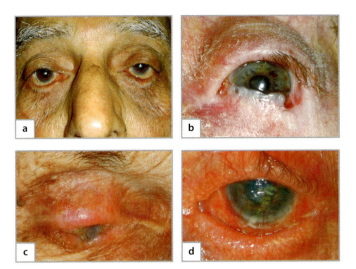

Figure 27.3 Cicatricial causes of eyelid malposition. (a) Lower lid retraction and lagophthalmos due to conjunctival forniceal contraction in ocular mucous membrane pemphigoid (OcMMP). (b) OcMMP resulting in obliteration of the inferior fornix, complete adhesion of the lower eyelid to the globe, and ocular surface exposure due to lagophthalmos. (c) Advanced OcMMP with complete obliteration of the conjunctival fornices and keratinization of the ocular surface. (d) Severe ocular complications of linear IgA disease: cicatricial lower eyelid entropion, lagophthalmos, and ocular surface failure (the fellow eye not shown, but similarly affected and being blind due to severe microbial keratitis).

intensity and duration of free radical scavengers (in the form of topical ascorbate and oral vitamin C), and prevention of ocular surface infection and glaucoma. However, such injuries often profoundly affect ocular surface anatomy and physiology, and subsequent visual rehabilitation can be challenging, requiring significant corneal and oculoplastics expertise. In general, corneal rehabilitation (which may include penetrating and non-penetrating keratoplasty, limbal stem cell grafting, and keratoprosthesis surgery) can only be considered once any associated eyelid or eyelash malposition has been corrected, and lagophthalmos has been addressed.

LACRIMAL DISEASE

In addition to providing essential corneal nutrients and oxygen to the cornea, the dynamic 'sweep' of tears to the medial canthus dilutes and removes toxic cytokines, cellular debris, and microbes from the ocular surface. Thus, any mechanical disorder that interferes with this process can lead to stagnation of the tear film and ocular surface toxicity. Such disorders include (i) any pathology that reduces the blink frequency (e.g. Parkinson's disease) or excursion (e.g. facial nerve palsy or paresis), (ii) impaired eyelid–globe apposition (e.g. ectropion, eyelid margin irregularity, and severe enophthalmos), and (iii) lacrimal outflow obstruction. Facial nerve palsy typically interferes with the first two of these processes, whereas stenosis of the lacrimal outflow pathways, including retained foreign bodies such as intracanalicular (or lacrimal duct) plugs and stents, can cause a buildup of stagnant debris on the ocular surface. The latter effect is further exacerbated where there is condensation of mucus and bacterial proliferation within the enlarged lacrimal sac (potentially leading to an infected mucocele). In the presence of a healthy cornea with an intact epithelium, ocular surface disease is uncommon, but where there are preexisting risk factors for corneal disease—such as SJS or lagophthalmos from any cause—chronic ocular surface inflammation and infection can occur. For this reason, all patients with surface failure require a careful lacrimal assessment if treatable risk factors are to be identified.

ORBITAL DISEASE

Any orbital pathology that causes proptosis, reduced globe elevation, and/or reduced corneal sensation can lead to corneal exposure. Pathologies therefore include all orbital apical inflammatory, vascular, and neoplastic processes that impair the function of the trigeminal nerve (corneal sensation) and/or the superior branch of the oculomotor nerve (elevation of the globe). Furthermore, where there is also exophthalmos due to a mass effect, lagophthalmos further contributes to the risk of corneal exposure. Finally, in thyroid eye disease, the most common causes for both unilateral and bilateral proptosis, upper and lower lid retraction, and reduced globe elevation (due to inferior rectus fibrosis) are major risk factors for severe exposure keratopathy.

True dry eye disease occurs very infrequently following lacrimal gland inflammation or surgery, although it can occur following the inadvisable practice of performing a lacrimal gland biopsy via the conjunctival fornix (in which the lacrimal ductules are often inadvertently injured). However, reduced tear production not uncommonly occurs following the treatment of lacrimal gland carcinoma with surgical excision and adjunctive high-dose radiotherapy to the lacrimal fossa. The latter can cause an ocular sicca syndrome, and frequent topical lubrication may be required indefinitely. Although excision of the lacrimal gland mass can be complicated by secondary ptosis, corrective surgery should be resisted because of the major risk of secondary corneal exposure and even perforation.

TRAUMATIC AND IATROGENIC CAUSES

Injury or surgery to the periocular region carries a risk of corneal exposure due to structural eyelid changes, blink function, and altered lacrimal physiology. Frequently, periocular injuries cause eyelid malpositions, lid margin notches or peaks (**Figure 27.4a**), reduced tissue compliance and/or innervation of the eyelids with incomplete blink cycle, lagophthalmos, and impaired lacrimal outflow (**Table 27.2**). Chemical injuries to the ocular surface can also result in corneal stem cell failure and lead to progressive surface scarring in addition to synechiae and impaired lid closure and even cryptophthalmos (**Figure 27.4b** and **27.4c**). Impaired dynamic function of the upper eyelid carries the highest risk of exposure keratopathy, and where there is reduced tear delivery to the ocular surface, the risk of corneal complications is even higher. Thus, despite surgical restoration of ocular anatomy, and correction of

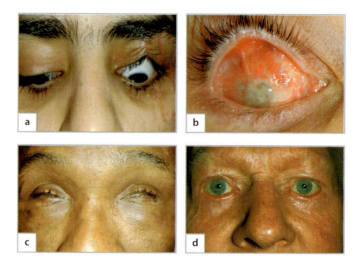

Figure 27.4 Traumatic and iatrogenic causes of ocular surface disease. (a) Upper eyelid laceration healing with vertical traction causing lid peaking and lagophthalmos. (b) Periocular scarring secondary to chemical injury (acetyl chloride, sustained during a chemistry class) leading to ocular surface failure. (c) Severe ocular chemical injury (battery acid) causing bilateral keratinization of the ocular surfaces. (d) Bilateral lower lid cicatricial ectropion due to chronic topical glaucoma mediation. The ectropion resolved with a change of medication.

entropion, trichiasis, or lagophthalmos, if the dynamic function of the eyelid remains impaired, subtle corneal surface exposure and troublesome lacrimal symptoms can persist.

Important iatrogenic causes of keratopathy include cicatricial ectropion secondary to chronic topical medication (**Figure 27.4d**), surgery or radiotherapy for orbital tumors (e.g. lacrimal gland tumors), systemic and topical drug reactions, and exposure of suture or other material on the posterior eyelid surface (**Table 27.2**). In particular, debulking of eyelid and orbital neurofibroma (Lee et al. 2004b) and dermolipomas (Economidis et al. 1978) are well known to carry a risk of postoperative dry eye (iatrogenic sicca syndrome), and the patient should always be warned of this unlikely but potentially serious complication. Surgery for the latter should be performed by an experienced surgeon with the use of an operating microscope, with attention given to removing a minimum of healthy conjunctiva, and avoidance of both the superolateral conjunctival fornix and fascial sheath over the lateral rectus muscle. Where high-dose orbital radiotherapy is indicated (e.g. after excision of a malignant lacrimal gland tumor), a degree of dry eye disease should be anticipated, frequent lubricants prescribed, and subsequent ptosis surgery be avoided if possible, for reasons discussed above.

REFERENCES

Auquier-Dunant A, Mockenhaupt M, Naldi L, et al. Severe cutaneous adverse reactions. Correlations between clinical patterns and causes of erythema multiforme majus, Stevens-Johnson syndrome, and toxic epidermal necrolysis: results of an international prospective study. *Arch Dermatol* 2002; **138**:1019–1024.

Chan LS, Ahmed AR, Anhalt GJ, et al. The first international consensus on mucous membrane pemphigoid: definition, diagnostic criteria, pathogenic factors, medical treatment, and prognostic indicators. *Arch Dermatol* 2002; **138**:370–379.

Collin JR. Congenital upper lid coloboma. *Aust N Z J Ophthalmol* 1986; **14**:313–317.

Economidis I, Tragakis M, Mangouritsas N, Papademetriou D. Keratoconjunctivitis sicca following excision of a dermolipoma of the lacrimal gland. *Ann Ophthalmol* 1978; **10**:1273–1278.

Elder MJ, Bernauer W, Leonard J, Dart JK. Progression of disease in ocular cicatricial pemphigoid. *Br J Ophthalmol* 1996; **80**:292–296.

Evans JR, Solomon AW. Antibiotics for trachoma. *Cochrane Database Syst Rev* 2011:CD001860.

Ezra DG, Beaconsfield M, Sira M, et al. Long-term outcomes of surgical approaches to the treatment of floppy eyelid syndrome. *Ophthalmology* 2010; **117**:839–846.

Khandekar R, Mohammed AJ, Courtright P. Recurrence of trichiasis: a long-term follow-up study in the Sultanate of Oman. *Ophthalmic Epidemiol* 2001; **8**:155–161.

Kim NM, Jung JH, Choi HY. The effect of epiblepharon surgery on visual acuity and with-the-rule astigmatism in children. *Korean J Ophthalmol* 2010; **24**:325–330.

Lee V, Currie Z, Collin JR. Ophthalmic management of facial nerve palsy. *Eye (Lond)* 2004a; **18**:1225–1234.

Lee V, Ragge NK, Collin JR. Orbitotemporal neurofibromatosis. Clinical features and surgical management. *Ophthalmology* 2004b; **111**:382–388.

Miserocchi E, Baltatzis S, Roque MR, Ahmed AR, Foster CS. The effect of treatment and its related side effects in patients with severe ocular cicatricial pemphigoid. *Ophthalmology* 2002; **109**:111–118.

Morax S, Hurbli T. The management of congenital malpositions of eyelids, eyes and orbits. *Eye* 1988; **2**:207–219.

Noda S, Hayasaka S, Setogawa T. Epiblepharon with inverted eyelashes in Japanese children. I. Incidence and symptoms. *Br J Ophthalmol*. 1989; **73**:126–127.

O'Donnell BA, Collin JR. Distichiasis: management with cryotherapy to the posterior lamella. *Br J Ophthalmol* 1993; **77**:289–292.

Oshry T, Rosenthal G, Lifshitz T. Argon green laser photoepilation in the treatment of trachomatous trichiasis. *Ophthal Plast Reconstr Surg* 1994; **10**:253–255.

Ponti G, de Leon MP. Muir-Torre syndrome. Lancet Oncol 2005; 6:980–987.

Price NC, Collin JR. Congenital horizontal tarsal kink: a simple surgical correction. *Br J Ophthalmol* 1987; **71**:204–206.

Ramos-Castellón C, Ortiz-Nieva G, Fresán F, et al. Ocular involvement and blindness secondary to linear IgA dermatosis. *J Ophthalmol* 2010; 2010:280396.

Rose GE. The giant fornix syndrome: an unrecognized cause of chronic, relapsing, grossly purulent conjunctivitis. *Ophthalmology* 2004; **111**:1539–1545.

Rossiter JD, Ellingham R, Hakin KN, Twomey JM. Corneal melt and perforation secondary to floppy eyelid syndrome in the presence of rheumatoid arthritis. *Br J Ophthalmol* 2002; **86**:483.

Savar A, Oellers P, Myers J, et al. Positive sentinel node in sebaceous carcinoma of the eyelid. *Ophthal Plast Reconstr Surg* 2011; **27**:e4–e6.

Saw VP, Dart JK, Rauz S, et al. Immunosuppressive therapy for ocular mucous membrane pemphigoid strategies and outcomes. *Ophthalmology* 2008; **115**:253–261.

Shields JA, Demirci H, Marr BP, Eagle RC Jr, Shields CL. Sebaceous carcinoma of the eyelids: personal experience with 60 cases. *Ophthalmology* 2004; **111**:2151–2157.

World Health Organization. The Global Burden of Disease: 2004 Update. Geneva: World Health Organization, 2008.

Chapter 28　Artificial tear substitutes

Nora Khatib, Penny A. Asbell

■ INTRODUCTION

Dry eye disease (DED) has been defined by the Report of the Definition and Classification Subcommittee of the International Dry Eye Workshop as a multifactorial disease of the tears and ocular surface that results in symptoms of discomfort, visual disturbance, and tear film instability, with potential damage to the ocular surface. It is accompanied by increased osmolarity of the tear film and inflammation of the ocular surface (International Dry Eye Workshop 2007a). Although there is significant interest and effort to develop pharmaceutical agents to treat DED, the mainstay of therapy continues to be the use of artificial tear solutions (Behrens et al. 2006, International Dry Eye Workshop 2007b). Several types of tear substitutes are available that vary in consistency, composition, and duration of action. This chapter covers the goals of therapy, efficacy of artificial tear solutions, the US Food and Drug Administration (FDA) approval process in the United States, variations in composition and ingredients in tear substitutes, and limitations of use.

■ NORMAL AND ABNORMAL TEAR FILM

The tear film is essential to the maintenance of a healthy ocular surface. Its functions are to lubricate the ocular surface, deliver nutrients to surface epithelial cells (mainly oxygen), form a smooth optical surface for clear visual acuity, and remove debris and harmful substances from contact with the eye. To optimally perform these functions, the tear film must have all components present, as well as normal tear dynamics and flow during the blink mechanism to preserve the ocular surface.

The normal tear film is a coating on the ocular surface epithelium composed of an outer lipid sealant overlying an aqueous mucin-containing gel. The corneal and conjunctival epithelial surfaces interact intimately with the tear film by producing its components and stabilizing the fluid layer. The apical surfaces of epithelial cells have multiple ridge-like folds termed microplicae from which proteins of the glycocalyx, an extracellular protein matrix coating the surface epithelium, are expressed (Cher 2007, Gipson et al. 2004). The major constituent of the glycocalyx is membrane-associated mucins (Gipson et al. 2004). These mucins extend directly into the mucoaqueous layer of the tear film and have weak, disadhesive interactions with secreted mucins to allow for fluid flow and movement. Two different types of mucins are secreted into the aqueous layer by the conjunctival goblet cells and lacrimal gland. Conjunctival goblet cells secrete large gel-forming mucins, while the lacrimal gland produces smaller soluble mucins (Gipson et al. 2004). The main role of mucins in the tear film is to remove debris and harmful pathogens from contact with the ocular surface with each blink. The aqueous, secreted from the main and accessory lacrimal glands, is a medium for the mucins and contains a decreasing gradient of mucins from the ocular surface

to the lipid layer (International Dry Eye Workshop 2007a). The outer lipid layer is produced by meibomian glands in the upper and lower tarsi of the lids (International Dry Eye Workshop 2007a, International Workshop on Meibomian Gland Dysfunction, 2011a). It consists of two layers, an outer non-polar lipid layer and an inner polar lipid layer, with intercalated proteins (International Workshop on Meibomian Gland Dysfunction, 2011b). The polar layer stabilizes the non-polar layer, which serves to retard evaporation of the tear film (International Workshop on Meibomian Gland Dysfunction, 2011b). The current view of the interpalpebral tear film reveals a complex fluid with multiple components derived from several different sources on the ocular surface and lid margins (**Figure 28.1**).

To encompass the entirety of the tear film, composed of the interpalpebral and retropalpebral portions, the neologism 'dacruon' was termed (Cher 2007, 2008). The dacruon represents the mucoaqueous layer and lipid sealant of the interpalpebral portion of the tear film as well as the opposing mucoaqueous reservoirs of the palpebral and conjunctival surfaces in the retropalpebral portion, which lacks an

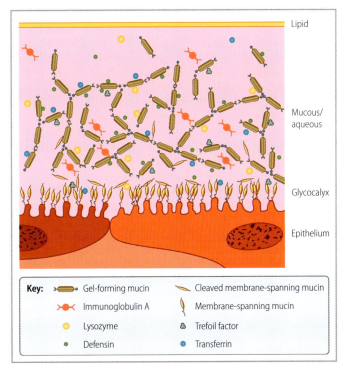

Figure 28.1 The normal tear film showing membrane-associated mucins interacting with microplicae of the epithelium and with secreted mucins in the aqueous layer. Numerous molecules, including lysozyme, immunoglobulin A, defensin, and transferrin, are also present in the normal tear film and protect the epithelium from harmful pathogens. Redrawn with permission from Gipson et al. (2004), Elsevier.

outer lipid layer. The dacruon is anchored to the underlying epithelial surfaces via the glycocalyx and membrane-associated proteins. In this view, the attachment of the tear film to the underlying epithelium implies that the eyelids are the main source of movement of the tear film during the blink mechanism. With each blink, shearing force generated by movement of the lids is dissipated by the central mucoaqueous layers, permitting frictionless movement of the lids (Cher 2007, 2008).

The tear film is a dynamic structure that is constantly changing during different phases of the blink mechanism. After blinking, the tear film initially undergoes a rapid buildup phase to form a smooth and stable tear film. Following the buildup phase, the tear film undergoes a gradual thinning and breaks up. The tear film thins at a greater rate at the center of the cornea than at the periphery, affecting optical clarity (Montés-Micó et al. 2010). Dry spots begin to form in the normal tear film 10–12 seconds postblink, resulting in a number of aberrations on the surface epithelium (Wander & Koffler 2009). The dynamic changes in the tear film occur at a faster rate in dry eye patients with inadequate tear films (Montés-Micó et al. 2010). The outer lipid coating also undergoes dynamic changes during the blink. The lipid layer is compressed during the blink and must redistribute to coat the new aqueous layer on lid opening. Lipid film spreading is rapid in normal eyes to protect the tear film from evaporation and occurs in 0.3 second (Montés-Micó et al. 2010). In DED, tear lipid film spreading is significantly slower, occurring at 3.5 and 2.2 seconds in patients with lipid and aqueous tear deficiency, respectively (Montés-Micó et al. 2010).

The layers of the tear film work as a single unit, and an abnormality in one component affects the others and compromises the normal function of the tear film as a whole. A deficiency in the lipid layer causes increased rates of evaporation of the aqueous layer and decreased tear break-up time, as in meibomian gland dysfunction (MGD). MGD is an alteration of glandular secretion, either hypersecretion, hyposecretion, or obstruction of the glands, that results in a change in lipid composition of meibomian secretions that can ultimately affect the normal tear film to result in ocular surface disease and irritation (International Workshop on Meibomian Gland Dysfunction 2011a). Correspondingly, a thin aqueous layer can be insufficient to support the normal lipid layer, resulting in its thinning and even disappearance in severe DED. To compensate for the shorter tear break-up time and rapid changes in the tear film, the blink rate is increased in patients with DED (Montés-Micó et al. 2010).

Regardless of the etiology of the abnormal tear film, the outcome and effect on the ocular surface are similar (Asbell 2006, International Dry Eye Workshop 2007a). Increased evaporation and decreased aqueous production create an unstable and hyperosmolar tear film (International Dry Eye Workshop 2007a). Tear hyperosmolarity stimulates the inflammatory cascade on the surface epithelium, including activation of inflammatory cytokines and matrix metalloproteinases (International Dry Eye Workshop 2007a). These inflammatory molecules damage the corneal and conjunctival epithelium by altering cell permeability and by degrading the cellular basement membrane, resulting in cellular injury and apoptosis (International Dry Eye Workshop 2007a). Hyperosmolarity of the tear film also alters the normal action of mucins, which diminishes ocular surface lubrication and leads to increased shear stress during the blink (Asbell 2006). The underlying cause of symptoms of DED has not been identified but likely results from one or a combination of tear hyperosmolarity, ocular surface inflammation, reduced mucin expression, shear stress between the lid and ocular surface, and hypersensitivity of ocular surface sensory nerves (International Dry Eye Workshop 2007a).

EFFICACY OF ARTIFICIAL TEAR SOLUTIONS

The first-line therapy for DED is the use of artificial lubricants. The goal of the use of artificial tear solutions is primarily to relieve the symptoms associated with DED and to re-establish a new equilibrium in a deficient tear film. Thus, an ideal artificial tear substitute will form a stable tear film with increased tear break-up time, protect the corneal and conjunctival epithelium from damage and microbial contamination, maintain optical clarity for adequate visual acuity, and provide relief of symptoms and comfort to the patient while being cost-effective (Asbell 2006).

DED causes symptoms that can significantly impact sufferers' daily activities, workplace productivity, and quality of life (Asbell 2006, International Dry Eye Workshop 2007c). Repeated exposure of the ocular surface epithelium due to tear deficiencies produces sensations of ocular discomfort, including foreign body sensation, irritation, burning, redness, and intermittent blurred vision. These symptoms can be debilitating and interfere with daily vision-related activities, such as driving, reading, and working with the computer, which negatively impact quality of life (**Table 28.1**) (Asbell 2006, Nelson et al. 2005). DED also causes contact lens intolerance and results in ineligibility for laser-assisted in situ keratomileusis (LASIK), which can negatively affect quality of life for contact lens wearers (International Dry Eye Workshop 2007c). To measure the degree to which DED affects quality of life, a utility assessment comparing the impact of various diseases on quality of life demonstrated that DED scored similar to moderate angina (International Dry Eye Workshop 2007c). This assessment indicates that the symptoms of DED are a real and chronic irritant to

Table 28.1 Effect of dry eye symptoms on daily life

Quality-of-life measure*	Patients (%)†
Feel less confident	38.6
Need to decrease leisure time	35.7
Frustrated with daily activities	34.3
Need to change daily activities	25.7
Feel unhappy or depressed	25.7
Need to decrease work time	11.4
Require help	14.3
Miss outings	12.9
Change work	7.1
Other	22.9
None of the above apply to me	27.1
Vision-related activity‡	
Driving at night	32.3
Reading	27.5
Working with computer	25.7
Watching television	17.9

Asbell (2006) and Nelson et al. (2005).
*Any impact of symptoms.
†Each patient indicated as many items as appropriate.
‡Symptoms interfered with activities most or all of the time.

patients. Many questionnaires have been developed and used to assess the severity and impact of DED on daily function and quality of life. Results of the Impact of Dry Eye on Everyday Life Survey administered to individuals with DED and those with normal tear films revealed that DED limited daily activities, caused bodily pain and discomfort, and diminished energy (International Dry Eye Workshop 2007c). The impact of DED on daily life became clinically significant in individuals suffering from moderate and more severe DED (International Dry Eye Workshop 2007c). In addition to the quality-of-life issues for DED sufferers, there are financial implications for the individual and society at large. A recent publication suggests that the medical cost for dry eye care per year in the United States is about US$800 per year, or about US$3.8 billion for all DED patients. However, if one includes the loss of productivity with reduced effort and/or missed work days, the societal burden is estimated to be about US$11,000 per DED patient or US$55 billion per year for all DED patients—obviously a significant economic burden for all (Yu et al. 2011).

Artificial tears reduce ocular symptomatology of DED, providing relief to patients. Although symptoms of DED are rarely eliminated, artificial tears aid in relieving discomfort to varying degrees and improving quality of life. Several studies have investigated the efficacy of artificial tear solutions in relieving ocular symptoms and its correlation with objective evidence of improvement of the ocular surface health with epithelial staining techniques and Schirmer's test. The results of these studies have been inconclusive and often demonstrate symptom relief without objective clinical evidence of disease improvement (International Dry Eye Workshop 2007c). However, installation of artificial lubricants has been shown to increase the interblink interval and tear break-up time (Montés-Micó et al. 2010). The duration of this effect is dependent on the viscosity of the artificial lubricant used (Gipson et al. 2004, Montés-Micó et al. 2010). Although there is controversial evidence that artificial tears improve ocular surface health, the use of artificial tears to improve patient symptoms and quality of life is an important goal of therapy.

Not only are artificial tears useful in symptomatic treatment of ocular surface disease, but they also play an important role in restoring and maintaining clear visual acuity. The precorneal tear film is the strongest and most anterior refractive medium of the eye and must be devoid of irregularities for an optically clear retinal image to be formed. A number of methods have been used to assess the contribution of the tear film to optical image clarity. The double-pass method, in which images are projected onto the retina after passing through ocular media twice, provides information on the clarity of foveal images. Videokeratoscopy takes advantage of the reflective characteristic of the tear film to obtain dynamic images of changes in the air–tear film surface. Wavefront aberrometry uses color-coded maps and polynomial expansions to qualitatively and quantitatively assess temporal fluctuations in the tear film and optical quality (**Figure 28.2**). Interferometry provides information on the thickness of the lipid layer by measuring the interference patterns of light reflected by the anterior aspect of the lipid layer and by the lipid–aqueous interface. Combined optical coherence tomography (OCT) and wavefront sensor technologies have been used to collect simultaneous measurements of the tear meniscus and wavefront aberrations to examine tear film stability and dynamics and their effects on optical quality (Koh et al. 2010, Tung et al. 2012). Videomeniscometry is a new technology, which digitally calculates the radius of the tear meniscus to evaluate tear volume and tear and eye drop turnover (Yokoi & Komuro 2004). The double-pass method and videokeratoscopy have demonstrated that abnormalities in the tear film occurring after tear break-up, similar to those seen in ocular surface disease, affect optical quality and result in deterioration of foveal images and reduction in contrast sensitivity

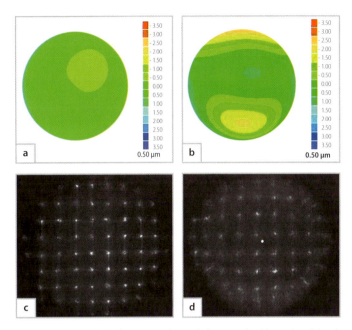

Figure 28.2 Wavefront aberration color-coded maps: a healthy patient (a) and a patient with dry eye disease (b). Pupil diameter of 6.0 mm. The left column shows the matrix of dots of the aberrometer image. With permission from Montés-Micó et al. (2010), Elsevier.

(Montés-Micó et al. 2010). These tear film aberrations increase with time after the blink, as shown by wavefront aberrometry, and occur more quickly in patients with DED (International Dry Eye Workshop 2007c, Montés-Micó et al. 2010). Following a blink, the lipid layer has been shown by interferometry to rapidly spread over the aqueous layer of the tear film to slow its evaporation. This rate is prolonged in dry eyes, which can further destabilize the tear film (International Dry Eye Workshop 2007a, Montés-Micó et al. 2010).

The use of artificial tears improves visual function in ocular surface disease, as evidenced by the methods previously mentioned. The instillation of artificial tears results in a significant decrease in surface irregularity and asymmetry, which leads to a more uniform tear film and stable refractive medium (Montés-Micó et al. 2010). Artificial tears have been shown to increase tear break-up time by 60%, indicating greater stability of the tear film (Montés-Micó et al. 2010). Decreased aberrations in the tear film result in significantly improved contrast sensitivity and visual acuity (Montés-Micó et al. 2010). Correspondingly, most patients with dry eye disease reported subjective improvement in visual function with the use of artificial tears. Simultaneous OCT and wavefront sensing has shown that different artificial tear solutions have varying effects on tear film stability and visual quality for varying durations following drop instillation. These effects were partly dependent on the severity of DED and likely due to greater instability of the lipid layer with more severe disease. This technology will be useful to further objectively evaluate the efficacy of various artificial tear solutions (Tung et al. 2012).

FDA APPROVAL PROCESS FOR ARTIFICIAL TEAR SOLUTIONS

All artificial tear solutions must be approved by the US FDA prior to sale and use. The FDA has published an ophthalmic monograph detailing labeling requirements and permissible ingredients, each with a concentration range that may be used in over-the-counter (OTC)

ophthalmic solutions (**Table 28.2**). The labeling requirements provide a list of approved indications or claims that can be listed on the drug label when marketing a tear solution and are specific for each class of active ingredients. New artificial tear formulations meeting the specified requirements are not required to undergo testing for clinical efficacy. Beyond these guidelines, there is little regulation on the inclusion of inactive ingredients (permissible concentration ranges) and even fewer on their permissible combinations.

There are five main categories in the ophthalmic monograph: astringents, demulcents, emollients, hypertonicity agents, and vasoconstrictors. Most applicable to the development of artificial tear solutions are the astringents, demulcents, and emollients. Astringents are agents that clear mucous from the ocular surface by precipitating

Table 28.2 FDA ophthalmic monograph

Astringents
Zinc sulfate (0.25%)

Demulcents
Cellulose derivatives • Carboxymethylcellulose sodium (0.2–2.5%) • Hydroxyethyl cellulose (0.2–2.5%) • Hypromellose (0.2–2.5%) • Methylcellulose (0.2–2.5%)
Dextran 70 (0.1%)
Gelatin (0.01%)
Polyols (liquid) • Polyethylene glycol 300 (0.2–1.0%) • Polyethylene glycol 400 (0.2–1.0%) • Polysorbate 80 (0.2–1.0%) • Propylene glycol (0.2–1.0%)
Polyvinyl alcohol (0.1–4.0%)
Povidone (0.1–2.0%)

Emollients
Lanolin preparations • Anhydrous lanolin (1–10% when used with one or more oleaginous emollients) • Lanolin (1–10% when used with one or more oleaginous emollients)
Oleaginous ingredients • Light mineral oil (up to 50% when combined with another emollient) • Mineral oil (up to 50% when combined with another emollient)
Paraffin (up to 5% when combined with another emollient)
Petrolatum (up to 100%)
White petrolatum (up to 100%)
White wax (up to 5% when combined with another emollient)
Yellow wax (up to 5% when combined with another emollient)

Hypertonicity agents
Sodium chloride (2–5%)

Vasoconstrictors
Ephedrine hydrochloride (0.123%)
Naphazoline hydrochloride (0.01–0.03%)
Phenylephrine hydrochloride (0.08–0.20%)
Tetrahydrozoline hydrochloride (0.01–0.05%)

Abelson et al. (2003) and US Food and Drug Administration (2004).
Active ingredients permitted for use in artificial tear solutions with allowable concentration ranges.

proteins. The demulcent category includes agents that lubricate and soothe the ocular surface. Up to three different demulcents may be used in one artificial tear substitute. For a discussion of the cellulose derivatives, liquid polyols, and polyvinyl alcohol (PVA), refer to Section 'Viscosity.' Dextran 70 is a high-molecular-weight polysaccharide that enhances demulcent properties of other compounds in this category but lacks inherent demulcent qualities. For this reason, it must be combined with at least one other demulcent, most commonly hydroxypropyl methylcellulose (HPMC). The emollients are agents applied to the ocular surface for protection and prevention of drying. The last two categories on the monograph, hypertonicity agents and vasoconstrictors, are mainly used for the treatment of corneal edema and conjunctival injection, respectively (Abelson et al. 2003, US Food and Drug Administration 2004).

Currently, if other ingredients not listed on the monograph for artificial tears are used, then the FDA is likely to require clinical trials for approval of the product. This process would require significant cost in both time and money to achieve a marketable product and is therefore not likely to be undertaken for an OTC artificial tear product.

COMPOSITION OF ARTIFICIAL TEAR SOLUTIONS

Artificial tear solutions are buffered solutions that vary in the type and concentration of viscosity agent, osmolarity, electrolyte composition, and presence of compatible solutes and preservatives.

Viscosity

Viscosity refers to the property of resisting flow, which in reference to artificial tear solutions serves to increase tear film duration in the conjunctival cul-de-sac. However, as viscosity is increased, the tear film becomes less optically clear, resulting in blurring of vision. In the development of tear substitutes, a balance must be reached with an optimal concentration of viscosity agents so that duration of action is maximized, with minimal interference with vision. Several different polymers are used in artificial tears to increase viscosity, including cellulose derivatives, PVA, liquid polyols, hydroxypropyl-guar (HP-guar), sodium hyaluronate (SH), and lipids.

The cellulose derivatives are viscoelastic polymers of polysaccharides, including HPMC, hydroxymethylcellulose, hydroxypropylcellulose, and carboxymethylcellulose (CMC). The most commonly used cellulose derivatives today are CMC and HPMC. CMC is an anionic macromolecule that binds to corneal epithelial cells via a glucose receptor on the apical surface, which enhances the duration of action of CMC (Garret et al. 2007). Conversely, HPMC is a neutral polysaccharide that has fewer interactions with charged molecules and mucins in the tear film. A comparison of ocular retention times of solutions of anionic CMC and neutral HPMC has shown that CMC has a longer duration of action, likely due to its anionic charge and ability to complex with other molecules on the ocular surface (International Dry Eye Workshop 2007b). Variations in the concentration of viscosity agents affect the consistency of the resulting formulation. CMC is typically used in a concentration range of 0.25–1.00%, with lower concentrations forming a more liquid solution and higher concentrations resulting in a solution with liquid and gel properties. Solutions with lower concentrations of viscosity agents are used for mild dry eye symptoms, whereas those with higher concentrations are reserved for more severe disease.

PVA and the liquid polyols are polymers with low viscosity that are often used in combination with other demulcents to yield solutions with greater viscosity and lubricating capability. PVA is a synthetic, non-toxic polymer, and the liquid polyols are sugar-like hydrogenated carbohydrates. Polyethylene glycol and propylene glycol are the most commonly used polyols. Two other polymers in this category are glycerin and polysorbate 80, which are commonly incorporated into oil emulsions.

HP-guar is a gelling agent that remains in a solution of low viscosity when stored in packaging at a pH of 7.0. On exposure to the tear film, it cross-links with borate and forms a bioadhesive gel that restores the inner mucous layer of the normal tear film. HP-guar may preferentially bind to more hydrophobic areas of the epithelium to form a protective coating over devitalized cells, which provides targeted therapy and may lead to greater symptom relief (International Dry Eye Workshop 2007b).

SH is a viscoelastic glycosaminoglycan that adheres to cell surfaces and binds water, allowing it to hold moisture on the ocular surface. SH was originally derived from comb structures of roosters, and today it is made in laboratories via recombinant DNA technology and microbial fermentation (Foulks 2011). It binds to the CD44 receptor on corneal and conjunctival epithelial cells, which interacts with cytoskeletal proteins, suggesting that SH may play a role in cellular adhesion and motility (Dogru & Tsubota 2011). Multiple studies comparing the efficacy of SH and CMC have shown contradictory results (International Dry Eye Workshop 2007b). SH is currently used in the most frequently prescribed artificial tear solution in Japan and is widely available in Europe; however, it has not yet been approved by the FDA for use in the United States as an active ingredient. It is currently used as an inactive ingredient in contact lens rewetting solutions and other ocular solutions in the United States (Foulks 2011). There is an interest in using SH as an active ingredient in artificial tear solutions, but it is unclear at this time whether the FDA will approve its use.

Artificial tear solutions that contain lipids in the form of castor oil and mineral oil are designed to retard evaporation of the tear film by reforming and mimicking the normal outer lipid layer of the tear film. Restoring a deficient lipid layer is as important as replenishing the mucous and aqueous components. Comparisons of tear formulations containing cellulose derivatives to mineral oil solutions demonstrated equal efficacy and relief of dry eye symptoms (Wang et al. 2007). Lipid-containing tear formulations may be of particular benefit to individuals with MGD.

Osmolarity

An important variable of artificial tear solutions is the osmolarity, which is further divided into the crystalloid osmolarity and colloidal osmolality. Crystalloid osmolarity refers to the concentration of molecules in the tear solution, and colloidal osmolality, also known as oncotic pressure, is based on the concentration of macromolecules within a solution. In DED, the inciting factor for inflammation is the hyperosmolar tear film. The use of hypo-osmolar tear solutions reduces the osmolarity of the tear film and may decrease damage to the ocular surface by decreasing the degree of inflammation. Evidence is controversial on whether a hypotonic or isotonic formulation is more beneficial in DED and has greater efficacy in reversing ocular surface damage (International Dry Eye Workshop 2007b, Lemp 2008).

Compatible solutes

Another method to protect the ocular surface epithelium from damage due to osmotic stress is by the incorporation of compatible solutes into tear formulations. In the presence of hyperosmolar tears, the corneal and conjunctival epithelial cells lose water following the osmotic gradient. To replenish internal water content, these cells increase their internal electrolyte concentration, many of which are harmful and can lead to further cellular damage. Compatible solutes, also called osmoprotectants, are small, non-ionic molecules, such as glycerin, erythritol, and levocarnitine. They protect epithelial cells by preventing an increase in potentially harmful electrolytes in response to the osmotic gradient, following cellular uptake of the osmoprotectants (Lemp 2008).

Electrolyte composition

Tear solutions that most closely mimic the electrolyte composition of normal tears are beneficial in healing and maintaining the ocular surface. The normal tear film contains numerous electrolytes, including potassium, chloride, bicarbonate, sodium, calcium, and magnesium. Of these, potassium and bicarbonate appear to be most important in maintaining the ocular surface. The normal tear film contains a higher concentration of potassium than serum. Its role is critical in maintaining normal corneal epithelial thickness, which may otherwise swell in a low potassium environment (Green et al. 1992). Bicarbonate is a buffer in the normal tear film that maintains a slightly alkaline environment on the ocular surface. Bicarbonate-containing solution promotes the repair of epithelial barrier function following damage to the corneal epithelium and is a factor in maintaining normal epithelial ultrastructure (Ubels et al. 1995). Of note, artificial tear preparations containing bicarbonate require special foil packaging, because on contact with air, bicarbonate turns into carbon dioxide, which easily diffuses through plastic packaging.

Preservatives

A key component of artificial tear solutions is preservatives, which are used to prevent contamination and microbial growth. The two main categories of preservatives are detergent and oxidative preservatives. Detergent preservatives act primarily by disrupting or dissolving lipids in cell membranes, resulting in alterations in cell membrane permeability. Oxidative preservatives are a newer category of preservatives that act by inducing oxidative reactions, which disrupt cellular metabolism. The effects of detergent and oxidative preservatives are generally non-specific and amount to injury in both microbial and normal ocular surface cells. To eliminate the risk of ocular surface damage, preservative-free tear solutions have been developed and are an appealing therapeutic option for patients with moderate-to-severe DED.

Two detergent preservatives used in ophthalmic solutions are benzalkonium chloride (BAK), the most widely used preservative in ophthalmic solutions, and polyquaternium-1 (Polyquad). BAK has a dual mechanism of action through its direct action on cells via detergent properties and indirectly by inducing inflammation, oxidative stress, and apoptosis. This dual effect makes BAK an efficacious preservative against microbial organisms and confers its bactericidal and fungicidal properties. However, this effect is non-specific and can result in damage to the conjunctival and corneal epithelia (International Dry Eye Workshop 2007b, Noecker & Miller 2011, Tressler et al. 2011). There is no doubt that in high concentrations, BAK causes ocular surface inflammation, loss of conjunctival goblet cells, increased corneal permeability, and cellular apoptosis (Noecker & Miller 2011, Tressler et al. 2011). Despite this known risk, BAK continues to be safely used as a preservative today because most ophthalmic solutions contain

BAK in low concentrations, ranging from 0.005 to 0.02%. Furthermore, BAK is rapidly diluted by the tear film following drop use. After instillation of a drop with 0.005% BAK, the concentration in the tear film was reduced 8-fold following 30 seconds and further to 16- and 36-fold at 1 and 3 minutes, respectively (Tressler et al. 2011). This rapid decrease in concentration of BAK on the ocular surface results in low levels in contact with the surface epithelium and a reduced risk of ocular surface damage. Long-term studies have shown that there is no higher incidence of adverse effects in healthy individuals (Noecker & Miller 2011, Tressler et al. 2011). However, laboratory and animal studies have shown that even very low concentrations of BAK are toxic to some degree to the conjunctival and corneal epithelia (Epstein et al. 2009, Noecker & Miller 2011, Tressler et al. 2011).

There have been few studies to date comparing the effects of BAK and preservative-free solutions in patients with preexisting ocular surface disease, and their outcomes are controversial. Currently, it remains unclear how toxic BAK-preserved drops are for patients who have already a compromised surface, such as patients with DED and/or patients on chronic drops, such as patients with glaucoma. Because these individuals may be more susceptible to toxic effects of BAK due to decreased tear production or delayed tear clearance, consideration of the use of alternatively preserved or preservative-free solutions is warranted (Noecker & Miller 2011, Tressler et al. 2011). Polyquad is a detergent preservative, which may be less toxic than BAK. Decreased toxicity can be attributed to its unique characteristic of attraction by bacterial cells and repulsion by epithelial cells, thereby minimizing potentially damaging interactions with the ocular surface while maximizing antimicrobial activity (Rosenthal et al. 2003). Despite this feature, Polyquad has been shown to cause superficial epithelial damage, mainly by decreasing conjunctival goblet cell density (Lopez & Ubel 1991).

The newer oxidative preservatives include the stabilized oxychloro complex (Purite) and sodium perborate. These second-generation preservatives have been termed the 'vanishing' preservatives because of their degradation in the tear film, which theoretically minimizes ocular toxicity. On exposure to ultraviolet light, Purite is degraded into water, oxygen, sodium, and chloride. The chlorine free radicals interfere with microbial intracellular processes and protein synthesis, causing microbial cell death. Similarly, sodium perborate decomposes on contact with the tear film and is converted into hydrogen peroxide, water, and oxygen. Hydrogen peroxide oxidizes bacterial cell membranes and alters cellular enzymes to impede intracellular protein synthesis. However, as with the detergent preservatives, individuals with DED may not have sufficient tear volume to result in complete degradation of the oxidative preservatives and may experience irritation (International Dry Eye Workshop 2007b).

A new preservative, sofZia, is an ionic buffer that is inactivated on exposure to cations in the normal tear film. It is composed of borate, sorbitol, propylene glycol, and zinc and decomposes into these molecules in the tear film. Similar to the oxidative preservatives, it prevents microbial contamination when packaged but minimizes ocular surface damage. It has been shown to have the same effect on the ocular surface as preservative-free drops (Tressler et al. 2011). Currently, this preservative is only being used in a formulation of the glaucoma medication travoprost.

Ethylenediaminetetra-acetic acid is a chelating agent used to inactivate heavy metals. Although it is does not have sufficient antimicrobial activity to be used as a preservative alone, it can be used in combination with other preservatives and allows for a lower concentration of more toxic preservatives.

Despite the development of less toxic preservatives, with frequent use almost all preserved tear solutions will cause some degree of ocular surface damage, especially in patients with preexisting ocular surface disease. For those with moderate-to-severe DED, preservative-free artificial tears may be helpful and at least not exacerbate ocular surface disease from frequent artificial tear applications. The disadvantage of preservative-free solutions is the FDA requirement for packaging in single-dose vials because of a lack of means to prevent microbial contamination. This constraint increases costs for manufacturers due to the need for additional packaging and subsequently leads to higher consumer prices. To deal with the concern of increased risk of infection, there are now preservative-free solutions with a unique mixture of ions and buffers to prevent microbial growth that have been shown to have similar efficacy as oxidative preservatives (Rosenthal et al. 2006).

Different packaging modalities are currently available to dispense preservative-free artificial tears in multidose containers. Reclosable multidose vials are convenient for use and reduce consumer costs. However, one study has demonstrated that reclosable multidose vials are more prone to microbial contamination, especially when used by patients with poor technique for drop instillation, which is associated with advanced age and fingertip touch (Kim et al. 2008). Recently, a multidose vial with a dispensing mechanism that prevents microbial growth has been approved by the FDA. The bottle dispenses drops through an airless antibacterial dispensing system, which contains an antibacterial silver coil in the tip and a valve to prevent air entry into the bottle. The cost of this product is similar to that of other preserved tear solutions.

In conclusion, preservative-free artificial tears are recommended for individuals with moderate-to-severe DED to minimize ocular surface toxicity until further research and the development of safer, effective preservatives is undertaken.

◾ OINTMENTS AND GELS

Ointments and gels are preparations with high viscosity and increased retention time that are suitable for managing severe DED. Ointments are thicker than gels and are composed of a mixture of petrolatum and mineral oil. Due to their high viscosity, ointments cause a significant amount of visual blurring and are best suited for nighttime use. Gels form a transparent, lubricating film on the epithelial surface of the eye with less visual blurring than ointments. The active ingredient in gels is carbomer, a high-molecular-weight polymer of acrylic acid. Carbomers swell on the ocular surface by absorbing and retaining water, and thereby thicken the tear film. Recently, a non-blurring carbomer-containing solution has been developed for daytime use. These gel tears are retained longer than traditional artificial tear solutions and have an effect on tear break-up time up to 60 minutes after use (Uchiyama et al. 2008). Gel tears reduce the frequency of drop instillation and maximize comfort for patients without interfering significantly with vision.

◾ INSERTS

Artificial tear inserts are small, preservative-free pellets of polymers of hydroxypropyl cellulose that are a long-acting therapy with low frequency of use. They are placed in the inferior fornix below the level of the tarsus and dissolve with the patient's tears to slowly release a small amount of hydroxypropyl cellulose and provide a constant amount of lubrication. Inserts have been found to be safe and effective for the treatment of moderate-to-severe DED. They provide relief of dry eye symptoms, increase tear break-up time and the tear meniscus, and decrease corneal and conjunctival staining (Wander & Koffler 2009). Long-term treatment with the inserts leads to a continued improvement in symptoms. The majority of patients who used both inserts and artificial tear solutions preferred the insert because of greater symptom relief (Wander & Koffler 2009). The most common side effect is blurring of vision, which is typically transient and likely due to an enlarged and more viscous tear meniscus. Other limitations, which affect <3% of users, include irritation of the lower lid and cornea, caking of the eyelashes, difficulty placing the insert in the inferior fornix, time needed for the practitioner to educate patients on use, and diminished efficacy for patients with severe DED due to a lack of tears necessary to melt the insert (Nguyen & Latkany 2011, Wander & Koffler 2009). Inserts are currently FDA-approved for use in treating DED; however, they are not available over the counter. Overall, inserts are a safe and convenient therapy recommended for moderate-to-severe DED.

SHORTCOMINGS

The tear film is a complex structure with numerous components serving different functions to maintain homeostasis on the ocular surface. The development of artificial tear solutions ideally aims to mimic the structure and function of the normal tear film, but tear substitutes are devoid of a large number of molecules normally present in the tear film and are not continuously produced and/or supplied to the tear film, unlike normal tears. This compromises the ability of artificial tears to fulfill all the functions of the normal tear film. Additionally, FDA requirements limit permissible ingredients and their combinations in artificial tear solutions, which can further hinder the development of solutions that mimic the normal tear film.

The first-line therapy for DED remains artificial tears, which are primarily a palliative measure; however, their role in treatment of DED may be expanding. Artificial tear solutions have been shown to relieve symptoms associated with DED and prevent further damage to the conjunctival and corneal epithelia. They have not been shown to reverse the pathology of or treat the underlying disease. Yet current work on artificial tear solutions is moving beyond merely demonstrating safety of the solution. It is aimed at showing efficacy and improvement in ocular surface disease with regular use by studying effects on tear break-up time and ocular surface staining. Recent research suggests that artificial tears may play a role in reducing ocular surface inflammation. Use of an artificial tear containing propylene glycol, polyethylene glycol, and HP-guar for 30 days led to a decrease in HLA-DR, an inflammatory biomarker, on the ocular surface (Raynor et al. 2010). Further research and development of newer artificial tear solutions may expand the role of artificial tears in ocular surface disease.

Currently, no artificial tear substitute has been proven to be clinically superior to others. Despite the large prevalence of DED, there has not been a large-scale, randomized clinical trial comparing the efficacy of multiple tear substitutes. There have been numerous randomized, controlled trials comparing the efficacy of up to two or three different tear substitutes, often with contradictory or equivocal results. This lack of research leaves clinicians and patients with the challenge of choosing an artificial tear substitute providing the greatest symptom relief. There are several different formulations of artificial tears with varying combinations of ingredients, and the effects of each on the ocular surface and degree of symptom relief vary from individual to individual. This variation in effect may in part be due to differing etiologies of ocular surface disease.

The development of new artificial tear solutions will likely be aimed at individualizing artificial tears and matching artificial tear solutions with a specific underlying ocular surface abnormality. For example, new tear solutions have incorporated a lipid component to address the alteration of the lipid layer in MGD. This form of personalized medicine requires further research into the etiology and pathology of tear film abnormalities. The future is likely to see continued new entries into the artificial tear market and increasing personalization of products to address needs specific to changes in the tear film in patients with DED to ultimately lead to improved management and symptom relief.

REFERENCES

Abelson MB, Kumar R, Sleeper A. All you need to make an artificial tear. Rev Ophthalmol 2003. http://www.revophth.com/content/d/therapeutic_topics/i/1338/c/25639/. (Last accessed September 30, 2011.)

Asbell PA. Increasing importance of dry eye syndrome and the ideal artificial tear: consensus views from a roundtable discussion. Curr Med Res Opin 2006; **22**:2149–2157.

Behrens A, Doyle JJ, Stern L, et al. Dysfunctional tear syndrome: a Delphi approach to treatment recommendations. Cornea 2006; **25**:900–907.

Cher I. Another way to think of tears: blood, sweat, and … 'dacruon.' Ocul Surf 2007; **5**:251–254.

Cher I. A new look at lubrication of the ocular surface: fluid mechanics behind the blinking eyelids. Ocul Surf 2008; **6**:79–86.

Dogru M, Tsubota K. Pharmacotherapy of dry eye. Expert Opin Pharmacother 2011; **12**:325–334.

Epstein SP, Ahdoot M, Marcus E, Asbell PA. Comparative toxicity of preservatives on immortalized corneal and conjunctival epithelial cells. J Ocul Pharmacol Ther 2009; **25**:113–119.

Foulks GN. Hyaluronic acid for the ocular surface. Eyecare Educators. http://www.eyecareeducators.com/site/hyaluronic_acid_for_the_ocular_surface.htm. (Last accessed December 29, 2011.)

Garret Q, Simmons PA, Xu S, et al. Carboxymethylcellulose binds to human corneal epithelial cells and is a modulator of corneal epithelial wound healing. Invest Ophthalmol Vis Sci 2007; **48**:1559–1567.

Gipson IK, Hori Y, Argüeso P. Character of ocular surface mucins and their alteration in dry eye disease. Ocul Surf 2004; **2**:131–148.

Green K, MacKeen DL, Slagle T, Cheeks, L. Tear potassium contributes to maintenance of corneal thickness. Ophthalmic Res 1992; **24**:99–102.

International Dry Eye Workshop. The definition and classification of dry eye disease: report of the Definition and Classification Subcommittee of the International Dry Eye Workshop (2007). Ocul Surf 2007a; **5**:75–92.

International Dry Eye Workshop. Management and therapy of dry eye disease: report of the Management and Therapy Subcommittee of the International Dry Eye Workshop (2007). Ocul Surf 2007b; **5**:163–178.

International Dry Eye Workshop. The epidemiology of dry eye disease: report of the Epidemiology Subcommittee of the International Dry Eye Workshop (2007). Ocul Surf 2007c; **5**:93–107.

International Workshop on Meibomian Gland Dysfunction. The International Workshop on Meibomian Gland Dysfunction: report of the definition and classification subcommittee. Invest Ophthalmol Vis Sci 2011a; **52**:1930–1937.

International Workshop on Meibomian Gland Dysfunction. The International Workshop on Meibomian Gland Dysfunction: report of the subcommittee on tear film lipids and lipid-protein interactions in health and disease. Invest Ophthalmol Vis Sci 2011b; **52**:1979–1993.

Kim MS, Choi CY, Chung HR, Woo HY. Microbial contamination of multiply used preservative-free artificial tears packed in reclosable containers. Br J Ophthalmol 2008; **92**:1518–1521.

Koh S, Tung C, Aquavella J, et al. Simultaneous measurement of tear film dynamics using wavefront sensor and optical coherence tomography. Invest Ophthalmol Vis Sci 2010; **51**:3441–3448.

Lemp MA. Management of dry eye disease. *Am J Manag Care* 2008; **14**:S88–S101.

Lopez B, Ubel J. Quantitative evaluation of the corneal epithelial barrier: effect of artificial tears and preservatives. *Curr Eye Res* 1991; **10**:645–656.

Montés-Micó R, Cerviño A, Ferrer-Blasco T, García-Lázaro S, Madrid-Costa D. The tear film and the optical quality of the eye. *Ocul Surf* 2010; **8**:185–192.

Nelson JD, Helms H, Fiscella R, et al. The relative burden of dry eye in patients' lives: comparisons to a U.S. normative sample. *Invest Ophthalmol Vis Sci* 2005; **46**:46–50.

Nguyen T, Latkany R. Review of hydroxypropyl cellulose inserts for treatment of dry eye. *Clin Ophthalmol* 2011; **5**:587–591.

Noecker R, Miller KV. Benzalkonium chloride in glaucoma medications. *Ocul Surf* 2011; **9**:159–162.

Raynor GS, Sheyman AT, Epstein SP, et al. Modulation of HLA-DR in dry eye subjects following 30 days of treatment with a novel artificial tear product. *Invest Ophthalmol Vis Sci* 2010; **51**:S6268.

Rosenthal R, Henry C, Stone R, Schlech B. Anatomy of a regimen: consideration of multipurpose solutions during non-compliant use. *Cont Lens Anterior Eye* 2003; **26**:17–26.

Rosenthal RA, Buck SL, Henry CL, Schlech BA. Evaluation of the preserving efficacy of lubricant eye drops with a novel preservative system. *J Ocul Pharmacol Ther* 2006; **22**:440–448.

Tressler CS, Beatty R, Lemp MA. Preservative use in topical glaucoma medications. *Ocul Surf* 2011; **9**:140–158.

Tung CI, Kottaiyan R, Koh S, et al. Noninvasive, objective, multimodal tear dynamics evaluation of 5 over-the-counter tear drops in a randomized controlled trial. *Cornea* 2012; **31**:108–14.

Ubels JL, McCartney MD, Lantz WK, et al. Effects of preservative-free artificial tear solutions on corneal epithelial structure and function. *Arch Ophthalmol* 1995; **113**:371–378.

Uchiyama E, Di Pascuale MA, Butovich IA, McCulley JP. Impact on ocular surface evaporation of an artificial tear solution containing hydroxypropyl (HP) guar. *Eye Contact Lens* 2008; **34**:331–334.

US Food and Drug Administration. Code of federal regulations, title 21, 2004. http://www.accessdata.fda.gov/scripts/cdrh/Cfdocs/cfCFR/CFRSearch.cfm. (Last accessed September 30, 2011.)

Wander AH, Koffler BH. Extending the duration of tear film protection in dry eye syndrome: review and retrospective case series study of the hydroxypropyl cellulose ophthalmic insert. *Ocul Surf* 2009; **7**:154–162.

Wang IJ, Lin IC, Hou YC, Hu FR. A comparison of the effect of carbomer-, cellulose- and mineral oil-based artificial tear formulations. *Eur J Ophthalmol* 2007; **17**:151–159.

Yokoi N, Komuro A. Non-invasive methods of assessing the tear film. *Exp Eye Res* 2004; **78**:399–407.

Yu J, Asche CV, Fairchild CJ. The economic burden of dry eye disease in the United States: a decision tree analysis. *Cornea* 2011; **30**:379–387.

Chapter 29

Anti-inflammatory therapy for dry eye disease: rationale and strategy

John D. Sheppard, Niraj S. Shah, Giovanni DiSandro, Jr., Brianne Anthony

MECHANISMS OF DRY EYE INFLAMMATION

Dry eye disease (DED) or keratoconjunctivitis sicca (KCS) is a prevalent, chronic, multifactorial condition convincingly coupled to inflammatory mechanisms of action (Sheppard 2003). DED has been classified into two particular forms based on the National Eye Institute/Industry Workshop on Clinical Trials in Dry Eyes: (a) tear-deficient and (b) evaporative. Although the entire disease process is multifactorial, the core mechanism of DED is believed to be related to two specific dysfunctions: tear hyperosmolarity (aqueous/tear-deficient) and tear film instability (evaporative).

It is believed that DED is strongly correlated with chronic inflammation of the lacrimal gland. The inflammatory change is the key factor leading to corneal and conjunctival cell damage, which often produces many of the signs and symptoms of DED (Lemp et al. 2007).

T-cell activation and elevation of proinflammatory cytokines

It is believed there are acute and chronic forms of irritation of the ocular surface that lead to T-cell activation. Acute irritation of the ocular surface due to hyperosmolarity, neurotrophic decadence, androgen senescence, viral, bacterial, or environmental factors leads to the presence of naive T-cell infiltration. The acute form of inflammation leads to expression of vascular endothelial proteins, which play a role in the diapedesis and extravasation of the T cells out of the vessels. High levels of intercellular adhesion molecule (ICAM-1) and lymphocyte function-association antigen (LFA-1) expression play a great role in this process. Inflammation of the lacrimal gland is due to the focal perivascular and periductal CD4 T-cell and B-cell infiltrates. These cellular infiltrates appear to focus around venules (Li et al. 2004). In contrast to the acute form of ocular surface irritation, the chronic form deals with primed or activated T cells that present to the ocular surface and lacrimal tissue. These activated T cells are the result of the activation and drainage of antigen-presenting cells (APCs) to the lymphatic organs of the body where they are presented to the naive T cells. The T cells are then primed, and they are then able to target specific proteins or antigens on the ocular surface and lacrimal stroma.

As with most immune responses, the activation of these inflammatory cells leads to the release of a subset of proinflammatory cytokines, mainly IL-1β, IL-2, TNF-α, and INF-γ. The increase in these proinflammatory tear cytokines leads to the destruction or apoptosis of the secretory stroma of the lacrimal gland and lacrimal ductules as well as dysfunction of the remaining tissue. Lymphocytic infiltration is also increased in conjunctival tissues, leading to decreased goblet cell density, tear film instability, and clinically positive signs such as lissamine staining and eventual keratinization in advanced cases. The combination of proinflammatory cytokine production and glandular dysfunction leads to a decrease in tear production (Luo et al. 2005).

Increased tear osmolarity

Aqueous tear deficiency implies that the main cause of DED is related to a lack of tear secretion, increased evaporative rate, or a combination of both. The general premise states that, compared to a normal initial tear film volume, a decrease in the aqueous portion of the tear film will lead to a higher tear film osmolarity. This phenomenon occurs whether aqueous loss is through evaporation or decreased secretion. The hyperosmolar tear film state leads to hyperosmolarity of the ocular surface epithelial cells, causing production and release of proinflammatory cytokines as described earlier. These proinflammatory cytokines (e.g. IL-1α, IL-1β, and TNF-γ) and metalloproteases such as MMP-9 proceed to induce an inflammatory cascade in the epithelial surface cells via the mitogen-activated protein (MAP) kinase and NFκB signaling pathways (De Paiva et al. 2006).

This inflammatory cascade leads to the apoptosis of the goblet cells and a direct decrease in mucus/mucin production. The pathological loss of goblet cells has been identified in all forms of dry eyes via decreased levels of secreted gel mucin (MUC5AC) in the tear film and membrane-associated mucins (MUC1 and MUC4). These mucins play a vital role in spreading the tear film, providing tear film adhesion to superficial corneal and conjunctival epithelial cells, binding the aqueous tear film layer to the ocular surface, and thereby lubricating the ocular surface. Progressive loss of secreted and membrane-associated mucins progresses and augments the cyclic positive feedback loop of DED.

In DED, conjunctival expression of inflammatory markers has been related to extravasation of fluid and protein due to increased vascular permeability. Expression of proinflammatory cytokines is enhanced in a hyperosmolar environment (Luo et al. 2007). Tear film osmolarity can now be quantitatively measured in the clinic with a commercially available device, requiring only 50 nL of tear (Sullivan et al. 2010) (**Figures 29.1** and **29.2**).

Conjunctival expression of inflammatory markers

There has been evidence to show that one of the functions of the conjunctival surface is to produce an immune quiescent environment, endowed with APCs but devoid of activated T cells. It has been demonstrated that even after direct stimulation by various pathogens no intracellular expression of Toll-like receptors (TLR-2 and TLR-4) has been identified. The initiation of the expression of the surface markers

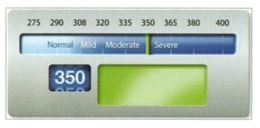

Figure 29.1 Tear film osmolarity report. The most sensitive threshold between normal and mild or moderate subjects was found to be 308 mOsms/L, while severe dry eye disease begins at 350 mOsms/L.

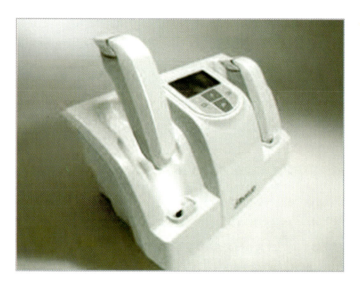

Figure 29.2 Tear lab station with two patient probes and charging device.

on the ocular surface begins with the loss of the barrier function of the endothelial cells. This allows for extravasation of proteins and fluid from these vessels. Within the tear film, proinflammatory cytokines (IL-1, IL-6, IL-8, and TNF-α) along with chemokines (IL-8) have been shown to impair epithelial cell proliferation, hinder the production of membrane-spanning molecules (Mucin-1), and cause goblet cell decimation, loss of accessory lacrimal gland tissues, T-cell infiltration, ocular surface keratinization, and angiogenesis of the corneal and conjunctival tissues (Barabino & Dana 2007).

Neurotrophic ocular surface disease

The densely innervated cornea predisposes the tissue to the heavy influence of nervous signaling in the regulation, normal cellular turnover, healing, and protection of the surface epithelium. The main glands associated with production of aqueous tear film (lacrimal), mucus (goblet cells), and oil (meibomian gland) of the tear film are also richly innervated. The majority of the innervation comes from the parasympathetic nervous system, with acetylcholine (Ach) and vasoactive intestinal peptide (VIP) being the main neurotransmitters. In addition to neurotransmitters, there is a great deal of hormonal influence on the lacrimal gland. This principle is manifested in individuals who are dealing with chronic low androgen states and aging. The influence of the chronic low androgen state and aging leads to a poorly functioning lacrimal gland (Dartt et al. 1996).

The Ach acts via muscarinic receptors to stimulate the lacrimal gland to produce water, protein, and electrolytes, whereas VIP, secreted from fibers around the basal membrane of the conjunctival epithelium, stimulates conjunctival goblet cells to secrete mucus. The third part of the tear film, the most external oily lipid layer, is secreted from the meibomian glands and then regularly distributed by the normal blinking mechanism. The mechanical motion of the blink reflex extrudes the oil from the meibomian gland orifices. The combination of proportionate oil, water, proteins, electrolytes, and mucin constitutes a stable tear film. A slight imbalance in the relative percentage of any of the tear film components can lead to tear film instability. Tear film instability then potentiates an environment of hyperosmolarity and thus the ocular surface insult required to initiate a deleterious cascade of events.

As the ocular surface begins to experience damage via osmotic imbalance, inflammatory cell infiltration, or mechanical stress from loss of surface lubrication, the lacrimal gland begins reflex secretion. The reflex stimulation of the lacrimal gland is promulgated by sensory stimulation from the trigeminal nerve, leading to an increased blink rate and increased lacrimal gland secretion.

Trigeminal nerves are located in proximity with acinar, ductal, and myoepithelial cells as well as blood vessels, and hence can control a wide variety of lacrimal gland functions. With initially increased lacrimal gland production, tear film components begin to lose the precise ratios, leading to tear film instability, and chronologically variable states of lubrication enhance the insult. The tear film instability leads to cellular ocular surface damage, as described previously, and downward spiral of inflammatory cascades and triggers, which continue to exert downward pressure and produce further mechanical damage, increasing the neurotrophic ocular surface disease that incited the cascade (Yoshino 1996, Zoukhri et al. 1994). The entire process deteriorates as initially responsive lacrimal acini progressively decrease in the number.

Concomitant lid margin disease

Lid margin disease such as blepharitis is a major comorbidity in patients with DED (DEWS Report 2007). Blepharitis is believed to be related to a bacterial infection, inflammation, parasitic colonization, dermatologic conditions, meibomian gland dysfunction (MGD), or combination of many factors. Furthermore, blepharitis can be divided into anterior and posterior forms, as well as precise diagnostic and therapeutic stages recently well delineated by the Meibomian Gland Workshop (Foulks & Nichols 2012). Anterior blepharitis is often related to staphylococcal infection or seborrheic inflammation, whereas posterior blepharitis is primarily related to MGD or mixed etiologies. Staphylococcal blepharitis is primarily an infectious condition related to colonization of the lid margin by normal skin flora, whereas seborrheic blepharitis and MGD have an inflammatory component with an immunological basis. The two forms of blepharitis tend to differ in their presentations.

Posterior blepharitis usually presents with the complaints of a chronic gritty irritation in eyes, progressively improved through the day. It is believed that irritation is due to a buildup of inflammatory mediators beneath the eyelids during sleeping. As the condition progresses, it worsens MGD, and in severe untreated cases, eventual progressive fibrosis of the meibomian glands occurs. The damage to the meibomian glands leads to an insufficiency of the oil component of the tear film. The unbalanced tear film leads to a higher evaporative state leading to worsening symptoms later in the day. This is believed to be the most common association with chronic DED.

Anterior blepharitis primarily presents as crusting and irritation at the base of the lashes, sometimes with erythema and edema of the adjacent skin. With chronic inflammation, trichiasis and madarosis or lash loss occur. With the seborrheic form, the crusting tends to be oily or greasy. This can lead to debris in the tear film, which then instigates damage to the corneal epithelium and triggers the cascade of proinflammatory mediators. In addition to damage to the corneal and conjunctival surface by debris in the tear film, there is a marked increased incidence of hyperosmolarity (Gilbard 1999).

Concomitant autoimmune diseases

Sarcoidosis is a chronic systemic disorder, characterized by the presence of noncaseating granulomas in multiple organs, most frequently involving the lungs. In addition to the lungs, involvement of other tissues can include the liver, lymph nodes, skin, kidneys, central nervous system, and salivary and lacrimal glands. Identification of granulomatous infiltration of the lacrimal gland and conjunctiva via blind biopsy has been used to confirm the diagnosis of sarcoidosis with atypical symptoms and work-up (Baughman et al. 2003).

Many of the patients afflicted with sarcoidosis suffer from DED, whereas as many as 25% may develop uveitis. The involvement of the salivary and lacrimal glands in sarcoidosis is one of the similarities between sarcoidosis and Sjögren's syndrome (SS). As with SS, sarcoidosis is a disease mediated by T-cell lymphocytic infiltrates and proinflammatory cytokines, including TNF-α, IL-1, and IL-6. These mediators are the same cytokines that lead to inflammatory changes that affect the function of the lacrimal gland, which in turn can promote an aqueous-deficient state and induce the downward spiral cycle seen in most patients with DED (Drosos et al. 1989, 1999, Ramos-Casals et al. 2004).

Chronic graft-versus-host disease

Graft-versus-host disease (GVHD) is a disease process that develops after hematopoietic stem cell transplantation performed on patients suffering from hematological malignancies. This disease can present clinically with either a slow or acute onset. Chronic GVHD usually develops about 100 days after transplantation and is characterized by signs and symptoms similar to autoimmune diseases. DED is the most frequent ocular complication associated with chronic GVHD occurring in 50–70% of cases, and can quickly assume severe status requiring aggressive interventions (Kansu 2004).

The histopathologic features of the lacrimal gland in chronic GVHD include prominent fibrosis and an increase in stromal fibroblasts. As in SS and sarcoidosis, chronic GVHD is a T-cell-driven disease with CD4+ and CD8+ T cells detected in periductal areas of the lacrimal gland and a disconnect in the regulation of cytokine production, with increased production of proinflammatory cytokines (Anderson & Regillo 2004, Calissendorff et al. 1989, Mencucci et al. 1997, Ogawa & Kuwana, 2003, Ogawa et al. 1999).

Current therapies for chronic GVHD-associated DED are still mainly symptomatic and anti-inflammatory. They include the use of preservative-free artificial tears, topical steroids, up to qid topical cyclosporine, systemic immunosuppressant medications, autologous serum eye drops, or punctual plug occlusion.

Aging

There is a high prevalence of the aqueous-deficient type of DED among the elderly. Studies in animals have shown that lacrimal gland secretion in response to several neural agonists decreases with increasing age (Ríos et al. 2005). Other studies have shown that, with age, the lacrimal gland undergoes dramatic structural changes highlighted by inflammation. Increased focal infiltration by T and B cells, increased numbers of mast cells, and increased accumulation of lipofuscin in the lacrimal gland occur with aging.

Aging is also associated with increased production of proinflammatory cytokines. Increased amounts of IL-1β and TNF-α were found in lacrimal glands of old, but not young mice. Additionally, as in SS, sarcoidosis, and chronic GVHD, the lacrimal gland from aged individuals demonstrates histopathological signs of atrophy and increased fibrosis (Dalzell 2003).

Infection

Lacrimal gland deficiency is associated with several other systemic and autoimmune diseases. Although the lacrimal gland is not the primary target in these diseases, inflammation of this gland is often seen. Chronic disease processes associated with DED include hepatitis C, acquired immunodeficiency syndrome due to infection by human immunodeficiency virus (HIV), thyroid eye disease (Eckstein et al. 2004), and diabetes (De Vita et al. 2002, Ramos-Casals et al. 2002).

The fact that both the lacrimal and salivary glands are involved in both hepatitis C and HIV infections reinforces the possible involvement of viruses in the pathogenesis of autoimmune diseases of the lacrimal gland. Indeed, it has been suggested that an initial infection and/or reactivation of Epstein–Barr virus, cytomegalovirus, or herpes virus-6, all of which have been detected in biopsies from patients with SS, might be a cause or potentiating agent of SS.

Primary and secondary SS

SS is an exocrine autoimmune process in which the lacrimal and salivary glands are targeted by activated T cells. The attack on the lacrimal and salivary glands leads to acinar and ductal cell death. The loss of the acinar and ductal cells creates aqueous hyposecretion as well as expression of autoantigens: Ro/SSA and La/SSB are expressed on the epithelial cell surface. Hyposecretion is amplified by a potentially reversible neurosecretory block. Neurotropic hyposecretion is thus due to the effects of locally released inflammatory cytokines or to the presence of circulating antibodies, such as anti-M3 antibody directed against muscarinic receptors within the glands.

Primary SS consists of the occurrence of aqueous-deficient DED, in combination with symptoms of dry mouth, in the presence of autoantibodies, evidence of reduced salivary secretion, and with a positive focus score on minor salivary gland biopsy (Vitali et al. 1993).

Secondary SS consists of the features of primary SS together with the features of an additional overt autoimmune connective disease, such as rheumatoid arthritis, which is the most common, or systemic lupus erythematosus, polyarteritis nodosa, Wegener's granulomatosis, systemic sclerosis, primary biliary sclerosis, or mixed connective tissue disease (Fox et al. 1986).

CURRENTLY AVAILABLE ANTI-INFLAMMATORY THERAPY

The argument for inflammation as a central mechanism, if not the primary cause of DED, is irrefutable. Thus, therapeutic strategies, particularly pharmacological, focus upon elimination, reduction, or modulation of the deleteriously upregulated immune response of patients with DED on the ocular surface and in the lacrimal gland. Multiple risk factors have been identified for predisposing individuals to DED, both modifiable and nonmodifiable. Nonmodifiable risk factors include female sex, older age, low body mass index, hypertension, and history of coronary artery disease (Sahai & Malik 2005). Modifiable risk factors include contact lens wear, smog exposure, use of visual display monitor such as a computer for extended periods, smoking, and medication use such as diuretics, antihistamines, antidepressants, and analgesics. Patients should be educated on curtailing these factors, particularly smoking, if at all possible. Environmental control and targeted reduction of modifiable risk factors can significantly reduce the requirements for induction and maintenance pharmacologic therapy for DED.

■ Topical calcineurin inhibitors

Calcineurin is an evolutionarily conserved serine/threonine protein phosphatase serving in multiple calcium-dependent signal transduction pathways in many biochemical processes (Rusnak & Mertz 2000). It serves numerous functions in the mammalian immune response, including T-lymphocyte activation and cytokine signaling, neutrophil chemokinesis, lymphocyte degranulation, apoptosis by mediating Fas ligand action, and macrophage function.

When the membrane-bound T-cell receptor is activated by an appropriate ligand, it causes a cascade of signals leading to intracytoplasmic calcium release. This stimulates calcineurin, which dephosphorylates the nuclear factor for activation of T cells (NF-AT). It is believed that NF-AT and calcineurin are transported into the nucleus and stimulate the transcription of IL-2 and other inflammatory cytokines (Fruman et al. 1992). IL-2 is then released and binds cell membrane receptors on T cells to stimulate propagation (Donnenfeld & Pflugfelder 2009). In addition to its activities in T-cell activation, calcineurin may be involved in signaling processes and cytokine production in other immune cells, including those of mast cells and eosinophils, as well as skeletal, cardiac, and epidermal tissues (Crabtree & Olson 2002).

Cyclosporine

Cyclosporine is a naturally produced compound of the fungi *Tolypocladium inflatum* and *Beauveria nevus* (Donnenfeld & Pflugfelder 2009). It binds to and complexes with cyclophilin A, and this complex in turn binds to and inhibits calcineurin by halting its dephosphorylation of NF-AT (Fruman et al. 1992). Cyclosporine must be bound to cyclophilin in order to be effective in inhibiting calcineurin, and because of its large surface area of interaction with the drug–immunophilin complex, cyclosporine has a specificity for its biological target that is equivalent to growth factor–receptor interactions (Ho et al. 1996, Klee et al. 1998). Of note, cyclosporine has also been shown to bind to cyclophilin D, and thereby plays a role in preventing programmed cell death (Waldmeier et al. 2003).

Systemic usage

Cyclosporine has been used systemically since 1983 to prevent rejection of solid organ transplants (DeBakey 1984). It later found multiple indications in lower doses for autoimmune diseases such as rheumatoid arthritis, inflammatory bowel disease, and psoriasis. Systemic cyclosporine has been used for various inflammatory ocular conditions, as in the prevention of rejection of limbal allografts after transplantation, severe chronic uveitis, and Behcet's disease (Binder et al. 1987, Dick et al. 1997). It has also been used along with chemotherapy in the treatment of retinoblastoma (Eckstein et al. 2005).

The most severe side effect of cyclosporine is nephrotoxicity (Stepkowski 2000). It is also known to cause hypertension, gingival hyperplasia, and susceptibility to opportunistic infections.

Topical formulation

Cyclosporine was initially formulated into a 2% topical ophthalmic solution by pharmacists and found success in the treatment of vernal keratoconjunctivitis. A wide variety of bases and emollients were employed, including peanut oil, castor oil, nanoparticles, liposomes, and olive oil. It was found to be both safe and effective. In addition, it significantly lowered the need for steroid therapy with its concomitant side effects (Hingorani et al. 1998). Further studies found success in treatment of herpes simplex stromal keratitis (Sheppard et al. 2009), superior limbic keratoconjunctivitis, childhood phlyctenular keratoconjunctivitis, Mooren's ulcer, Thygeson's superficial punctate keratitis, SS, and corneal allograft rejection (Doan et al. 2006, Perry et al. 2003).

Topical cyclosporine has been primarily used for the treatment of KCS. The 0.05% ophthalmic emulsion of cyclosporine has been approved by the Food and Drug Administration (FDA) and commercially available for dry eye therapy since 2003 under the brand name Restasis (Allergan 2010), and has become a mainstay in the treatment of DED in the United States (**Figure 29.3**).

Pharmacology in the eye

HLA-DR, a marker of immunologic activation, as well as CD40 and Fas, both markers of apoptosis, has been found to be elevated in the conjunctival epithelia of patients with DED. Topical cyclosporine has been found to reduce concentrations of these inflammatory markers (Brignole 2001) and has been shown to reduce apoptosis of conjunctival epithelial cells and prevent goblet cell loss in animal models of DED. It has been shown to nearly double conjunctival goblet cell density in phase 3 drug trials (Sall et al. 2000, Strong et al. 2005). Ocular surface changes, such as squamous metaplasia, are also noted in patients with DED; epithelial cell turnover of the conjunctival epithelium is decreased after treatment with topical cyclosporine, thus decreasing metaplasia (Kunert et al. 2002). Because corneal epithelial damage can interrupt signaling of corneal nerves and inhibit feedback to the lacrimal glands and central nervous system, cyclosporine may preserve some neurogenic tear production. This could in part explain why many patients with DED continue to garner improvement in dry eye symptoms months after cessation of cyclosporine.

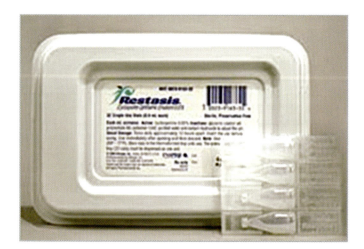

Figure 29.3 Topical cyclosporine 0.05% emulsion (Restasis) is supplied in two sealed plastic tubs for 1 month of treatment, each tub containing 30 preservative-free twist-off cap single-dose units.

The tear film itself may be considered one facet of the pathogenesis of inflammatory DED, and therefore one focus of therapy. Elevated proinflammatory cytokines, such as IL-6, have been shown to be elevated in the tears of patients with DED, and these levels fall after treatment with topical cyclosporine (Pflugfelder et al. 1999, Turner et al. 2000). Moreover, an association with decreased tear turnover has been shown in DED (Pflugfelder et al. 2004). Occlusion of lacrimal drainage pathways via punctual plugs has been observed to decrease aqueous tear production in patients without DED (Yen et al. 2001). In addition, treatment of patients with SS with topical anti-inflammatory medications has shown greater improvement in DED than punctual occlusion alone. It may be that controlling ocular inflammation prior to punctual occlusion can provide greater benefit in the treatment of DED by preventing the ocular surface from being bathed in a proinflammatory cytokine-filled tear solution. Thus, considering pretreatment with topical cyclosporine or other anti-inflammatory agents prior to performing punctual occlusion may be rational.

Clinical effects of topical cyclosporine in keratoconjunctivitis sicca

Topical cyclosporine 0.05% was FDA approved in 2004 to improve tear production in cases of KCS where the presumed etiology is ocular inflammation. In clinical trials, patients documented rapid improvement in blurred vision due to amelioration of ocular surface dryness. However, other beneficial effects can take months to fully manifest. Schirmer's testing improved significantly at 3 months, and more so at 6 months for the entire cohort. Over half the patients studied experienced a statistically significant improvement in Schirmer's testing: 59% >5 mm improvement and 15% >10 mm improvement. According to phase 3 trials, corneal staining did not significantly decrease from controls for 4 months (Sall et al. 2000).

Clinical effects in post-LASIK DED

Patients who have undergone laser-assisted in situ keratomileusis (LASIK) may develop DED postoperatively, and those with preexisting DED may have worsened symptoms. Presumably, damage to the sensory nerves during creation of the corneal flap (Kim & Kim 1999) disrupts a feedback loop between the cornea and the lacrimal gland (Perez-Santonja et al. 1999). The lipid layer of the tear film is also thinner post-LASIK (Patel et al. 2001). Treating patients with DED with topical cyclosporine 1 month prior to LASIK, cessation of the drug for a few days postoperatively, and resumption for 3 months thereafter improve Schirmer's scores significantly compared to artificial tears alone (Salib et al. 2006). The postoperative refractive spherical equivalents of these patients were also closer to their intended target.

Clinical use in contact lens intolerance

A sensation of dryness is the most common cause complaint in contact lens wearers. These patients may demonstrate decreased tear production, breakup time, and goblet cell density, as would any patient with DED (Cakmak et al. 2003). Contact lens users with DED also have elevated inflammatory marker tear levels, such as IL-6, which become undetectable after cessation of contact lens wear (Schultz & Kunert 2000). Cyclosporine decreases surface dryness and need for rewetting drops, and increases the daily amount of time wearers can tolerate their lenses.

Clinical use in posterior blepharitis and MGD

Bacterial flora of the lid margins produces lipases that partially degrade meibomian secretions and alter their solubility, thereby causing them to block meibomian gland orifices and hinder their ability to prevent aqueous evaporation (Shimazaki et al. 1995). Hence, treatment of blepharitis and MGD are mainstays of dry eye therapy.

Topical cyclosporine significantly improves clinical findings, especially meibomian gland inclusions, but not subjective symptoms such as burning or itching (Doan et al. 2006, Perry et al. 2003). Studies have shown significantly more improvement in posterior blepharitis in patients treated with cyclosporine compared to patients treated with tobramycin and dexamethasone (Rubin & Rao 2006).

Side effects of topical cyclosporine

Histologic animal studies have shown sufficiently effective concentrations of cyclosporine in surface ocular tissues but minimal concentrations intraocularly when applied topically (Acheampong et al. 1999). Studies on human patients using commercially available concentrations of cyclosporine have found no detectable levels of the drug in plasma. Presumably, minimal if any systemic absorption of cyclosporine would present essentially none of the side effects of systemic cyclosporine therapy, and clinical trials have supported this (Sall et al. 2000, Strong et al. 2005).

Ocular side effects of topical cyclosporine are generally mild and well tolerated. The most common side effect is a burning sensation in about 15% of patients. This can be made significantly more tolerable, however, by induction therapy with loteprednol etabonate for 2 weeks prior to initiating cyclosporine (Sheppard et al. 2011). Other adverse effects are discharge, fetal bovine serum, hyperemia, or pain in 1–3% of patients. According to phase 3 trials, only 2.5% of patients had to discontinue therapy due to adverse effects.

Given the immunosuppressive effects of cyclosporine, one might presume it would increase the prevalence of infectious keratitis; in phase 3 trials, however, this did not occur in any of the treated patients. In fact, animal studies have shown a possible decrease in corneal bacterial cultures after successful cyclosporine treatment (Salisbury et al. 1995). It may be that severe DED poses a greater risk of infectious keratitis due to inadequacy of the tear film and its resident antibacterial compounds to decrease bacterial load on the ocular surface, as well as inflammatory damage to the corneal epithelium. There has been evidence that a combination of topical cyclosporine and topical steroids can precipitate an infectious keratitis, or prolong the course of one that has not been fully treated and is not sterile (Chou & Prabhu 2011). Caution must be exercised in these cases, and cyclosporine is contraindicated in eyes with active bacterial infections. Because cyclosporine possesses innate antifungal activity, its use as an adjunctive anti-inflammatory agent in active fungal infections may be beneficial but remains controversial.

Clinical use and dosing

Cyclosporine is commercially available in preservative-free single-use vials for twice-daily administration. Patients must be counseled to use topical cyclosporine as a scheduled medication, since they may be self-administered instead as an 'as needed' application similar to artificial tears. Patients should be counseled about side effects. The bid dosing is on label, but increased frequency up to qid has been recommended for severe DED, GVHD, fungal keratitis, and atopic keratoconjunctivitis.

Tacrolimus (FK-506)

Tacrolimus is a macrolide produced by a *Streptomyces* strain of bacteria (Kino et al. 1987). It is structurally unrelated to cyclosporine but shares with it the quality of lipophilicity, which complicates efforts to find a suitable clinical vehicle (Bierer et al. 1993, Zhai et al. 2011).

Tacrolimus has a similar mode of action to cyclosporine in that it works to prevent transcription of IL-2 in T lymphocytes (Reinhard et al. 2002). It binds to an intracellular class of molecules designated FK-506-binding proteins (FKBPs), namely FKBP-12 (Harding et al. 1989). This complex binds calcium, calmodulin, and calcineurin, thereby inhibiting the activation of NF-AT. Tacrolimus also prevents histamine release by mast cells and basophils, and blocks the synthesis of prostaglandins. Because of a large surface area of interaction of the drug–immunophilin complex with calcineurin, FK-506 and cyclosporine both have a specificity for their biologic targets that is equivalent to growth factor–receptor interactions (Ho et al. 1996).

Systemic usage

Tacrolimus was originally used to prevent rejection in solid organ transplant as a cocktail with corticosteroids, mycophenolate, and IL-2 inhibitors, and was found to be more effective in doing so than cyclosporine (Jensik 1998, O'Grady et al. 2002). It has also been used orally in lower doses to treat systemic autoimmune disorders such as rheumatoid arthritis, psoriasis, and inflammatory bowel disease.

In ocular disease, there have been extensive case reports of DED due to chronic GVHD, resolving with systemic tacrolimus administration (Aoki 2005). It has also been used systemically for ocular inflammatory conditions such as limbal allograft rejection, Behcet's, and severe uveitis.

Topical formulation

Tacrolimus has found great success as a topical ointment in treating dermatologic immune pathology, particularly atopic dermatitis, with fewer adverse effects than corticosteroids (Zhai et al. 2011). Formulations for topical use in the eye were attempted with castor oil, olive oil, and dextrin, which caused significant irritation. Other vehicles have been investigated, such as liposomes and cyclodextrin, and may offer good ocular distribution and penetration.

Ocular pharmacology

Tacrolimus has a much larger ability to suppress inflammation than cyclosporine, as well as greater corneal and conjunctival penetration (Reinhard et al. 2002).

Reconstituted topical tacrolimus 0.03%, used dermatologically for atopic eczema, has found off-label use for eczematous eyelid disease and atopic keratoconjunctivitis, as well as DED (Tam et al. 2010). Animal models show high absorption of topically applied tacrolimus in conjunctival and corneal tissue but low concentrations in blood, suggesting that few systemic side effects might be expected (Fujita et al. 2008).

Topically applied tacrolimus decreases expression of multiple cell markers during active inflammation as well as inflammatory cytokines. It also decreases infiltration of lymphocytes, and helps preserve goblet and epithelial cells in the conjunctiva. Neuroprotective properties have also been described both in vivo and in vitro. It is conceivable that these properties may mitigate corneal nerve damage and thereby improve neurogenic production of tears.

Clinical effects

Tacrolimus has been shown to be effective for immunosuppression in a myriad of ophthalmic conditions, particularly prevention of corneal allograft rejection (Joseph et al. 2007). It has also found success in treating other conditions including ocular pemphigoid, uveitis,

vernal keratoconjunctivitis, atopic keratoconjunctivitis, and Mooren's ulcer (Zhai 2011).

Allogenic stem cell transplantation to treat leukemia and lymphoma can have the unfortunate complication of GVHD. About half of these patients suffer from ocular complications, the most common being DED and MGD. There is associated infiltration of the lacrimal gland with T cells and secretory epithelial inflammation and dysfunction (Tichelli et al. 1996). Eventually, fibrosis of lacrimal tissue develops with a resultant DED resembling SS. This often does not respond to systemic GVHD treatment. However, systemically administered tacrolimus has successfully treated this secondary DED (Ogawa et al. 2001). Moreover, case studies have shown topical tacrolimus 0.03% ointment to be successful in treating recalcitrant DED related to systemic GVHD (Tam et al. 2010). Given cyclosporin's benefit to dry eye therapy, it is conceivable that tacrolimus would have similar effects on Sjögren and non-Sjögren's KCS. Further study is warranted in this area.

Adverse effects

Side effects due to systemic administration of tacrolimus can be severe, the most common of which is nephrotoxicity, seen throughout the calcineurin inhibitor class. This renal vasculopathy leads to systemic hypertension. Also seen are neurotoxicity, metabolic abnormalities, and susceptibility to infection.

The most common ocular side effect from topical tacrolimus is burning immediately after application, but this is typically tolerable (Wyrsch et al. 2009). One small study suggested an increased risk of herpetic epithelial disease while on tacrolimus; this connection warrants further investigation (Joseph et al. 2007). No systemic drug absorption has been measured following ocular administration.

It should be noted that commercially available topical tacrolimus for dermatologic use, as well as the similar drug pimecrolimus, carries an FDA-mandated black box warning due to a potential for development of skin cancers and lymphoma. One case of systemic tacrolimus use possibly causing conjunctival intraepithelial neoplasia has been reported; however, no large study has described ocular malignancies due to tacrolimus use systemically or topically (Pournaras et al. 2007).

Pimecrolimus

Pimecrolimus is also a macrolide, primarily used topically in the treatment of atopic eczema. Like tacrolimus, it binds to FKB-12 to inhibit the calcineurin-mediated inflammatory cascade (Birnbaum et al. 2007a, 2007b). Its binding to FDBP-12 and its potency, however, are threefold weaker than those of tacrolimus. Like the other macrolide calcineurin inhibitors, pimecrolimus inhibits the production of numerous inflammatory cytokines as well as mast cell activation. Animal studies have shown 1% pimecrolimus ointment to be as safe and more effective than cyclosporine ointment in controlling KCS.

Ocular pharmacology

Topical pimecrolimus ointment has been used with some success for blepharitis, where 1% formulations applied to the eyelids of patients with blepharitis showed improvement in primary blepharitis symptoms as well as associated symptoms including DED (Auw-Hadrich & Reinhard 2009). Other small studies have suggested direct benefits for DED. One study evaluated different concentrations of pimecrolimus ophthalmic suspensions on corneal staining, showing 0.3% to have a significant benefit (Ousler et al. 2005). Oral pimecrolimus, 30 mg twice daily, has also been studied. This treatment was safe and suggested an improvement, albeit a statistically nonsignificant one due to small sample size (Tomsic et al. 2005). Further investigation of pimecrolimus in the treatment of inflammatory DED is warranted.

Adverse effects

There has been some suggestion that pimecrolimus displays significantly less toxicity compared to cyclosporine and tacrolimus, in that it allows the primary sensitization immune response to occur, but inhibits the secondary manifestations leading to hypersensitivity. Therefore, it may have a more selective mechanism of immunomodulation, which could reduce some side effects (Meingassner et al. 2003).

Pimecrolimus, like tacrolimus, carries a black box warning for a potential relationship to the development of certain cancers with dermatologic use. No extensive studies have been carried out to evaluate the potential for tumorigenesis in ocular tissues, however.

▮ Voclosporin

Voclosporin is a relatively new calcineurin inhibitor that is being tested as a steroid-sparing oral therapeutic agent for the treatment of noninfectious posterior uveitis (Anglade et al. 2008). In vitro studies have shown it to be more potent than cyclosporine as an immunosuppressive, and systemic administration has shown efficacy for treatment of panuveitis (Gregory et al. 2004). In 2010 an application for marketing approval of systemic voclosporin was submitted in Europe; it was withdrawn the following year, however, because of development of systemic hypertension among some study participants. As of this writing, voclosporin is being studied in the treatment of uveitis at 60 centers. The manufacturer expects the results of these studies to be the basis for a successful resubmission to the Food and Drug Administration (2006) (Deuter 2010).

Topical voclosporin solutions are currently being investigated for the treatment of KCS. Like the other cyclosporine analogues, topical formulations should mitigate the risk of systemic adverse effects. Given the success of other calcineurin analogues in treating DED, one can expect eventual and hopefully fruitful investigations into voclosporin efficacy on the ocular surface.

Topical corticosteroids

Corticosteroids comprise a large group of anti-inflammatory drugs used in a variety of pathologies and organ systems. In a typical inflammatory cascade, phospholipase A converts cell membrane phospholipids to arachidonic acid, which eventually leads to the production of prostaglandins, thromboxane, prostacyclins, and leukotrienes. Corticosteroids inhibit this process far upstream by inhibiting phospholipase A. They have also been shown to decrease matrix metalloproteinase-9, which is an enzyme activated by inflammatory cytokines and contributes to potential corneal epithelial irregularities and stromal degradation.

Topical steroids are very useful for rapid improvement of inflammatory symptoms, including those of DED (Yang et al. 2006). They can also be used in conjunction with other dry eye therapies to increase efficacy of treatment. For example, as mentioned earlier, loteprednol can be useful in the induction of cyclosporine treatment to decrease stinging sensation from the latter. Another study showed a significantly better effect on corneal staining when topical steroids were used prior to punctual occlusion as opposed to punctual occlusion alone. Short courses have been used off-label to interrupt inflammation and break the inflammatory cycle.

Systemic steroids are the mainstays of treating some pathologic mechanisms causing DED, namely GVHD (Riemens et al. 2010). In this section, however, we focus primarily on topical application of corticosteroids.

Steroids are known for causing several ocular side effects, particularly cataracts, intraocular pressure elevation, inhibition of wound healing, corneal thinning, and decrease in innate defense against infectious keratitis. Particular brands and preparations of corticosteroid formulations have different profiles of penetration into the ocular structures, and so have varying degrees of severity of these adverse effects (Yang et al. 2006).

Nonpreserved topical methylprednisolone has been used in the past for Sjögren-associated dry eye therapy, and may be beneficial as a short-term treatment course. A pulse therapy, consisting of treatment four times per day for 2 weeks followed by tapering every 2 weeks, resulted in improvement in ocular signs for several weeks to months, with only 20% recurrence. A second pulse therapy in these patients resulted in only one recurrence (Hong et al. 2007).

While successful, methylprednisolone treatment has complications typical of 'hard' topical corticosteroids such as elevated intraocular pressure and development or worsening of posterior subcapsular cataracts (Marsh & Pflugfelder 1999). One small-population study showed no complications occurring during 2 weeks of pulse therapy, but occurring nevertheless with more prolonged treatment courses.

Prednisolone acetate is a topical steroid that is used with success in treating intraocular inflammation as well as surface processes, and may have some use in the treatment of DED. It has been shown to decrease nerve growth factor (NGF), which is elevated in the tears of patients with DED. Another small-population study evaluated its use in chronic GVHD; although improvement in cicatricial conjunctivitis was seen, dry eye symptoms remained (Robinson et al. 2004). Compared to hyaluronic acid drops, topical prednisolone is about equally effective in improving symptoms and tear breakup time, and significantly more effective after 1 month. It also improves cell morphology by impression cytology (Lemp 2008). Given its intraocular absorption, chronic use can cause cataract formation, intraocular pressure elevation, herpetic reactivation, delayed wound healing, and other adverse events typical of topical steroids.

Loteprednol etabonate

To avoid ocular side effects, some practitioners prefer the use of so-called smart steroids, which have less intraocular penetration or are rapidly metabolized to inactive metabolites. One frequently used steroid with these softer characteristics is loteprednol etabonate. It shares a basic core structure with prednisolone but has an ester at carbon-20 rather than a ketone. It is metabolized by ubiquitous constitutive esterase enzymes to an inactive carboxylic acid after topical application or drainage into the nasolacrimal system, thereby decreasing the likelihood of untoward effects (Pavesio & DeCory 2008). Moreover, the carbon-20 ketone of other corticosteroids is believed to be associated with cataract formation, while the carbon-20 ester of loteprednol makes it less likely to contribute to cataractogenesis. Animal studies have shown high levels of loteprednol and inactive metabolites in the cornea after topical administration, substantial permeation into the iris and ciliary body, and very low levels in the aqueous (Druzgala et al. 1991). There is very little systemic absorption of the active drug.

Loteprednol has been shown to improve subjective and objective signs of DED, and has shown efficacy in dry eye treatment in patients who display a greater degree of inflammatory component to DED, such as conjunctival hyperemia and central corneal fluorescein staining (Pflugfelder et al. 2004). This is particularly beneficial because central staining correlates with surface irregularity and visual acuity changes related to DED.

Loteprednol has a much lower incidence of side effects compared to some other topical corticosteroids, particularly prednisolone acetate and difluprednate. Loteprednol is metabolized to inactive compounds fairly quickly (Pflugfelder et al. 1999). A summation of the randomized studies used for FDA approval showed that, overall, a course of loteprednol therapy lasting longer than a month resulted in only a 2% incidence of intraocular pressure elevation, compared to a 7% incidence with prednisolone acetate. When those clinical trial patients using loteprednol with soft contact lenses were eliminated from this analysis, the incidence of intraocular pressure (IOP) rise with loteprednol was reduced markedly, equivalent statistically to placebo. This may be a result of the prolonged residence time of loteprednol when accompanied by a contact lens acting as a drug depot on the ocular surface. One large-population study found that an IOP elevation of 10 mmHg occurred in 1.7% of patients taking loteprednol compared to 0.5% taking vehicle and 6.7% taking prednisolone. Finally, an evaluation of patients treated for several years on loteprednol 0.2% for allergic conjunctivitis found no change in mean IOP from baseline, and no cataract formation (Ilyas et al. 2004, Novack et al. 1998). Of patients who do experience intraocular pressure elevation on loteprednol, 28% had preexisting open-angle glaucoma or ocular hypertension. The average pressure increase was just >9 mmHg, and mean duration of loteprednol treatment required to raise the IOP was 55 days (Rajpal et al. 2011). Bartlett et al. (1993) showed that the IOP rise on loteprednol when given to known glaucoma steroid responder subjects was less than half than that of subjects treated with prednisolone acetate.

Loteprednol is potent relative to other topical corticosteroids (Samudre 2004), and is available in four commercial preparations: topical suspensions at 0.2% and 0.5% concentrations, a topical 0.5% suspension in combination with 0.3% tobramycin, and a topical 0.5% preservative free ointment. The 0.5% suspension (Lotemax, Bausch & Lomb, Rochester NY) is typically used for the treatment of ocular inflammation, such as post-operatively. This concentration is also indicated on the label for acute anterior uveitis (Loteprednol Etabonate US Uveitis Study Group 1999), seasonal allergic conjunctivitis, and chronic papillary conjunctivitis. The other topical preparation is a 0.2% suspension used to treat ocular surface conditions such as allergic conjunctivitis and DED. There is also a combination of 0.5% loteprednol and 0.3% tobramycin (Pavesio & DeCory 2008). It can be used four times daily for DED believed to have some inflammatory component (Pflugfelder et al. 2004). Loteprednol can also be used in conjunction with cyclosporine as a temporary induction agent to prevent surface irritation and side effects of cyclosporine, as recommended by the results of a prospective, randomized, placebo-controlled multicenter clinical trial. The protocol suggests beginning loteprednol therapy 14 days before starting cyclosporine and tapering it after the latter's initiation (Sheppard et al. 2011).

Loteprednol is often used as a second-line therapy in place of other corticosteroids that have caused adverse effects. One study of patients suffering from IOP elevation due to prednisolone therapy who were subsequently changed to loteprednol found that IOP was decreased an average of 33% at 3 weeks and 45% at 39 weeks with no effect in anti-inflammatory response (Holland et al. 2009).

Fluorometholone

Fluorometholone is another topical steroid that is used for various inflammatory ocular diseases. It significantly improves signs and symptoms of DED compared to flurbiprofen, a topical nonsteroidal anti-inflammatory drug, or artificial tears alone; it is also better at preserving numbers of goblet cells (Avunduk et al. 2003, Behrens et al. 2006). It has been shown to improve subjective symptoms and objective signs of DED as quickly as 1 week after treatment inception in patients for whom artificial tears have not provided improvement (Yang et al. 2006). No steroid-associated adverse effects were noted to occur within 1 month of treatment initiation. Thus, fluorometholone may continue to gain popularity as a 'soft' steroid for use in the treatment of DED.

Essential fatty acids

Polyunsaturated fatty acids (PUFAs) play a large role in parts of the inflammatory cascade. As mentioned in previous sections, arachidonic acid is derived from cellular membrane lipids and is oxygenated to produce inflammatory factors, including thromboxanes, leukotrienes, and prostaglandins; these in turn lead to pain, vasodilation, and inflammatory cell chemotaxis. The production of arachidonic acid, which is an omega-6 fatty acid, is inhibited by corticosteroids. Non-steroidal anti-inflammatory drugs and aspirin inhibit the formation of downstream inflammatory mediators (Cortina & Bazan 2011).

Omega-3 and omega-6 fatty acids have drawn considerable attention over the past several years as our understanding of their functions in the balancing of pro- and anti-inflammatory mediators in the body has improved. A major proving ground of their activity has been in ocular surface disease, particularly inflammatory DED. Topical and dietary formulations of these fatty acids have been shown to be beneficial for ocular inflammation and dry eye signs and symptoms. Animal models have shown improvement in corneal staining and a decrease in certain inflammatory cells and cytokines, including TNF-α after treatment with topical omega-3 fatty acids (Rashid et al. 2008). Supplementation with g-linolenic acid (GLA) and omega-3 (n-3) polyunsaturated fatty acids has been found to decrease expression of disease-relevant ocular surface inflammatory mediators that are implicated in the pathogenesis of chronic DED, concomitant to improvement in dry eye symptoms and the stabilization of ocular surface irregularity (Sheppard et al. 2012).

In addition, there are relatively new families of anti-inflammatory lipid-derived mediators that play a role in the natural change from inflammation to resolution after injury. These are the arachidonic acid-derived lipoxins, the omega-3-derived resolvins and protectins, and maresins (Cortina & Bazan 2011). These agents attenuate inflammation, in part by decreasing polymorphonuclear leukoctye (PMN) infiltration and promoting macrophage cleanup, while at the same time failing to induce immunosuppression (Serhan 2010). For example, a lipoxygenase produced by corneal epithelial cells converts the omega-3 fatty acid docosahexaenoic acid (DHA) into neuroprotectin D1 (NPD1), which has neuroprotective and antiapoptotic effects, and increases corneal re-epithelialization in an animal model. Topical DHA supplementation has been shown to promote significant corneal nerve regeneration after lamellar keratectomy in an animal model, but only when combined with pigment epithelial-derived factor, which is one of many factors that can activate the synthesis of NPD1 from DHA (Cortina & Bazan 2011).

Similarly, eicosapentaenoic acid (EPA) is converted to resolvin E1, which, when applied topically, increased tear flow, improved epithelial health, decreased COX-2 expression, and decreased macrophage infiltration in a mouse dry eye model (Li et al. 2010). Of note, a synthetic analogue of resolvin E1 has completed phase 2 clinical trials, showing statistically significant improvements in treated patients with DED (NCT00799552). These data suggest that the promotion of resolution pathways in addition to the suppression of inflammatory ones may be another step in the treatment of DED (De Paiva et al. 2012).

Recent research suggests that the relative concentration of a specific family of PUFA (omega-3 versus omega-6), or even a specific type of omega-6 fatty acid, can affect the balance of inflammation. Generally speaking, omega-3 fatty acid metabolism produces more anti-inflammatory products as compared to the more proinflammatory products of omega-6 fatty acids (Rand & Asbell 2011). Certain combinations of these, however, can be beneficial. Supplementation with high concentrations of omega-3 fatty acids and the specific omega-6 fatty acid linoleic acid can decrease tear film osmolarity and dry eye symptoms (Larmo et al. 2010). SS patients treated with omega-6 supplements consisting of linoleic acid and GLA have an increase in anti-inflammatory eicosanoid concentration and an improvement in dry eye symptoms and corneal staining (Aragona et al. 2005). Also, combinations of fatty acids show some benefit; dietary supplementation with combined omega-3 fatty acids (DHA and EPA) and omega-6 fatty acids (GLA and LA) provided improvement in dry eye symptoms, corneal staining, Schirmer's testing, and tear breakup time (Creuzot et al. 2006). It is possible that GLA, the product of the omega-6 linoleic acid, may promote the production of less inflammatory prostanoids and thereby reduce the synthesis of the more inflammatory omega-6 arachidonic acid products.

Aside from specific omega-6 fatty acid precursors, the balance between inflammatory and anti-inflammatory mediators can be altered by modifying the intake of specific PUFAs. A large cross-sectional study of women showed that those with higher dietary omega-3 fatty acid intake had 68% less incidence of DED. In addition, women with a dietary ratio of omega-6 to omega-3 of 15:1 or greater were 2.5 times more likely to suffer from DED (Milijanovic et al. 2005)

High dietary intake of the omega-3 fatty acids (α-linolenic acid, EPA, and DHA) can 'tip the scales' of production of anti-inflammatory versus inflammatory factors. It is presumed to do this via competitive inhibition, with more omega-3 derivatives being formed relative to the more inflammatory omega-6 arachidonic acid derivatives. Competitive inhibition is thought to take place when dietary PUFA intake has an omega-6 to omega-3 ratio of 4:1 or lower (Cortina & Bazan 2011, James et al. 2000). Interestingly, it has been hypothesized that early humans' diets consisted of an omega-6 to omega-3 fatty acid ratio of 1:1. Some sources state that the current Western diet provides a ratio as high as 16:1, however, suggesting that a more 'paleolithic' diet could promote less systemic inflammation than modern fare (Simopoulos 2002).

Dosing

Most of the essential fatty acid (EFA) supplements on the market today are not regulated by the FDA, making it difficult to recommend a standardized dosage. Many commercially available preparations of fish oil contain 300 mg of EPA and DHA in each 1000 mg capsule (Rand & Asbell 2011). There is a commercially available prescription supplement for hypertriglyceridemia that contains 840 mg of DHA and EPA in each 1000 mg capsule.

The FDA has provided no formal recommendations for dietary consumption of EFAs for DED or other ocular diseases, nor has the 2007 International Dry Eye Workshop. The American Heart Association recommends two servings of omega-3 fatty acid-rich fish per week to help mitigate cardiovascular risk. One or more large-scale studies would be extraordinarily beneficial in setting standards for supplemental dosages of EFAs for the treatment of DED.

◼ Doxycycline

It has been well demonstrated that matrix metalloproteinase-9 (MMP-9), an inflammatory enzyme upregulated by inflammatory cytokines, is elevated in the tears of patients with DED. It can alter corneal epithelial morphology and permeability, and decreases apical cell density (Beardsley et al. 2008). MMP-9 is inhibited by doxycycline (as well as by corticosteroids), which thereby decreases corneal surface irregularity. In addition to improving corneal epithelium irregularity, doxycycline has been shown to improve symptoms of irritation and increase tear film stability in patients with ocular rosacea (Frucht-Pery et al. 1993). Oral doxycycline can be used in doses as high as 100 mg PO bid, and as low as 20 mg PO qid. The anti-inflammatory effect requires far lower tissue and blood levels than the anti-microbial effect, and is thus less potentially toxic. Although many patients fare extremely well on long-term oral tetracyclines for ocular and cutaneous diseases, several precautions are in order. First, gastrointestinal irritation is common, particularly if taken on an empty stomach as so many pharmacists seem to insist. Patients should take doxycycline only when there is food in the stomach. Second, photosensitivity precautions must be taken, particularly at higher altitudes, more equatorial latitudes, and in fair-skinned patients. Third, tetracycline derivatives are absolutely contraindicated during pregnancy, breastfeeding, and until dentition is fully formed in order to prevent irreversible staining of the enamel. Finally, some data may indicate that there is an increased risk of breast cancer in susceptible women taking long-term antibiotics (Garcia-Rodriguez & Gonzalez-Perez 2005).

◼ ANTI-INFLAMMATORY DRUG PIPELINE FOR DED

The acceleration of research focused on DED over the past several decades has led to an increase in knowledge regarding the pathophysiology of the disease. The pipeline for DED is now brimming with innovation, from investigational therapies to pioneering clinical models, study designs, and technologies.

Because eye care providers wait for the approval of additional options for the treatment of DED, it is of utmost importance that we continue to learn more about the pathologic processes at work and strive to develop novel methods and models to understand the disease better.

Sarcode

Several new dry eye drug candidates are currently under evaluation and show great potential. SAR1118 (SARCode) is a novel selective small-molecule lymphocyte function-associated antigen-1 (LFA-1) antagonist, inhibiting T-cell migration, proliferation, adhesion, and cytokine release, thus preventing T-cell-mediated chronic inflammation (Murphy et al. 2011). In a phase 3 study, the efficacy of SAR1118 (5.0%) preservative-free ophthalmic solution was compared with placebo in the treatment of DED fully enrolled in early 2012.

Sarcode Bioscience's phase 2 clinical study on the ophthalmic solution SAR1118, a small-molecule integrin antagonist, demonstrated statistically significant results in signs and symptoms of DED. SAR1118 (recently adopted name Lifitegrast) inhibits T-cell inflammation by blocking the binding interaction between two proteins LFA-1 and ICAM-1. Pharmacokinetic studies showed the small molecule to have adequate exposure on the ocular surface with minimal systemic concerns (Semba et al. 2011).

Sarcode recently announced the OPUS-1 pivotal phase 3 trial results using Lifitegrast 5.0% BID compared to placebo BID. The multicenter, randomized, double-masked and placebo controlled study showed statistically significant improvement in both signs (corneal fluorescein staining) and symptoms (ocular irritation and ocular dryness), particularly in the patient subset using artificial tears prior to study enrollment (Sheppard 2013). The clinical trials access number for OPUS-1 is NCT01421498.

Regenerex

Regenerex has an exciting approach for treating DED. Thymosin β 4 (Tβ4) is a synthetic copy of a naturally occurring 43-amino acid peptide having both anti-inflammatory and wound healing properties. Previous murine models of Tβ4 have evaluated and demonstrated that it promotes and accelerates corneal ocular surface defect healing in DED. In data presented at ARVO 2011, RGN-259 reduced ocular surface damage associated with DED in rats (Dunn 2010). RGN-259 performed better than Restasis in reducing corneal damage in one arm of the experiment.

In November 2011, phase 2 results of the clinical trial were released. Although primary endpoints were not met, the study of 72 patients did show that RGN-259 had statistically significant benefits over placebo: reduction from baseline in central corneal fluorescein staining; reduction in exacerbation of superior corneal fluorescein staining; and reduction in exacerbation of ocular discomfort at day 28 during a 75-minute challenge in a controlled adverse environment. The clinical trial locator is NCT01387347.

■ Mimetogen: Mimetogen/MIM-D3

It has been known that patients with DED have reduced mucin within the tear film, creating tear film instability. Mimetogen has developed a small-molecule compound that stimulates mucin properties: MIM-D3. The small molecule targets mucin receptors to improve tear quality by mechanism similar to that of naturally occurring NGF. In murine studies, MIM-D3 showed statistically significantly decreased corneal staining compared to vehicle (Jain et al. 2011).

Mimetogen has developed a family of small-molecule tyrosine kinase receptor agonists that are powerful mucin secretagogues that have been shown to stimulate MUC 5AC secretion from conjunctival goblet cells. MIM-D3 is a small-molecule mimetic of NGF and has completed a phase 2 study designed to compare the safety and efficacy of 1% MIM-D3 and 5% MIM-D3 with placebo for the treatment of the signs and symptoms of DED. The clinical trial access number is NCT0125707.

Alcon: ESBA105

Alcon has just completed a phase 2 clinical trial (NCT01338610) for severe DED utilizing ESBA105, a monoclonal anti-TNF-α variable fragment in a 10 mg/mL ophthalmic solution acquired by Alcon from ESBATech. Topically administered ESBA105 quickly reaches therapeutic levels in both the anterior and posterior segments without any need for penetration enhancers. Drug penetration and ocular biodistribution patterns with topical application appear highly attractive for clinical use to treat TNF-dependent ocular diseases (Ottiger et al. 2009). The unique properties of this topical biologic agent include an anterior segment half-life of 5 hours, a nonvitrectomized posterior segment half-life of, and a very low systemic drug exposure, reducing the risk of serious side effects common with this class of drug. The randomized, double-blind study for severe DED concluded in February 2012. The

bioavailability of this drug suggests that severe ocular surface diseases could benefit greatly from this therapy. ESBA105 has also been explored in other conditions such as acute anterior uveitis.

Santen: DE-101

Santen is exploring rivoglitazone for the treatment of corneal and conjunctival epithelial disorders associated with DED. Interestingly, this chemical entity is an effective systemic hypoglycemic agent with a well-established safety profile (Uchiyama et al. 2011). The results of phase 2a clinical trials in the United States and Japan have led the company to conduct a phase 2b clinical trial in Japan and phase 1 and phase 2 clinical trials in the United States with higher dosages. Currently, a phase 2, multicenter, randomized, 6-month long study is assessing the safety and efficacy of two concentrations of DE-101 ophthalmic suspension compared to placebo, qid, for the treatment of DED. The primary endpoint is tear volume increase from baseline. The estimated enrollment number for this study is 165, with completion date being targeted for the end of 2012. The clinical trial identification number is NCT01468168.

■ Selective glucocorticoid receptor agonists

Selective glucocorticoid receptor agonists (SEGRAs) provide the molecular efficacy of corticosteroids while theoretically bypassing their side effects by acting directly upon the nuclear target of mRNA synthesis. This new anti-inflammatory drug category promises advances in dermatology, rheumatology, and neurology as well as ophthalmology.

Santen: DE-110 SEGRA

In addition to its rivoglitazone protocols, Santen Pharmaceutical recently completed a 12-week randomized, multicenter phase 2 trial of DE-110 for the treatment of DED. DE-110 is one of the SEGRA initiatives that, with the nonsteroidal and anti-allergic properties, make it the key for the treatment of DED (Kato et al. 2011). The phase 2 was completed in October 2011, with the estimated enrollment number of 160. The study compared two doses of DE-110 to placebo dosed qid. The clinical trial identification number is NCT01239069.

Bausch & Lomb: Mapracorat

Currently, the SEGRA entity closest to FDA approval is Mapracorat, now under investigation for ocular surface and postoperative inflammation. Increase in osmolarity of tears is possibly the main component of discomfort and visual disturbances caused by DED (Bron et al. 2009). Previous studies assessed the anti-inflammatory effects of Mapracorat in an in vitro osmotic stress model (Megan et al. 2010), and another study showed that Mapracorat inhibited hyperosmolarity-induced proinflammatory cytokines, with efficacy and potency comparable to dexamethasone (Zhang et al. 2009). Mapracorat (BOL-303242-X) is a novel glucocorticoid receptor agonist currently undergoing formal clinical investigations for the treatment of DED. In June 2011, a phase 2 study to identify the concentration and frequency of dosing of BOL-303242-X ophthalmic suspension commenced (NCT01163643). Additional trials are anticipated.

Eyegate: EGP-437

Eyegate Pharmaceuticals is currently investigating a novel yet historically well-documented method to increase a charged drug's bioavailability: iontophoresis. Dexamethasone phosphate, a potent corticosteroid, has established efficacy and safety profiles for ophthalmic indications. Dexamethasone phosphate is being evaluated in clinical trials due to its profile and charged character, enabling iontophoretic mobility. The delivery system uses a small electrical current that charges the proprietary preparation of the dexamethasone molecule and subsequently enhances the bioavailability of the drug by penetrating further through the surface and into the anterior segment.

Ocular iontophoresis treatments with EGP-437 showed improvements in dry eye signs and symptoms relative to the placebo group in a phase 2 efficacy study (Patane et al. 2011). In April 26, 2011, the drug's phase 3 trial was completed (NCT01129856). This drug–device combination trial showed statistically significant improvements in several signs and symptoms of DED in the treatment groups; however, the primary endpoints were not achieved. Additional trials for ocular surface disease are anticipated. Furthermore, this same technology shows considerable promise in clinical trials for acute noninfectious anterior uveitis, noninfectious scleritis, and postcataract inflammation control.

ISTA: bromfenac

ISTA Pharmaceuticals was purchased by Bausch & Lomb, effective April 2012. According to the company's website, ISTA Pharmaceuticals plans to file a new drug application with the FDA for Prolensa in the treatment of postoperative inflammation and pain following cataract extraction (Silverstein et al. 2011). Commercial launch is set for early 2013, pending approval.

Prolensa is a low-dose formulation of the active ingredient of Xibrom and Bromday—bromfenac. ISTA has announced positive results from a proof-of-concept phase 2 clinical study in subjects with DED (NCT01212471). The study achieved statistical significance in objective primary endpoints of fluorescence and lissamine corneal staining. Patients also achieved statistically significant improvements in subjective symptoms. A phase 3 dose-ranging study to evaluate safety and efficacy of bromfenac ophthalmic solution in DED commenced in 2011. Unfortunately, results of Remura (low-dose bromfenac for the treatment of DED) have proven to be no better than artificial tear product at reducing the signs and symptoms of DED.

ISTA: ecabet sodium

ISTA has also announced positive results of ecabet sodium for the treatment of DED. Ecabet sodium is mucin secretagogue (Nakamura et al. 1997). The results are from a phase 2b clinical study that showed a positive trend of tear breakup time as well as Schirmer's scores compared to placebo, indicating potential efficacy. The next steps for this drug would be moving forward to phase 3 studies and a new drug application (NCT00667004 & NCT00370747).

Resolvyx

RX-10045 (Resolvyx) is a synthetic resolvin analogue formulated for topical application to treat diseases of the eye and is being investigated for the treatment of DED (De Paiva et al. 2012). In a phase 2 trial, RX-10045 produced dose-dependent improvement in both the signs and symptoms of DED, and was generally shown to be safe and well tolerated (NCT00799552). In 2011, Resolvyx and Celtic Therapeutics announced that they would be entering into a final agreement under which Celtic had acquired and licensed rights to RX-10045.

Allergan

Also on the docket and of obvious interest is Allergan's Restasis X, a new variation of cyclosporine, which is listed in phase 2 clinical trials. Variable concentrations and vehicles are available (Baiza-Duran et al. 2010), and adjustments may enhance clinical responses comparable to the currently available 0.05% emulsion (Restasis, Allergan).

Rebamipide

Acucela and Otsuka have partnered to initiate a phase 3 clinical trial with a 2% concentration of the topical mucin secretagogue, Rebamipide (NCT01319773). Rebamipide is currently approved in Japan under the trade name Mucosta. Previous studies showed an increase of mucin-like substance with the initiation of the 1% concentration topical solution. The 1% concentration also showed improvement in corneal Rose Bengal scores (Urashima et al. 2012).

Many other agents remain in the laboratory or the early pipeline. A litany of novel agents are capable of regulating the inflammatory response without the potential side effects seen with corticosteroids for example. One of these advances is Tβ4. Previous studies suggest that it not only regulates the inflammatory response but enhances corneal re-epithelialization without the side effects seen in corticosteroids (Sosne et al. 2010).

The need for continued research and development of new therapeutic agents is crucial for the introduction of more varied and effective prescription solutions for the patient with DED. Application of current therapies is still limited, and thus management of the disease will only be further transformed as new studies are developed, aiding in the understanding of pathogenesis, thus expanding our approach to patient care. Nevertheless, this multifaceted and complex disease will continue to require a multitude of therapeutic approaches.

■ REFERENCES

Acheampong A, Shackleton M, Tang-Liu D. Distribution of cyclosporin A in ocular tissues after topical administration to albino rabbits and beagle dogs. *Curr Eye Res* 1999; **18**:91–103.

Allergan, Inc. Restasis package insert. http://www.allergan.com/assets/pdf/restasis_pi.pdf, 2010. (Last accessed April 17, 2013.)

Anderson NG, Regillo C. Ocular manifestations of graft versus host disease. *Curr Opin Ophthalmol* 2004; **15**:503–507.

Anglade E, Aspeslet L, Weiss S. A new agent for the treatment of noninfectious uveitis: rationale and design of three LUMINATE (Lux Uveitis Multicenter Investigation of a New Approach to Treatment) trials of steroid-sparing voclosporin. *Clin Ophthalmol* 2008; **2**:693–702.

Aoki S, Mizote H, Minamoto A, et al. Systemic FK506 improved tear secretion in dry eye associated with chronic graft versus host disease. *Br J Ophthalmol* 2005; **89**:243–244.

Aragona P, Bucolo C, Camicione P. Systemic omega-6 essential fatty acid treatment and pge1 tear content in Sjögren's syndrome patients. *Investig Ophthalmol Visual Sci* 2005; **46**:4474–4479.

Auw-Hadrich C, Reinhard T. Treatment of chronic blepharokeratoconjunctivitis with local calcineurin inhibitors. *Das Ophthalmologe* 2009; **106**:635–638.

Avunduk A, Avunduk M, Varnell E, Kaufman H. The comparison of efficacies of topical corticosteroids and nonsteroidal anti-inflammatory drops on dry eye patients: a clinical and immunocytochemical study. *Am J Ophthalmol* 2003; **136**:593–602.

Baiza-Duran L, Medrano-Palafox J, Hernandez-Quintela E, Lozano-Alcazar J, Alaniz-de La OJF. Comparative clinical trial of the efficacy of two different aqueous solutions of cyclosporine for the treatment of moderate to severe dry eye syndrome. *Br J Ophthalmol* 2010; 210–216.

Barabino S, Dana MR. Dry eye syndrome. Immune response and the eye. *Chem Immunol Allergy* 2007; **92**:176–184.

Bartlett JD, Horwitz B, Laibovitz R, Howes JF. Intraocular pressure response to loteprednol etabonate in known steroid responders. *J Ocul Pharmacol* 1993; **9**:157–165.

Baughman RP, Lower EE, du Bois RM. Sarcoidosis. *Lancet* 2003; **361**:1111–1118.

Beardsley R, DePaiva C, Power D, Pflugfelder S. Desiccating stress decreases apical corneal epithelial cell size—modulation by the metalloproteinase inhibitor doxycycline. *Cornea* 2008; **27**:935–940.

Behrens A, Doyle J, Stern L. Dysfunctional tear syndrome: a Delphi approach to treatment recommendations. *Cornea* 2006; **25**:900–907.

Bierer B, Hollander G, Fruman D, Burakoff S. Cyclosporin A and FK506: molecular mechanisms of immunosuppression and probes for transplantation biology. *Curr Opin Immunol* 1993; **5**:763–773.

Binder A, Graham E, Sanders M. Cyclosporin A in the treatment of severe Behcet's uveitis. *Br J Rheumatol* 1987; **26**:285–291.

Birnbaum F, Reis A, Reinhard T. Topical immunosuppressives after penetrating keratoplasty. Ophthalmologe 2007a; **104**:381–387.

Birnbaum F, Schwartzkopff J, Scholz C, Reinhard T. Topical pimecrolimus does not prolong clear graft survival in a rat keratoplasty model. *Graefes Arch Clin Exp Ophthalmol* 2007b; **245**:1717–1721.

Brignole F, Pisella PJ, De Saint Jean M, et al. Flow cytometric analysis of inflammatory markers in KCS: 6-month treatment with topical cyclosporin A. *Investig Ophthalmol Visual Sci* 2001; **42**:90–95.

Bron AJ, Yokoi N, Gafney E, Tiffany JM. Predicted phenotypes of dry eye: proposed consequences of its natural history. *Ocul Surf* 2009; **7**:78–92.

Cakmak S, Unlu M, Karaca C, Nergiz Y, Ipek S. Effects of soft contact lenses on conjunctival surface. *Eye Contact Lens* 2003; **29**:230–233.

Calissendorff B, el Azazi M, Lönnqvist B. Dry eye syndrome in long-term follow-up of bone marrow transplanted patients. *Bone Marrow Transplant* 1989; **4**:675–678.

Chou T, Prabhu S. Clinical course and management of postoperative methicillin-resistant Staphylococcus aureus keratitis in immunocompromised patients: two case reports. *Clin Ophthalmol* 2011; **5**:1789–1793.

Cortina MS, Bazan HE. Docosahexaenoic acid, protectins, and dry eye. *Curr Opin Clin Nutr Metab Care* 2011; **14**:132–137.

Crabtree GR, Olson EN. NFAT signaling: choreographing the social lives of cells. *Cell* 2002; **109**:S67–S79.

Creuzot C, Passemard M, Viau S. Improvement of dry eye symptoms with polyunsaturated fatty acids. *J French Ophthalmol* 2006; **29**:868–873.

Dalzell MD. Dry eye: prevalence, utilization, and economic implications. *Managed Care* 2003; **12**:9–13.

Dartt DA, Kessler TL, Chung EH, et al. Vasoactive intestinal peptide-stimulated glycoconjugate secretion from conjunctival goblet cells. *Exp Eye Res* 1996; **63**:27–34.

DeBakey M. Cyclosporin A: a new era in organ transplantation. *Compr Ther* 1984; **10**:7–15.

De Paiva CS, Corrales RM, Villareal AL, et al. Cosrticosteroid and doxycycline suppress MMP-9 and inflammatory cytokine expression, MAPK activation, in the corneal epithelium in experimental dry eye. *Exp Eye Res* 2006; **83**:526–535.

De Paiva CS, Schwartz CE, Gjörstrup P, Pflugfelder SC. Resolvin E1 (RX-10001) reduces corneal epithelial barrier disruption and protects against goblet cell loss in a murine model of dry eye. *Cornea* 2012; **31**:1299–1303.

Deuter C. Systemic voclosporin for uveitis treatment. *Ophthalmology* 2010; **107**:672–675.

De Vita S, Damato R, De Marchi G, et al. True primary Sjögren's syndrome in a subset of patients with hepatitis C infection: a model linking chronic infection to chronic sialadenitis. *Isr Med Assoc J* 2002; **4**:1101–1105.

DEWS Report. The definition and classification of dry eye disease: report of the Definition and Classification Subcommittee of the International Dry Eye Workshop (2007). *Ocul Surf* 2007; **5**:75–92.

Dick A, Azim M, Forrester J. Immunosuppressive therapy for chronic uveitis: optimizing therapy with steroids and cyclosporin A. *Br J Ophthalmol* 1997; **81**:1107–1112.

Doan S, Gabison E, Gatinel D, et al. Topical cyclosporine A in severe steroid-dependent childhood phlyctenular keratoconjunctivitis. *Am J Ophthalmol* 2006; **141**:62–66.

Donnenfeld E, Pflugfelder S. Topcial ophthalmic cyclosporine: pharmacology and clinical uses. *Surv Ophthalmol* 2009; **54**:321–338.

Drosos AA, Constantopoulos SH, Psychos D, et al. The forgotten cause of sicca complex: sarcoidosis. *J Rheumatol* 1989; **16**:1548–1551.

Drosos AA, Voulgari PV, Psychos DN, et al. Sicca syndrome in patients with sarcoidosis. *Rheumatol Int* 1999; **18**:177–180.

Druzgala P, Wu W, Bodor N. Ocular absorption and distribution of loteprednol etabonate, a soft steroid, in rabbit eyes. *Curr Eye Res* 1991; **10**:933–937.

Dunn SP, Heidemann DG, Chow CY, et al. Treatment of chronic non-healing neurotrophic corneal epithelial defects with thymosin beta 4. *Arch Ophthalmol* 2010; **128**:636–638.

Eckstein AK, Finkenrath A, Heiligenhaus A, et al. Dry eye syndrome in thyroid-associated ophthalmopathy: lacrimal expression of TSH receptor suggests involvement of TSHR-specific autoantibodies. *Acta Ophthalmol Scand* 2004; **82**:291–297.

Eckstein L, VanQuill K, Bui S. Cyclosporin A inhibits calcineurin/nuclear factor of activated T-cells signaling and induces apoptosis in retinoblastoma cells. *Investig Ophthalmol Visual Sci* 2005; **46**:782–790.

Food and Drug Administration. FDA approves updated labeling with boxed warning and medication guide for two eczema drugs, Elidel and protopic. FDA News Release 2006; 06–09.

Foulks GN, Nichols KK. Improving awareness, identification and management of meibomian gland dysfunction. *Ophthalmology* 2012; **119**:S1–S12.

Fox RI, Robinson CA, Curd JG, et al. Sjogren's syndrome. Proposed criteria for classification. *Arthritis Rheumatol* 1986; **29**:477–585.

Frucht-Pery J, Sagi E, Hemo I, Ever-Hadani P. Efficacy of doxycycline and tetracycline in ocular rosacea. *Am J Ophthalmol* 1993; **116**:88–92.

Fruman D, Klee C, Bierer B, Burakoff S. Calcineurin phosphatase activity in T lymphocytes is inhibited by FK 506 and cyclosporin A. *Proc Natl Acad Sci U S A* 1992; **89**:3686–3690.

Fujita E, Teramura Y, Shiraga T, et al. Pharmacokinetics and tissue distribution of tacrolimus (FK506) after a single or repeated ocular instillation in rabbits. *J Ocul Pharmacol Ther* 2008; **24**:309–319.

Garcia-Rodriguez LA, Gonzalez-Perez A. Use of antibiotics and risk of breast cancer. *Am J Epidemiol* 2005; **161**:616–619.

Gilbard JP. Dry eye, blepharitis and chronic eye irritation: divide and conquer. *J Ophthalmic Nurs Technol* 1999; **18**:109–115.

Gregory CR, Kyles AE, Bernsteen L, et al. Compared with cyclosporine, ISATX247 significantly prolongs renal allograft survival in a nonhuman primate model. *Transplantation* 2004; **78**:681–685.

Harding M, Galat A, Uehling D. A receptor for the immunosuppressand FK 50 is a cis trans peptidyl-prolyl isomerase. *Nature* 1989; **341**:758–760.

Hingorani M, Moodaly L, Calder VL, Buckley RJ, Lightman S. A randomized, placebo-controlled trial of topical cyclosporin a in steroid-dependent atopic keratoconjunctivitis. *Ophthalmology* 1998; **105**:1715–1720.

Ho S, Clipstone N, Timmermann L, et al. The mechanism of action of cyclosporin A and FK506. *Clin Immunol Immunopathol* 1996; **80**:S40–S45.

Holland E, Djalilian A, Sanderson J. Attenuation of ocular hypertension with the use of topical loteprednol etabonate 0.5% in steroid responders after corneal transplantation. *Cornea* 2009; **28**:1139–1143.

Hong S, Kim T, Chung S, Kim E, Seo K. Recurrence after topical nonpreserved methylprednisolone therapy for keratoconjunctivitis sicca in Sjögren's syndrome. *J Ocul Pharmacol Ther* 2007; **23**:78–82.

Ilyas H, Slonim C, Braswell G, Favetta J, Schulman M. Long-term safety of loteprednol etabonate 0.2% in the treatment of seasonal and perennial allergic conjunctivitis. *Eye Contact Lens* 2004; **30**:10–13.

Jain P, Li R, Lama T, et al. An NGF mimetic, MIM-D3, stimulates conjunctival cell glycoconjugate secretion and demonstrates therapeutic efficacy in a rat model of dry eye. *Exp Eye Res* 2011; **93**:503–512.

James M, Gibson R, Cleland L. Dietary polyunsaturated fatty acids and inflammatory mediator production. *Am J Clin Nutr* 2000; **71**:343S–348S.

Jensik S. Tacrolimus (FK 506) in kidney transplantation: three-year survival results of the US multicenter, randomized, comparative trial. FK 506 Kidney Transplant Study Group. *Transpl Proc* 1998; **30**:1216–1218.

Joseph A, Raj D, Shanmuganathan V, et al. Tacrolimus immunosuppression in high-risk corneal grafts. *Br J Ophthalmol* 2007; **91**:51–55.

Kansu E. The pathophysiology of chronic graft-versus-host disease. *Int J Hematol* 2004; **79**:209–215.

Kato M, Hagiwara Y, Oda T, et al. Beneficial pharmacological effects of selective glucocorticoid receptor agonist in external eye. *J Ocul Pharmacol Ther* 2011; **27**:353–360.

Kim W, Kim J. Change in corneal sensitivity following laser in situ keratomileusis. *J Cataract Refractive Surg* 1999; **25**:368–373.

Kino T, Hatanaka H, Hashimoto M, et al. FK-506, a novel immunosuppressant isolated from a streptomyces: I. Fermentation, isolation, and physico-chemical and biological characteristics. *J Antibiotics* 1987; **40**:1249–1255.

Klee CB, Ren H, Wang X. Regulation of the calmodulin-stimulated protein phosphatase, calcineurin. *J Biol Chem* 1998; **273**:13367–13370.

Kunert K, Tisdale A, Gipson I. Goblet cell numbers and epithelial proliferation in the conjunctiva of patients with dry eye syndrome treated with cyclosporine. *Arch Ophthalmol* 2002; **120**:330–337.

Larmo P, Jarvinen R, Sertala N. Oral sea buckthorn oil attenuates tear film osmolarity and symptoms in individuals with dry eye. *J Nutr* 2010; **140**:1462–1468.

Lemp M. Management of dry eye. *Am J Managed Care* 2008; **14**:88–101.

Lemp MA, Baudouin C, Baum J, et al. The definition and classification of dry eye disease: report of the definition and classification subcommittee of the international dry eye workshop. *Ocul Surf* 2007; **65**–90.

Li QD, Chen Z, Song EJ, et al. Stimulation of matrix metalloproteases by hyperosmolarity by JNK pathway in human corneal epithelial cells. *Invest Ophthalmol Visual Sci* 2004; **45**:4302–4311.

Li N, He J, Scwartz C. Resolvin E1 improves tear production and decreases inflammation In a dry eye mouse model. *J Ocul Pharmacol Therap* 2010; **26**:431–439.

Loteprednol Etabonate US Uveitis Study Group. Controlled evaluation of loteprednol etabonate and prednisolone acetate in the treatment of acute anterior uveitis. *Am J Ophthalmol* 1999; **127**:537–544.

Luo L, Li QD, Carrales RM, Pflugfelder SC. Hyperosmoler saline is a proinflammatory stress on the mouse ocular surface. *Eye Contact Lens* 2005; **31**:186–193.

Luo L, Li DQ, Pflugfelder SC. Hyperosmolarity-induced apoptosis in human corneal epithelial cells is mediated by cytochrome c and MAPK pathways. *Cornea* 2007; **26**:452–460.

Marsh P, Pflugfelder S. Topical nonpreserved methylprednisolone therapy for keratoconjunctivitis sicca in Sjogren syndrome. *Ophthalmology* 1999; **106**:811–816.

Megan EC, Harrington KL, Ward KW, Zhang J-Z. Mapracorat, a novel selective glucocorticoid receptor agonist, inhibits hyperosmolar-induced cytokine release and MAPK pathways in human corneal epithelial cells. *Mol Vis* 2010; **16**:1791–1800.

Meingassner J, Fahrngruber H, Bavandi A. Pimecrolimus Inhibits the elicitation phase but does not suppress the sensitization phase in murine contact hypersensitivity, in contrast to tacrolimus and cyclosporine A. *J Investig Dermatol* 2003; **121**:77–80.

Mencucci R, Rossi Ferrini C, Bosi A, et al. Ophthalmological aspects in allogenic bone marrow transplantation: Sjögren-like syndrome in graft-versus-host disease. *Eur J Ophthalmol* 1997; **7**:13–18.

Milijanovic B, Rivedi K, Dana M. Relationship between dietary n-3 and n-6 fatty acids and clinically diagnosed dry eye. *Am J Clin Nutr* 2005; **82**:887–893.

Murphy CJ, Bentley E, Miller PE, et al. The pharmacologic assessment of a novel lymphocyte function-associated antigen-1 antagonist (SAR1118) for the treatment of keratoconjunctivitis sicca in dogs. *Invest Ophthalmol Vis Sci* 2011; **52**:3174–3180.

Nakamura M, Endo K, Nakata K, Hamano T. Gefarnate stimulates secretion of mucin-like glycoproteins by corneal epithelium in vitro and protects corneal epithelium from desiccation in vivo. *Exp Eye Res* 1997; **65**:569–574.

Novack G, Howes J, Crockett R, Sherwood M. Change in intraocular pressure during long-term use of loteprednol etabonate. *J Glaucoma* 1998; **7**:266–269.

Ogawa Y, Okamoto S, Kuwana M, et al. Successful treatment of dry eye in two patients with chronic graft-versus-host disease with systemic administration of FK506 and corticosteroids. *Cornea* 2001; **20**:430–434.

Ogawa Y, Kuwana M. Dry eye as a major complication associated with chronic graft-versus-host disease after hematopoietic stem cell transplantation. *Cornea* 2003; **22**:S19–S27.

Ogawa Y, Okamoto S, Wakui M, et al. Dry eye after haematopoietic stem cell transplantation. *Br J Ophthalmol* 1999; **83**:1125–1130.

O'Grady J, Burroughs A, Hardy P. Tacrolimus versus microemulsified ciclorporin in liver transplantation: the TMC randomised control trial. *Lancet* 2002; **360**:1119–1125.

Ottiger M, Thiel MA, Feige U, Lichtlen P, Urech DM. Efficient intraocular penetration of topical anti-TNF-single-chain antibody (ESBA105) to anterior and posterior segment without penetration enhancer. *Invest Ophthalmol Vis Sci* 2009; **50**:779–786.

Ousler GW, Haque R, Weichselberger A, et al. Comparison of pimecrolimus 1%, 0.3% and 0.1% with vehicle for the treatment of dry eye in the controlled adverse environment (CAE) model. *Assoc Res Vision Ophthalmol* 2005.

Patane MA, Cohen A, From S, et al. Ocular iontophoresis of EGP-437 (dexamethasone phosphate) in dry eye patients: results of a randomized clinical trial. *Clin Ophthalmol* 2011; **5**:633–643.

Patel S, Perez-Santonja J, Alio J, Murphy P. Corneal sensitivity and some properties of the tear film after laser in situ keratomileusis. *J Refractive Surg* 2001; 17:17–24.

Pavesio C, DeCory H. Treatment of ocular inflammatory conditions with loteprednol etabonate. *Br J Ophthalmol* 2008; **92**:455–459.

Perez-Santonja J, Sakla H, Cardona C, Chipont E, Alio J. Corneal sensitivity after photorefractive keratectomy and laser in situ keratomileusis for low myopia. *Am J Ophthalmol* 1999; **127**:497–504.

Perry H, Doshi-Carnevale S, Donnenfeld E, Kornstein H. Topical cyclosporine A 0.5% as a possible new treatment for superior limbic keratoconjunctivitis. *Ophthalmology* 2003; **110**:1578–1581.

Pflugfelder S, Jones D, Ji Z, Afonso A, Monroy D. Altered cytokine balance in the tear fluid and conjunctiva of patients with Sjögren's syndrome keratoconjunctivitis sicca. *Curr Eye Res* 1999; **19**:201–211.

Pflugfelder S, Maskin SL, Anderson B, et al. A randomized, double-masked, placebo-controlled, multicenter comparison of loteprednol etabonate ophthalmic suspension, 0.5%, and placebo for treatment of keratoconjunctivitis sicca in patients with delayed tear clearance. *Am J Ophthalmol* 2004; **138**:444–457.

Pournaras J, Chamot L, Uffer S, Zografos L. Conjunctival intraepithelial neoplasia in a patient treated with tacrolimus after liver transplantation. *Cornea* 2007; **26**:1261–1262.

Rajpal RK, Digby D, D'Aversa G, et al. Intraocular pressure elevations with loteprednol etabonate: a retrospective chart review. *J Ocul Pharmacol Ther* 2011; **27**:305–308.

Ramos-Casals M, Brito-Zerón P, García-Carrasco M, et al. Sarcoidosis or Sjögren syndrome? Clues to defining mimicry or coexistence in 59 cases. *Medicine* 2004; **83**:85–95.

Ramos-Casals M, García-Carrasco M, Brito Zerón MP, et al. Viral etiopathogenesis of Sjögren's syndrome: role of the hepatitis C virus. *Autoimmun Rev* 2002; **1**:238–243.

Rand A, Asbell P. Nutritional supplements for dry eye syndrome. *Curr Opin Ophthalmol* 2011; **22**:279–282.

Rashid S, Jin Y, Ecoiffier T, et al. Topical omega-3 and omega-6 fatty acids for treatment of dry eye. *Arch Ophthalmol* 2008; **126**:219–225.

Reinhard T, Reis A, Mayweg S, et al. Topical Fk506 in inflammatory corneal and conjunctival diseases. A pilot study. *Klin Monbl Augenheilkd* 2002; **219**:125–131.

Riemens A, Boome LT, Imhof S, Kuball J, Rothova A. Current insights into ocular graft versus-host disease. *Curr Opin Ophthalmol* 2010; **21**:485–494.

Ríos JD, Horikawa Y, Chen LL, et al. Age-dependent alterations in mouse exorbital lacrimal gland structure, innervation and secretory response. *Exp Eye Res* 2005; **80**:477—491.

Robinson M. et al. Topical corticosteroid therapy for cicatricial conjunctivitis associated with chronic graft-versus-host disease. Bone Marrow Transpl 2004; 33:1031–1035.

Rubin M, Rao S. Efficacy of topical cyclosporin 0.05% in the treatment of posterior blepharitis. *J Ocul Pharmacol Ther* 2006; **22**:47–53.

Rusnak F, Mertz P. Calcineurin: form and function. *Physiol Rev* 2000; **80**:1483–1521.

Sahai A, Malik P. Dry eye: prevalence and attributable risk factors in a hospital-based population. *Indian J Ophthalmol* 2005; **53**:87–91.

Salib G, McDonald M, Smolek M. Safety and efficacy of cyclosporine 0.05% drops versus unpreserved artificial tears in dry-eye patients having laser in situ keratomileusis. *J Cataract Refractive Surg* 2006; **32**:772–778.

Salisbury M, Kaswan R, Brown J. Microorganisms isolated from the corneal surface before and during topical cyclosporine treatment in dogs with keratoconjunctivitis sicca. *Am J Vet Res* 1995; **56**:880–884.

Sall K, Stevenson O, Mundorf T, Reis B. Two multicenter, randomized studies of the efficacy and safety of cyclosporine ophthalmic emulsion in moderate to severe dry eye disease. *Ophthalmology* 2000; **107**:631–639.

Samudre S, Lattanzio F, Williams P, Sheppard J. Comparison of topical steroids for acute anterior uveitis. *J Ocul Pharmacol Ther* 2004: **20**:533–547.

Schultz C, Kunert K. Interleukin-6 levels in tears of contact lens wearers. *J Interferon Cytokine Res* 2000; **20**:309–310.

Semba CP, Swearingen D, Smith VL, et al. Safety and pharmacokinetics of a novel lymphocyte function-associated antigen-1 antagonist ophthalmic solution (SAR1118) in healthy adults. *J Ocul Pharmacol Ther* 2011; **27**:99–104.

Serhan C. Novel lipid mediators and resolution mechanisms in acute inflammation: to resolve or not? *Am J Pathol* 2010; **177**:1576–1591.

Sheppard JD. Guidelines for the treatment of chronic dry eye disease. *Manag Care* 2003; **12**:20–25.

Sheppard JD, Wertheimer ML, Scoper SV. Modalities to decrease stromal herpes simplex keratitis reactivation rates. *Arch Ophthalmol* 2009; **127**:852–856.

Sheppard JD, Scoper SV, Samudre SS. Topical loteprednol pretreatment reduces cyclosporine stinging in chronic dry eye disease. *J Ocular Pharmacol Therap* 2011; **27**:23–27.

Sheppard JD, Pflugfelder SC, Singh R, et al. Long-term treatment with nutritional supplements containing gamma linolenic acid and omega 3 fatty acids improve moderate to severe keratoconjunctivitis sicca. *Invest Ophthalmol Vis Sci* 2012; 53:ARVO abstract 581.

Sheppard JD, Semba CP. Phase 3 randomized double-masked placebo-controlled trial of Lifitegrast in dry eye in patients previously on artificial tears. ASCRS 2013, Chicago.

Shimazaki J, Sakata M, Tsubota K. Ocular surface changes and discomfort in patients with meibomian gland dysfunction. *Arch Ophthalmol* 1995; **113**:1266–1270.

Silverstein SM, Cable MG, Sadri E, et al. Once daily dosing of bromfenac ophthalmic solution 0.09% for postoperative ocular inflammation and pain. *Curr Med Res Opin* 2011; **27**:1693–1703.

Simopoulos A. The importance of the ratio of omega-6/omega-3 essential fatty acids. *Biomed Pharmacother* 2002; **56**:365–379.

Sosne G, Qiu P, Kurpakus-Wheater M, Matthew H. Thymosin beta4 and corneal wound healing: visions of the future. *Ann N Y Acad Sci* 2010; **1194**:190–198.

Stepkowski SM. Molecular targets for existing and novel immunosuppressive drugs. *Expert Rev Mol Med* 2000; **2**:1–23.

Stern MA. T Cell staining of conjunctival and lacrimal gland specimens in chronic dry eye disease. *J Biol Sci* 1998; **4**:211–214.

Strong B, Farley W, Stern M, Pflugfelder SC. Topical cyclosporine inhibits conjunctival epithelial apoptosis in experimental murine keratoconjunctivitis sicca. *Cornea* 2005; **24**:80–85.

Sullivan BD, Whitmer D, Nichols KK, et al. An objective approach to dry eye disease severity. *Invest Ophthalmol Vis Sci* 2010; **51**:6125–6130.

Tam P, Young A, Cheng L, Lam P. Topical 0.03% tacrolimus ointment in the management of ocular surface inflammation in chronic GVHD. *Bone Marrow Transpl* 2010; **45**:957–958.

Tichelli A, Duell T, Weiss M, et al. Late-onset keratoconjunctivitis iscca syndrome after bone marrow transplantation: incidence and risk factors. *Bone Marrow Transpl* 1996; **17**:1105–1111.

Tomsic M, Gekkieva M, Weichselberger A, Yannoulis N. Evaluation of pimecronlimus tablets 30 mg bid for the treatment of dry eye in primary Sjögren's syndrome patients. *Assoc Res Vision Ophthalmol* 2005.

Turner K, Pflugfelder SC, Ji Z, et al. Interleukin-6 levels in the conjunctival epithelium of patients with dry eye disease treated with cyclosporine ophthalmic emulsion. *Cornea* 2000; **19**:492–496.

Uchiyama M, Koda H, Fischer T, et al. In vitro metabolism of rivoglitazone, a novel peroxisome proliferator-activated receptor γ agonist, in rat, monkey, and human liver microsomes and freshly isolated hepatocytes. *Drug Metab Dispos* 2011; **39**:1311–1319.

Urashima H, Takeji Y, Okamoto T, Fujisawa S, Shinohara H. Rebamipide increases mucin-like substance contents and periodic acid Schiff reagent-positive cells density in normal rabbits. *J Ocul Pharmacol Ther* 2012; **28**:264–270.

Vitali C, Bombardieri S, Moutsopoulos HM, et al. Preliminary criteria for the classification of Sjogren's syndrome: results of a prospective concerted action supported by the European Community. *Arthritis Rheumatol* 1993; **36**:340–347.

Waldmeier P, Zimmermann K, Qian T, Tintelnot-Blomley M, Lemasters J. Cyclophilin D as a drug target. *Curr Med Chem* 2003; **10**:1485–1506.

Wyrsch S, Thiel M, Becht C. Safety of treatment with tacrolimus ointment for anterior segment inflammatory diseases. *Klinsche Monbl Augenheilkd* 2009; **226**:234–236.

Yang C, Sun W, Gu Y. A clinical study of the efficacy of topical corticosteroids on dry eye. *J Zheijiang Univ Sci* 2006; **7**:675–678.

Yen M, Pflugfelder S, Feuer W. The effect of punctal occlusion on tear production, tear clearance, and ocular surface sensation in normal subjects. *Am J Ophthalmol* 2001; **131**:314–323.

Yoshino K, Monroy D, Pflugfelder SC. Cholinergic stimulation of lactoferrin and epidermal growth factor secretion by the human lacrimal gland. *Cornea* 1996; **15**:617–621.

Zhai J, Gu J, Yuan J, Chen J. Tacrolimus in the treatment of ocular diseases. *Biodrugs* 2011; **25**:89–103.

Zhang JZ, Cavet ME, VanderMeid KR, et al. BOL-303242-X, a novel selective glucocorticoid receptor agonist, with full anti-inflammatory properties in human ocular cells. *Mol Vis* 2009; **15**:2606–2616.

Zoukhri D, Hodges RR, Dicker DM, et al. Role of protein kinase C in cholinergic stimulation of lacrimal gland protein secretion. *FEBS Lett* 1994; **351**:67–72.

Chapter 30 — Blood-derived eye drops

Francisco C. Figueiredo, Oliver J. Baylis

■ INTRODUCTION

The tear film is complex both physically and chemically. It has many roles such as lubrication, protection, nourishment, and defense. Most therapeutic agents, such as a lubricant, anti-inflammatory, or antibiotic, have one specific role. However, even when used in combination, these therapeutic agents fall far short of the natural properties of the normal tear film.

A number of therapies are available for the treatment of ocular surface diseases, and should be tailored to address the individual patient's needs. This includes using artificial tear drops, increasing the secretion of or conserving tears, or targeting the associated inflammation in the ocular surface.

The ideal therapeutic eye drop would be similar to normal healthy tears. It should have excellent wetting and lubrication properties, the correct biochemical makeup, and the optimum level of growth factors, cytokines, and vitamins to support the ocular surface epithelium and maintain health. It should have no effect on vision, and be acceptable to use in terms of convenience and comfort. There should be no infection risk or toxicity, and the drop should be synthetically mass-produced economically.

Serum manufactured from blood and related products offer several of the above-mentioned properties that are not currently possible with manufactured products. Fox et al. (1984) used autologous serum therapeutically to treat 15 patients with keratoconjunctivitis sicca, and showed that after treatment patients had significantly less Rose Bengal staining as well as improved symptoms compared with their prior medication with ocular lubricants alone. Since then, the use of autologous serum for ocular surface disorders has become widespread. Blood-derived eye drops are an additional topical treatment option that should be considered in more severe cases. They are particularly useful for patients who do not respond to conventional pharmaceutical eye drops. They may be prepared from the patient's own serum, as described by Fox et al. (1984), or from other sources (i.e. allogeneic serum, platelet-enriched plasma, umbilical cord serum, and albumin).

Blood-derived eye drops contain growth factors, immunoglobulins, and nutrients, mimicking the natural tears. They have been shown to be clinically beneficial in healing and maintaining the ocular surface, in addition to reducing patient's discomfort/pain and improving visual performance.

■ Indications

The great majority of patients for whom blood-derived eye drops, in particular autologous serum eye drops (ASEs), will be applied for are those with severe dry eye disease (DED), such as that associated with Sjögren's syndrome. They have also been used to treat ocular surface disorders secondary to connective tissue diseases such, as rheumatoid arthritis, or due to viral keratitis, chemical or thermal burns, fifth nerve palsy, drug toxicity, limbal stem cell deficiency, and iatrogenic procedures, such as corneal transplantation. There are other specific indications in which blood-derived eye drops have been proved to be beneficial (Table 30.1).

In the UK, the NHS Blood and Transplant (NHSBT) Tissue Services has provided an ASE manufacturing service to ophthalmologists since 2003. More information regarding this service is available on the NHSBT website at http://www.nhsbt.nhs.uk/tissueservices/products/eyes/autologous/. Unfortunately, there are no national or international guidelines (i.e. the National Institute for Health and Clinical Excellence in the UK) on this highly specialized form of treatment. Blood-derived eye drops are prepared using specific manufacturing conditions as defined by current pharmaceutical Good Manufacturing Practice guidelines.

Initial treatment with any form of blood-derived eye drops may be provided for a 3- to 6-month trial period following well-defined indication criteria (Table 30.2). However, existing patients who are

Table 30.1 Blood-derived eye drop indications with cited references

Indication	Source of product	References
Dry eye disease (Sjögren's and non-Sjögren's syndrome)	ASE	Fox et al. (1984) Tananuvat et al. (2001) Noble et al. (2000) Kojima et al. (2005) Lee and Chen (2008)
Persistent corneal epithelial defects	ASE	Tsubota et al. (1999) Jeng and Dupps (2009)
	ASLE	Chiang et al. (2009)
	UCSE	Vajpayee et al. (2003)
	Albumin	Unterlauft et al. (2009)
Recurrent corneal erosions	ASE	Benitezdel Castillo et al. (2002) Ziakas et al. (2010)
	UCSE	Yoon et al. (2011)
Graft-versus-host disease (following bone marrow transplantation)	ASLE	Chiang et al. (2007)
	UCSE	Yoon et al. (2007)
Corneal ulceration	PRP	Koffler (2006) Alio et al. (2007)
Neurotrophic keratopathy	PRP	Geremicca et al. (2010)
Keratopathy in diabetes mellitus	ASE	Schulze et al. (2006)
Superior limbic keratoconjunctivitis	ASE	Goto et al. (2001)
Postsurgery, for example, penetrating keratoplasty	ASE	Chen et al. (2010)
Limbal stem cell deficiency/chemical or thermal burn	ASE	Kolli et al. (2010)
	PRP	Marquez De Aracena Del Cid and Montero De Espinosa (2009)

ASE, autologous serum eye drops; ASLE, allogeneic serum eye drops; UCSE, umbilical cord serum eye drops; PRP, platelet-enriched plasma (eye drops).

well established on treatment and obtain significant benefit are likely to continue to require this form of treatment for a prolonged period. Significant benefit is often defined as a substantial improvement in symptoms of dryness, irritation, pain, and photophobia. In some patients there may be also an improvement in visual function.

AUTOLOGOUS SERUM

Manufacture

Autologous serum is produced when the whole blood of the patient is allowed to clot, and then the cellular components and clots are removed. ASEs are generally produced in dilutions of 20–100%, and they may also contain antibiotic agents, depending on the manufacturing protocol.

There is no universally accepted protocol for the production of autologous serum drops, and there is variation in the literature and debate as to the best method. Production factors that may vary include the length of clotting time, the centrifugal force used, the duration of centrifugation, the dilution, and the diluents. Variations in these factors have been shown to alter the concentration of biochemical factors within the serum (Liu et al. 2005).

In the UK, the NHS Blood and Transplant Service is a service for individual patients. The donation of blood follows the same procedures as for normal allogenic blood donations. The blood is clotted for 2–3 days at 4°C followed by centrifugation to produce 200 mL of serum. This is diluted with 50% normal saline under sterile conditions and then aliquoted into 3 mL vials. Some are used for quality control and the others supplied to the patient. Following delivery to the patients, all blood-derived eye drop bottles must be stored frozen, in a domestic freezer or the freezer compartment of a domestic refrigerator. Approximately 130 units are produced per donation (NHSBT website; Noble et al. 2000).

Laboratory evidence

Serum has pH and osmolality similar to those of tears. It contains multiple factors, such as cytokines, vitamins, and growth factors, which allow it to support epithelial cells and ocular surface homeostasis

Table 30.2 Indications and patient requirements to prescribe blood-derived eye drops

1.	Severe and/or disabling and constant ocular surface disease not responding to high frequency of non-preserved conventional therapy
2.	Treatment and control of all associated eye disease (e.g. blepharitis, lid mal position, trichiasis, and allergy)
3.	Control of environmental effects (e.g. low relative humidity and occupational) and systemic medications (e.g. beta-blockers).
4.	Poor Schirmer's 1 score (indicating very severe aqueous tear deficiency): ≤2 mm in 5 minutes
5.	Punctal occlusion (i.e. cautery and/or punctal plugging), to conserve tears by preventing tear drainage
6.	The patient meets criteria as a potential blood donor (autologous and allogeneic) in order that serum can be safely donated for drop manufacture
7.	The patient agrees to store (freeze) aliquoted blood-derived eye drops at home and to use it as prescribed by the treating ophthalmologist
8.	The patient understands the severity of eye condition, lack of response to conventional treatment, and the need to use blood-derived products

(Yamada et al. 2008). Two growth factors that have particular significance in ASEs are epidermal growth factor (EGF) and transforming growth factor-β (TGF-β).

EGF is a mitogenic factor for epithelial cells, which causes DNA synthesis, extracellular matrix generation, and proliferation. It also facilitates cell motility and delays terminal differentiation. EGF is secreted in the tears, and EGF receptors are found throughout the cornea. It is important for corneal epithelial turnover and regeneration in disease.

TGF-β is also important for ocular surface homeostasis and is found in the cornea and tears. It modulates the action of EGF and inhibits epithelial cell growth, although it has a stimulatory effect on extracellular matrix and fibroblasts (Klenkler & Sheardown 2004). TGF-β concentration is approximately five times higher in serum than in tears, and because of this, some groups opt to use 20% diluted serum for ASEs (Yamada et al. 2008).

Many other growth factors are present in the anterior segment of the eye, where they have a variety of roles. Of note is nerve growth factor, important for both epithelial homeostasis and nerve regrowth following injury, which in turn is beneficial for epithelial health. A full review of growth factors in the eye has been given by Klenkler and Sheardown (2004).

Liu et al. (2006) investigated the effects of serum (as well as other blood products) on corneal epithelial cells in culture and compared the levels of important nutrients. Serum was the best product tested at supporting epithelial proliferation, differentiation, and migration—all necessary properties for ocular surface regeneration.

Clinical evidence

Of the studies in the literature, most are case reports or series. On the whole, these report favorable outcomes. However, caution must be exercised when interpreting the results as demonstrated by the fact that one of the first blood products to be used in the eye was fibronectin, which had initial promise in case series, but did not show benefit as part of a controlled study (Gordon et al. 1995).

Most patients have 'conventional treatment' before trying ASEs. This is usually topical, although punctual occlusion and bandage contact lenses may be used. The actual treatment protocol varies as does the compliance with it. This does provide some element of study control, in which serum drops are added 'compared to the maximum treatment,' which is taken as a baseline.

Other treatments may confound results when analyzing autologous serum efficacy, although they may well be clinically appropriate, such as the use of punctal occlusion. Even in studies that do have control groups and/or randomize to treatment, nearly all fall short of a true double-masked randomized control study. One reason for this is that it is easy to identify serum drops from other ocular lubricants.

A useful review of ASEs is given by Yamada et al. (2008).

Dry eye disease

Fourteen studies have been published on the treatment of ocular surface disease in the form of severe DED, with autologous serum. The underlying pathology included DED, Sjögren's syndrome, graft-versus-host disease, ocular mucous membrane pemphigoid, aniridia, and hypovitaminosis A. In all but one of these studies, there was an improvement in outcomes, although the measures used varied. The most frequently reported outcomes were patient symptoms, staining using fluorescein and/or Rose Bengal, and tear break-up time.

A few controlled studies have been published.

Tananuvat et al. (2001) randomized ASEs to one eye and normal saline to the other of 12 patients with DED. While both treatment and control groups significantly improved from baseline, there was no statistical difference between the two.

Noble et al. (2000) reported on 31 eyes of 16 patients with DED that were randomized to receive either ASEs or conventional treatment for 3 months and then crossed over for 3 months. ASEs significantly improved subjective symptoms and impression cytology findings (e.g. squamous metaplasia and goblet cell density) during the ASE treatment phase. It should be noted that the study was not masked and 10 other patients did not complete it.

Kojima et al. (2005) found significant improvement in fluorescein and Rose Bengal staining scores, tear break-up time, and pain scores when 37 eyes of 20 patients with DED were randomized to receive ASEs rather than artificial tears only. Objective assessments performed were masked.

Many of the published studies have relatively short follow-up; however, Lee and Chen (2008) treated recalcitrant DED due to a variety of underlying conditions, in 23 patients for a follow-up period of 17 months. There was subjective improvement in 76%, reduction in fluorescein staining in 74%, and a reduced use of lubricants in 70%—and no significant complications.

Persistent epithelial defects

Persistent epithelial defects may be caused by a variety of underlying pathologies, and can give rise to a host of complications such as pain, secondary infection, inflammation, scar formation, corneal melting, and perforation (Chen et al. 2010).

Schulze et al. (2006) performed a randomized trial of ASEs versus sodium hyaluronate drops for patients with diabetes who required iatrogenic epithelial debridement during the course of vitrectomy surgery. These patients often had poor corneal epithelial healing. Epithelial defects healed in 4.3 days in the ASE group, significantly faster than compared to 7.1 days in the control group.

Chen et al. (2010) compared epithelial healing in 165 eyes that had undergone penetrating keratoplasty between one cohort of patients who received ASEs and another cohort who received non-serum-based topical treatment (surgical protocols were otherwise similar). The main finding was that epithelialization was faster with ASEs: this was particularly significant for patients with diabetes and those receiving large-diameter grafts that tend to epithelialize more slowly.

While these studies show benefit with ASEs for epithelialization in patients with slower healing, there are other patients who have more severe disease and persistent defects that last many months despite treatment. Tsubota et al. (1999) treated 16 patients who had persistent epithelial defects for an average of 7.2 months. They received 20% ASEs six times per day: 43% healed within 2 weeks and 60% within 1 month. Similar results were reported by Jeng and Dupps (2009), who treated 25 patients with persistent epithelial defects in neurotrophic corneas: 68% healed in 4 weeks, 88% in 8 weeks, and one at 18 weeks. Jeng and Dupps (2009) also observed that the time to heal was proportional to the total defect duration.

These data suggest that not only is autologous serum very useful in healing epithelial defects, but early treatment is also beneficial, to improve healing and avoid complications. It is worth persisting with ASEs in cases that are slow to respond as well as considering adjuvant therapy.

Facilitating the healing of corneal epithelium also has other benefits such as improving visual acuity, improving corneal sensation, and reducing corneal scarring.

Recurrent corneal erosion

ASEs produce excellent results when used to treat recurrent corneal erosion. Benitezdel Castillo et al. (2002) reported a reduction in recurrence episodes from 2.2 per month to 0.03 per month for 11 patients with refractory disease. These patients were treated with a tapering course of ASEs for 3 months and followed up for a mean period of 9 months. There were no recurrences during the actual treatment period. Ziakas et al. (2010) treated 33 patients who had failed with other treatments with autologous serum for 6 months and then reported mean follow-up of 30 months. There were no recurrences during the treatment phase, and only five patients (15%) had a single recurrence during the follow-up period. These results are impressive, but there have been no controlled studies to date.

Other ocular surface diseases

Goto et al. (2001) treated 22 eyes of 11 patients with superior limbal keratitis who had not responded to lubricants or topical corticosteroids; 82% responded well, with subjective improvement and a significant reduction in ocular surface staining with Rose Bengal and fluorescein drops. Also, limbal squamous metaplasia was shown to reduce by impression cytology. Other diseases treated with ASEs are listed in **Table 30.1**.

Autologous ASEs in combination with other treatments

ASEs are also useful when combined with other treatments. Cases have been published in which non-healing ulcers and corneal melts have been treated with ASEs in addition to other medications. In these cases, it has been the ASEs, when added into the treatment regimen, that seem to have made the difference.

Many authors have used ASEs as an adjuvant therapy to surgical treatment protocols, such as ocular reconstruction, involving penetrating keratoplasty, limbal allografting, and amniotic membrane transplantation, in which they are reported to be critical to success. In addition, ASEs are also important for the success of ex vivo cultured autologous limbal stem cell transplants (Kolli et al. 2010).

▮ Risks and benefits of autologous ASEs

Autologous ASEs are preservative-free, and many studies have published encouraging clinical results in a wide range of difficult-to-treat conditions. The ASE has favorable physical and chemical properties to replace tears and support the ocular surface. The success of ASE treatment, however, depends on the serum containing adequate nutrients and not being toxic in itself. Bradley et al. (2008) found no significant difference between multiple growth factors in serum in patients with DED compared to healthy age-matched controls. Phasukkijwatana et al. (2011) compared EGF, TGF-β1, TGF-β2, and fibronectin levels between patients with chronic Stevens–Johnson syndrome and non-immune-mediated DED, and again found no significant differences. However, in autoimmune and other systemic inflammatory diseases, general blood cytokine levels can be altered and upregulated (Szodoray et al. 2007); also, the potential presence of autoantibodies in the serum against antigens in the lacrimal tissue can lead to further tissue damage and consequently aggravate the DED. This could potentially reduce the effectiveness of ASEs or seriously compromise even further the ocular surface.

However, there are also drawbacks and limitations. First of all, it has to be produced on a patient-by-patient basis; thus, the availability relies on local funding arrangements. Patients should be able to give blood on a regular basis (up to every 3 months) for chronic conditions. There are potential risks of infection. Leite et al. (2006) found contaminating organisms in 6 out of 11 bottles of ASEs when kept in domestic fridges and freezers, and there has been a case report of bilateral corneal ulcers secondary to contaminated ASEs in a patient with impaired immunity. Weisbach et al. (2007) found previously undiscovered hepatitis B and C viruses in 2.3% of patients referred for ASEs. It is possible to transmit hepatitis and human immunodeficiency (HIV) viruses from a single drop of serum. Therefore, not only is there a risk of contamination for the patient, but also risk to others who may mistakenly administer the eye drops, which is likely to be a higher risk outside a controlled healthcare setting.

Although autologous serum has had miraculous benefits for certain conditions, it is not an ideal therapy to use in the wider population.

ALLOGENEIC ASEs

Since the original report by Fox et al. (1984), autologous ASEs have been widely used for the treatment of severe ocular surface disorders with very favorable outcomes. However, the use of autologous serum is contraindicated in patients not medically fit to donate their own blood for preparation of autologous ASEs. To that effect, Chiang et al. (2007 and 2009) were the first to propose the use of topical allogeneic serum eye drops (ALSEs) as a safe and effective alternative therapeutic option to autologous ASEs for the treatment of severe ocular surface diseases not responding to conventional therapy.

There are only two reports in the literature regarding the use of ALSEs from the same group in Taiwan. Chiang et al. (2007) reported the beneficial use of ALSEs to treat two patients with ocular surface disease caused by chronic graft-versus-host disease. The two patients did not respond to conventional treatment and were not fit to donate their own blood for autologous ASE preparation. The authors prepared ALSEs from blood donated by close relatives (either spouse or close blood relations). In both cases, the authors reported a significant benefit after a 10-month follow-up period. The ocular surface was completely stable without complications in the first case, and the second case showed a considerable improvement in clinical signs of ocular surface inflammation; better patient's comfort was reported when compared to the beginning of treatment with ALSEs.

Subsequently, Chiang et al. (2009) went on to report a larger retrospective case series from a single center using ALSEs in 36 patients with persistent corneal epithelial defects, who did not respond to conventional treatment and could not donate their own blood for preparation of autologous ASEs. The blood was obtained from close healthy relatives after performing standard serological investigation used in blood transfusion, including blood-borne viral diseases (i.e. HIV, hepatitis B and hepatitis C viruses). Patients were instructed to use ALSEs hourly while awake and were followed up for a median of 14.6 months (range 3–20 years). The epithelial defects healed completely within 2 weeks of treatment in 15 patients (41.7%). Eleven other patients (30.5%) took up to 2 months to completely heal their epithelial defect. The remaining 10 patients (27.8%) showed no improvement after 2 weeks and underwent treatment with amniotic membrane transplantation at this stage. The authors reported no adverse events in any of the 36 patients for the duration of the study. The authors also reported no significant difference in treatment response between patients treated with non-consanguineous ALSEs (from spouses) and those treated with consanguineous ALSEs ($p = 0.35$).

Julian et al. (2010) from Denmark at the World Corneal Congress VI in Boston reported further use of ALSEs to treat 22 patients with severe DED refractory to conventional therapy. ALSEs were obtained from regular male volunteer donors. The serum drops were supplied frozen and were ABO matched to the recipients. Patients were instructed to use the allogeneic serum drops six times per day for a period of 2–4 weeks. All patients completed the study and no side effects were reported. Fourteen patients (63%) reported beneficial effects on subjective symptoms, and improvement in ocular surface changes was observed in 12 patients (55%) at slit-lamp examination.

■ Risks and benefits of allogeneic ASEs

There is some evidence supporting the topical use of ALSEs as an alternative treatment option in severe ocular surface disease, for patients unable to donate their own blood due to medical contraindications. The three reported case series described previously clearly demonstrate the potential benefits and safety of ALSEs. None of the patients in these series had adverse reactions to allogeneic ASEs or developed secondary infections during the course of the studies. However, any allogeneic blood donation carries a risk of disease transmission, although this is significantly reduced by careful donor selection and screening.

This treatment will allow certain patients to greatly benefit from topical ASEs. ALSEs can be prepared prospectively from a donor volunteer and be readily available frozen upon request. It must be emphasized, however, that all published studies to date are essentially case reports. This highlights the need for studies with a larger sample size and a randomized controlled clinical trial to be performed.

PLASMA: PLATELET-RICH PLASMA EYE DROPS

Circulating platelets contain α-granules that store many active molecules, such as growth factors and cytokines. These are released when the platelets are activated, for example when a blood clot is formed, thus aiding tissue regeneration. In vitro studies have demonstrated that platelet lysate has much higher concentrations of growth factors than serum (Liu et al. 2006). Since growth factors are essential to corneal epithelial cell health and regeneration, various groups have attempted to use platelets and the growth factors they contain as part of therapeutic eye drops.

By taking whole blood and concentrating the platelets by centrifugation, platelet-rich plasma (PRP) can be manufactured that has a concentration of platelets 5–20 times greater than that in peripheral blood, as well as all the other necessary factors. Several authors have investigated the therapeutic use of autologous PRP. This can be either administered as an eye drop for ocular surface disease or activated by calcium to form an enriched fibrin clot that can be used surgically (Alio et al. 2007).

In clinical studies, PRP eye drops healed 50% and significantly improved 42% of 24 eyes with chronic corneal ulcers, with two eyes showing no change (Alio et al. 2007). There was also significant improvement when PRP eye drops were used for patients with symptomatic DED and those who had ongoing ocular surface symptoms following penetrating keratoplasty (PKP). Geremicca et al. (2010) reported the successful treatment of 120 eyes with epithelial and stromal defects secondary to neurotrophic keratopathy and trauma.

Koffler (2006) used platelet-enriched plasma gel to form therapeutic growth factor-enriched fibrin clots, which were successfully used to heal six chronic non-healing neurotrophic ulcers. This technique was also used postoperatively following PKP in high-risk corneal ulcer patients, who had suffered from repeated corneal transplant melting, with promising results. Alio et al. (2007) combined this technique with amniotic membrane transplantation to treat or prevent threatened corneal perforation in 14 eyes, all of which were either completely healed or significantly improved.

Marquez de Aracena Del Cid & Montero De Espinosa (2009) described the subconjunctival injection of enriched plasma for the treatment of acute chemical burns, which led to improved outcomes.

Risks and benefits of PRP eye drops

The clinical benefits and safety of PRP eye drops have been demonstrated previously. So far, there have been no clinical controlled studies to compare PRP therapy with ASEs or other treatments. In theory, PRP eye drops have the advantage of containing a higher concentration of growth factors than ASEs. There is an additional method of administration to produce an enriched fibrin clot that is used surgically.

PRP eye drops can be autologous or allogeneic. The use of allogeneic fresh frozen plasma and platelets is well established in other clinical fields, and both products are widely available from blood banks. Thus, their use may circumvent several problems of producing ASEs or ALSEs on an individual patient basis. Further work is needed in this area.

UMBILICAL CORD ASEs

Umbilical cord blood can be extracted from the umbilical cord and/or placenta after uncomplicated cesarean sections. Ang et al. (2011) compared cytokine levels in umbilical cord serum, adult serum as well as fetal calf serum and found the highest levels in umbilical cord serum. Umbilical cord serum outperformed all other preparations in the support of limbal and conjunctival cell cultures in vitro, and it is effective at a fraction of the concentration of the other preparations such as adult serum.

The indications for umbilical cord serum eye drop (UCSE) use are very similar to those for ALSEs, essentially in the context of patients unable to donate their own blood due to medical contraindications and not responding to conventional treatment. In addition, UCSEs contain additional factors to ASEs, and may offer greater clinical benefits for certain patients.

Vajpayee et al. (2003) were the first to report a randomized controlled clinical trial evaluating the therapeutic efficacy of UCSEs. Sixty eyes of 59 patients were divided into two groups receiving treatment with either ASEs or UCSEs. Patients with persistent epithelial defect not responding to conventional treatment were included. After 3 weeks of treatment, the authors reported significantly faster healing of the corneal epithelial defect in patients using the UCSEs ($p < 0.05$) compared to the ASEs.

Subsequently, Yoon et al. from South Korea published four separate case series, evaluating the treatment of persistent corneal epithelial defect, DED, neurotrophic keratopathy, and recurrent corneal erosions with UCSEs. In the first series, 14 patients (14 eyes) with persistent epithelial defect not responding to conventional treatment were treated with 20% UCSEs six times a day. The epithelial defect completely healed within 4 weeks in 85.8% of the patients. In the second series, 12 patients (24 eyes) with severe DED were treated with UCSEs. After 6 months of treatment, the symptom score, corneal sensitivity, tear break-up time, and corneal epithelial score improved significantly ($p < 0.01$). In the third series, 28 patients (28

eyes) suffering from neurotrophic keratopathy were treated with UCSEs 6–10 times per day. The epithelial defect healed within 4 weeks in 22 eyes (78.6%) and after 4 weeks in the remaining 6 eyes (21.4%). In the most recently published series (Yoon et al. 2011), a controlled, parallel-group study compared UCSEs as well as artificial tears to artificial tears only on the frequency of recurrence of corneal erosions in 35 patients (35 eyes). The mean frequency of recurrence was 0.5 (SD 0.79) in the first treatment group and 2.24 (SD 1.09) in the second group ($p < 0.01$). Of note, no significant complication or adverse reaction was observed in these series.

Yoon et al. (2007) published a prospective case-control study, comparing the therapeutic effect between ASEs and UCSEs in the treatment of severe DED. Forty-eight patients (92 eyes) with severe DED were treated with ASEs (41 eyes of 21 patients) or UCSEs (51 eyes of 27 patients). At 2 months, symptoms and the corneal epithelial score improved significantly in the UCSE treatment group compared with the ASE group ($p \leq 0.04$).

Risks and benefits of umbilical cord ASEs

USCEs have been shown to be safe and effective in the treatment of acute and chronic severe ocular surface diseases, such as acute chemical injury, neurotrophic keratopathy, and DED. However, the current evidence is limited to just a few publications from two centers, and randomized, controlled, clinical trials with large sample size are still lacking.

No significant complication or adverse reaction was observed in the reported clinical trials. However, similarly to ALSEs, UCSEs also carries a risk of disease transmission, although this is significantly reduced by careful donor selection and screening.

Perhaps the main obstacle to research and ultimately clinical use for USCE is the availability. While umbilical cord blood is generated at every birth and is otherwise disposed of, convincing beneficial evidence, ethical approval, validated and regulated processing systems, and sensitive approaches to mothers are all required before UCSEs can become more widely used.

ALBUMIN

Albumin is the main protein within tears, and it can be extracted and purified from donated blood and made into eye drops. It has many effects, such as buffering pH, binding toxins, and supporting tissue growth. Human albumin is available commercially as a pharmaceutical product normally used for infusion, which can be used to produce small aliquots for topical use (unlicensed use). Unterlauft et al. (2009) reported the use of 5% albumin eye drops for ocular surface disease in patients unsuitable for ASEs; 22 eyes with persistent epithelial defects and 9 eyes with punctate epitheliopathy were treated. Twenty-eight of these showed benefit after an average of 6.5-week treatment, deemed to be due to the albumin eye drops.

Risks and benefits of albumin eye drops

As with other blood-derived products, there has been some success reported in the limited studies conducted so far. Albumin as an infusion product has been safely used for many years and is thus widely available. However, the purity is only 95% and there is still some infection risk. Also, albumin eye drops lack many of the beneficial components such as growth factors. However, there are likely to be groups of patients who do benefit from albumin eye drops, if further studies support its use.

CONCLUSIONS

Currently, there is great interest in using blood derivatives in the management of a variety of ocular surface diseases resistant to conventional medical treatment. The rationale for this more expensive topical treatment is not completely elucidated yet, but it is based on the principles, similar to ASEs, that all other blood derivatives contain growth factors (i.e. EGF, FGF, NGF, TGF-β, and other growth factors), cytokines, and vitamins essential for the proliferation, differentiation, and maturation of the normal ocular surface epithelium.

At present, most published studies demonstrate the safety and efficacy of topical use of blood-derived products, including ASEs, ALSEs, UCSEs, PRP, and albumin for the management of severe ocular surface diseases. However, there is a need for further randomized controlled clinical trials comparing the different types of ASEs, including different concentrations.

Finally, the ultimate source of therapeutic eye drops is synthetically produced and promptly available at a reasonable cost, which contains all the necessary components at the correct concentrations or even customized for optimum benefit, without the potential drawbacks and risks of blood-derived products.

REFERENCES

Alio JL, Abad M, Artola A, et al. Use of autologous platelet-rich plasma in the treatment of dormant corneal ulcers. *Ophthalmology* 2007; **114**:1286. e1–1293.e1.

Ang LPK, Do TP, Thein ZM, et al. Ex vivo expansion of conjunctival and limbal epithelial cells using cord blood serum-supplemented culture medium. *Invest Ophthalmol Vis Sci* 2011; **52**:6138–6147.

Benitezdel Castillo JM, Martinezde la Casa JM, CuiñaSardiña RC, et al. Treatment of recurrent corneal erosions using autologous serum. *Cornea* 2002; **21**:781–783.

Bradley JC, Bradley RH, McCartney DL, Mannis MJ. Serum growth factor analysis in dry eye syndrome. *Clin Experiment Ophthalmol* 2008; **36**:717–720.

Chen YM, Hu FR, Huang JY, et al. The effect of topical autologous serum on graft re-epithelialization after penetrating keratoplasty. *Am J Ophthalmol* 2010; **150**:352.e352–359.e352.

Chiang CC, Lin JM, Chen WL, Tsai YY. Allogeneic serum eye drops for the treatment of severe dry eye in patients with chronic graft-versus-host disease. *Cornea* 2007; **26**:861–863.

Chiang CC, Lin JM, Chen WL, Tsai YY. Allogeneic serum eye drops for the treatment of persistent corneal epithelial defect. *Eye* 2009; **23**:290–293.

Fox RI, Chan R, Michelson JB, Belmont JB, Michelson PE. Beneficial effect of artificial tears made with autologous serum in patients with keratoconjunctivitis sicca. *Arthritis Rheum* 1984; **27**:459–461.

Geremicca W, Fonte C, Vecchio S. Blood components for topical use in tissue regeneration: evaluation of corneal lesions treated with platelet lysate and considerations on repair mechanisms. *Blood Transfus* 2010; **8**:107–112.

Gordon JF, Johnson P, Musch DC. Topical fibronectin ophthalmic solution in the treatment of persistent defects of the corneal epithelium. Chiron Vision Fibronectin Study Group. *Am J Ophthalmol* 1995; **119**:281–287.

Goto E, Shimmura S, Shimazaki J, Tsubota K. Treatment of superior limbic keratoconjunctivitis by application of autologous serum. *Cornea* 2001; **20**:807–810.

Jeng BH, Dupps WJ Jr. Autologous serum 50% eyedrops in the treatment of persistent corneal epithelial defects. *Cornea* 2009; **28**:1104–1108.

Julian HO, Olesen HB, Hansen MB, Harritshøj L. Poster: ready-made allogeneic serum eye drops for severe dry eye disease. World Cornea Congress VI. Boston, 2010.

Klenkler B. Sheardown H. Growth factors in the anterior segment: role in tissue maintenance, wound healing and ocular pathology. *Exp Eye Res* 2004; **79**:677–688.

Koffler BH. Autologous serum therapy of the ocular surface with novel delivery by platelet concentrate gel. *Ocular Surface* 2006; **4**:188–195.

Kojima T, Ishida R, Dogru M, et al. The effect of autologous serum eyedrops in the treatment of severe dry eye disease: a prospective randomized case-control study. *Am J Ophthalmol* 2005; **139**:242–246.

Kolli S, Ahmad S, Lako M, Figueiredo F. Successful clinical implementation of corneal epithelial stem cell therapy for treatment of unilateral limbal stem cell deficiency. *Stem Cells* 2010; **28**:597–610.

Lee GA, Chen SX. Autologous serum in the management of recalcitrant dry eye syndrome. *Clin Exp Ophthalmol* 2008; **36**:119–122.

Leite SC, de Castro RS, Alves M, et al. Risk factors and characteristics of ocular complications, and efficacy of autologous serum tears after haematopoietic progenitor cell transplantation. *Bone Marrow Transplant* 2006; **38**:223–227.

Liu L, Hartwig D, Harloff S, et al. An optimised protocol for the production of autologous serum eyedrops. *Graefes Arch Clin Exp Ophthalmol* 2005; **243**:706–714.

Liu L, Hartwig D, Harloff S, et al. Corneal epitheliotrophic capacity of three different blood-derived preparations. *Invest Ophthalmol Vis Sci* 2006; **47**:2438–2444.

Marquez De Aracena Del Cid R, Montero De Espinosa I. Subconjunctival application of regenerative factor-rich plasma for the treatment of ocular alkali burns. *Eur J Ophthalmol* 2009; **19**:909–915.

Noble BA, Loh RS, MacLennan S, et al. Comparison of autologous serum eye drops with conventional therapy in a randomized controlled crossover trial for ocular surface disease. *Br J Ophthalmol* 2000; **88**:647–652.

Phasukkijwatana N, Lertrit P, Liammongkolkul S, Prabhasawat P. Stability of epitheliotrophic factors in autologous serum eye drops from chronic Stevens-Johnson syndrome dry eye compared to nonautoimmune dry eye. *Curr Eye Res* 2011; **36**:775–781.

Schulze SD, Sekundo W, Kroll P. Autologous serum for the treatment of corneal epithelial abrasions in diabetic patients undergoing vitrectomy. *Am J Ophthalmol* 2006; **142**:207–211.

Szodoray P, Alex P, Chappell-Woodward CM, et al. Circulating cytokines in Norwegian patients with psoriatic arthritis determined by a multiplex cytokine array system. *Rheumatology* 2007; **46**:417–425.

Tananuvat N, Daniell M, Sullivan LJ, et al. Controlled study of the use of autologous serum in dry eye patients. *Cornea* 2001; **20**:802–806.

Tsubota k, Goto E, Shimmura S, Shimazaki J. Treatment of persistent corneal epithelial defect by autologous serum application. *Ophthalmology* 1999; **106**:1984–1989.

Unterlauft JD, Kohlhaas M, Hofbauer I, Kasper K, Geerling G. Albumin eye drops for treatment of ocular surface diseases. *Ophthalmologe* 2009; **106**:932–937.

Vajpayee RB, Mukerji N, Tandon R, et al. Evaluation of umbilical cord serum therapy for persistent corneal epithelial defects. *Br J Ophthalmol* 2003; **87**:1312–1316.

Weisbach V, Dietrich T, Kruse FE, Eckstein R, Cursiefen C. HIV and hepatitis B/C infections in patients donating blood for use as autologous serum eye drops. *Br J Ophthalmol* 2007; **91**:1724–1725.

Yamada C, King KE, Ness PM. Autologous serum eyedrops: literature review and implications for transfusion medicine specialists. *Transfusion* 2008; **48**:1245–1255.

Yoon KC, Choi W, You IC, Choi J. Application of umbilical cord serum eyedrops for recurrent corneal erosions. *Cornea* 2011; 30744–748.

Yoon KC, Jeong IY, Im SK, et al. Therapeutic effect of umbilical cord serum eyedrops for the treatment of dry eye associated with graft-versus-host disease. *Bone Marrow Transplant* 2007; **39**:231–235.

Ziakas NG, Boboridis KG, Terzidou C, et al. Long-term follow up of autologous serum treatment for recurrent corneal erosions. *Clin Exp Ophthalmol* 2010; **38**:683–687.

Chapter 31

Secretagogues, mucolytics, and anticollagenolytics for dry eye disease treatment

Eduardo M. Rocha, Ana P. Cotrim, Davi Lazarini Marques, Peter S. Reinach, Monica Alves

■ INTRODUCTION

Dry eye disease (DED) is a complex disease with multifactorial causes. Such complexity limits the efficacy of any single treatment. In such a situation, well-known medications used for treating inflammatory, neurological, and other types of diseases can be used effectively for attenuating DED clinical features. Such a strategy to treat DED has been ongoing in several other medical fields for more than three decades. Other than artificial tears, it has resulted in generating the major part of the DED therapeutic arsenal (Akpek et al. 2011).

In this chapter, we provide a critical overview of three examples of classes of drugs initially developed for other purposes, but have also proven to be somewhat efficacious in the treatment of some clinical DED features. These groups are secretagogues, mucolytics, and anticollagenolytics. The general characteristics, mechanism of action, representative drugs, presentation, administration, and clinical efficacy of these groups are discussed here. For further reading, see Ashburn and Thor (2004) and Cade-Jorge et al. (2009).

■ SECRETAGOGUES

Secretagogues are medications that mimic neurotransmitters. They are agonists of exocrine secretion that stimulate tear formation by a group of glands in the lacrimal system (**Table 31.1**).

Their mechanism of action was initially thought to be limited to acting as a simple compensatory agent, to supplement neural input to impaired exocrine glands. However, their effects are now thought to be more complex. They may act (a) to suppress the inhibitory effects of inflammatory mediators rather than supplement neurotransmitter

action (Zoukhri & Kublin 2001), (b) as competitors of autoantibody interactions with muscarinic receptors (Bacman et al. 2001), and (c) as surrogates for impaired autonomic function by neurotransmitter mimicry. These possible roles are necessary for proper exocrine gland development and function and probably also for a balanced inflammatory response (Kam & Sullivan 2011, Knox et al. 2010) (**Figure 31.1**).

Among these, the most studied secretagogue is pilocarpine, originally obtained from an Amazonian plant and used in phytotherapy by the ancient natives in Brazil. It has been, for a long time, the first choice for antiglaucoma topical medication (Murube 2005). This parasympathetic mimetic can be prepared in capsules, but it is also commercially available.

The ideal indication for its usage would be in cases of 7th nerve palsy involving the lacrimal nerve or trigeminal lesion leading to neurotrophic ocular surface diseases and/or damage to the terminal efferent portion of parasympathetic nerves to the lacrimal system (**Table 31.2**). In these situations, it is effective because this muscarinic agonist provides neurotransmitter replacement. However, in other clinical studies involving massive inflammation and/or extensive tissue destruction, such as seen in Sjögren's syndrome and sicca syndrome post radiotherapy, its effectiveness is limited even though systemic treatment is convenient because it lessens dryness in other organs (Fox et al. 1991, Gorsky et al. 2004).

Available clinical data reveals that pilocarpine has therapeutic efficacy. In partitioned doses, from 5 to 20 mg/day, it improves comfort and reduces lubricant eye drops frequency, decreases Rose Bengal staining, quality, number of conjunctival surface cells, and tear film break-up time (TBUT), in a few weeks. However, it does not increase tear flow measured with Schirmer's test in Sjögren's syndrome patients

Table 31.1 Summary of secretagogues used in dry eye disease treatment

Drug	Doses, route	Mechanism of action	Effect	Commercial name	Contraindications/side effects
Pilocarpine hydrochloride	5 mg, po, qid	M3 agonist	Muscarinic	Salagen (Novartis)	Asthma, narrow-angle glaucoma, sweating, urinary urgency, intestinal discomfort
Cevimeline hydrochloride	30 mg, po tid	M3 agonist	Muscarinic	Evoxac (Daiichi)	
Bethanechol (carbamic ester of beta-methylcholine)	10 mg, po, qid	Analog of acetylcholine, cholinesterase resistant	Nicotinic and muscarinic effects	Urecholine	
Anethole, Anetholtrithione	25 mg, po, tid	Undetermined	Non-muscarinic	Felviten, Sulfarlem	Abdominal discomfort
Eledoisin	0.1% of eledoisin aqueous solution as eye drop	Analog of substance P	Cholinergic and/or irritating secretion stimulation	Eloisin	Non-reported

po, per oral; qid, four times a day; tid, three times a day.

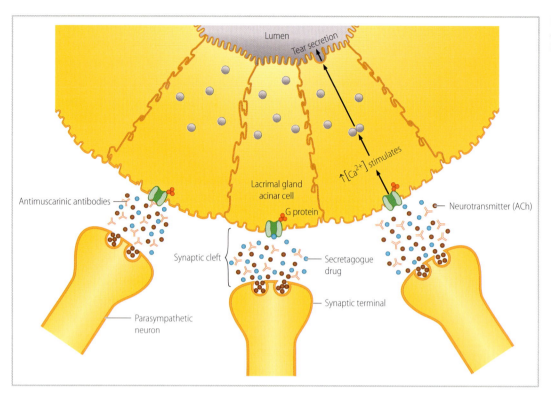

Figure 31.1 Mechanism of action of secretagogues on lacrimal glands.

(Aragona et al. 2006, Tsifetaki et al. 2003). Nevertheless, there are concerns about its usage because of side effects such as headache, increased sweating, palpitations, increased urinary frequency, and intestinal tract distress. Moreover, interaction with beta-blockers may potentiate side effects. Since the studies were conducted only from 1 to 5 months, it is unknown whether drug tolerance could become an issue after a longer period.

Cemiveline is a newer commercially available medication for sicca syndrome, used from 20 to 90 mg/day. Its mechanism and side effects are similar to those of pilocarpine, but it has a longer half-life. Different clinical studies have shown contradictory data about objective signs, such as those in the Schirmer's test, but they agree about comfort improvement (Ono et al. 2004, Venables 2004, Weber & Keating 2008).

Bethanechol is a drug available for postoperative and postpartum urinary retention. When it was investigated for use in dry mouth secondary to radiotherapy, salivary secretions increased to levels similar to those seen with pilocarpine, but the drug had side effects (Gorsky et al. 2004).

Eledoisin is a drug that is being investigated for topical use in DED patients for the last four decades in Europe. It is derived from an extract of salivary gland of an octopus from the Mediterranean Sea. Although

Table 31.2 Neurogenic diseases with compromised autonomic system and dry eye disease that would be treatable with oral cholinergic agonists

Diseases
VII nerve (facial) palsy
V nerve (trigeminus) palsy
Riley day syndrome (familial dysautonomia)
Neuropathy secondary to diabetes mellitus
Neuropathy secondary to hanseniasis
Anticholinergic side effects of medications

it demonstrated an ability to increase tear flow when topically applied, it is not known whether it is a genuine secretagogue or just induces reflex tearing due to an irritating effect (Göbbels et al. 1991).

Anethole was investigated in the 1980s for systemic use in Sjögren's syndrome; however, subsequent clinical trials did not reveal substantial benefit in using it for improving xerostomia (Malmström et al. 1988, Schiødt et al. 1986). A few years ago, a study addressing its effect in DED revealed that Anethole was beneficial in improving some DED symptoms based on a comparison of pre- and post-treatment signs, and those in a placebo-treated group. It is more efficacious in moderate to severe cases, over a 4-week usage period.

In conclusion, despite many available secretagogue options, pilocarpine and cemiveline remain the most accepted for use in DED therapy. Despite their major limiting systemic side effects, they could also be advantageous for treatment of other organ dryness. For further reading see Tracey (2007) and Weber and Keating (2008).

■ MUCOLYTICS

Figure 31.2 provides a diagrammatic representation of tear film structure and the action of mucolytics. Bromhexine is a synthetic derivative of vasicine, an alkaloid drug with secretomimetic and mucolytic effects; therefore, it fits into both drug categories presented here. It was initially developed for respiratory disorder treatment, but also investigated in the 1980s for systemic treatment of Sjögren's syndrome symptoms, including DED (**Table 31.3**).

Ambroxol, its metabolite, stimulates surfactant synthesis and inhibits Na^+ channels. It has a clinical effect similar to that of bromhexine, and some analgesic and anti-inflammatory effects (Malerba & Ragnoli 2008).

Small clinical trials revealed that both medications could improve symptoms or signs of DED; however, in other studies, ambroxol did not show any improvement in Sjögren's syndrome patients' DED (Avisar et al. 1981, Ichikawa et al. 1988, Manthorpe et al. 1984).

Taken together, these results suggest that bromhexine, in adequate doses, is superior to its metabolite for DED treatment.

N-acetylcysteine (NAC) is a major mucolytic agent used initially to liquefy bronchial secretions. In the last four decades, topical presentation has been investigated for its effectiveness in the treatment of filamentary keratitis, DED, and other ocular surface diseases such as alkaline burn and vernal keratoconjunctivitis (Absolon & Brown 1968) (**Table 31.3**).

Its proposed mechanism is to act as an (1) antioxidant, (2) inhibitor of collagenases, and (3) anti-inflammatory agent, besides having mucolytic activity by breaking the disulfide bonds between mucoproteins present in mucus.

In a recent study with patients with chronic blepharitis, oral intake of NAC, 100 mg tid, to complement the traditional treatment (warm compress, antibiotic, and corticosteroids), improved several parameters including fern test and tear film break-up time (Yalçin et al. 2002).

The main observation from preclinical studies is that topical formulations of NAC at doses of 20% or higher are toxic to the cornea (Sugar & Waltman 1973). At concentrations from 0.3 to 20% for topical application, or 100–300 mg/day for oral use, also including different vehicles, NAC has proven to be efficacious in reducing tissue levels of inflammatory cytokines, removing mucous filaments, hastening corneal epithelial healing, and reducing corneal neovascularization. However, none of those results were striking enough to lead to further clinical studies or to make it an obligatory therapeutic adjuvant in DED or keratoconjunctivitis (Kubota et al. 2011, Manthorpe et al. 1984).

A possible explanation for this limited effectiveness is that mucous filaments are a result of diverse conditions that are generally continuously injurious to corneal epithelia with variable intensity (Tanioka et al. 2009).

Therefore, there are no documented promising results suggesting that NAC has any potential therapeutic value, besides reducing, for a limited time over a defined dose range, corneal mucous filament formation and/or modestly improving tear film stability. However, such effects may only be temporary, since higher doses or extended use can be toxic to cornea epithelia.

In conclusion, neither mucolytic agent has been incorporated into the broad therapeutic options for DED, probably due to the modest as well as conflicting reports on their efficacy.

■ ANTICOLLAGENOLYTICS

Tetracyclines comprise a group of antibiotics that have been used to improve ocular surface inflammation and meibomian gland dysfunction (MGD). Their mechanism of action as protein synthesis inhibitor impacts on matrix metalloproteinase expression and lipid secretion composition.

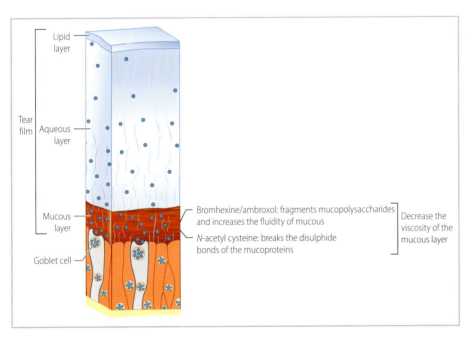

Figure 31.2 Mechanism of action of mucolytics on ocular surface.

Table 31.3 Characteristics of mucolytics used in dry eye disease treatment

Drug	Doses, route of administration	Mechanism of action	Effect	Commercial name
Bromhexine	20–48 mg/day tablets or oral solution	Increases serous secretion and activates ciliary epithelial secretions	Increases tear volume and fluidity	Bisolvon, Benadryl
Ambroxol	120–135 mg/day tablets	Similar to bromhexine	Similar to bromhexine	Mucosolvan, Lasolvan, Mucoangin
NAC	Topical eye drops 0.3–10%	Mucolytic	Removes mucous filaments from cornea	NAC
NAC	Tablets 600 mg	Antioxidant and mucolytic	Improves TBUT	Fluimucil, Mucomyst
NAC, N-acetylcysteine; TBUT, tear film break-up time.				

In this context, tetracycline or its semisynthetic derivatives are being currently prescribed for a broad number of patients around the world. It is also being investigated in clinical and experimental studies to revert MGD keratinization and prevent corneal damage due to dryness and/or other adverse effects, such as persistent epithelial defect, neovascularization, and systemic symptoms of Sjögren´s syndrome or rheumatoid arthritis (i.e. dry mouth, arthritis, and fatigue). Those studies addressed issues of doses, routes of administration (i.e. topical or systemic), and efficacy and benefit of combination with other drugs such as corticosteroids (Beardsley et al. 2008, Perry et al. 1986).

Currently, tetracycline or its derivatives are useful as adjuvant systemic therapy for MGD and corneal epitheliopathy as they are helpful in epithelium healing, reducing inflammation and dryness. Its effects on the MGD may take several weeks to become perceptible; therefore, a treatment plan lasting for at least 8 weeks should be planned, but appearance of side effects should be monitored during this period. The major contraindications are related to pregnancy and childhood because tetracyclines affect growth of teeth and bones (Dréno et al. 2004) (Table 31.4). For further reading see Paiva and Pflugfelder (2008) and Federici (2011).

Table 31.4 Summary of anticollagenolytics used in dry eye disease treatment

Drug	Oral doses	Effect	Contraindications or side effects
Tetracycline	250 mg qid or 500 mg bid	Antiphotolytic and anti-inflammatory	Avoid during pregnancy and childhood: affects fetus bone growth and causes permanent teeth discoloration. Avoid with meals to prevent its inactivation. Photosensivity
Doxycycline	100 mg qid		Impairs the effectiveness of many types of hormonal contraceptives. Skin photosensitivity
Minocycline	50 mg bid		Vestibular disturbances, skin photosensitivity

bid, two times a day; qid, once a day; qid, four times a day.

REFERENCES

Absolon MJ, Brown CA. Acetylcysteine in kerato-conjunctivitis sicca. *Br J Ophthalmol* 1968; **52**:310–316.

Akpek EK, Lindsley KB, Adyanthaya RS, et al. Treatment of Sjögren's syndrome-associated dry eye an evidence-based review. *Ophthalmology* 2011; **118**:1242–1252.

Aragona P, Di Pietro R, Spinella R, Mobrici M. Conjunctival epithelium improvement after systemic pilocarpine in patients with Sjogren's syndrome. *Br J Ophthalmol* 2006; **90**:166–170.

Ashburn TT, Thor KB. Drug repositioning: identifying and developing new uses for existing drugs. *Nat Rev Drug Discov* 2004; **3**:673–683.

Avisar R, Savir H, Machtey I, et al. Clinical trial of bromhexine in Sjögren's syndrome. *Ann Ophthalmol* 1981; **13**:971–973.

Bacman S, Berra A, Sterin-Borda L, Borda E. Muscarinic acetylcholine receptor antibodies as a new marker of dry eye Sjögren syndrome. *Invest Ophthalmol Vis Sci* 2001; **42**:321–327.

Beardsley RM, De Paiva CS, Power DF, Pflugfelder SC. Desiccating stress decreases apical corneal epithelial cell size–modulation by the metalloproteinase inhibitor doxycycline. *Cornea* 2008; **27**:935–940.

Cade-Jorge F, Cade-Jorge I, Kusabara AA, Rocha EM. Perspectives in therapeutic innovation in ocular surface disorders and dry eye syndrome. *Recent Patents on Endocrine, Metabolic & Immune Drug Discovery* 2009; **3**:194–199.

Dréno B, Bettoli V, Ochsendorf F, et al. European recommendations on the use of oral antibiotics for acne. *Eur J Dermatol* 2004; **14**:391–399.

Federici TJ. The non-antibiotic properties of tetracyclines: clinical potential in ophthalmic disease. *Pharmacol Res* 2011; **64**:614–623.

Fox PC, Atkinson JC, Macynski AA, et al. Pilocarpine treatment of salivary gland hypofunction and dry mouth (xerostomia). *Arch Intern Med* 1991; **151**:1149–1152.

Gorsky M, Epstein JB, Parry J, et al. The efficacy of pilocarpine and bethanechol upon saliva production in cancer patients with hyposalivation following radiation therapy. *Oral Surg Oral Med Oral Pathol Oral Radiol Endod* 2004; **97**:190–195.

Göbbels M, Selbach J, Spitznas M. Effect of eledoisin on tear volume and tear flow in humans as assessed by fluorophotometry. *Graefes Arch Clin Exp Ophthalmol* 1991; **229**:549–552.

Ichikawa Y, Tokunaga M, Shimizu H, et al. Clinical trial of ambroxol (Mucosolvan) in Sjögren's syndrome. *Tokai J Exp Clin Med* 1988; **13**:165–169.

Kam WR, Sullivan DA. Neurotransmitter influence on human meibomian gland epithelial cells. *Invest Ophthalmol Vis Sci* 2011; **52**:8543–8548.

Knox SM, Lombaert IM, Reed X, et al. Parasympathetic innervation maintains epithelial progenitor cells during salivary organogenesis. *Science* 2010; **329**:1645–1647.

Kubota M, Shimmura S, Kubota S, et al. Hydrogen and N-acetyl-L-cysteine rescue oxidative stress-induced angiogenesis in a mouse corneal alkali-burn model. *Invest Ophthalmol Vis Sci* 2011; **52**:427–433.

Malerba M, Ragnoli B. Ambroxol in the 21st century: pharmacological and clinical update. *Expert Opin Drug Metab Toxicol* 2008; **4**:1119–1129.

Malmström MJ, Segerberg-Konttinen M, Tuominen TS, et al. Xerostomia due to Sjögren's syndrome. Diagnostic criteria, treatment and outlines for a continuous dental care programme and an open trial with Sulfarlem. *Scand J Rheumatol* 1988; **17**:77–86.

Manthorpe R, Petersen SH, Prause JU. Mucosolvan in the treatment of patients with primary Sjögren's syndrome. Results from a double-blind cross-over investigation. *Acta Ophthalmol (Copenh)* 1984; **62**:537–541.

Murube J. Pilocarpine and tear secretion. *Ocul Surf* 2005; 3:119–125.

Ono M, Takamura E, Shinozaki K, Tsumura T, et al. Therapeutic effect of cevimeline on dry eye in patients with Sjögren's syndrome: a randomized, double-blind clinical study. *Am J Ophthalmol* 2004; **138**:6–17.

Paiva CS, Pflugfelder SC. Rationale for anti-inflammatory therapy in dry eye syndrome. *Arq Bras Oftalmol* 2008; **71**:89–95.

Perry HD, Kenyon KR, Lamberts DW, et al. Systemic tetracycline hydrochloride as adjunctive therapy in the treatment of persistent epithelial defects. *Ophthalmology* 1986; **93**:1320–1322.

Schiødt M, Oxholm P, Jacobsen A. Treatment of xerostomia in patients with primary Sjögren's syndrome with sulfarlem. *Scand J Rheumatol Suppl* 1986; **61**:250–252.

Sugar A, Waltman SR. Corneal toxicity of collagenase inhibitors. *Invest Ophthalmol* 1973; **12**:779–782.

Tanioka H, Yokoi N, Komuro A, et al. Investigation of the corneal filament in filamentary keratitis. *Invest Ophthalmol Vis Sci* 2009; 50:3696–3702.

Tracey KJ. Physiology and immunology of the cholinergic antiinflammatory pathway. *J Clin Invest* 2007; **117**:289–296.

Tsifetaki N, Kitsos G, Paschides CA, et al. Oral pilocarpine for the treatment of ocular symptoms in patients with Sjögren's syndrome: a randomised 12 week controlled study. *Ann Rheum Dis* 2003; **62**:1204–1207.

Venables PJ. Sjögren's syndrome. *Best Pract Res Clin Rheumatol* 2004; **18**:313–329.

Weber J, Keating GM. Cevimeline. *Drugs* 2008; **68**:1691–1698.

Yalçin E, Altin F, Cinhüseyinoglue F, Arslan MO. N-acetylcysteine in chronic blepharitis. *Cornea* 2002; **21**:164–168.

Zoukhri D, Kublin CL. Impaired neurotransmitter release from lacrimal and salivary gland nerves of a murine model of Sjögren's syndrome. *Invest Ophthalmol Vis Sci* 2001; **42**:925–932.

Chapter 32 Immunosuppressants and biologic therapy

Cheryl A. Arcinue, Diana Isabel Pachón Suárez, C. Stephen Foster

INTRODUCTION

Ocular surface disorders can be potentially vision threatening if not recognized and treated early. They can lead to scarring, vascularization, ulceration, corneal perforation, and eventual blindness and loss of the eye. Infections, malignancy, trauma, inflammatory disorders, and anatomical and congenital abnormalities may cause ocular surface disruption and damage. It is therefore important to address the underlying cause of the disorder to break the vicious cycle. If the cause is proven to be inflammatory in nature, then adequate control of inflammation is mandatory prior to attempting any form of eyelid or conjunctival surgery and visual rehabilitation with a corneal transplant or keratoprosthesis.

Many ocular surface disorders are associated with systemic conditions that need to be controlled systemically. You must treat the underlying systemic condition, in addition to the ocular disorder, in order to entirely battle the disease. Ocular surface disorders and associated systemic conditions that may require immunosuppressants and biologic therapy are listed in **Table 32.1**.

IMMUNOMODULATORY THERAPY

An essential modality in the treatment of ocular surface disorders is corticosteroids. However, the potential side effects of long-term corticosteroid therapy are well known and serious, and include osteoporosis, weight gain, hyperglycemia and diabetes, increased susceptibility to infection, cataracts, increased intraocular pressure, and glaucoma. Once the clinician knows that corticosteroids are needed for a long period of time to bring the patient's condition into remission, early employment of corticosteroid-sparing immunomodulatory therapy is advised, which results in superior outcomes and less drug toxicity. The goal is remission with no inflammation, off all corticosteroids, and without drug-induced problems. A list of drugs used in immunomodulatory therapy, their recommended dosages and routes of administration, and the most common potential side effects associated with each drug are given in **Table 32.2**.

Patients and clinicians alike have faced the dilemma of deciding whether the benefits of immunosuppressive therapy outweigh the risks associated with it. One particular concern is whether these drugs cause an increased risk of overall mortality and cancer. Accurate information about the long-term risks of immunomodulatory therapy is needed for informed clinical decision making. The Systemic Immunosuppressive Therapy for Eye Diseases (SITE) cohort study (Kempen et al. 2009) was a retrospective cohort study evaluating overall and cancer mortality in relation to immunosuppressive drug exposure among patients with ocular inflammatory diseases. Patients who used methotrexate (MTX), azathioprine, mycophenolate mofetil (MMF), cyclosporine, systemic corticosteroids, or dapsone had overall and cancer mortality similar to that of patients who never took immunosuppressive drugs. In patients who used cyclophosphamide, overall mortality was not

increased and cancer mortality was non-significantly increased. Tumor necrosis factor (TNF) inhibitors were associated with an increase in overall and cancer mortality (although these results were less robust and additional evidence is needed).

Antimetabolites
Methotrexate

MTX has been widely used in the treatment of rheumatological and autoimmune diseases because of its efficacy, acceptable safety profile, low cost, and ease of administration. It inhibits purine and pyrimidine synthesis by acting as a folic acid analog and inactivating the enzyme dihydrofolate reductase. Extensive evidence has demonstrated that the anti-inflammatory effects of MTX are mediated by an increase in adenosine, which inhibits neutrophil chemotaxis and decreases endothelial permeability. It also inhibits the production of TNF-α, as

Table 32.1 Ocular surface disorders requiring immunosuppressive therapy and biologics

Ocular surface disorder	Associated systemic disease
Dry eye disease, keratoconjunctivitis sicca	Sjögren's syndrome (SS) Scleroderma
Atopic keratoconjunctivitis	Atopic dermatitis Atopy Eczema
Chronic cicatrizing conjunctivitis	Stevens–Johnson syndrome Toxic epidermal necrolysis Rosacea Eczema Scleroderma Lichen planus Sarcoidosis SS
Ocular cicatricial pemphigoid (OCP)	Mucous membrane pemphigoid (MMP)
Scleritis	Systemic lupus erythematosus (SLE) HLA-B27-associated disorders Rheumatoid arthritis (RA) Relapsing polychondritis Granulomatosis with polyangiitis (Wegener) Polyarteritis nodosa (PAN)
Peripheral ulcerative keratitis	RA Granulomatosis with polyangiitis (Wegener) PAN SLE Rosacea Atopy Sarcoidosis

Table 32.2 Immunomodulatory therapy

Drug class	Dose	Route of administration	Potential side effects
ANTIMETABOLITES			
Methotrexate	7.5–50 mg/week	PO, SQ, IV	Bone marrow suppression, hepatotoxicity
Azathioprine	1–3 mg/kg/day	PO	Bone marrow suppression
Mycophenolate mofetil	2 g/day	PO	Bone marrow suppression
Cytarabine	100–200 mg/week	IV	Bone marrow suppression, GI disturbances
CALCINEURIN INHIBITORS			
Cyclosporine	2–5 mg/kg/day	PO	Hypertension, nephrotoxicity
Tacrolimus	0.05–0.15 mg/kg/day	PO, IV	Hypertension, nephrotoxicity, neurological problems
Sirolimus	2 mg/day	PO	GI disturbances, increased risk of infection
ALKYLATING AGENTS			
Cyclophosphamide	1–3 mg/kg/day or 1 g/m^2 (initial dose)	PO or pulsed IV (every 2 weeks)	Bone marrow suppression, hemorrhagic cystitis, increased risk of bladder cancer, sterility
Chlorambucil	0.15 mg/kg/day (initial dose)	IV	Bone marrow suppression, sterility

GI, gastrointestinal; IV, intravenous; PO, per orem (oral); SQ, subcutaneous.

well as interleukin (IL)-6, IL-8, IL-10, IL-12, and macrophage inflammatory protein-1α. It also downregulates both cellular and humoral immune responses (Chan & Cronstein 2002, Tian & Cronstein 2007).

Studies have found MTX to be effective in scleritis (Jachens & Chu 2008, Shah et al. 1992), bullous pemphigoid (Kjellman et al. 2008), ocular cicatricial pemphigoid (OCP), and drug-induced OCP (McCluskey et al. 2004). The SITE cohort study (Gangaputra et al. 2009) suggests that adding MTX to an anti-inflammatory regimen is moderately effective in controlling inflammation and achieving corticosteroid-sparing success, although many months may be required for the therapeutic effect to be seen. MTX is also useful as an alternative option when a second or third agent is needed to achieve better control of inflammation (Bom et al. 2001).

The effect on DNA synthesis is also responsible for the potential side effects that may occur with MTX, including bone marrow suppression, liver toxicity, and stomatitis. Folic acid supplementation (1 mg once a day) helps to prevent these toxicities. MTX is given in doses of 7.5–50.0 mg once a week. It is available in oral, subcutaneous, and intravenous (IV) forms. Regular screening with a complete blood count (CBC) and liver enzymes (aspartate aminotransferase [AST], alanine aminotransferase [ALT]) is required at 6-week intervals. Liver enzymes twice the normal values warrant cessation of therapy; the levels usually return to normal rapidly. It can then be restarted at a lower dose. Patients are advised to abstain from all alcohol consumption. MTX is absolutely contraindicated in women who may become pregnant and anyone with liver disease. Renal clearance is the principal mechanism of excretion of MTX, and its use in renal insufficiency is hazardous, although not absolutely contraindicated.

Azathioprine

Azathioprine is a prodrug. Following oral ingestion, it is metabolized into active 6-mercaptopurine. Azathioprine is better absorbed and less likely to be inactivated by liver enzymes than 6-mercaptopurine. It is a purine analog and acts as a chain terminator during nucleic acid synthesis and inhibits proliferation of lymphocytes; T and B lymphocytes are particularly susceptible to the action of azathioprine. It may be used alone or in combination with other immunosuppressants in autoimmune diseases such as rheumatoid arthritis and Crohn's disease, and in organ transplantation.

The SITE cohort study (Pasadhika et al. 2009) also evaluated the success of azathioprine for non-infectious ocular inflammatory disease. Approximately 43% of MMP patients and 20% of scleritis patients had control of their ocular inflammation within 6 months of treatment. Patients with MMP also achieved corticosteroid-tapering success. The study reported that prior use of other antimetabolites was associated with an approximate 60% lower likelihood of control of inflammation with azathioprine, but prior use of alkylating agents was not associated with a significantly different likelihood of success. Patients with an associated systemic inflammatory disease did not tend to fare as well (but the difference observed was not statistically significant). Higher dosages of azathioprine (≥125 mg per day) did not affect the chance of achieving treatment success to a significant degree.

Azathioprine is prescribed orally in doses of 1–3 mg/kg per day. The main potential side effect to be monitored is bone marrow suppression. Azathioprine should not be used with other purine analogs, such as allopurinol, because it may cause severe pancytopenia. Other potential side effects include gastrointestinal (GI) symptoms, such as nausea and vomiting. Acute pancreatitis can also occur in patients with Crohn's disease. The drug undergoes hepatic metabolism, and patients should be screened for bone marrow suppression and hepatotoxicity with regular CBC and liver enzymes.

The enzyme thiopurine S-methyltransferase (TPMT) inactivates 6-mercaptopurine. Genetic polymorphisms of TPMT occur in the population. Patients with impaired TPMT activity are at risk of potential life-threatening neutropenia with azathioprine therapy. Assays of serum TPMT are available and should be obtained prior to commencing therapy.

Mycophenolate mofetil

MMF is an immunosuppressive drug that has been reported to be effective in the treatment of solid organ transplant rejection and multiple autoimmune diseases. It is a prodrug that is metabolized to mycophenolic acid. It reversibly inhibits inosine-5-monophosphate dehydrogenase in the purine synthesis pathway. MMF does not affect the salvage pathway of purine nucleotide synthesis; thus, it results in selective inhibition of replicating T and B lymphocytes. This may account for fewer side effects with MMF compared with other antimetabolites. It also disrupts cellular adhesion to the vascular endothelium.

MMF has been found to be effective in OCP, atopic keratoconjunctivitis (AKC), prevention of graft rejection after penetrating keratoplasty, and quiet (not active) cases of scleritis and posterior scleritis (Zierhut et al. 2005). MMF may be useful as a corticosteroid-sparing agent in patients with controlled scleral disease who are taking prednisone; however, it did not seem helpful in patients with active scleral inflammation requiring additional immunosuppression, even if given at higher daily dosages (Sen et al. 2003). It was also reported as a treatment for patients with scleritis and uveitis refractory to or intolerant of MTX (Sobrin et al. 2008). Similar to azathioprine, patients were less likely to experience corticosteroid-sparing success with MMF if they had used other immunosuppressive drugs previously (Thorne et al. 2005). However, in this study (Choudhary et al. 2006), MMF appears to be a safe and effective second- or third-line adjunct or alternative immunosuppressant in refractory cases and works well in combination with cyclosporine, tacrolimus, and anti-TNF agents. It has potential as a first- or second-line agent and can be considered at a dose of 3 g per day in refractory cases.

MMF is prescribed orally at a dosage of 1 g, twice per day, on an empty stomach, not to exceed doses of >3 g per day to avoid potential toxicity. It is usually well tolerated and has similar side effects as the other antimetabolites, namely, bone marrow suppression, GI symptoms, and increased risk of infection. Regular monitoring with CBC and liver enzymes is mandatory, and we usually do this every 6 weeks.

Cytosine arabinoside

Cytosine arabinoside, or cytarabine, is used mainly in the treatment of hematological malignancies. It is an antimetabolite that interferes with DNA synthesis. Its mechanism of action is due to its rapid conversion into cytosine arabinoside triphosphate, which disrupts DNA in the S phase of the cell cycle.

Cytarabine has been reported to be effective in some rheumatological conditions that have associated ocular complications, such as rheumatoid arthritis (McCune & Friedman 1993). We have also used this for some cases of chronic cicatrizing conjunctivitis associated with OCP.

Cytarabine is rapidly deaminated in the body into its inactive metabolite uracil arabinoside; thus, it is often given by IV infusion at doses of 100–200 mg every week. It is ineffective via the oral route, and subcutaneous or intramuscular injections result in lower plasma levels when compared with IV infusion. The side effect profile of cytarabine is similar to that of the other antimetabolites: myelosuppression and GI disturbances (associated with rapid IV infusion). A unique toxicity associated with this drug is cerebellar toxicity, when it is given in high doses.

◼ Calcineurin inhibitors

Calcineurin is a calcium- and calmodulin-dependent phosphatase that is involved in T-cell signaling and activation. It activates nuclear factor of activated T cell (NFAT), a transcription factor, which is then translocated into the nucleus, where it upregulates the transcription and expression of IL-2, which acts primarily on T-helper cell response. The calcineurin–NFAT pathway is the target of this class of drugs known as calcineurin inhibitors.

Cyclosporine

Cyclosporine, or cyclosporin A, is an immunosuppressive agent that is a natural product of a fungus. It binds to an immunophilin (cyclophilin), which prevents activation of calcineurin. It has been used extensively in rheumatological and autoimmune diseases, uveitis, and organ transplantation. One of the advantages of cyclosporine is that its therapeutic effect starts to show within a few days, as compared to several weeks for other immunosuppressive agents.

Cyclosporine was found to be effective in several cases of active necrotizing scleritis and keratolysis associated with rheumatoid arthritis. These cases had failed to respond to disease-modifying agents or immunosuppressive therapy, but their ocular and arthritic disease subsequently responded to cyclosporine (McCarthy et al. 1992). It has also been found to be effective for the treatment of OCP, with improvement in patients' quality of life, resolution of conjunctival and corneal lesions, as well as marked decrease in the cellular infiltrates and antibody deposition in subsequent biopsies (Alonso et al. 2006). It may also be used in atopic dermatitis and AKC (Anzaar et al. 2008).

Cyclosporine is given orally in doses of 2–5 mg/kg per day, either as a single dose or as twice-daily regimen. The twice-daily dose is preferred to prevent large spikes in cyclosporine levels in the serum, which can predispose to renal toxicity. This drug is metabolized in the liver by the cytochrome P-450 microsomal enzyme system; agents that interfere with cytochrome P-450 activity (e.g. ketoconazole, oral contraceptives, erythromycin, and grapefruit juice) can cause changes in cyclosporine levels and should be avoided. The potential side effects of cyclosporine are mainly dose-dependent. Nephrotoxicity and hypertension are the two most important side effects to watch out for. The serum creatinine must not rise above 30% from baseline. A decrease in the dose by 50–100 mg per day at a time is advised; abrupt cessation may cause a rebound of the ocular inflammation. Other side effects include hepatotoxicity, hypertrichosis, gingival hypertrophy, neuropathy, and GI disturbances.

Tacrolimus

Tacrolimus (FK506) is a macrolide antibiotic derived from the bacterium *Streptomyces tsukubaensis*. It has essentially the same mechanism of action as cyclosporine but it binds to the immunophilin FK-506-binding protein 12 (FKBP12) instead of cyclophilin.

Tacrolimus was found to be only partially effective in a minority of OCP patients refractory to conventional immunosuppressive agents (Letko et al. 2001). Like cyclosporine, it has been successful in the treatment of atopic dermatitis and AKC (Anzaar et al. 2008).

Tacrolimus is given at doses of 0.05–0.15 mg/kg per day and can be given through the oral or IV routes. The therapeutic dose of tacrolimus is lower compared to cyclosporine, but with the same toxic effects. Hypertension and nephrotoxicity should be closely monitored. Neurological symptoms, such as headache, neuropathy, seizures, and meningitis-like symptoms, as well as GI symptoms such as nausea and abdominal pain may occur. It is also metabolized by the cytochrome P-450 system.

Sirolimus

Sirolimus, also known as rapamycin, is a macrolide antibiotic derived from isolates of *Streptomyces hygroscopicus*. It is similar in structure to tacrolimus but it has a different mechanism of action than other calcineurin inhibitors. It also binds to the same immunophilin as tacrolimus (FKBP12) but blocks the mammalian target of rapamycin (mTOR) instead of inhibiting calcineurin. It blocks the proliferative signals of transduction in T cells; this blockage prevents the expression of IL-2, IL-4, and IL-6. It inhibits the response to IL-2, but does not affect its production. Its effect occurs later in the cell cycle (G1 to S phase transition) as compared with cyclosporine or tacrolimus. It can be used synergistically with cyclosporine, since they have different mechanisms of action; however, tacrolimus and sirolimus would competitively inhibit each other, since they bind to the same immunophilin.

Sirolimus has been reported to be effective in controlling experimental autoimmune uveoretinitis in rats, in combination with tacrolimus (Ikeda et al. 1997) and cyclosporine (Martin et al. 1995). No reports to date have been published for the use of sirolimus on ocular surface disorders.

Sirolimus is given in doses of 2 mg per day. It is given as a tablet or solution, taken orally, once a day. Potential side effects include GI disturbances, skin problems, pneumonitis, and increased risk of infection.

Alkylating agents

Alkylating agents interfere with DNA replication by cross-linking nucleic acids, causing abnormal base pairing and subsequent chain termination.

Cyclophosphamide

The cytotoxic activity of cyclophosphamide is directed against lymphocytes undergoing cell division. It effectively controls inflammation in scleritis and OCP (Pujari et al. 2010). Cyclophosphamide is especially useful in recalcitrant and severely progressive cases associated with life-threatening systemic conditions, such as granulomatosis with polyangiitis (Wegener), rheumatoid arthritis, polyarteritis nodosa, and relapsing polychondritis. It can be combined with high-dose corticosteroids for immediate or rapid control of inflammation and continued as a corticosteroid-sparing agent.

It can be given orally in doses of 1–3 mg/kg per day or as pulsed IV therapy with an initial dose of 1 g/m^2, with subsequent doses titrated individually based on the clinical response, patient tolerance, and hemodynamic profile. Infusions are typically given every 2–4 weeks. It has considerable myelosuppressive effects, which can be used as a guide for determining dosing adjustments. The goal is to bring the white blood cell count to 3000–4500, with an absolute neutrophil count of ≥1000. Monitoring of the white blood cell count is extremely important as the patient is at increased risk of opportunistic infections; Pneumocystis carinii pneumonia prophylaxis with an antibiotic such as trimethoprim and sulfamethoxazole may be started three times per week. Bladder toxicity and increased risk of bladder cancer from acrolein, its metabolite, may be decreased with intermittent pulsed IV therapy and premedication with 2-mercaptoethane sulfonate. It is teratogenic and can cause sterility in both men and women in a dose-dependent manner (total cumulative dose).

Chlorambucil

Chlorambucil interferes with DNA replication by translocating alkyl groups for hydrogen, targeting dividing lymphocytes, and conse-

quently causing immunosuppression. It is commonly used for hematological malignancies, but it is not as widely studied for ocular diseases as cyclophosphamide. It has been found to be effective in some cases of non-infectious uveitis, and also in Sjögren´s syndrome (SS) (Kingsmore et al. 1993).

It can be given in low doses over a long-term period or it can be given as a high-dose, short-term therapy over 3–6 months with gradually increasing doses each week. We usually start with an initial dose of 0.15 mg/kg per day with subsequent doses titrated based on the clinical response, patient tolerance, and hemodynamic profile. It has similar side effects to cyclophosphamide, except for hemorrhagic cystitis that does not occur with chlorambucil. We also monitor the white blood cell count of the patient to gauge the therapeutic effect and to monitor for severe leukopenia.

BIOLOGICS/BIOLOGICAL RESPONSE MODIFIERS

More specific treatments with biological properties have emerged recently, such as monoclonal antibodies and soluble cytokine receptors; these are known as biologics or biological response modifiers (BRMs). In rheumatological diseases, there is a misbalance between endogenous anti-inflammatory cytokines (such as IL-4, IL-10, IL-11, and IL-13) and proinflammatory cytokines (such as TNF-α, IL-1, IL-6, IL-8, and IL-12). Inhibiting the action of cytokines causes communication between cells to be interrupted, which stops the predominant proinflammatory response. Although traditional immunomodulatory therapies such as antimetabolites and alkylating agents have been a great advancement for ocular surface diseases, targeting specific cytokines with BRMs holds promise as an effective treatment, particularly in refractory cases. A list of commonly used BRMs, their recommended dosages and routes of administration, and the most common potential side effects associated with each drug are given in **Table 32.3**.

Etanercept

Etanercept is an engineered recombinant dimeric protein generated by the fusion of ligand-binding portion of human TNF type 2 receptor (TNFR-2) linked to the Fc portion of human IgG1. It acts by competitively inhibiting the binding of TNF-α and TNF-β to their cell surface receptors.

It is Food and Drug Administration (FDA)-approved for rheumatoid arthritis, ankylosing spondylitis, psoriatic arthritis, and plaque psoriasis. There has been some conflicting evidence regarding its use in ocular surface diseases, such as scleritis (Michalova & Lim 2008), OCP (Canizares et al. 2006), and SS (Sankar et al. 2004).

Table 32.3 Biological response modifiers

Drug class	Dose	Route of administration	Potential side effects
Etanercept	25 mg 2×/week	SQ	Injection site reactions, increased risk of infection, drug-induced lupus
Infliximab	5 mg/kg	IV	Increased risk of infection, headache, rash, GI symptoms, drug-induced lupus
Adalimumab	40 mg every 2 weeks	SQ	Injection site reactions, increased risk of infection, drug-induced lupus
Anakinra	100 mg/day	SQ	Injection site reactions
Interferon-α	150 IU/day	SQ	Flu-like symptoms, fatigue
Rituximab	375 mg/m^2	IV	Infusion reactions, arrhythmias, increased risk of infection
Daclizumab	1 mg/kg every 2 weeks	IV	Increased risk of infection, headaches, nausea, skin reactions
GI, gastrointestinal; IV, intravenous; PO, per orem (oral); SQ, subcutaneous.			

Etanercept is given at a dose of 25 mg twice per week, subcutaneously. The expected onset of action is between 1 and 8 weeks. Side effects include increased risk of infection and cancer, and drug-induced lupus. It is important to be aware of other complications such as tuberculous uveitis. However, the most common side effect of etanercept is a reaction at the injection site, which can affect 37% of patients (Rodrigues et al. 2009).

Infliximab

Infliximab is a chimeric human immunoglobulin IgG1 with a mouse Fv variable fragment with high TNF-α affinity and neutralizing capacity. It binds to both the transmembrane and soluble form of human TNF-α. It induces apoptosis of T cells, monocytes, and macrophages.

It is FDA-approved for the treatment of rheumatoid arthritis, ankylosing spondylitis, psoriatic arthritis, ulcerative colitis, and Crohn's disease. Several case series reports have been published on the off-label use of infliximab in scleritis (Murphy et al. 2004, Sobrin et al. 2007), peripheral ulcerative keratitis (PUK) (Galor & Thorne 2007, Odorcic et al. 2009), OCP (Rodrigues et al. 2009), and SS (Cordero-Coma et al. 2007, Heffernan & Bentley 2006).

The initial dose is an IV infusion of 5 mg/kg every 6–8 weeks with a maximum dose of 10 mg/kg every 4 weeks. The expected onset of action is between 1 and 8 weeks. The most common potential side effects are respiratory infections, headache, rash, coughing, and abdominal pain. It is also associated with an increased risk of infection and cancer, and drug-induced lupus.

Adalimumab

Adalimumab is a fully human recombinant monoclonal antibody composed of two κ light chains and two IgG1 heavy chains. This medication neutralizes TNF-α by blocking its binding to p55 and p75 cell-surface receptors.

The FDA has approved adalimumab for the treatment of rheumatoid arthritis and psoriatic arthritis. There is one case report of a patient with scleritis, who responded to adalimumab (Restrepo & Molina 2010).

The usual dose of adalimumab in ocular inflammatory disorders is 40 mg, subcutaneously, every 2 weeks. Its side effect profile is similar to that of infliximab and etanercept.

Anakinra

Anakinra is a recombinant, human IL-1RA (receptor antagonist) prepared from cultures of *Escherichia coli*. IL-1 mediates inflammatory and immunological reactions and shares many properties with TNF-α.

Anakinra has been FDA-approved for rheumatoid arthritis. Some cases have been reported on patients with scleritis (Botsios et al. 2007). Experimental studies suggest that IL-1 plays a role in SS (Solomon et al. 2001) and allergic eye diseases (Keane-Myers et al. 1999), but anakinra's use on these diseases is yet to be investigated.

Its dose is 100 mg daily, subcutaneously. The most common side effects are reactions at the site of injection. Risk of lymphoma has been reported in patients with rheumatoid arthritis; however, lymphoma incidence is increased per sé in these patients. Also, a randomized clinical trial did not show a significant increase in serious side effects with the use of anakinra (Mertens & Singh 2009).

INTERFERON-α

Interferon-α is an antiviral and immunomodulatory cytokine produced by leukocytes infected by virus. It is commonly used for hematologic malignancies. A randomized study in patients with SS showed a decrease in ocular dryness symptoms (Cummins et al. 2003).

The dose for ocular surface disorders is 150 IU per day. The most common potential side effects are flu-like symptoms and fatigue. However, these symptoms tend to diminish with repeated injections and may be managed with analgesics.

Rituximab

Rituximab is a chimeric murine and human monoclonal IgG1 antibody against CD20, which regulates the activation and differentiation of B cells. It is thought to inhibit T-cell activation through the reduction of antigen-presentation by B cells or by inducing lysis of peripheral B lymphocytes.

Rituximab is approved for patients with non-Hodgkin's lymphoma and rheumatoid arthritis. It has been successful in reported cases of scleritis (Taylor et al. 2009, Iaccheri et al. 2010), OCP (Foster et al. 2010, Ross et al. 2009), PUK (Albert et al. 2011, Huerva et al. 2010), and dry eye disease related to SS (Pijpe et al. 2005, Seror et al. 2007).

Rituximab is given as an IV infusion, 375 mg/m², every week for 6 weeks, and then monthly for 4 months. The most frequent adverse events are infusion reactions and arrhythmias. Neutropenia, human antichimeric antibodies, and multifocal leukoencephalopathy have also been reported in some cases.

Daclizumab

Daclizumab is a humanized IgG monoclonal antibody produced by recombinant DNA technology that specifically binds CD25 of the human IL-2 receptor that is expressed on activated T lymphocytes. It selectively inhibits activated but not resting T cells. It is FDA-approved to prevent rejection in renal transplant patients.

Some have reported its efficacy in patients with OCP, chronic cicatrizing conjunctivitis, and Stevens–Johnson syndrome refractory to conventional therapy (Fiorelli et al. 2010). Daclizumab is given intravenously at a dose of 1 mg/kg every 2 weeks with an onset of action within days. Potential side effects include headaches, nausea, lymphadenopathy, and skin reactions.

INTRAVENOUS IMMUNOGLOBULIN

Intravenous immunoglobulin (IVIg) was initially used for the treatment of patients with immunodeficiencies. IVIg is sterile, purified IgG, produced from pooled human plasma, with trace amounts of IgA or IgM. Its actions include modulation of complement activation, suppression of idiotypic antibodies, saturation of Fc receptors on macrophages, and suppression of inflammatory mediators (cytokines, chemokines, metalloproteinases).

Off-label use of IVIg in rheumatoid arthritis, systemic lupus erythematosus, granulomatosis with polyangiitis (Wegener), Behcet's disease, Vogt-Koyonagi-Harada, and other forms of uveitis have been reported. It has also been found to be effective in OCP (Foster

& Ahmed 1999, Sami et al. 2004) and in arresting progression of OCP compared to conventional immunosuppressive therapy (Letko et al. 2004). Combination of IVIg with rituximab was also found to be successful in recalcitrant OCP cases (Foster et al. 2010). It has been used with success in patients with Stevens–Johnsons syndrome and toxic epidermal necrolysis (French et al. 2006).

Patients with IgA deficiency may develop severe anaphylactic reactions to IVIg. Laboratory tests include the following: liver and renal function tests, CBC with differential, hepatitis screen to assess for possible disease transmission by IVIg, immunoglobulin levels to exclude IgA deficiency (If no IgA antibodies are found, then anti-IgA antibody titers should be obtained), and rheumatoid and cryoglobulin levels (IVIg can cause hematologic complications). The infusions are given over a period of 2–3 days and the cycle is repeated monthly for an indefinite period of time depending on the response to treatment.

FUTURE THERAPY
Voclosporin

Voclosporin is a next-generation calcineurin inhibitor that was developed by modifying the functional group of cyclosporine. It exhibits a favorable safety profile, a strong correlation between pharmacokinetic and pharmacodynamic response, and a wide therapeutic window. The LUMINATE (Lux Uveitis Multicenter Investigation of a New Approach to TrEatment) clinical development program was initiated in 2007 to assess the safety and efficacy of voclosporin for the treatment, maintenance, and control of all forms of non-infectious uveitis. If LUMINATE is successful, voclosporin would be the first FDA-approved corticosteroid-sparing agent for this condition (Anglade et al. 2008).

Rilonacept (IL-1 Trap)

Rilonacept, also known as IL-1 Trap, is a dimeric fusion protein consisting of the extracellular domain of human IL-1 receptor and the FC domain of human IgG1 that binds and neutralizes IL-1. It was FDA-approved in 2008 as an orphan drug for cryoporin-associated periodic syndromes, which are autoinflammatory diseases (i.e. the body spontaneously produces substances that cause inflammation without the formation of antibodies) that have symptoms of recurrent fever, rash, and joint pain. This may be useful for other inflammatory diseases as well wherein IL-1 plays a major role.

CONCLUSIONS

Ocular surface disorders are potentially vision threatening and can ultimately lead to loss of the eye if not recognized and treated early. Our ultimate goal is to achieve remission, without any inflammation, off all corticosteroids, and without any associated drug toxicity. As with any therapy, the risks and benefits must be weighed and the clinician and patient are both involved in the informed clinical decision-making process. If used correctly and the patients monitored regularly for any drug toxicity, immunomodulatory therapy and biologics are safe and effective treatment options for patients with ocular surface disorders needing long-term systemic immunosuppression to avoid the devastating and well-known corticosteroid side effects.

FURTHER READING

Chan RY, Foster CS. A step-wise approach to ocular surface rehabilitation in patients with ocular inflammatory disease. *Int Ophthalmol Clin* 1999; **39**:83–108.

Jabs DA, Rosenbaum JT, Foster CS, et al. Guidelines for the use of immunosuppressive drugs in patients with ocular inflammatory disorders: recommendations of an expert panel. *Am J Ophthalmol* 2000; **130**:492–513.

Lee FF, Foster CS. Pharmacotherapy of uveitis. *Expert Opin Pharmacother* 2010; **11**:1135–1146.

REFERENCES

Albert M, Beltran E, Martinez-Costa L. Rituximab in rheumatoid arthritis-associated peripheral ulcerative keratitis. *Arch Soc Esp Oftalmol* 2011; **86**:118–120.

Alonso A, Bignone ML, Brunzini M, Brunzini R. Ocular autoimmune pemphigoid and cyclosporin A. *Allergol Immunopathol (Madr)* 2006; **34**:113–115.

Anglade E, Aspeslet LJ, Weiss SL. A new agent for the treatment of noninfectious uveitis: rationale and design of three LUMINATE (Lux Uveitis Multicenter Investigation of a New Approach to Treatment) trials of steroid-sparing voclosporin. *Clin Ophthalmol* 2008; **2**:693–702.

Anzaar F, Gallagher MJ, Bhat P, et al. Use of systemic T-lymphocyte signal transduction inhibitors in the treatment of atopic keratoconjunctivitis. *Cornea* 2008; **27**:884–888.

Bom S, Zamiri P, Lightman S. Use of methotrexate in the management of sight-threatening uveitis. *Ocul Immunol Inflamm* 2001; **9**:35–40.

Botsios C, Sfriso P, Ostuni PA, Todesco S, Punzi L. Efficacy of the IL-1 receptor antagonist, anakinra, for the treatment of diffuse anterior scleritis in rheumatoid arthritis. Report of two cases. *Rheumatology (Oxford)* 2007; **46**:1042–1043.

Canizares MJ, Smith DI, Conners MS, Maverick KJ, Heffernan MP. Successful treatment of mucous membrane pemphigoid with etanercept in three patients. *Arch Dermatol* 2006; **142**:1457–1461.

Chan ES, Cronstein BN. Molecular action of methotrexate in inflammatory diseases. *Arthritis Res* 2002; **4**:266–273.

Choudhary A, Harding SP, Bucknall RC, Pearce IA. Mycophenolate mofetil as an immunosuppressive agent in refractory inflammatory eye disease. *J Ocul Pharmacol Ther* 2006; **22**:168–175.

Cordero-Coma M, Anzaar F, Sobrin L, Foster CS. Systemic immunomodulatory therapy in severe dry eye secondary to inflammation. *Ocul Immunol Inflamm* 2007; **15**:99–104.

Cummins MJ, Papas A, Kammer GM, Fox PC. Treatment of primary Sjogren's syndrome with low-dose human interferon alfa administered by the oromucosal route: combined phase III results. *Arthritis Rheum* 2003; **49**:585–593.

Fiorelli VM, Dantas PE, Jackson AT, Nishiwaki-Dantas MC. Systemic monoclonal antibody therapy (daclizumab) in the treatment of cicatrizing conjunctivitis in Stevens-Johnson syndrome, refractory to conventional therapy. *Curr Eye Res* 2010; **35**:1057–1062.

Foster CS, Ahmed AR. Intravenous immunoglobulin therapy for ocular cicatricial pemphigoid: a preliminary study. *Ophthalmology* 1999; **106**:2136–2143.

Foster CS, Chang PY, Ahmed AR. Combination of rituximab and intravenous immunoglobulin for recalcitrant ocular cicatricial pemphigoid: a preliminary report. *Ophthalmology* 2010; **117**:861–869.

French LE, Trent JT, Kerdel FA. Use of intravenous immunoglobulin in toxic epidermal necrolysis and Stevens-Johnson syndrome: our current understanding. *Int Immunopharmacol* 2006; **6**:543–549.

Galor A, Thorne JE. Scleritis and peripheral ulcerative keratitis. *Rheum Dis Clin North Am* 2007; **33**:835–854.

Gangaputra S, Newcomb CW, Liesegang TL, et al. Systemic Immunosuppressive Therapy for Eye Diseases Cohort Study. Methotrexate for ocular inflammatory diseases. *Ophthalmology* 2009; **116**:21882198.e1.

Heffernan MP, Bentley DD. Successful treatment of mucous membrane pemphigoid with infliximab. *Arch Dermatol* 2006; **142**:1268–1270.

Huerva V, Sanchez MC, Traveset A, Jurjo C, Ruiz A. Rituximab for peripheral ulcerative keratitis with wegener granulomatosis. *Cornea* 2010; **29**:708–710.

Iaccheri B, Androudi S, Bocci EB, et al. Rituximab treatment for persistent scleritis associated with rheumatoid arthritis. *Ocul Immunol Inflamm* 2010; **18**:223–225.

Ikeda E, Hikita N, Eto K, Mochizuki M. Tacrolimus-rapamycin combination therapy for experimental autoimmune uveoretinitis. *Jpn J Ophthalmol* 1997; **41**:396–402.

Jachens AW, Chu DS. Retrospective review of methotrexate therapy in the treatment of chronic, noninfectious, nonnecrotizing scleritis. *Am J Ophthalmol* 2008; **145**:487–492.

Keane-Myers AM, Miyazaki D, Liu G, et al. Prevention of allergic eye disease by treatment with IL-1 receptor antagonist. *Invest Ophthalmol Vis Sci* 1999; **40**:3041–3046.

Kempen JH, Daniel E, Dunn JP, et al. Overall and cancer related mortality among patients with ocular inflammation treated with immunosuppressive drugs: retrospective cohort study. BMJ 2009; 39:b2480.

Kingsmore SF, Silva OE, Hall BD, et al. Presentation of multicentric Castleman's disease with sicca syndrome, cardiomyopathy, palmar and plantar rash. *J Rheumatol* 1993; **20**:1588–1591.

Kjellman P, Eriksson H, Berg P. A retrospective analysis of patients with bullous pemphigoid treated with methotrexate. *Arch Dermatol* 2008; **144**:612–616.

Letko E, Ahmed AR, Foster CS. Treatment of ocular cicatricial pemphigoid with tacrolimus (FK 506). *Graefes Arch Clin Exp Ophthalmol* 2001; **239**:441–444.

Letko E, Miserocchi E, Daoud YJ, et al. A nonrandomized comparison of the clinical outcome of ocular involvement in patients with mucous membrane (cicatricial) pemphigoid between conventional immunosuppressive and intravenous immunoglobulin therapies. *Clin Immunol* 2004; **111**:303–310.

Martin DF, DeBarge LR, Nussenblatt RB, Chan CC, Roberge FG. Synergistic effect of rapamycin and cyclosporin A in the treatment of experimental autoimmune uveoretinitis. *J Immunol* 1995; **154**:922–927.

McCarthy JM, Dubord PJ, Chalmers A, Kassen BO, Rangno KK. Cyclosporine A for the treatment of necrotizing scleritis and corneal melting in patients with rheumatoid arthritis. *J Rheumatol* 1992; **19**:1358–1361.

McCluskey P, Chang JH, Singh R, Wakefield D. Methotrexate therapy for ocular cicatricial pemphigoid. *Ophthalmology* 2004; **111**:796–801.

McCune WJ, Friedman AW. Immunosuppressive drug therapy for rheumatic disease. *Curr Opin Rheumatol* 1993; **5**:282–292.

Mertens M, Singh JA. Anakinra for rheumatoid arthritis. Cochrane Database Syst Rev 2009; CD005121.

Michalova K, Lim L. Biologic agents in the management of inflammatory eye diseases. *Curr Allergy Asthma Rep* 2008; **8**:339–347.

Murphy CC, Ayliffe WH, Booth A, et al. Tumor necrosis factor alpha blockade with infliximab for refractory uveitis and scleritis. *Ophthalmology* 2004; **111**:352–356.

Odorcic S, Keystone EC, Ma JJ. Infliximab for the treatment of refractory progressive sterile peripheral ulcerative keratitis associated with late corneal perforation: 3-year follow-up. *Cornea* 2009; **28**:89–92.

Pasadhika S, Kempen JH, Newcomb CW, et al. Azathioprine for ocular inflammatory diseases. *Am J Ophthalmol* 2009; **148**:500.e2–509.e2.

Pijpe J, Van Imhoff GW, Spijkervet FK, et al. Rituximab treatment in patients with primary Sjogren's syndrome: an open-label phase II study. *Arthritis Rheum* 2005; **52**:2740–2750.

Pujari SS, Kempen JH, Newcomb CW, et al. Cyclophosphamide for ocular inflammatory diseases. *Ophthalmology* 2010; **117**:356–365.

Restrepo JP, Molina MP. Successful treatment of severe nodular scleritis with adalimumab. *Clin Rheumatol* 2010; **29**:559–561.

Rodrigues EB, Farah ME, Maia M, et al. Therapeutic monoclonal antibodies in ophthalmology. *Prog Retin Eye Res* 2009; **28**:117–144.

Ross AH, Jaycock P, Cook SD, Dick AD, Tole DM. The use of rituximab in refractory mucous membrane pemphigoid with severe ocular involvement. *Br J Ophthalmol* 2009; **93**:421–422, 548.

Sami N, Letko E, Androudi S, et al. Intravenous immunoglobulin therapy in patients with ocular-cicatricial pemphigoid: a long-term follow-up. *Ophthalmology* 2004; **111**:1380–1382.

Sankar V, Brennan MT, Kok MR, et al. Etanercept in Sjogren's syndrome: a twelve-week randomized, double-blind, placebo-controlled pilot clinical trial. *Arthritis Rheum* 2004; **50**:2240–2245.

Sen HN, Suhler EB, Al-Khatib SQ, et al. Mycophenolate mofetil for the treatment of scleritis. *Ophthalmology* 2003; **110**:1750–1755.

Seror R, Sordet C, Guillevin L, et al. Tolerance and efficacy of rituximab and changes in serum B cell biomarkers in patients with systemic complications of primary Sjogren's syndrome. *Ann Rheum Dis* 2007; **66**:351–357.

Shah SS, Lowder CY, Schmitt MA, et al. Low-dose methotrexate therapy for ocular inflammatory disease. *Ophthalmology* 1992; **99**:1419–1423.

Sobrin L, Christen W, Foster CS. Mycophenolate mofetil after methotrexate failure or intolerance in the treatment of scleritis and uveitis. *Ophthalmology* 2008; **115**:1416–1421.

Sobrin L, Kim EC, Christen W, et al. Infliximab therapy for the treatment of refractory ocular inflammatory disease. *Arch Ophthalmol* 2007; **125**:895–900.

Solomon A, Dursun D, Liu Z, et al. Pro- and anti-inflammatory forms of interleukin-1 in the tear fluid and conjunctiva of patients with dry-eye disease. *Invest Ophthalmol Vis Sci* 2001; **42**:2283–2292.

Taylor R, Salama AD, Joshi L, Pusey CD, Lightman SL. Rituximab is effective in the treatment of refractory ophthalmic Wegener's granulomatosis. *Arthritis Rheum* 2009; **60**:1540–1547.

Thorne JE, Jabs DA, Qazi FA, et al. Mycophenolate mofetil therapy for inflammatory eye disease. *Ophthalmology* 2005; **112**:1472–1477.

Tian H, Cronstein BN. Understanding the mechanisms of action of methotrexate: implications for the treatment of rheumatoid arthritis. *Bull NYU Hosp Jt Dis* 2007; **65**:168–173.

Zierhut M, Stübiger N, Siepmann K, Deuter CM. MMF and eye disease. *Lupus* 2005; **14**:s50–s54.

Chapter 33 Hormonal therapies

Austin K. Mircheff, Samuel C. Yiu

INTRODUCTION

It is widely appreciated that lacrimal gland physiological function decreases and ocular surface homeostasis generally deteriorates as women and men age and that both dry eye disease (DED) associated with Sjögren's syndrome and idiopathic DED are more prevalent in women.

Most of the reports on hormonal influences in DED etiopathogenesis have revolved around the concepts that both lacrimal gland physiological dysfunction and ocular surface inflammation stem from autoimmune processes; that androgens are generally protective, while estrogens favor autoimmune disease development; and that androgens promote optimal meibomian gland function. Testosterone is the biosynthetic precursor of dihydrotestosterone (DHT), which binds with higher affinity to androgen receptors. Testosterone is also the biosynthetic precursor of estrone, estradiol, and progesterone. Thus, testosterone is produced in the ovaries as well as in the testes, and it has been inferred that the higher estrogen–androgen ratio accounts for the greater prevalence of DED in women than in men during the reproductive years.

Most of the testosterone in the body is produced in an intracrine way, by conversion of the adrenal steroids, dihydroepiandrosterone (DHEA), and dihydroepiandrosterone sulfate (DHEAS). Because adrenal androgen production decreases with age in women and men, it has been inferred that age-related decreases in adrenal androgen production account for age-related increases in the prevalence of idiopathic DED in both genders.

The cessation of gonadal steroid production at menopause causes further, abrupt decreases in circulating levels of free testosterone, total testosterone, DHT, and estradiol (Rothman et al. 2011). While early clinical studies focused on presumed roles of estrogens and progestogens (Metka et al. 1991), it now seems more likely that the loss of ovarian androgen production at menopause contributes to a further increase in the prevalence of DED (Versura & Campos 2005).

The hormonal changes associated with the normal progress of the female reproductive cycle and life cycle also seem consistent with the theory that Sjögren's pathogenesis begins during the reproductive years, and is promoted by completing pregnancies to term, but often remains subclinical until the menopause.

The concept that estrogens favor lacrimal gland and DED development seemed to be supported by an analysis of data from the Women's Health Study (Schaumberg et al. 2001), which indicated that severe DED is more prevalent in postmenopausal women who used estrogen replacement therapy (OR = 1.69) or estrogen–progestogen replacement therapy (OR = 1.29). Studies showing that the prevalence of DED is increased in women with complete androgen insensitivity syndrome and in men using antiandrogen therapy for prostate cancer provided additional evidence for the concept that the androgens play protective and supportive roles (Cermak et al. 2003). Moreover, clinical laboratory studies indicated that serum levels of testosterone and testosterone metabolites are lower in women with Sjögren's syndrome (Sullivan et al. 2003), and basic laboratory studies showed that administration of DHT suppressed lacrimal gland inflammatory autoimmune activity in several of the murine models for Sjögren's syndrome (Sullivan et al. 1999).

EVOLVING VIEWS ON SYSTEMIC HORMONE REPLACEMENT

Interest in systemic hormonal therapies decreased dramatically after an analysis of data from the Women's Health Initiative (Rossouw et al. 2002) demonstrated the possibility that the benefits of estrogen–progestogen replacement therapy in decreasing risks for colorectal cancer, endometrial cancer, and hip fracture were outweighed by increased risks for coronary heart disease, breast cancer, and stroke. Moreover, an epidemiological study seemed to indicate that androgens increase the risk for breast cancer (Wierman et al. 2006). However, opinions are being revised in view of subsequent findings that the overall benefit–risk ratio of estrogen–progestogen replacement depends on the amount of time that elapses between the menopause and the implementation of therapy. If initiated early, replacement therapy significantly reduces hot flushes, urogenital atrophy, coronary artery disease, and overall mortality (Santen et al. 2010). More recent work has also shown that androgen supplementation provides significant benefits to women for whom estrogen–progestogen replacement does not adequately control hot flushes. It remains controversial, but studies suggest that it has a favorable safety profile (Liu et al. 2011).

Because the number of women electing estrogen–progestogen replacement therapy for climacteric symptoms is again increasing, it should be considered anew how hormonal therapies might impact DED pathogenesis and ask whether certain regimens may be effective modalities for DED therapy and, potentially, prophylaxis.

OPHTHALMIC EXPERIENCE WITH HORMONAL THERAPIES

Principal findings from epidemiological, observational, and interventional studies of hormonal therapies are summarized in **Tables 33.1** and **33.2**.

Estradiol

Seemingly in accord with the findings reported by Schaumberg et al. (2001), Uncu et al. (2006) found that a 12-month course of transdermal estradiol without progestogen decreased Schirmer's scores by 20% in women who had not presented with DED complaints at the outset of the study.

Table 33.1 Impact of estrogen and estrogen–progestogen therapies on the ocular flow, tear flow; path, ocular surface pathology; SX, symptoms.

Author	Intervention	Months	Subjects/study type	Years postmenopausal or (age)	SX	MGD	Flow	TBUT	Path	Location	Hottest temperature (°C)/ humidity (%)	Coldest temperature (°C)/ humidity (%)
Schaumberg	Estrogen		Epidemiological		↑					USA; diverse		
Uncu	Estrogen	6	Non-DED/prospective	(51 ± 2.3)			–			Gorukle Bursa, Turkey	31°C/65%	2°C/75%
		12					→					
Schaumberg	Estrogen–progestogen		Epidemiological		↑					USA; diverse		
Jensen	Estrogen–progestogen		Observational		→		←			Baltimore, MD, USA	33°C/52%	–2°C/66%
Uncu	Estrogen–progestogen	6	Non-DED/prospective	(48 ± 0.6)			–			Gorukle Bursa, Turkey	31°C/65%	2°C/75%
		12				←	→					
Erdem	Estrogen–progestogen	3	Non-DED/prospective	1.4 ± 1.2		←	–	–		Ankara, Turkey	30°C/41%	–4°C/79%
Taner	Estrogen–progestogen	6	Non-DED/prospective	4.3 ± 4.4			–	–	–	Ankara, Turkey	30°C/41%	–4°C/79%
Kuscu	Estrogen–progestogen	6	Non-DED/prospective	(50 ± 4.9)		→	–	–		Manisa, Turkey	35°C/41%	3°C/74%
Pelit	Estrogen–progestogen	3	Non-DED/prospective	3.0 ± 1.0			–	←	→	Ankara, Turkey	30°C/41%	–4°C/79%
Moon	Estrogen–progestogen	1	Non-DED/prospective		→		–	←	→	Incheon, Korea	29°C/79%	–5°C/62%
		3			→		–	←	→			
Affinito	Estrogen–progestogen	3	Non-DED/prospective	4.1 ± 2.7	↑		←			Naples, Italy	29°C/63%	6°C/71%
		6			↑		←					
Altintas	Estrogen–progestogen	2	Non-DED/prospective	(47 ± 3.4)			←	–		Izmit, Turkey	30°C/41%	
Guaschino	Estrogen–progestogen	12	Non-DED/prospective	(60 ± 5.4)			←			Trieste, Italy	28°C/59%	3°C/67%
Okon	Estrogen–progestogen	12	Non-DED/prospective	<1			–	–		Lodz, Poland	23°C/74%	–4°C/88%
				1–5			←	←				
				>5			←	←				
Erdem	Estrogen–progestogen	3	DED/prospective*	3.2 ± 2.2		–	–	–		Ankara, Turkey	30°C/41%	–4°C/79%
Sator	Estrogen–progestogen	4	DED/prospective	3.9 ± 1.4	–	–	–			Vienna, Austria	25°C/66%	–4°C/77%
Chaikittisilpa	Estrogen–progestogen	3	DED/prospective	4.1 ± 1.4	–		←			Bangkok, Thailand	30°C/77%	20°C/74%
Metka	Estrogen–progestogen	3	DED/prospective		→		←			Vienna, Austria	25°C/66%	–4°C/77%
		12			→		←					
Sator	Estrogen–progestogen–estrogen†	4	DED/prospective	3.2 ± 1.3	→		←			Vienna, Austria	25°C/66%	–4°C/77%

–, no change.
DED, dry eye disease; MGD, meibomian gland dysfunction; TBUT, tear film break-up time.
*No use of artificial tear substitutes.
†Supplemented with topical ophthalmic estrogen.

Table 33.2 Impact of estrogen–antiandrogen; estrogen–androgen; and androgen therapies on the ocular surface

Authors	Intervention	Months	Subjects/study type	Years postmenopausal or (age)	SX	MGD	Flow	TBUT	Path	Location	Hottest temperature (°C)/humidity (%)	Coldest temperature (°C)/humidity (%)
Coksuer	Estrogen–drospirenone	6	Non-DED/prospective	(52 ± 5.1)	→		←	←		Kutahya, Turkey	29°C/54%	–3°C/80%
Taner	Estrogen–progestogen–tibolone	6	Non-DED/prospective	4.4 ± 3.5			←	←	–	Ankara, Turkey	30°C/41%	–4°C/79%
Scott	Estrogen–methyltestosterone		DED/retrospective		→					Los Angeles, CA, USA	24°C/55%	7°C/49%
Uncu	Tibolone	6	Non-DED/prospective	(52 ± 1.6)			–			Gorukle Bursa, Turkey	31°C/65%	2°C/75%
		12					→					
Sartore	Tibolone	3	Sjögren's syndrome/case report		→		←			Trieste, Italy	28°C/59%	3°C/67%
		12			→		←					
Pillemer	DHEA	6	Sjögren's syndrome/prospective		–		–		–	Bethesda, MD, USA	31°C/53%	–1°C/58%
Drosos	Nandrolone	6	Sjögren's syndrome/prospective.		–		–		–	Ioannina, Greece	31°C/54%	0°C/77%
Worda	Testosterone*	3	DED/case report	(male)	→		–	←		Vienna, Austria	25°C/66%	–4°C/77%

–, no change.
DED, dry eye disease; DHEA, dihydroepiandrosterone; MGD, meibomian gland dysfunction; TBUT, tear break-up time.
*Topical, applied to eyelid skin.

Estrogens and progestogens
Menopausal women without DED

A survey of menopausal women found that those taking hormone replacement therapy had fewer ophthalmic complaints and higher Schirmer's scores (Jensen et al. 2000). Studies of women without DED who began estrogen–progestogen replacement have yielded contradictory findings. Uncu et al. (2006) found that a 12-month course of estrogen–progestogen replacement decreased Schirmer's scores. Erdem et al. (2007) found that a 3-month course of estrogen–progestogen replacement increased meibomian gland dysfunction (MGD) scores (from 0.3 ± 0.2 to 1.3 ± 0.4) in 11 out of 18 subjects. Taner et al. (2004) found that a 6-month course of estrogen–progestogen failed to alter Schirmer's scores, tear break-up time (TBUT), or conjunctival signs. Kuscu et al. (2003) also found that estrogen–progestogen replacement had no impact on Schirmer's scores or TBUT, but they reported that it decreased meibomian gland inflammation. Pelit et al. (2003) found that a 3-month course failed to alter Schirmer's scores, but they reported that it significantly increased TBUT and conjunctival goblet cell density. Moon et al. (2010) also found that a 3-month course failed to alter Schirmer's scores but increased TBUT and decreased fluorescein staining; moreover, they reported that it also decreased symptoms. Affinito et al. (2003) found that a 6-month course of transdermal estrogen and oral progestogen increased Schirmer's scores and decreased symptoms. Altıntaş et al. (2004) and Guaschino et al. (2003) found that estrogen and progestogen for 2 and 12 months, respectively, increased Schirmer's scores. Okoń et al. (2001) stratified participants into three groups: women who were menopausal for <1 year; women who were menopausal for 1–5 years; and women who were menopausal >5 years. Prior to initiation of estrogen–progestogen replacement, Schirmer's scores and TBUT were significantly decreased in the second group and further decreased in the third group. The 12-month course of estrogen–progestogen replacement had no significant impact on Schirmer's scores or TBUT in the first group, suggesting that it was neither deleterious nor beneficial to ocular surface homeostasis if the ocular surface was already healthy. However, the regimen increased Schirmer's scores and TBUT in the second and third groups, suggesting that it improved lacrimal gland function and ocular surface homeostasis if they had deteriorated but not yet become pathophysiological.

It is worthwhile to consider that differences in study design and uncontrolled environmental variables might have contributed to discrepancies between these findings. Erdem et al. (2007), who found that estrogen–progestogen replacement increased MGD, examined participants after 3 months; the women were 1.4 ± 1.2 years postmenopausal; and the study was done in Ankara, Turkey. Kuscu et al. (2003), who found that estrogen–progestogen replacement decreased MGD, examined participants after 6 months; the women's mean age was 50 ± 4.9 years; and the study was done in Manisa, Turkey. The hottest month in Ankara (30°C, 41% humidity) would seem less adverse than the hottest month in Manisa (35°C, 41% humidity) because increasing temperature increases the rate of evaporation at any humidity. On the other hand, Ankara winters (−4°C, 79% humidity) may be more adverse than Manisa winters (3°C, 74% humidity) because indoor heating decreases humidity. A more compelling hypothesis, however, is that the longer duration of treatment accounted for the decrease in MGD found by Kuscu et al.

Uncu et al. (2006) found that estrogen–progestogen replacement decreased Schirmer's scores after 12 months but not after 6 months. The women's mean age was 48 ± 0.6 years; and the study was done in Gorukle Bursa, Turkey. Altıntaş et al. (2004), who found estrogen–pro-

gestogen replacement increased Schirmer's scores, evaluated subjects after 2 months. The women's mean age was 47 ± 3.4 years; and the study was done in Izmit, Turkey. Historical temperature and humidity data for Izmit were not available to us, but one might provisionally infer that the longer duration of the hormone replacement regimen contributed to the adverse influence on lacrimal gland physiological function found by Uncu et al.

Affinito et al. (2003), who found that estrogen–progestogen replacement increased Schirmer's scores, evaluated subjects after 3 and 6 months. The women's mean age was 54 ± 5.9 years; and the study was done in Naples, Italy. Guaschino et al. (2003), who also found that estrogen–progestogen replacement increased Schirmer's scores, evaluated subjects after 12 months. The women's mean age was 60 ± 5.4 years, and the study was done in Trieste, Italy. High temperatures and humidities in summer and low temperatures and humidities in winter do not differ greatly between Gorukle Bursa, Naples, and Trieste. Therefore, one might infer that while not diseased, lacrimal gland physiological function had deteriorated more in the relatively older participants studied in Naples and Trieste than in the relatively younger participants studied in Gorukle Bursa. Thus, these findings are consistent with the inference that if lacrimal gland physiological function has not deteriorated substantially, estrogen–progestogen replacement affects it adversely; while if lacrimal gland function has deteriorated but not become pathological, estrogen–progestogen replacement improves it. This inference is consistent with the findings of Okoń et al. (2001) summarized above, although it should be noted that high temperatures and humidities in summer appear especially benign for the ocular surface in Lodz, Poland, where Okoń et al. worked, and that the outcome might be different in excessively hot, arid environments.

Although there may be biologically plausible explanations for the apparently discrepant findings, they nevertheless seem to pose a quandary: estrogen–progestogen replacement decreases lacrimal gland physiological function in the recently menopausal women for whom it can be implemented with the least risk of adverse cardiovascular events, and it improves lacrimal gland physiological function in the older women for whom it would confer significant risks of adverse cardiovascular events.

Menopausal women with DED

The small number of studies of women who had been menopausal for several years and who had clinically significant DED seems to suggest that estrogen–progestogen replacement in therapy is either benign or beneficial to ocular surface homeostasis. Erdem et al. (2007) found that a 3-month course had no impact on MGD, fluid production, or TBUT in patients who were instructed to not use artificial tear replacement. Sator et al. (1998) found that a 4-month course had no impact on symptoms or Schirmer's scores; however, they found that additional administration of topical ophthalmic estradiol decreased symptoms and increased Schirmer's scores. Chaikittisilpa et al. (2000) found that a 3-month course had no impact on symptoms but improved Schirmer's scores. Metka et al. (1991) found that after 3 and 12 months, estrogen–progestogen replacement decreased symptoms and improved Schirmer's scores.

Estradiol and drospirenone in women without DED

Drospirenone is a spironolactone derivative that has progestogen activity, but antiandrogen and antimineralocorticoid activities. It is included in some oral contraceptive formulations, and its antiandrogen activity is seemingly effective in reducing acne. As part of an estrogen combination therapy, its antimineralocorticoid activity reduces blood pressure; thus, it may obviate the cardiovascular risks associated with implementing estrogen–progestogen replacement after women have been menopausal for several years. Coksuer et al. (2011) found that a 6-month course of estrogen and drospirenone for women aged 52 ± 5.1 years significantly decreased ocular surface disease index (OSDI) score, from 28.5 to 21.5; significantly increased TBUT, from 8.6 to 10.3; and significantly increased Schirmer's scores, from 15.6 to 17.2.

Androgen–estrogen combinations

Tibolone has estrogenic, progestrogenic, and androgenic actions. Taner et al. (2004) found that a 6-month course of estrogen–progestogen replacement combined with tibolone resulted in slight but significant improvements in Schirmer's scores and TBUT in women without DED who had been menopausal for 4.4 ± 3.5 years.

Methyltestosterone binds to androgen receptors with high affinity without having to be converted to more potent metabolites (Friedel et al. 2006). Estratest combines esterfied equine estrogens with methyl-testosterone at either 1.25 mg estrogens/2.5 mg methyltestosterone or 0.625 mg estrogens/1.25 mg methyltestosterone. A review of the histories of 11 patients who began taking Estratest after they were diagnosed with severe DED indicated that 10 of these patients experienced at least slight symptomatic improvement and 8 showed some clinical improvement. Schirmer's test values for four of the patients were available; they improved bilaterally in three patients and unilaterally in one patient (Scott et al. 2005). Our subsequent clinical experience with the lower dose regimen has been consistent with these findings; when prescribed and supervised by a gynecologist or gynecological endocrinologist conversant with the risks and contraindications, it can be a useful treatment modality.

ANDROGENS

Uncu et al. (2006) found that a 12-month course of tibolone decreased Schirmer's scores by 20% in menopausal women aged 52 ± 1.6 years who did not have DED. In contrast, Sartore et al. (2003) reported the case of a menopausal woman with Sjögren's syndrome who experienced decreased symptoms and increased Schirmer's scores after 3 and 12 months on Tibolone.

The realization that most testosterone and DHT are generated by intracrine conversion from DHEA or DHEAS led to a preliminary, controlled trial of DHEA for Sjögren's syndrome patients; the study did not find DHEA to significantly improve salivary gland or lacrimal gland function (Pillemer et al. 2004). This finding does not necessarily contradict that of Sartore et al. (2003) because salivary gland conversion of DHEA to DHT is deficient in Sjögren's syndrome patients (Spaan et al. 2009). However, Drosos et al. (1988) found that nandrolone, a potent androgen with significant anabolic activity, failed to alter symptoms, Schirmer's scores, or ocular surface pathology in women with Sjögren's syndrome.

A patent claims that a testosterone-containing cream applied to the external palpebra is effective (US 6,659,985B2). Worda et al. (2001) reported that such a preparation was highly efficacious in the case of a 54-year old man who presented with severe DED. A patent (US 5,620,921) claims that topical ophthalmic androgen formulations are efficacious for patients with Sjögren's syndrome, and a patent application (US 2006/0211660 A1) claims that topical ophthalmic

formulations combining androgens estrogens are efficacious. The US Clinical Trials Database (ClinicalTrials.gov Identifier: NCT00755183) indicates that a trial of topical ophthalmic testosterone therapy for meibomian gland dysfunction was completed in 2009, but results have not been posted.

PHYSIOLOGY AND PATHOPHYSIOLOGY

In attempting to understand how hormonal therapies might impact the physiological functions of lacrimal glands with diminished or pathologically low functional capacities, it is helpful to think of the lacrimal gland as an effector organ in a physiological system. Many physiological systems function to maintain homeostatic set points; when they detect deviation from their set points, sometime referred to as error signals, they initiate neural signals that activate functions that work to eliminate the error signals. Apart from this formalism, the systems approach has the merit of accommodating the possibility that different components may respond differently to the same hormonal intervention (Sullivan et al. 2009).

Sensory and central neural components

Rosenthal and Borsook (2012) have reviewed the sensory mechanisms that elicit sensations of discomfort and initiate the autonomic secre-tomotor signals that acutely regulate lacrimal gland function. Cold receptors detect evaporation, initiating the baseline level of autonomic neurotransmission that maintains lacrimal gland fluid production when the eyes are opened. Nociceptors detect mechanical irritants, chemical irritants, and inflammatory mediators released by surface epithelial cells when injured or stressed by hyperosmolarity. In a sense, the heat loss of evaporation provides an error signal that is detected instantaneously, and it may obviate tear film osmolarity increases that would cause inflammation and initiate nociceptor signaling. In hot environments, absorption of heat can offset evaporative heat loss and, thereby, decrease baseline fluid production and allow tear film and meniscus osmolarity to increase. Thus, if lacrimal fluid continues to be produced at normal rates while osmolarity is increased, it would mean that one or more components of the system must be functioning insufficiently. In cases where discomfort is sensed, the functional insufficiency might be in the central circuits that process incoming nociceptor signals, in the parasympathetic and sympathetic nerves that carry the motor signals to the lacrimal glands, or in the lacrimal glands' intracellular signal transduction mechanisms or fluid production apparatus.

Conjunctiva and goblet cells

Autonomic neurotransmission activates goblet cell mucin secretion. Circulating estrogen and progesterone do not appear to influence mucin expression, at least in mice (Lange et al. 2003), but they may influence its functional status. The conjunctival epithelium undergoes a cycle of maturation index changes, which parallels the cycle of changes in the vaginal mucosa. Other ocular surface parameters also vary over the menstrual cycle (Versura et al. 2007). OSDI score is highest during the luteal phase, but, at the same time, TBUT is highest, and measures of squamous metaplasia and inflammation are lowest. These findings might suggest that the higher progesterone levels during the luteal phase promote a low-grade corneal allodynia.

After menopause, the maturation index remains low in the conjunctiva, as in the vaginal mucosa. However, a persistently low maturation index is associated with frank mucosal atrophy of the vaginal mucosa, while generalized, age-related atrophic changes appear not to occur in the conjunctival epithelium before the age of 70 (Abdel-Khalek et al. 1978), and goblet cell numbers remain unchanged, except in cases of DED. Severe nasal and temporal conjunctivochalasis (lid parallel conjunctival folding) becomes highly prevalent after the age of 40, more so in women than in men (Fodor et al. 2010). It is associated with DED, but it is not clear whether it is an etiopathogenic factor or a sequela of DED.

Meibomian glands

The combination of non-polar and polar lipids in the superficial, lipid phase of the tear film decreases surface tension and delays tear break-up. The lipid phase also creates a diffusion that impedes evaporation from the film. Most of the lipids are produced by the meibomian glands. Meibomian gland changes increase with age, and there is evidence that glands that appear grossly normal may nevertheless be obstructed (Blackie et al. 2010). MGD plausibly accounts for age-related increases in the rate of water evaporation from the tear film (Guillon & Maïssa 2010) and, therefore, for age-related decreases in TBUT (Ozdemir & Temizdemir 2010) and increases in tear film and tear meniscus osmolarity (Mathers et al. 1996). Tamer et al. (2006) found that levels of DHEA, DHEAS, and bioavailable testosterone (i.e. testosterone not bound to sex-hormone-binding globulin) are lower in individuals of both sexes who have MGD. Knop et al. (2011) have reviewed the further considerable evidence that androgens both support the meibomian glands' anatomic integrity and enhance their functional profile, while the estrogens exert opposing influences.

Lacrimal glands
A system within a system

If the lacrimal gland is an effector organ in a physiological system, each lacrimal gland is a system in its own right. Its secretory epithelium is organized into at least two components with different functions: the acini secrete an isotonic fluid, rich in Na^+ and Cl^-, and the ducts secrete an isotonic fluid, rich in K^+, Na^+, and Cl^-. Its stromal spaces are populated by diverse immune cells—not only plasmacytes but also $CD8^+$ T cells, $CD4^+$ T cells, double negative T cells (presumably including natural killer T cells), cells of the monocyte–macrophage–dendritic cell lineage, and mast cells—and the immune cells interact with the epithelia to accomplish several normal physiological functions.

At least in rats, mast cells respond to autonomic secretomotor signals by releasing histamine and serotonin, which may then act in paracrine fashion to potentiate epithelial cell electrolyte and fluid secretion, as histamine released from enteroendocrine-like cells potentiates acid secretion in the stomach. T cells cooperate with epithelial cells to maintain the lacrimal gland's resident plasmacyte population, which normally produce dimeric IgA (dIgA). The acinar and ductal epithelia then use polymeric immunoglobulin receptors (pIgR) to transfer dIgA into the nascent ocular surface fluid as secretory IgA. Our unpublished experiments indicate that acinar cells secrete CCL2, which recruits T cells and monocyte lineage cells. T cells secrete CCL28, which recruits immature plasmablasts. Ductal cells secrete

transforming growth factor (TGF)-β, and T cells secrete both TGF-β and interleukin (IL)-6. The combination of TGF-β and IL-6 induces plasmablasts to differentiate as mature plasmacytes. Epithelial cells also secrete prolactin and APRIL, and T cells also secrete BAFF; together with IL-6, these cytokines provide mitogenic signals that support ongoing survival of the mature plasmacytes and, presumably, other resident immune cells.

Hormone influences on functional capacity and acute functions

In rats, the higher androgen levels in males promote accumulation of larger numbers of IgA^+ plasmacytes and higher levels of epithelial cell pIgR expression (Hann et al. 1988). These actions may be species-specific, however, as tear IgA levels in humans have been reported to be higher in women than in men (Sen et al. 1978). In female rabbits, both DHT and estradiol support plasmacyte survival (Azzarolo et al. 2003). Lacrimal gland plasmacytes enter apoptosis within 2 hours after ovariectomy, and this phenomenon can be prevented by administration of either DHT or diethylstilbesterol (DES), an estrogen receptor agonist. The fact that apoptosis begins so rapidly after ovariectomy suggests that plasmacyte survival is determined by a balance between constitutive proapoptotic signals and hormone-dependent mitogenic signals. It is possible that the proapoptotic signals are carried by epithelial-cell- and T-cell-TGF-β, but they might also be generated by intrinsic programs characteristic of bone-marrow-derived cells.

In addition to supporting expression of mitogenic factors that, in turn, support plasmacyte survival, the androgens also appear to exert generalized trophic influences on the epithelium. Ovariectomy models natural menopause imperfectly because it does not mimic the gradual, age-related decline of adrenal steroid hormone production, sometimes referred to as adrenopause. Ovariectomizing sexually mature female rabbits caused a partial (i.e. 20%) regression of the lacrimal glands, and this gross regression was roughly paralleled by decreases in the total numbers of b-adrenergic receptors and total Na,K-ATPase activity (Azzarolo et al. 1997). DHT prevented the changes, and DES exacerbated them. Na,K-ATPase is the molecular engine that powers the secretion of Na^+, K^+, and Cl^- and, thus, generates the osmotic driving force for lacrimal fluid production. Therefore, DHT would seem to support the lacrimal gland's capacity to produce fluid. DHT treatment increased cholinergically induced fluid production by more then 60%, from 8 mL/min to 13 mL/min. This finding accords with the hypothesis that androgens support the lacrimal gland's capacity to produce fluid. However, DHT treatment suppressed baseline fluid production by half, from 2 mL/min to 1 mL/min. Because fluid production was measured under general anesthesia, it appears that this influence was exerted at the level of paracrine signaling or intracellular signal transduction, rather than at the level of sensory signal generation, sensory signal processing, or autonomic secretomotor signal generation.

DHT has been shown to exert mitogenic influences in ex vivo acinar cell models (Schönthal et al. 2000). Intracrine conversion of DHEA and DHEAS to testosterone and DHT in the lacrimal gland might account for the finding that Schirmer's scores are not changed in women with premature ovarian failure, even though DED symptoms and ocular surface pathology are increased (Smith et al. 2004). On the other hand, the atrophic changes that occur with normal aging and the cessation of ovarian steroid production at menopause may be more severe than the atrophic changes that follow surgical menopause. Acinar atrophy, distal ductal stenosis, proximal ductal dilatation, and interstitial fibrosis are highly prevalent in the lacrimal glands of elderly women and men (Obata et al. 1995), but gross anatomic atrophy appears to be considerably more prevalent in women (Ueno et al. 1996). It has been suggested that these changes are enduring sequelae of previous inflammatory processes. However, a plausible competing hypothesis is that they are unrelated to inflammation, but, rather, triggered by adrenopause-related losses of DHEA and DHEAS and menopause-related losses of testosterone and DHT. Likewise, residual gonadal testosterone production in men may be as important for the support it provides for lacrimal gland anatomic integrity and functional capacity as for its presumed ability to protect against autoimmune activation.

Paracrine influences on functional capacity and acute functions

In Sjögren's syndrome, large areas of intact-appearing epithelial tissue coexist with discrete lymphocytic foci, yet physiological dysfunction may be nearly absolute. Experiments with ex vivo labial salivary gland acinar cell preparations indicate that both nitric oxide (Caulfield et al. 2009) and IgG autoantibodies against the M_3 muscarinic cholinergic receptor (Dawson et al. 2006) suppress cholinergically induced elevations of cytosolic Ca^{2+}, a key intracellular signal in the activation of fluid production. However, the work of Ding and colleagues indicates that the functional defect in autoimmune dacryoadenitis is not limited to intracellular signal transduction but, rather, extends to include decreased expression of several ion transport and water channel proteins (e.g. Nandoskar et al. 2012).

Sjögren's dacryoadenitis is not the only immunopathological process that can occur in the lacrimal glands. The example of Mikuliscz's disease, which is characterized by extensive IgG_4 plasmacyte infiltration, demonstrates that not all immune cell infiltrates impair lacrimal gland fluid production (Tsubota et al. 2000). Waterhouse (1963) reported that focal lymphocytic infiltrates are present in more than 60% of lacrimal gland of women over the age of 64. Because this proportion exceeds estimates of the prevalence of DED by nearly a factor of 2, it suggests that some age-related infiltrates are associated with physiological dysfunction, while others are not. Moreover, our recent study (Mircheff et al. 2011) suggests that some of the lymphocytic infiltrates that accumulate may be associated with an adaptive immunoregulatory response, rather than with inflammatory immunopathology. The presumed immunoregulatory infiltrates appear to be induced by exposure to desiccating environmental conditions, but positive feedback interactions localized within individual glands are associated with idiosyncratic variations in their activities. Their increasing activities are characterized by high levels of CD8 mRNA and IL-10 mRNA, which suggests the recruitment of IL-10-expressing CD8+ regulatory cells, and by high levels of mRNAs for IL-1a, IL-1b, and IL-6, but normal levels of tumor necrosis factors-a mRNA and markedly decreased levels of interferon-g mRNA.

Of the cytokines that appear to participate in the lacrimal gland's adaptive immunoregulatory response, IL-1a, IL-b, and IL-6 are of particular interest because they decrease lacrimal gland functional capacity. Moreover, it appears that steroid reproductive hormone levels influence the formation or activity of the presumed immunoregulatory infiltrates because transcript abundances are much higher in glands from sexually mature virgin females than in glands from juvenile animals that have experienced the same environmental conditions.

POSSIBLE MECHANISMS TO ACCOUNT FOR THE CLINICAL FINDINGS

The recent advances summarized above suggest several new insights. First, not all lacrimal gland physiological dysfunction is caused by autoimmune inflammatory processes. Some cases of age-related dysfunction may result from atrophic changes that are secondary to loss of hormonal support for local expression of mitogenic paracrine mediators. It well may be that the beneficial responses seen in prospective studies of estrogen–progestogen replacement, estrogen–progestogen replacement supplemented with Tibolone, estrogen replacement supplemented with drospirenone, and estrogen replacement supplemented with methyltestosterone reflect reversals of such atrophic changes.

Second, some cases of lacrimal physiological dysfunction in women of reproductive age and in women recently menopausal may result from neither atrophic changes nor autoimmune inflammatory processes, but, rather, from high levels of IL-1a, IL-1b, and IL-6 associated with activation of the adaptive immunoregulatory response to excessively high levels. Therefore, the variations in Schirmer's test scores that have been so frustrating to diagnosticians and researchers—between normal individuals, between an individual's OS and OD, and between different measurements for the same eye—may result from variations in the level of activation of the adaptive immunoregulatory response. Estrogen–progestogen replacement in recently menopausal women who do not have DED may decrease lacrimal gland physiological function by providing increased support for the adaptive immunoregulatory response, rather than by promoting a local inflammatory autoimmune process. Administration of tibolone to menopausal women who do not have DED might also enhance the adaptive immunoregulatory response and, thereby, decrease lacrimal gland physiological function. In contrast, administration of tibolone to menopausal women with Sjögren's syndrome and administration of estrogens and methyltestosterone to women with severe DED might suppress inflammatory autoimmune activity and, thereby, improve lacrimal gland physiological function.

These inferences are biologically plausible, but they need to be tested. The seemingly promising findings with estrogens, progestogens, and tibolone; with estrogens and drospirenone; and with estrogens and methyltestosterone should be pursued. The design of such studies should be made keeping in mind the diverse mechanisms that cause lacrimal gland physiological dysfunction, the roles desiccating humidities play in activating the adaptive lacrimal gland immunoregulatory response, and the roles desiccating humidities and excessive temperatures play in initiating inflammatory autoimmune responses that may propagate from the ocular surface tissues to the lacrimal glands. Their informative value will increase as they address ocular surface homeostasis and lacrimal gland physiological function comprehensively, assessing tear film osmolarity and meibomian gland status, as well as the more common measures of tear film stability, lacrimal gland fluid production, and corneal and conjunctival inflammation.

◼ REFERENCES

Abdel-Khalek LMR, Williamson J, Lee WR. Morphological changes in the human conjunctival epithelium. I. In the normal elderly population. *Br J Ophthalmol* 1978; **62**:792–799.

Affinito P, Di Spiezio Sardo A, Di Carlo C, et al. Effects of hormone replacement therapy on ocular function in postmenopause. *Menopause* 2003; **10**:482–487.

Altintaş O, Caglar Y, Yüksel N, Demirci A, Karabaş L. The effects of menopause and hormone replacement therapy on quality and quantity of tear, intraocular pressure and ocular blood flow. *Ophthalmologica* 2004; **218**:120–129.

Azzarolo AM, Eihausen H, Schechter J. Estrogen prevention of lacrimal gland cell death and lymphocytic infiltration. *Exp Eye Res* 2003; **77**:347–354.

Azzarolo AM, Mircheff AK, Kaswan RL, et al. Androgen support of lacrimal gland function. Endocrine 1997; **6**:39–45.

Blackie CA, Korb DR, Knop E, et al. Nonobvious obstructive Meibomian gland dysfunction. *Cornea* 2010; **29**:1333–1345.

Caulfield VL, Balmer C, Dawson LJ, Smith PM. A role for nitric oxide-mediated glandular hypofunction in a non-apoptotic model for Sjögren's syndrome. *Rheumatology (Oxford)* 2009; **48**:727–733.

Cermak JM, Krenzer KL, Sullivan RM, Dana MR, Sullivan DA. Is complete androgen insensitivity syndrome associated with alterations in the meibomian gland and ocular surface? *Cornea* 2003; **22**:516–521.

Chaikittisilpa S, Tulvatana W, Taechakraichana N, Panyakhamlerd K, Limpaphayom K. Hormone replacement therapy and tear volume in postmenopausal women with dry eye. *Thai J Obstetrics Gynaecology* 2000; **12**:135–139.

Coksuer H, Ozcura F, Oghan F, Haliloglu B, Coksuer C. Effects of estradiol-drospirenone on ocular and nasal functions in postmenopausal women. *Climacteric* 2011; **14**:482–487.

Dawson LJ, Stanbury J, Venn N, et al. Antimuscarinic antibodies in primary Sjögren's syndrome reversibly inhibit the mechanism of fluid secretion by human submandibular salivary acinar cells. *Arthritis Rheum* 2006; **54**:1165–1173.

Drosos AA, van Vliet-Dascalopoulou E, Andonopoulos AP, et al. Nandrolone decanoate (deca-durabolin) in primary Sjögren's syndrome: a double blind pilot study. *Clin Exp Rheumatol* 1988; **6**:53–57.

Erdem U, Ozdegirmenci O, Sobaci E, et al. Dry eye in post-menopausal women using hormone replacement therapy. *Maturitas* 2007; **56**:257–262.

Fodor E, Barabino S, Montaldo E, Mingari MC, Rolando M. Quantitative evaluation of ocular surface inflammation in patients with different grade of conjunctivochalasis. *Curr Eye Res* 2010; **35**:665–669.

Friedel A, Geyer H, Kamber M, et al. 17beta-hydroxy-5alpha-androst-1-en-3-one (1-testosterone) is a potent androgen with anabolic properties. *Toxicol Lett* 2006; **165**:149–155.

Guaschino S, Grimaldi E, Sartore A, et al. Visual function in menopause: the role of hormone replacement therapy. *Menopause* 2003; **10**:53–57.

Guillon M, Maïssa C. Tear film evaporation—effect of age and gender. *Cont Lens Anterior Eye* 2010; **33**:171–175.

Hann LE, Allansmith MR, Sullivan DA. Impact of aging and gender on the Ig-containing cell profile of the lacrimal gland. *Acta Ophthalmol (Copenh)* 1988; **66**:87–92.

Jensen AA, Higginbotham EJ, Guzinski GM, Davis IL, Ellish NJ. A survey of ocular complaints in postmenopausal women. *J Assoc Acad Minor Phys* 2000; **11**:44–49.

Knop E, Knop N, Millar T, Obata H, Sullivan DA. The international workshop on Meibomian gland dysfunction: report of the subcommittee on anatomy, physiology, and pathophysiology of the Meibomian gland. *Invest Ophthalmol Vis Sci* 2011; **52**:1938–1978.

Kuscu NK, Toprak AB, Vatansever S, Koyuncu FM, Guler C. Tear function changes of postmenopausal women in response to hormone replacement therapy. *Maturitas* 2003; **44**:63–68.

Lange C, Fernandez J, Shim D, et al. Mucin gene expression is not regulated by estrogen and/or progesterone in the ocular surface epithelia of mice. *Exp Eye Res* 2003; **77**:59–68.

Liu J, Allgood A, Derogatis LR, et al. Safety and efficacy of low-dose esterified estrogens and methyltestosterone, alone or combined, for the treatment of hot flashes in menopausal women: a randomized, double-blind, placebo-controlled study. *Fertil Steril* 2011; **95**:366–368.

Mathers WD, Lane JA, Zimmerman MB. Tear film changes associated with normal aging. *Cornea* 1996; **15**:229–234.

Metka M, Enzelsberger H, Knogler W, Schurz B, Aichmair H. Ophthalmic complaints as a climacteric symptom. *Maturitas* 1991; **14**:3–8.

Mircheff AK, Wang Y, Thomas PB, et al. Systematic variations in immune response-related gene transcript abundance suggest new questions about environmental influences on lacrimal gland immunoregulation. *Curr Eye Res* 2011; **36**:285–294.

Moon JH, Jung JW, Shin KH, Paik HJ. Effect of hormone replacement therapy on dry eye syndrome in postmenopausal women: a prospective study. *J Korean Ophthalmol Soc* 2010; **51**:175–179.

Nandoskar P, Wang Y, Wei R, et al. Changes of chloride channels in the lacrimal glands of a rabbit model of Sjögren syndrome. *Cornea* 2012; **31**:273–279.

Obata H, Yamamoto S, Horiuchi H, Machinami R. Histopathologic study of human lacrimal gland. Statistical analysis with special reference to aging. *Ophthalmology* 1995; **102**:678–686.

Okoń A, Jurowski P, Goś R. The influence of the hormonal replacement therapy on the amount and stability of the tear film among peri- and postmenopausal women. *Klin Oczna* 2001; **103**:177–181.

Ozdemir M, Temizdemir H. Age- and gender-related tear function changes in normal population. *Eye* 2010; **24**:79–83.

Pelit A, Bağiş T, Kayaselçuk F, et al. Tear function tests and conjunctival impression cytology before and after hormone replacement therapy in postmenopausal women. *Eur J Ophthalmol* 2003; **13**:337–342.

Pillemer SR, Brennan MT, Sankar V, et al. Pilot clinical trial of dehydroepiandrosterone (DHEA) versus placebo for Sjögren's syndrome. *Arthritis Rheum* 2004; **51**:601–604.

Rosenthal P, Borsook D. The corneal pain system. Part I: the missing piece of the dry eye puzzle. *Ocul Surf* 2012; **10**:2–14.

Rossouw JE, Anderson GL, Prentice RL, et al. Risks and benefits of estrogen plus progestin in healthy postmenopausal women: principal results From the Women's Health Initiative randomized controlled trial. *JAMA* 2002; **288**:321–333.

Rothman MS, Carlson NE, Xu M, et al. Reexamination of testosterone, DHT, estradiol and estrone levels across the menstrual cycle and in postmenopausal women measured by liquid chromatography-tandem mass spectrometry. *Steroids* 2011; **76**:177–182.

Santen RJ, Allred DC, Ardoin SP, et al. Postmenopausal hormone therapy: an Endocrine Society scientific statement. *J Clin Endocrinol Metab* 2010; **95**:s1–s66.

Sartore A, Grimaldi E, Guaschino S. The treatment of Sjögren's syndrome with tibolone: a case report. *Am J Obstet Gynecol* 2003; **189**:894.

Sator MO, Joura EA, Golaszewski T, et al. Treatment of menopausal keratoconjunctivitis sicca with topical oestradiol. *Br J Obstet Gynaecol* 1998; **105**:100–102.

Schaumberg DA, Buring JE, Sullivan DA, Dana MR. Hormone replacement therapy and dry eye syndrome. *JAMA* 2001; **286**:2114–2119.

Schönthal AH, Warren DW, Stevenson D, et al. Proliferation of lacrimal gland acinar cells in primary culture. Stimulation by extracellular matrix, EGF, and DHT. *Exp Eye Res* 2000; **70**:639–649.

Scott G, Yiu SC, Wasilewski D, Song J, Smith RE. Combined esterified estrogen and methyltestosterone treatment for dry eye syndrome in postmenopausal women. *Am J Ophthalmol* 2005; **139**:1109–1110.

Sen DK, Sarin GS, Mathur GP, Saha K. Biological variation of immunoglobulin concentrations in normal human tears related to age and sex. *Acta Ophthalmol (Copenh)* 1978; **56**:439–444.

Smith JA, Vitale S, Reed GF, et al. Dry eye signs and symptoms in women with premature ovarian failure. *Arch Ophthalmol* 2004; **122**:151–156.

Spaan M, Porola P, Laine M, et al. Healthy human salivary glands contain a DHEA-sulphate processing intracrine machinery, which is deranged in primary Sjögren's syndrome. *J Cell Mol Med* 2009; **13**:1261–1270.

Sullivan DA, Bélanger A, Cermak JM, et al. Are women with Sjögren's syndrome androgen-deficient? *J Rheumatol* 2003; **30**:2413–2419.

Sullivan DA, Jensen RV, Suzuki T, Richards SM. Do sex steroids exert sex-specific and/or opposite effects on gene expression in lacrimal and meibomian glands? *Mol Vis* 2009; **15**:1553–1572.

Sullivan DA, Wickham LA, Rocha EM, et al. Androgens and dry eye in Sjögren's syndrome. *Ann N Y Acad Sci* 1999; **876**:312–324.

Tamer C, Oksuz H, Sogut S. Androgen status of the nonautoimmune dry eye subtypes. *Ophthalmic Res* 2006; **38**:280–286.

Taner P, Akarsu C, Atasoy P, Bayram M, Ergin A. The effects of hormone replacement therapy on ocular surface and tear function tests in postmenopausal women. *Ophthalmologica* 2004; **218**:257–259.

Tsubota K, Fujita H, Tsuzaka K, Takeuchi T. Mikulicz's disease and Sjögren's syndrome. *Invest Ophthalmol Vis Sci* 2000; **41**:1666–1673.

Ueno H, Ariji E, Izumi M, et al. MR imaging of the lacrimal gland. Age-related and gender-dependent changes in size and structure. *Acta Radiol* 1996; **37**:714–719.

Uncu G, Avci R, Uncu Y, Kaymaz C, Develioğlu O. The effects of different hormone replacement therapy regimens on tear function, intraocular pressure and lens opacity. *Gynecol Endocrinol* 2006; **22**:501–505.

Versura P, Campos EC. Menopause and dry eye. A possible relationship. *Gynecol Endocrinol* 2005; **20**:289–298

Versura P, Fresina M, Campos EC. Ocular surface changes over the menstrual cycle in women with and without dry eye. *Gynecol Endocrinol* 2007; **23**:385–390.

Waterhouse JP. Focal adenitis in lacrimal and salivary glands. *Proc R Soc Med* 1963; **56**:911–918.

Wierman ME, Basson R, Davis SR, et al. Androgen therapy in women: an Endocrine Society Clinical Practice guideline. *J Clin Endocrinol Metab* 2006; **91**:3697–3710.

Worda C, Nepp J, Huber JC, Sator MO. Treatment of keratoconjunctivitis sicca with topical androgen. *Maturitas* 2001; **37**:209–212.

Chapter 34 | Therapeutic contact lenses

Perry Rosenthal

■ INTRODUCTION

Unlike all other contact lenses, scleral lenses are supported entirely by the sclera, thereby enabling them to retain a fluid-filled chamber over and avoid all contact with the corneal surface. In effect, this device immerses the corneal surface in a pool of oxygenated artificial tears (**Figure 34.1**). Its fluid reservoir offers the following benefits: (1) masks irregular corneal astigmatism, (2) serves as a protective liquid corneal 'bandage,' (3) optimizes the hydration of the corneal epithelium, and (4) provides a vehicle for delivering drugs to the cornea and sustaining their surface residence time. The latter three functions are considered in this chapter.

Although its fluid compartment is the working part of a scleral lens, the design of its scleral bearing surface determines its wearing tolerance. Excessive focal scleral compression (as indicated by underlying vascular blanching) causes congestion and chemosis of the limbal conjunctiva (**Figure 34.2a**), thereby limiting its wearing comfort. Moreover, circumferential scleral compression promotes lens suction that can cause profound corneal edema and necessitate an urgent trip to an emergency clinic to pry the device off the eye (**Figure 34.2b**). On the other hand, failure to accommodate scleral toricity increases scleral compression over the flatter meridia and facilitates the intrusion of air bubbles and tear debris into the fluid chamber over the steeper scleral meridian (**Figure 34.2c**). Therefore, its design is governed by the need to (1) avoid any corneal contact and (2) align the shape of the bearing surface of the device with that of the underlying sclera in order to distribute its compressive force uniformly and avoid focal scleral compression (**Figure 34.2d**).

■ SCLERAL LENS VERSUS SOFT BANDAGE LENS

The therapeutic objectives of these modalities are to enhance the environment of the corneal surface, protect it from the friction of blinking and exposure to the evaporative environment, and maintain optimal corneal hydration. The advantages of soft contact lenses include widespread availability, minimal cost, ease of fitting, and high oxygen transmissibility. Nevertheless, they suffer from two major limitations. The first is adhesion. Although their transitional surfaces are highly wettable while in contact with water, they become hydrophobic when

exposed to air. This, combined with their tendency to dehydrate in vivo and the virtual absence of a tear pump, promotes their becoming bound to the underlying cornea with mucins—especially during overnight wear when tear production is normally attenuated. Moreover, as their exposed surface dries and becomes less lubricious, the friction generated as the upper lid slides over the lens during each blink amplifies the shear forces transmitted to the corneal surface. This effect is exacerbated by the accelerated dehydration associated with dry eyes. The corneal surface shear forces generated by blinking and lens removal are especially problematic when the corneal epithelium is fragile or loosely adherent to underlying Bowman's membrane. Added to these challenges, overnight wear of hydrogel contact lenses has been shown to reduce corneal epithelial adhesion (Madigan & Holden 1992). Below a certain level of tear deficiency, the available water can be insufficient to maintain adequate lens hydration. The competition between the cornea and lens for available tears is avoided by scleral lenses.

More worrisome is the stress imposed by overnight wear when tear production is virtually shut down. If eyes are dry during waking hours, the corneas become even more vulnerable to developing bacterial keratitis during overnight wear (Lemp 1990)—especially in the presence of epithelial defects. Nevertheless, the challenge faced by inexperienced patients or caregivers in inserting and removing soft contact lenses from fragile corneas usually makes extended wear mandatory. On the other hand, soft bandage lenses are useful as a protective barrier to corneal trauma caused by diseased superior tarsal conjunctiva and lid margins if basal tear secretion is sufficient to maintain their functional hydration (Ambroziak et al. 2004). And if worn overnight to resurface refractory corneal epithelial defects, the lenses should be saturated in vivo with sterile saline prior to removing them. Note: topical medications used during soft contact lens wear should be preservative-free since they can accumulate in the hydrogel matrix and cause toxic stress to the diseased corneas.

In contrast to soft bandage lenses, the rigidity of scleral lenses can be exploited to provide sufficient clearance over the cornea to avoid amplification of surface shear forces and facilitate the development of adhesion. On the other hand, the retention of a semistagnant pool of fluid over vulnerable corneal surfaces is a risk factor for the development of bacterial keratitis during overnight wear of scleral lenses, especially in the presence of epithelial defect. This should be mitigated by using prophylactic, dilute, non-preserved antibiotics in the lens reservoir.

■ ROLE OF SCLERAL LENSES IN MANAGING OCULAR SURFACE DISEASE

■ Protecting the corneal surface from exposure

Corneal exposure due to impaired lid function caused by neurological deficits, scarring, and/or loss of lid tissue are ideally managed by the

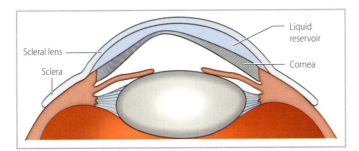

Figure 34.1 Scleral lens.

liquid corneal bandage of the scleral lens. There are two categories of lagophthalmos, each of which requires a somewhat different management strategy.

Extreme exposure

Extreme exposure refers to cases in which there is insufficient lid tissue to accommodate a tarsorraphy, such as in patients with third- and fourth-degree facial burns. These injuries often lead to corneal ulceration and perforation despite intensive around-the-clock eye lubrication and amniotic membrane onlays (Lin et al. 2011). The scleral lens is capable of preserving the integrity of these eyes (Schein et al. 1990, Williams & Aquavella 2007). Because these corneas are always exposed to the environment, oxygen deprivation is not a limiting factor. Therefore, scleral lenses can be worn continuously and safely on these eyes if they are removed every 24 hours for corneal examination and replaced with disinfected devices that contain fresh sterile, non-preserved artificial tears medicated with a dilute non-preserved antibiotic.

Corneal exposure occurring during waking hours

Eyes with lagophthalmos sufficient to cause daytime corneal exposure and corneal surface desiccation, in which the lids can be closed by tape tarsorraphy during sleep, are excellent candidates for scleral lens protection during waking hours (Rosenthal & Croteau 2005). In addition to providing vision and avoiding cosmetic disfigurement, these devices are more effective than surgical tarsorraphy, which should be reserved for urgent situations when scleral lenses are not available.

Lid-induced corneal trauma

Protecting the cornea from traumatic friction during blinking caused by diseased upper tarsal conjunctivae and lid margins, such as keratinization and distichiasis, strikingly mitigates corneal pain and photophobia and improves the health of the corneal surface (Romero-Rangel et al. 2000).

■ Healing refractory corneal epithelial defects

The environment of the corneal surface provided by scleral lenses accelerates the healing of otherwise refractory epithelial defects (Pullum et al. 2005). Those associated with corneal stem cell deficiency and sustained by metaplastic changes in the lid margins and tarsal conjunctiva are especially challenging to heal and may require a series of consecutive periods of continuous wear. The device should be removed at 24-hour intervals to monitor the cornea and exchange the scleral lens with one that has been disinfected. One drop of a non-preserved antibiotic such as moxifloxacin must be added to the saline in the fluid reservoir to prevent the development of bacterial keratitis. Overnight wear should be continued for 24 hours after the corneal defect has resurfaced before transitioning to daily wear. The effectiveness of these devices is illustrated in **Figure 34.3**. This patient's persistent epithelial defect in a penetrating keratoplasty performed for scarring caused by Stevens–Johnson syndrome had persisted for 8 months despite aggressive treatments. It resurfaced within 6 days of continuous scleral lens wear during which time the device was used according to the regimen described above. The practitioner should expect to see hypoxic corneal edema, which resolves when the patient is transitioned to daily wear.

■ Management of the neurotrophic cornea

Scleral lens wear during waking hours with nighttime corneal lubrication is an unmatched therapeutic and prophylactic strategy for preserving the surface integrity of neurotrophic corneas that have exhibited at least one episode of spontaneous epithelial breakdown.

■ Congenital corneal anesthesia

Congenital corneal anesthesia is most often associated with familial dysautonomia (FD), also known as Riley Day syndrome, which is primarily (but not exclusively) a genetic disease of Ashkenazi Jews. Congenital corneal anesthesia can also occur sporadically and unilaterally as isolated cases. Once the diagnosis of FD is made, the eyes of these infants and children should be closely monitored by their caregivers who are instructed in the use of fluorescein strips and blue filtered flashlight, since significant corneal epithelial breakdown can be present in white and quiet eyes. Moreover, they should be instructed to look for corneal exposure during the child's sleep and protect their eyes from inadvertent self-mutilation when awake.

Scleral lenses should be fitted as soon as the first corneal defect is discovered or preferably when the diagnosis of FD is made. Age is no barrier: our youngest patient, 5 months old, presented with a corneal ulcer in a dense scar in her right cornea and demonstrated early corneal epithelial breakdown in the left one. Both corneas rapidly resurfaced under scleral lenses and the corneal scar OD was barely visible 1 year later. Moreover, she was able to fixate with her right eye when OS was occluded after a period of intermittent patching OS. Her eyes continue to do well at age 3. The challenge in managing infants with this disease is working around their irregular sleep patterns. The rule of thumb that we follow is that devices are worn approximately 12 hours of every 24-hour period.

Acquired neurotrophic cornea

Scleral lens is the gold standard for managing these eyes (Visser et al. 2007). In contrast to those associated with corneal stem cell deficiencies, persistent epithelial defects in neurotrophic corneas generally heal rapidly under a scleral lens and overnight wear may not be necessary. Daily wear should be continued indefinitely to preserve the integrity of the corneal surface. Interestingly, we have sometimes observed striking remodeling of recently scarred corneal stroma under a scleral lens over time (**Figure 34.3a** and **34.3b**).

■ DRY EYE DISEASE

Defining dry eye disease (DED) has been problematic. Nevertheless, with rare exceptions, the one common feature that defines DED is the presence of chronic symptoms that mimic those associated with dry eyes (Begley et al. 2003). Therefore, it is reasonable to classify these patients into two categories: desiccating dry eye disease (DDED), in which the intensity of symptoms match the signs of ocular surface desiccation, and non-desiccating dry eye disease (NDDED), much more prevalent and in which the cause of DED-like symptoms is not obvious. Since symptoms are the cornerstone of NDDED, it is helpful to remind ourselves that virtually all the corneal nerves (C and Aδ fibers) are designed to carry pain signals (nociceptors). Moreover, the density of their terminals in the human cornea is 20–40-fold greater than dental pulp and most are strategically located between the apical

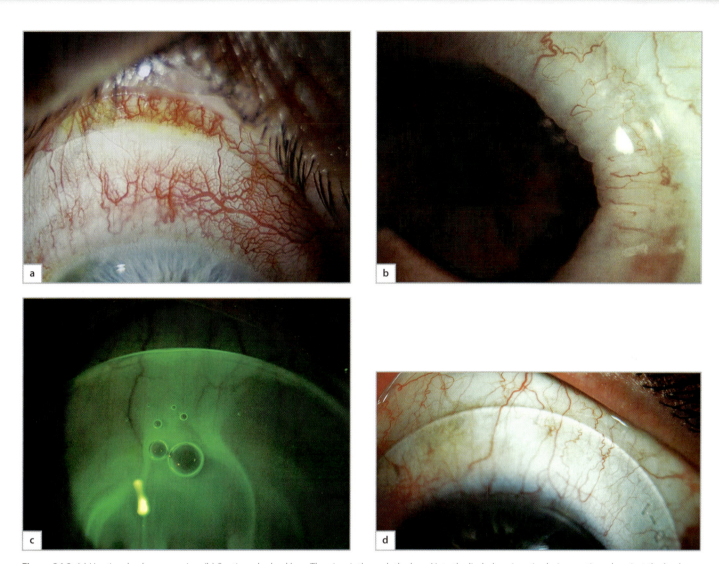

Figure 34.2 (a) Haptic scleral compression. (b) Suctioned scleral lens. The view is through the lens. Note the limbal conjunctiva being suctioned against the back surface of the device. The intense corneal edema is not visible. (c) Rotationally symmetrical haptic on a toric sclera. The increased inflow of tears brings air bubbles and debris under the lens optic and increases its compression along the flatter axis. (d) Red-enhanced photo of an aligned haptic. Note that the blood vessels coursing under the haptic are uninterrupted.

cells of the corneal epithelium (Mueller et al. 1997). Thus, the human cornea is both the body's most powerful pain generator and the most vulnerable to being activated and damaged by noxious stimuli. The inference is that all corneal sensations (including those of dry eyes) are variants of pain (Belmonte 2007). Substituting 'pain' for 'dry' in describing corneal symptoms shifts the focus to the corneal pain (nociceptive) system.

Desiccating dry eye disease

On the surface, DDED seems straightforward. Ocular surface drying causes corneal epithelial inflammation and the release of proinflammatory cytokines that reduce the activation thresholds of the nociceptive transducers, thereby increasing their sensitivity and responsiveness to noxious stimuli. This defines the state of hyperalgesia. Since the optical tear layer is the eyes' most powerful focusing lens and evaporation is the greatest threat to its integrity, it is not surprising that many of the corneal nerve sensors are tuned to this omnipresent

threat to vision. Sensitization of the tear-evaporation-sensitive nociceptive terminals (thermoreceptors and osmoreceptors) causes them to become hypersensitive to the surrogate markers of tear evaporation: a dynamic drop in temperature and elevated osmolarity (Belmonte & Gallar 2011, Hirata & Meng 2010). This, in turn, increases the thickness of the tear layer required to avoid their activation. Nociceptor sensitization can rise to the level in which the only method capable of suppressing their activity is by totally blocking tear evaporation such as covering the cornea with a (vapor-proof) scleral lens. This explains why inserting this device on eyes with desiccated surfaces instantly and completely suppresses DED symptoms, including photophobia. Although hyperalgesic corneas can be hypersensitive to fumes (chemicals), protons (acid), and mechanical stimuli in some cases, the dominant symptom of corneal inflammation is evaporative hyperalgesia and the gold standard treatment for DDED and non-desiccating DED is reducing tear evaporation or blocking it with scleral lenses. Reversal of signs of desiccating corneal epitheliopathy by scleral lens hydration can happen rapidly (**Figure 34.4a** and **34.4b**). Nevertheless, this is not

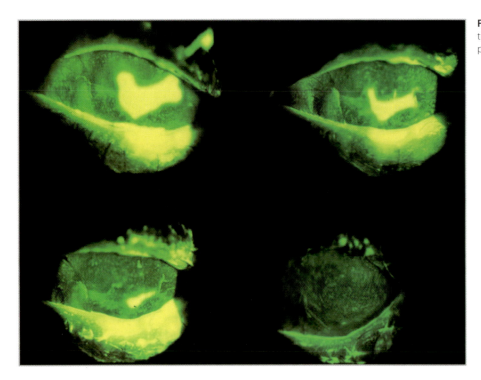

Figure 34.3 Persistent corneal defect refractory to treatment resolved in 6 days with the extended wear protocol describe herein.

accompanied by significant mitigation of symptoms of corneal hyperalgesia when the devices are not worn (personal experience). This type of corneal hyperalgesia (and the putative underlying subclinical inflammation) appears to have become hard-wired , thus representing a chronic disease in its own right.

Non-desiccating dry eye disease

The presence of subclinical corneal inflammatory evaporative hyperalgesia provides a more robust explanation for the enigmatic disparity between symptoms and signs in NDDED. Conventional wisdom explains this prevalent disease as due to hyperevaporation of tears associated with meibomian gland dysfunction (MGD). Although MGD increases the rate of tear evaporation, the many exceptions (patients who suffer from this lid disease but are asymptomatic, and others who suffer from NDDED but have normal-appearing meibomian glands) suggest the presence of a more fundamental pathoetiology. The clue was the identification of increased levels of cytokines in the tears of symptomatic patients with white and quiet eyes (Enriquez-de-Salamanca et al. 2010) that point to the presence of subclinical inflammation, nociceptor sensitization, and hypersensitivity to tear evaporation. This can explain why eyes do not have to be dry to feel dry and why the DED-like symptoms in non-dry eyes can be mitigated by conventional dry eye treatments.

Chronic spontaneous corneal pain

Just as symptoms of evaporative hyperalgesia are identified by their acute suppression on insertion, their persistence during scleral lens

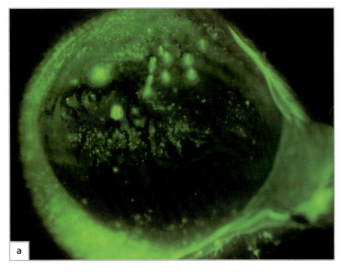

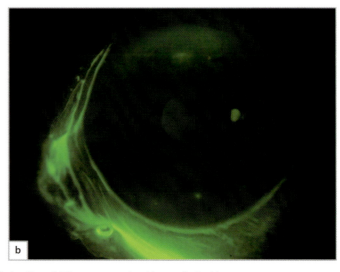

Figure 34.4 (a) Desiccating dry eye with staining and filaments prior to insertion of scleral lens. (b) The same eye after 4 hours of scleral lens wear.

wear (which suppresses symptoms of evaporative hyperalgesia) points to the presence of spontaneous (unprovoked) pain. Spontaneous corneal and cornea-projected pain can be the consequence of activity of unstable ectopic pain generators expressed by pathological regeneration of corneal neurons and sustained and amplified by sensitization of the central pain signaling pathways. Typically, these corneas show attrition of nerve fibers and sensory deficit (hypoesthesia) in addition to being the source of pain (provoked and spontaneous).

Neuropathic central sensitization

How do the corresponding synapses in the brain respond to intense and ongoing afferent pain signals? This is a critical question because its answer determines whether effective suppression of corneal hyperalgesia with scleral lenses alone can extinguish chronic corneal pain or whether therapeutic central neuromodulation interventions are also required.

Although cornea-projected centralized pain is often triggered by peripheral nerve injuries (of which LASIK is the classical model), it can also be caused by intrinsic axonopathies such as those associated with diabetes, infections such as herpes zoster, and certain neurological diseases including multiple sclerosis, non-length-dependent small fiber neuropathy, Guillain-Barré disease, and autoimmune disorders. In such cases of centralized corneal neuropathic pain, scleral lenses would only be helpful in suppressing symptoms of evaporative hyperalgesia, if any. Rarely, cornea-projected pain appears to originate in the central pain circuitry as suggested by the presence of comorbid signs and symptoms involving the innervation territory of non-ophthalmic branches of the trigeminal and other cranial nerves in the absence of signs of corneal neuropathy (Rosenthal & Borsook 2012). The value of scleral lenses in treating corneal centralized pain is determined by the contribution of evaporative corneal hyperalgesia in the pain mix and whether it has evolved to increase the sensitivity of the bulbar conjunctiva.

Extramural comorbid symptoms

In some patients with centralized corneal pain, symptoms can spread beyond the receptive field of the ophthalmic branch of the trigeminal nerve and project to the face, jaw, ear, and head. Some patients also report tinnitus, and hyperacusis, and can suffer from focal dystonias such as blepharospasm and Meige's syndrome (Borsook & Rosenthal 2011). Comorbid changes in affective and cognitive functions include depression, catastrophizing, difficulties in word retrieval, and impairment of working memory. Of special interest to ophthalmologists is the tendency of these patients to experience more intense pain of longer duration following surgery involving the territory of neuropathic pain (personal observations).

Chronic corneal pain and multisystem disorders

Corneal neuropathic pain affects women predominantly (Liverman et al. 2009), as do autoimmune disorders that are associated with a higher incidence of peripheral neuropathies. For example, DED-like symptoms can be associated with fibromyalgia, systemic lupus, rheumatoid arthritis and primary and secondary Sjögren's syndrome (SS), interstitial cystitis, chronic fatigue syndrome, multiple chemical sensitivities, and so on (Rosenthal & Borsook 2012).

Although SS is generally considered a classical example of DDED, many of these patients develop evaporative corneal hyperalgesia long before signs of ocular surface desiccation appear. This is consistent with the proclivity of SS patients to develop peripheral neuropathies

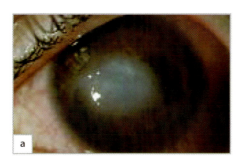

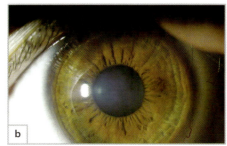

Figure 34.5 Left panel shows neurotrophic cornea 4 weeks after the epithelium has resurfaced. Right panel is the same eye 4 years later after daily scleral lens wear.

and ganglionopathies (Griffin et al. 1990). In many cases, ocular surface desiccation represents a late stage of SS. Nevertheless, many patients with Sjögren's syndrome and fibromyalgia suffer from dry eye-like symptoms in the absence of signs of dry eyes which are suppressed by scleral lenses.

◼ SCLERAL LENSES AS A VEHICLE FOR SUSTAINED DELIVERY OF TOPICAL CORNEAL DRUGS

The expanded fluid reservoir of scleral lenses can be used as a means of delivering topical non-preserved corneal medications over longer periods. Because it extends their corneal surface resident times with slow dilution during the wearing period, this off-label drug delivery system can be strikingly effective as a means of delivering dilute, non-toxic concentrations of drugs. Moreover, large molecules with limited corneal penetrance that are largely ineffective when used in the form of drops, such as bevacizumab, can be efficacious when delivered in the reservoir of scleral lenses (Jacobs et al. 2009). Other non-preserved drugs that we have used off-label in this manner to good advantage include dexamethasone (0.001%), subanesthetic concentrations of sodium channel blockers (lidocaine and ropivacaine 0.005%) and antibiotic (moxifloxacin 0.05%). Note: the efficacy of this drug delivery system is dependent on the lens design, particularly the ability to align the shape of the haptic bearing surface with that of the underlying sclera. For example, failure to accommodate scleral toricity can substantially increase the rate of tear flow beneath the devices, thereby accelerating drug dilution and the accumulation of tear debris under the devices.

◼ CONCLUSIONS

The modern scleral lens has proven to be a powerful therapeutic tool for managing a wide range of severe ocular surface diseases and continues to make a significant contribution to our understanding of the many manifestations of corneal neuropathic pain or DED.

■ REFERENCES

Ambroziak AM, Szaflik JP, Szaflik J. Therapeutic use of a silicone hydrogel contact lens in selected clinical cases. *Eye Contact Lens* 2004; **30**:63–67.

Begley CG, Chalmers RL, Abetz L, et al. The relationship between habitual patient-reported symptoms and clinical signs among patients with dry eye of varying severity. *Invest Ophthalmol Vis Sci* 2003; **44**:4753–4761.

Belmonte C. Eye dryness sensations after refractive surgery: impaired tear secretion or phantomcornea? *J Refract Surg* 2007; **23**:598–602.

Belmonte C, Gallar J. Cold Thermoreceptors, unexpected players in tear production and ocular dryness sensations. *Invest Ophthalmol Vis Sci* 2011; **52**:3888–3892.

Borsook D, Rosenthal P. Chronic (neuropathic) corneal pain and blepharospasm: five case reports. *Pain* 2011; **152**:2427-2431.

Chapman CR. Painful multi-symptom disorders: a systems perspective In: Kruger L, Light AR (eds). *Translational Pain Research: From Mouse to Man.* Boca Raton, FL: CRC Press; 2010.

Enriquez-de-Salamanca A, Castellanos E, et al. Tear cytokine and chemokine analysis and clinical correlations in evaporative-type dry eye disease. *Mol Vis* 2010; **16**:862–873.

Griffin JW, Cornblath DR, Alexander E, et al. Ataxic sensory neuropathy and dorsal root ganglionitis associated with Sjogren's syndrome. *Ann Neurol* 1990; **27**:304–315.

Hirata H, Meng ID. Cold-sensitive corneal afferents respond to a variety of ocular stimuli central to tear production: implications for dry eye disease. *Invest Ophthalmol Vis Sci* 2010; **51**:3969–3976.

Hirata H, Okamoto K, Tashiro A, Bereiter DA. A novel class of neurons at the trigeminal subnucleus interpolaris/caudalis transition region monitors ocular surface fluid status and modulates tear production. *J Neurosci* 2004; **24**:4224–4232.

Jacobs DS, Lim M, Carrasquillo KG, Rosenthal P. Bevacizumab for corneal neovascularization. *Ophthalmology* 2009; **116**:592–593; author reply 593–594.

Lemp MA. Is the dry eye contact lens wearer at risk? Yes. *Cornea* 1990; **9**:S48–S50; discussion S54.

Lin A, Patel N, Yoo D, DeMartelaere S, Bouchard C. Management of ocular conditions in the burn unit: thermal and chemical burns and Stevens-Johnson syndrome/toxic epidermal necrolysis. *J Burn Care Res* 2011; **32**:547–560.

Liverman CS, Brown JW, Sandhir R, et al. Oestrogen increases nociception through ERK activation in the trigeminal ganglion: evidence for a peripheral mechanism of allodynia. *Cephalalgia* 2009; **29**:520–531.

Madigan MC, Holden BA. Reduced epithelial adhesion after extended contact lens wear correlates with reduced hemidesmosome density in cat cornea. *Invest Ophthalmol Vis Sci* 1992; **33**:314–323.

Mueller LJ, Vresesn GF, Pels L, Cardozo BN, Willekens B. Architecture of human corneal nerves. *Invest Ophthalmol Vis Sci* 1997; **38**:985–994.

Okamoto K, Tashiro A, Chang Z, Bereiter DA. Bright light activates a trigeminal nociceptive pathway. *Pain* 2010; **149**:235–242.

Pullum KW, Whiting, MA, Buckley RJ. Scleral contact lenses: the expanding role. *Cornea* 2005; **24**:269–277.

Romero-Rangel T, Stavrou P, Cotter J, et al. Gas-permeable scleral contact lens therapy in ocular surface disease. *Am J Ophthalmol* 2000; **130**:25–32.

Rosenthal P, Borsook D. The corneal pain system. Part 1: the missing piece of the dry eye puzzle. *Ocul Surf* 2012; **10**:2–14.

Rosenthal P, Croteau A. Fluid-ventilated, gas-permeable scleral contact lens is an effective option for managing severe ocular surface disease and many corneal disorders that would otherwise require penetrating keratoplasty. *Eye Contact Lens* 2005; **31**:130–134.

Schein OD, Rosenthal P, Ducharme C. A gas-permeable scleral contact lens for visual rehabilitation. *Am J Ophthalmol* 1990; **109**:318–322.

Visser ES, Visser R, van Lier HJ, Otten HM. Modern scleral lenses part I: clinical features. *Eye Contact Lens* 2007; **33**:13–20.

Williams ZR, Aquavella JV. Management of exposure keratopathy associated with severe craniofacial trauma. *J Cataract Refract Surg* 2007; **33**:1647–1650.

Woolf CJ, Wiesenfeld-Hallin Z. The systemic administration of local anaesthetics produces a selective depression of C-afferent fibre evoked activity in the spinal cord. *Pain* 1985; **23**:361–374.

Chapter 35 | Antibiotic, antifungal, and antiviral drugs

Nambi Nallasamy, Terrence P. O'Brien

ANTIBIOTICS

Antibiotics have both antimicrobial and non-antimicrobial functions in the treatment of ocular surface disease. Common infectious ocular surface diseases include bacterial conjunctivitis and bacterial keratitis, while non-infectious ocular surface diseases that can be treated with antibiotics include blepharitis, meibomianitis, ocular rosacea, and dry eye disease (DED).

Blepharitis and meibomianitis

Blepharitis is commonly accompanied by crusting of the eyelid margin, conjunctival injection and irritation, and pruritus. Three of the six clinical classifications of blepharitis involve meibomian gland dysfunction (MGD). Alterations in normal triglyceride fatty acid composition in meibomian glands are considered to be a central feature of MGD and blepharitis. A recent study demonstrated that minocycline, a tetracycline antibiotic, improved tear break-up time while decreasing branched-chain fatty acid content in the meibum of human subjects with refractory MGD (Aronowicz et al. 2006). At present, studies indicate that the effects of tetracycline therapy for MGD are not secondary to reduction of bacterial growth, but are rather due to inhibition of bacterial lipase activity (Federici 2011). This reduction in bacterial lipase activity is thought to reduce the production of free fatty acids that exacerbates MGD. Today, patients with refractory blepharitis are commonly treated with doxycycline 50 mg PO bid, or minocycline 50 mg PO daily for 2 weeks, followed by doxycycline 20 mg PO daily until resolution of symptoms occurs. A promising new approach to refractory blepharitis involves the use of azithromycin 1% solution bid for 2 days, followed by daily application to the eyelids for 28 days (Veldman & Colby 2011). In a recent open-label study, patients treated with this regimen demonstrated a significant reduction in meibomian gland plugging, eyelid margin redness, palpebral conjunctival redness, and ocular discharge, with persistence of the results 4 weeks post-treatment (Haque et al. 2010). While patient symptoms of foreign body sensation, ocular dryness, and ocular burning also demonstrated a significant improvement during this open-label study, no randomized controlled trial has been performed to date to corroborate this evidence.

Ocular rosacea

Ocular rosacea often manifests as blepharoconjunctivitis and meibomianitis, and may include corneal neovascularization, corneal scarring, and keratitis. Several studies have demonstrated the effects of tetracyclines on clinical findings such as tear break-up time, bulbar injection, papillary hypertrophy, and corneal erosions in patients with ocular rosacea (Bartholomew et al. 1982). In two large studies, 3- to 6-month courses of 100 mg doxycycline PO daily or 250 mg tetracycline PO daily resulted in resolution of symptoms and signs in 85% of each of the tested populations (Quarterman et al. 1997, Seitsalo et al. 2007). While the effects on blepharoconjunctivitis, meibomianitis, and tear break-up time are likely secondary to the same alteration in fatty acid content described above, the mechanism for resolution of other manifestations of ocular rosacea secondary to treatment with tetracyclines remains unclear.

Keratoconjunctivitis sicca

Keratoconjunctivitis sicca or DED is generally the result of either an elevated rate of tear evaporation, often secondary to tear film composition abnormalities, or a diminished rate of tear secretion. The dehydration of the ocular surface and increase in tear film osmolality seen in DED have been demonstrated to lead to initiation of an inflammatory cascade, with activation of CD4+ T cells and production of proinflammatory cytokines such as TNF-α. These proinflammatory cytokines lead to MAP kinase activation and increased matrix metalloproteinase (MMP) expression. In animal models, doxycycline has been demonstrated to decrease MMP-9 expression and MMP-2 activity in addition to decreasing corneal permeability and improving corneal smoothness (Burns et al. 1989, De Paiva et al. 2006, Seedor et al. 1987). However, no clinical trials support the use of doxycycline for DED at present, with one randomized controlled trial demonstrating no symptomatic improvement in patients with Sjögren's syndrome on 20 mg doxycycline PO daily (Seitsalo et al. 2007).

Non-gonococcal conjunctivitis

Bacterial conjunctivitis in adults is generally caused by *Staphylococcus* species and *Streptococcus pneumoniae*. In children, *Haemophilus influenzae* and *Moraxella catarrhalis* are the most common causes of bacterial conjunctivitis, while contact lens wearers are often subject to infection with Gram-negative organisms such as *Pseudomonas aeruginosa*. To date, 10 randomized controlled trials have been published, comparing the use of antibiotics in bacterial conjunctivitis against placebo, all but two of which demonstrated a higher rate of microbial and clinical cure with antibiotic administration. The two studies that failed to demonstrate better outcomes with antibiotic use involved fusidic acid and chloramphenicol, while the fluoroquinolones—levofloxacin, ciprofloxacin, ofloxacin, norfloxacin, and besifloxacin—and the macrolide azithromycin have all been demonstrated to be superior to placebo in bacterial conjunctivitis (Hutnik & Mohammad-Shahi 2010, Rietveld et al. 2005, Rose et al. 2005).

Numerous randomized controlled trials have been performed to compare the efficacies of antibiotics in the treatment of bacterial conjunctivitis. To date, no single preferred antibiotic has emerged, with several trials demonstrating no differences in cure rates or time in clinical or microbial cure among various sets of antibiotics. Generally, a broad-spectrum, bactericidal topical antibiotic is recommended for treatment of bacterial conjunctivitis until Gram stain, culture results, or other classifying data can be obtained. Once a bacterial etiology can be determined with some confidence, coverage can be narrowed as appropriate.

In total, five classes of topical antibiotic are commonly available for use in bacterial conjunctivitis. These classes include the aforementioned fluoroquinolones and macrolides, in addition to peptides (polymyxin B combinations and bacitracin), aminoglycosides, and sulfas. Fluoroquinolones generally have a broader spectrum of coverage and a cleaner side-effect profile than the other classes mentioned. Besifloxacin, a relatively new fourth-generation fluoroqinolone, improves further upon the Gram-positive coverage of the fluoroquinolones, while maintaining their Gram-negative activity and tid dosing to achieve the needed concentration for efficacy in bacterial conjunctivitis. In a prospective, randomized controlled trial, besifloxacin was recently shown to be non-inferior to moxifloxacin in the treatment of bacterial conjunctivitis (McDonald et al. 2009). Polymyxin B combinations have broad-spectrum coverage similar to that of the fluoroquinolones, while maintaining a similarly favorable side-effect profile. The aminoglycosides can cause corneal ulceration with prolonged use and provide relatively weak streptococcal coverage, but are effective against Gram-negative organisms. Sulfa drugs, while providing good Gram-positive coverage, are limited in their use by patient allergy.

Despite the often self-limiting course of bacterial conjunctivitis, antibiotic therapy is important not only for its acceleration of recovery, but also for its prevention of progression to conditions such as anterior uveitis and bacterial keratitis.

■ Gonococcal conjunctivitis

Gonococcal conjunctivitis is a hyperacute form of conjunctivitis characterized by a rapid onset of profuse purulent secretion, ocular injection, and chemosis. Due to concern for fluoroquinolone resistance, gonococcal conjunctivitis is generally treated with a loading dose of 1 g intramuscular (IM) ceftriaxone, followed by a subsequent 1 g intravenous (IV) dose 12–24 hours later. Upon completion of these two doses, antibiotic coverage for non-gonococcal coinfection may be added with either erythromycin 250–500 mg PO daily, tetracycline 250–500 mg PO daily, or doxycycline 100 mg PO bid.

■ Bacterial keratitis

Bacterial keratitis can be difficult to distinguish from other forms of microbial keratitis and non-infectious keratitis. The clinician should be able to clinically estimate a likelihood of bacterial keratitis based on corneal signs, such as the status of the epithelium, the type of stromal inflammation, and the pattern of stromal involvement, as well as the patient's history, the clinical setting, and locally predominant pathogens. The treatment for a suspected bacterial keratitis depends on several factors, including the severity of infection, the aforementioned clinical signs, and local antibiotic resistance patterns. Depending on the clinical picture, the treating physician may consider one of the following three avenues: deferring treatment until laboratory evidence is obtained, initiating broad-spectrum antibiotic treatment, or initiating narrow-spectrum antibiotic treatment.

The traditional approach to treatment of bacterial keratitis focuses on achieving eradication of the causative organism. The tissue concentration necessary to rapidly eliminate the causative organism makes toxicity a central consideration in therapy for bacterial keratitis (O'Brien 2003). The use of parenteral antibiotics is generally avoided without impending perforation, intraocular spread, or systemic spread

due to the toxicity associated with the high serum levels necessary to achieve the required corneal tissue concentrations. The frequency of dosing also makes the question of inpatient or outpatient therapy a consideration. For patients with severe bacterial keratitis and those with poor compliance, the required antibiotic dosing frequency may make inpatient therapy more appropriate.

Several routes of administration are available to the clinician treating bacterial keratitis. Topical drop formulations remain the most widely used, but topical gels and ointments are also available. While antibiotic gels and ointments offer inherent lubrication, the need for dissolution of these agents in the precorneal tear film slows the process of achieving the desired tissue concentration. In addition to the aforementioned topical and parenteral formulations, subconjunctival injections, continuous lavage devices, polymer inserts, and transcorneal iontophoresis offer means to administer therapy for bacterial keratitis. While subconjunctival injections can aid in the treatment of the non-compliant patient or the patient with impending corneal perforation, they are generally avoided due to their ability to cause pain, subconjunctival hemorrhage, and conjunctival scarring. Continuous lavage, although offering the ability to achieve high tissue antibiotic concentrations and mechanical irrigation, is generally avoided due to expense, need for patient immobilization, and potential for epithelial trauma.

As with bacterial conjunctivitis, choosing an antibiotic with the appropriate spectrum of coverage is paramount. In polymicrobial keratitis or bacterial keratitis in which laboratory data is unavailable, a broad spectrum of coverage is desirable. Combined Gram-positive and Gram-negative coverage has traditionally been achieved with multiple agents, but can be achieved with a single agent as well. Agents commonly used in bacterial keratitis are listed in **Table 35.1**. Due to the prevalence of penicillinase-resistant *Staphylococcus* species, cephalosporins such as cefazolin are the most commonly used drugs for broad Gram-positive coverage. In patients unable to tolerate cephalosporins, vancomycin offers an alternative for Gram-positive coverage. The aminoglycoside antibiotics are generally preferred for achieving broad Gram-negative coverage. Gentamicin was commonly the aminoglycoside of choice for Gram-negative coverage, but has been superseded by tobramycin due to the development of gentamicin-resistant *P. aeruginosa* strains. (microbial keratitis secondary to *P. aeruginosa* infection is depicted in **Figure 35.1**) Accordingly, fortified drops of cefazolin (50 mg/mL) or vancomycin (50 mg/mL), in combination with tobramycin (13.6 mg/mL), represent the commonly used regimen for severe bacterial keratitis with unidentified causative organism(s). The fluoroquinolones offer an alternate means of achieving broad Gram-negative and Gram-positive coverage, with gatifloxacin, levofloxacin, and moxifloxacin all in common use at their commercial concentrations, given their relatively high potency. A new fluoroquinolone, besifloxacin, has been demonstrated to have greater potency against Gram positives than existing fluoroquinolones. In particular, besifloxacin has been demonstrated to have an eightfold lower minimum inhibitory concentration than gatifloxacin and moxifloxacin against methicillin-resistant *Staphylococcus aureus* in animal models, and may be appropriate for infections occurring in the hospital setting (Sanders et al. 2009, 2010).

More specific therapies can be applied after the identification of the causative organism(s). In streptococcal keratitis, Penicillin G 100,000 U/mL is the drug of choice. Gonococcal keratitis, like gonococcal conjunctivitis, is generally treated with ceftriaxone due to the emergence of penicillin-resistant strains of *Neisseria gonorrhoeae*. Nocardial keratitis

Table 35.1 Topical antibiotics used in the treatment of bacterial conjunctivitis

Antibiotic	Class	Coverage	Mechanism	Availability
Azithromycin	Macrolide	Broad spectrum	Bacteriostatic	Azasite 1% (Inspire Pharmaceuticals Inc)
Besifloxacin	Fluoroquinolone	Broad spectrum	Bactericidal	Besivance 0.6% (Bausch and Lomb)
Chloramphenicol	Chloramphenicol	Broad spectrum	Bacteriostatic	Topical drops not marketed in US; Optrex Infected Eyes 0.5% in UK
Ciprofloxacin	Fluoroquinolone	Broad spectrum	Bactericidal	Ciloxan 0.3% (Alcon Laboratories Inc) ointment or drops
Fusidic acid	Protein synthesis inhibitor	Primarily Gram positive	Bacteriostatic	Not available in US; Fucithalmic 1% (Leo Pharma) in Canada and UK
Gatifloxacin	Fluoroquinolone	Broad spectrum	Bactericidal	Zymar 0.3% (Allergan Inc)
Gentamicin	Aminoglycoside	Primarily Gram negative	Bactericidal	Generic 0.3% drops
Levofloxacin	Fluoroquinolone	Broad spectrum	Bactericidal	Iquix 1.5% (Vistakon Pharmaceuticals)
Lomeofloxacin	Fluoroquinolone	Broad spectrum	Bactericidal	Not available in US
Moxifloxacin	Fluoroquinolone	Broad spectrum	Bactericidal	Vigamox 0.5% (Alcon Laboratories Inc)
Neomycin-polymyxin B-gramcidin	Aminoglycoside	Broad spectrum	Bactericidal	Neosporin (King Pharmaceuticals Inc)
Netilimicin	Aminoglycoside	Primarily Gram negative	Bactericidal	Not available in US
Norfloxacin	Fluoroquinolone	Broad spectrum	Bactericidal	Chibroxin 0.3% (Merck and Co Inc); not available in US
Ofloxacin	Fluoroquinolone	Broad spectrum	Bactericidal	Generic 0.3% eye drops
Povidone-iodine		Broad spectrum	Bactericidal	Betadine 5% (Alcon Laboratories Inc)
Rifamycin	Rifamycin	Broad spectrum	Bactericidal	Not available in US
Tobramycin	Aminoglycoside	Primarily Gram negative	Bactericidal	Tobrex 0.3% (Alcon Laboratories Inc) ointment or drops

Adapted from Hutnik and Mohammad-Shahi (2010).

can be effectively treated with trimethoprim-sulfamethoxazole drops, with doses of 61 mg/mL and 80 mg/mL, respectively. Non-tuberculous mycobacterial keratitis, such as that caused by *Mycobacterium fortuitum* or *Mycobacterium chelonae*, has traditionally been treated with topical amikacin 10–20 mg/mL. The prevalence of amikacin-resistant mycobacterial strains has led to the use the fluoroquinolones ofloxacin, ciprofloxacin, gatifloxacin, and moxifloxacin. For those mycobacterial strains demonstrating resistance to fluoroquinolones, topical formulations of the macrolides clarithromycin (10–40 mg/mL) and azithromycin (2 mg/mL) are now used.

Once the choice of antibiotic has been made, 'loading' is performed to achieve a bactericidal tissue concentration rapidly. This process involves applying one antibiotic drop every 2 minutes for five applications. Once this process has been completed, antibiotic drops are administered every 30 minutes for the first 24–72 hours, alternating drugs when multiple antibiotics are used. If the patient appears to be responding clinically, the frequency of antibiotic administration can begin to be tapered. This commonly occurs within 36–48 hours of initiation of effective bactericidal therapy, with halting of keratitis progression by 48–72 hours from initiation of treatment. These processes are marked by a halting of the progression of stromal infiltrates and the initiation of re-epithelialization.

ANTIFUNGALS

Of the fungal infections of the ocular surface, only fungal keratitis is a well-defined clinical entity. Accordingly, this section will focus on the use of antifungal medications (see **Table 35.2**) in the treatment of fungal keratitis.

Antifungal therapy for fungal keratitis

Fungal keratitis often occurs in one of three clinical scenarios—trauma, superinfection of a prior bacterial infection, and immunosuppression. The most common of these scenarios is trauma involving fungus-contaminated plant material. In fungal keratitis related to trauma, the most common causative organisms are filamentous fungi such as *Fusarium* and *Aspergillus*. In fungal superinfection of the cornea or fungal keratitis in the setting of immunosuppression, *Candida* species are the most common causative agents. Also, less likely, contact lens wearers using contaminated cleaning or storage solutions may develop fusarium keratitis. Due to the relatively slow growth of the filamentous fungi, keratitis secondary to *Fusarium* and *Aspergillus* infection may go unrecognized and untreated for days or weeks. For mild to moderate infections, topical antifungals are generally used. Topical natamycin (50 mg/mL) is used for hyphal forms, while topical amphotericin B (1.0–2.5 mg/mL) is recommended for yeast forms. Recently, miconazole 10 mg/mL and voriconazole 1% have been used as well. Each of these topical antifungals is applied for 24–72 hours, at which point the frequency of dosing can be tapered slowly if clinical improvement begins to occur. Tissue concentrations of topical antifungals can be increased through debridement of the corneal epithelium (Kalkanci & Ozdek 2011). Severe infections can be treated with the addition of a sunconjunctival, intracameral, or systemic antifungal. Miconazole is administered either subconjunctivally (1.2 mg daily for 3 weeks) or parenterally (90 mg daily for 3 weeks), while ketoconazole (200–400 mg PO daily to tid), itraconazole, fluconazole (800 mg PO loading, 400 mg daily maintenance), and voriconazole

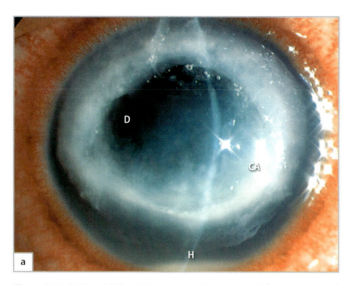
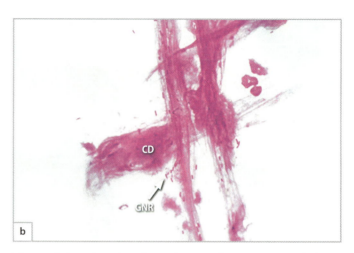

Figure 35.1 (a) Microbial keratitis in a contact lens wearer. Soft contact lenses (especially extended wear lenses) predispose the eye to Gram-negative microbial keratitis. Epithelial hypoxia or other trauma may enable Pseudomonas species to attach to and penetrate the corneal epithelium, rapidly destroy the corneal stroma, and cause perforation. (b) Gram-negative rods (red) are seen in the corneal scrape. CA, cellular abscess; CD, cellular debris; GNR, Gram-negative rods; H, hypopyon. Adapted from David J, Spalton DJ, Hitchings RA, Hunter PA (eds), Atlas of clinical ophthalmology, 3rd edn. Oxford: Elsevier Ltd, 2005.

can be administered orally. Amphotericin B is administered either parenterally (1 mg/kg over 6 hours) or intracamerally.

ANTIVIRALS

Among the viral infections commonly affecting the ocular surface are herpes simplex virus (HSV1 and HSV2), varicella zoster virus (VZV), and various enteroviruses and adenoviruses. While HSV and VZV infections commonly result in keratitis, enteroviruses and adenoviruses can cause conjunctivitides with varying levels of severity. The management of ocular viral infections is complicated by the existence of multiple disease states, the use of anti-inflammatory and immunomodulatory medications, and changing demographics in the face of vaccination (Gordon 2000).

Antiviral therapy for herpes simplex virus infection

HSV infection is a common cause of corneal blindness, but has many ocular manifestations, from eyelid to optic nerve. Ocular surface manifestations include conjunctivitis, episcleritis, scleritis, and keratitis of varying depths (Wilhelmus 2010). Therapy for HSV corneal disease is dependent upon both the phase of the disease (primary, latent, or recurrent) and the depth of the infection (epithelial, stromal, or endothelial). Commonly used antivirals are depicted in **Figure 35.2**. Primary infection with HSV is often subclinical, and most ocular manifestations are seen as the result of recurrent disease. Since conjunctivitis secondary to HSV is difficult to distinguish from other viral conjunctivitides, HSV ocular surface disease is generally diagnosed and characterized by the nature of its corneal involvement.

HSV epithelial keratitis

HSV keratitis involving the corneal epithelium can have several manifestations, including superficial punctate lesions, decreased corneal sensation, and, classically, dendritic lesions. Ulceration along dendritic lesions (depicted in **Figure 35.3a**) is common, and can progress to form geographic ulcers.

Today, the standard therapy for epithelial keratitis includes debridement of the involved epithelium and a topical nucleoside analog (trifluridine or vidarabine) and/or an oral antiviral (acyclovir, famciclovir, or valacyclovir). Trifluridine is a deoxyuridine analog that is generally used six to nine times per day for 5–7 days or until the ulcer begins to heal, and subsequently reduced in frequency to five times per day for 1–2 weeks. Reduction in trifluridine frequency upon evidence of improvement of corneal ulceration is performed to avoid epithelial toxicity and possible allergic reaction, both of which have been documented with topical use (Holdiness 2001). Trifluridine has largely replaced idoxuridine as the deoxyuridine analog of choice for the treatment of HSV epithelial keratitis due to its comparatively less toxicity in regenerating corneal epithelium, empirically greater efficacy (95% vs. 75% in one multicenter trial) (Laibson et al. 1977), and the lack of documented resistance (whereas HSV strains resistant to idoxuridine have been noted) (Coleman et al. 1968). While trifluridine is formulated as a drop, its alternative, vidarabine, is available commercially only as a 3% ointment. In guttate form, vidarabine is less effective than both trifluridine and idoxuridine (Pavan-Langston et al. 1979). Vidarabine in ointment form, however, has been shown to be significantly more effective than guttate idoxuridine, though significantly less effective than guttate trifluridine (Wilhelmus 2010).

Oral antivirals such as acyclovir (400 mg PO tid), famciclovir (250 mg PO daily), and valacyclovir (500 mg PO bid), can be used for 2–3 weeks in place of or in conjunction with topical therapy. A recent meta-analysis of several studies of HSV epithelial keratitis found no significant difference in efficacy or time to healing between topical therapy alone and combined topical and oral antiviral therapy, and no significant difference in efficacy or time to healing between topical and oral therapy (Wilhelmus 2010). In particular, no significant difference was found between efficacy and time to healing between topical therapy with topical trifluridine and oral acyclovir. Accordingly, the choice between oral and topical therapy (or a combination of the two) is largely dependent upon patient factors, such as the ease and effectiveness with which eye drops can be instilled.

Additional antiviral medications have begun to be studied for use in HSV epithelial keratitis, including ganciclovir, foscarnet,

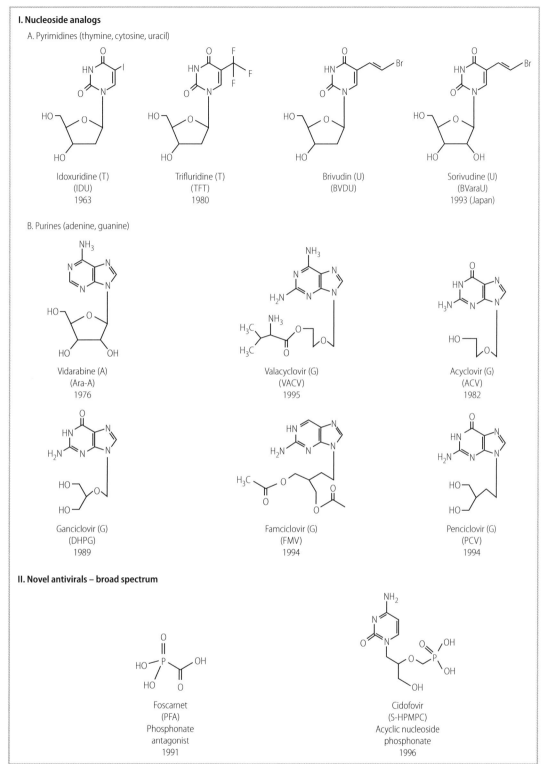

Figure 35.2 Commonly used ophthalmic antivirals. The single letter within the parentheses represents the natural base for each antiviral nucleoside analog. The year indicates date of FDA approval. A, adenine; T, thymine; G, guanine; U, uracil. Adapted from Gordon (2000).

I. Nucleoside analogs

A. Pyrimidines (thymine, cytosine, uracil)

Idoxuridine (T)
(IDU)
1963

Trifluridine (T)
(TFT)
1980

Brivudin (U)
(BVDU)

Sorivudine (U)
(BVaraU)
1993 (Japan)

B. Purines (adenine, guanine)

Vidarabine (A)
(Ara-A)
1976

Valacyclovir (G)
(VACV)
1995

Acyclovir (G)
(ACV)
1982

Ganciclovir (G)
(DHPG)
1989

Famciclovir (G)
(FMV)
1994

Penciclovir (G)
(PCV)
1994

II. Novel antivirals – broad spectrum

Foscarnet
(PFA)
Phosphonate
antagonist
1991

Cidofovir
(S-HPMPC)
Acyclic nucleoside
phosphonate
1996

and cidofovir. Ganciclovir, like acyclovir, is a viral thymidine kinase inhibitor and has been shown to be as safe and effective as acyclovir (Hoh et al.1996, Tabbara & Al Balushi 2010, Wilhelmus 2010). Unlike acyclovir, ganciclovir has been shown to rapidly induce apoptosis in virus-infected cells, which may manifest itself as improved healing time as further studies are performed (Shaw et al. 2001). Foscarnet and cidofovir, both of which are potent inhibi-

tors of HSV replication, remain to be studied in sufficient detail for conclusions to be made regarding their efficacy in the treatment of HSV epithelial keratitis.

Finally, as adjuncts to antiviral therapy, both debridement of epithelial lesions and interferon therapy appear to decrease healing time (68% vs. 53% and 84% vs. 43% at 7 days, respectively), but do not appear to increase overall efficacy (Wilhelmus 2010).

HSV disciform keratitis

Disciform keratitis refers to a self-limited process involving a disc-shaped area of stromal edema, keratic precipitates, and Descemet's folds, with or without endotheliitis, thought to be the result of a cell-mediated immune reaction. Debate continues, however, as to whether disciform keratitis is accompanied by low-level stromal viral replication (Kaufman 2000). Accordingly, the mainstay of treatment for disciform keratitis is not antiviral, but anti-inflammatory (topical prednisolone phosphate 0.12–1.0% daily to qid, with subsequent taper). Antiviral therapy, generally with topical trifluridine daily or acyclovir

Table 35.2 Drugs used in the treatment of fungal keratitis

Group	Mode of action	Antifungals
Azole	Azole derivatives bind to heme moiety of cytochrome P450 and interfere with certain mixed oxidase functions. Fungal a-1-4 demethylation of lanosterol is inhibited, blocking formation of ergo sterol and the accumulation of a-1-4 methyl sterols.	Econazole
		Clotrimazole
		Miconazole
		Itraconazole
		Fluconazole
		Bifonazole
		Ketoconazole
		Oxiconazole
Polyenes	Bind with sterols in fungal cell wall, principally ergosterol, causing leakage of cell contents and ultimately cell death	Amphotericin B
		Collagen shield presoaked with amphotericin B
		Amphotericin B methyl ester
		Natamycin

Adapted from Shukla PK, Kumar M, Keshava GBS. Mycotic keratitis: an overview of diagnosis and therapy. Mycoses 2008; 51:183–199. doi: 10.1111/j.1439-0507.2007.01480.x.

400 mg PO bid, is added in the presence of epithelial involvement or as prophylaxis when treating with steroid doses greater than 0.12% prednisolone phosphate bid.

HSV stromal keratitis

The pathogenesis of HSV stromal keratitis (HSK), depicted in **Figure 35.3b**, is related to a combination of immune complex deposition, cell-mediated immune reaction, and a cytokine-mediated inflammatory cascade (Gordon 2000). In necrotizing forms of the disease, HSV DNA, antigen, and intact virions have been found in the affected corneas, pointing squarely at a role of active HSV replication in pathogenesis in herpetic necrotizing stromal keratitis (HNSK) (Brik et al. 1993, Holbach et al. 1990a, 1990b). The landmark study in the treatment of acute HSK remains the Herpetic Eye Disease Study (HEDS), which demonstrated the value of a 10-week course of 1% prednisolone phosphate combined with topical trifluridine (Wilhelmus et al. 1994). Combined steroid and trifluridine therapy was shown to reduce the duration and rate of progression of HSK, with no increased risk of recurrent HSV infection versus placebo. Addition of oral acyclovir to this regimen provided no improvement in outcomes (Barron et al. 1994). However, HEDS did not differentiate between necrotizing and non-necrotizing HSK, and more recent studies indicate a role for tailored therapies in better-differentiated cases. In patients with non-necrotizing HSK, intolerant of or unresponsive to steroids, three prospective studies have indicated that topical cyclosporin A (CsA) is effective in treating non-necrotizing HSK (combined 83% HSK resolution rate, with 64% resolution rate of prior neovascularization) (Gündüz & Ozdemir 1997, Heiligenhaus & Steuhl 1999, Rao 2006). No significant adverse effects have been seen when using Restasis or artificial tear-based formulations of CsA. Multiple studies have begun to examine a role of amniotic membrane transplant (AMT) in HNSK by potentially reducing inflammation and lessening the likelihood of perforation in severely affected corneas. While in vitro and animal subject data indicate a possible role for AMT in treating HNSK through a combination of anti-inflammatory

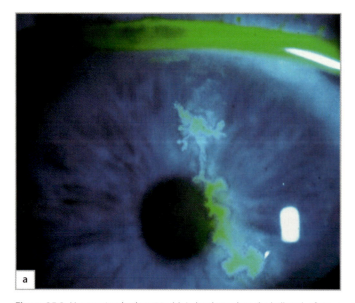

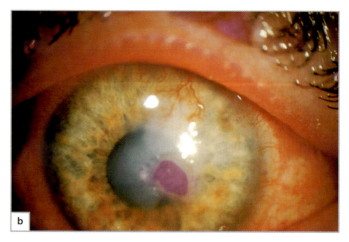

Figure 35.3 Herpes simplex keratitis. (a) A dendritic ulcer, the hallmark of recurrent corneal herpetic epithelial keratitis. Fluorescein stains the area of epithelial cell loss; disease is limited to the epithelium. Dendritic ulcers generally heal within 7 days of initiation of an effective topical antiviral agent. (b) Chronic active stromal herpes simplex keratitis, which involves reactivation of viral replication in the stroma with an associated immune response. This patient has an area of ulceration surrounded by stromal edema and infiltrate in an old herpetic scar, as well as an area of superficial corneal vascularization. Adapted from David J, Spalton DJ, Hitchings RA, Hunter PA (eds), Atlas of clinical ophthalmology, 3rd edn. Oxford: Elsevier Ltd, 2005.

factors (interleukin (IL)-10, IL-1ra, activin, and protease inhibitors), inhibition of neutrophil and macrophage chemotaxis, inhibition of endothelial cell proliferation and migration, and promotion of T- and B-lymphocyte apoptosis (Heiligenhaus et al. 2001, Mencucci et al.2011), no prospective clinical studies support the use of AMT for HNSK to date.

Recurrent HSV keratitis

While inducing resolution of active infection is paramount, the prevention of recurrence or progression of one form of HSV keratitis to a more dangerous form is essential for the long-term visual health of a patient. On this front, the HEDS II provided important results, demonstrating that long-term therapy with acyclovir 400 mg bid significantly reduced the 1-year recurrence rate of all forms of ocular HSV (18% vs. 30%) and was particularly effective in reducing the recurrence rate of HSK (8% vs. 13%), while being less effective in reducing the recurrence of HSV epithelial keratitis (9% vs. 11%) (The Herpetic Eye Disease Study Group 1997). However, treatment of epithelial herpetic disease with oral acyclovir combined with a topical antiviral did not reduce the likelihood of developing stromal disease.

Prevention of HSV keratitis is of particular importance in patients who will undergo or have already undergone penetrating keratoplasty (PK). Although HEDS II demonstrated the efficacy of oral acyclovir in reducing recurrence of HSK, the study excluded those patients who had undergone PK. Recent studies have examined the efficacy of both oral and topical antivirals postoperatively in patients undergoing PK. The use of topical antivirals as prophylaxis against recurrent disease is generally avoided due to findings of epithelial toxicity, delayed wound healing, and persistent epithelial defects with long-term therapy. In addition, topical antiviral prophylaxis has not been found to reduce the incidence of graft failure after PK (Moyes et al. 1994). Multiple studies confirm the benefit of using an oral systemic antiviral postoperatively to reduce both the rate of disease recurrence and the rate of graft failure. Questions remain, however, as to the best oral antiviral to use, the optimal dosage of that antiviral, and the optimal duration of prophylactic treatment post-PK. Most studies performed on this topic have involved the use of oral acyclovir, and have demonstrated up to a 70% reduction in risk of graft failure at 5 years (Goodfellow et al. 2011), often utilizing a regimen of 400 mg PO acyclovir bid. Recently, valacyclovir has been studied for this purpose as well, and has been found to be at least as effective as acyclovir as post-PK prophylaxis. Oral antiviral prophylaxis post-PK has been shown to improve 5-year graft survival rates with as little as 6 months of treatment (Jansen et al. 2009), despite traditional recommendations of greater than 1 year of treatment post-PK (Garcia et al. 2007, van Rooij et al. 2003, Tambasco et al. 1999).

New approaches to treatment of recurrent HSV keratitis

In addition to the use of oral antivirals in the treatment of recurrent HSV disease, vaccines, ganglionic blockers, and immunomodulatory medications have been used with varying levels of success. To date, several inactivated whole virus vaccines have been attempted, but none of them have shown beneficial results in controlled trials. New vaccination approaches including live attenuated virus vaccines, disabled single-cycle virus vaccines, subunit vaccines, and plasmid DNA vaccines are currently in development and represent promising new approaches to the suppression or prevention of ocular HSV disease (Bernstein & Stanberry 1999, Krause & Straus 1999). In addition,

blockade of the reactivation of HSV at the ganglionic level while in the latent state offers an intuitively appealing means for viral suppression. Thymidine kinase inhibitor 9-(4-hydroxybutyl)-N2-phenylguanine, topical bromfenac sodium, intraperitoneal geldanamycin, IM AMP, alpha-blockers thymoxamine and corynanthine, and beta-blocker propranolol have all been demonstrated to reduce reactivation of latent HSV-1 in animal models (Gebhardt et al. 1996, Kaufman et al. 1996). The efficacy of these medications in clinical practice remains to be studied.

■ Antiviral therapy for herpes zoster keratitis

Ocular surface involvement in Herpes zoster ophthalmicus (HZO) is a potentially blinding condition. Prior to the initiation of use of oral acyclovir in 1982, topical antivirals such as idoxuridine and vidarabine had failed to demonstrate therapeutic efficacy in HZO. The introduction of oral acyclovir created a new standard of care in management of HZO. In 1986, a landmark trial demonstrated that oral acyclovir reduced dendritic keratitis, episcleritis, and iritis during the acute phase of infection, and reduced the rate of development of subsequent chronic stromal keratitis (McKendrick et al. 1986). The subsequent development of thymidine kinase negative acyclovir-resistant VZV has been handled with IV foscarnet.

The introduction of the oral antivirals famciclovir (prodrug of penciclovir) and valacyclovir (prodrug of acyclovir) in the mid-1990s once again changed the standard of care in the management of zoster. The prodrug formulation of these drugs allowed for achievement of increased serum concentrations and, ultimately, simpler dosing regimens. In addition, both drugs have been demonstrated to be superior to acyclovir in the resolution of acute pain in zoster (Beutner et al. 1995, Tyring et al. 1995). Accordingly, currently suggested regimens for acute HZO include acyclovir 800 mg PO five times daily, famciclovir 500 mg PO tid, or valacyclovir 1 g PO tid, each for 7–10 days. Ideally, each should be started within 72 hours of rash onset, with the addition of steroids, cycloplegics, and IOP reduction as necessary. While oral antivirals more potent than acyclovir, famciclovir, and valacyclovir have been developed, such as sorivudine, safety concerns regarding these more potent antivirals have prevented their adoption (Bell et al. 1997, Gnann et al. 1998).

Today, widespread vaccination of children against VZV has changed the landscape of disease secondary to VZV. Despite its original development in Japan in 1974, adoption of the vaccine in the United States only occurred in 1995. In addition to concerns regarding the long-term efficacy of the vaccine, adoption in the United States was delayed as a result of concerns that infant vaccination may increase rates of adult herpes zoster due to expected decreases in periodic adult exposure to children infected with varicella, which is thought to boost cell-mediated immunity (CMI) against VZV in adults. The effectiveness of the VZV vaccine in preventing initial infection with varicella has thus created a need for effective means of boosting VZV-specific CMI. A booster vaccine for this purpose is approved only for adults over 60 at present. In the very long term, however, the varicella vaccine virus (VVV) will likely replace wild-type VZV at the population level, and as VVV has a significantly lower risk of reactivation than wild-type VZV, the risk of herpes zoster is expected to decline overall (Liesegang 2008). Accordingly, given the currently available vaccination techniques, a rise in herpes zoster rates is expected in the coming decades, followed by a significant decline.

Therapy for ocular adenoviral infections

Adenoviral infections of the ocular surface have a wide range of natural histories, but most tend to be highly contagious, with virus shed for up to 2 weeks after symptom onset. Over 50 different strains of adenoviridae are known to cause conjunctivitis. Epidemic keratoconjunctivitis (EKC) is a particularly contagious conjunctivitis caused primarily by adenovirus type 8 (Ad8), Ad19, and Ad37. The common form of EKC is a severe conjunctivitis that may be accompanied by fibrin pseudomembranes, hemorrhage, epithelial keratitis, and severe pain. The epithelial keratitis may progress to a subepithelial infiltration that may become persistent. While adenoviral ocular infections are generally considered self-limiting, with active treatment (if any) focusing on reducing the ocular inflammatory response, several drugs have been studied with regard to their ability to decrease the duration of viral shedding and symptoms in EKC and other adenoviral ocular infections.

The topical antivirals idoxuridine, vidarabine, trifluridine, and acyclovir have demonstrated no clinical efficacy in adenoviral ocular infections to date. However, topical and IV formulations of cidofovir have been noted in case reports to promote resolution of symptoms and possible prophylaxis against infection in the contralateral eye (Skevaki et al. 2011). Topical 1% N-chlorotaurine has been shown to reduce the duration of illness in one study of 33 patients (Teuchner et al. 2005), while a mixture of 0.4% povidone iodine and 0.1% dexamethasone daily for 5 days was shown to promote clinical resolution and reduce viral titers in a study of five patients (Pelletier et al. 2009). In vitro results indicate potential roles for the nucleoside analog reverse transcriptase inhibitors (NARTIs) zalcitabine and stavudine in the treatment of ocular adenoviral infections. An additional approach with promising in vitro results thus far is the conjugation of sialic acid to non-polar tails, which prevents the binding to and infection of conjunctival cells by adenoviral virions (Aplander et al. 2011).

Therapy for enterovirus infections

Enteroviridae can create a hemorrhagic conjunctivitis like that caused by adenoviridae. However, no clinically effective therapies are known for enterovirus infections. In vitro evidence has been gathered supporting possible roles for arildone, interferon-α, benzimidazoles, and most recently, siRNA against the EV70 viral polymerase 3D gene (Jun et al. 2011, Langford et al. 1985, 1995).

Therapy for other viral infections

Common viruses with ocular manifestations other than those already mentioned include Epstein–Barr virus (EBV), measles, mumps, and rubella. While EBV is known to cause a distinctive stromal keratitis, no specific treatment exists for the ocular EBV infection. Ocular manifestations of measles, mumps, and rubella, likewise, have no specific therapies. Unlike EBV, infection with these three viruses can be effectively prevented with vaccination.

REFERENCES

Aplander K, Marttila M, Manner S, et al. Molecular wipes: application to epidemic keratoconjunctivitis. *J Med Chem* 2011; **54**:6670–6675.

Aronowicz JD, Shine WE, Oral D, Vargas JM, McCulley JP. Short term oral minocycline treatment of meibomianitis. *Br J Ophthalmol* 2006; **90**:856–860.

Barron BA, Gee L, Hauck WW, et al. Herpetic Eye Disease Study. A controlled trial of oral acyclovir for herpes simplex stromal keratitis. *Ophthalmology* 1994; **101**:1871–1882.

Bartholomew RS, Reid BJ, Cheesbrough MJ, Macdonald M, Galloway NR. Oxytetracycline in the treatment of ocular rosacea: a double-blind trial. *Br J Ophthalmol* 1982; **66**:386–388.

Bell WR, Chulay JD, Feinberg JE. Manifestations resembling thrombotic microangiopathy in patients with advanced human immunodeficiency virus (HIV) disease in a cytomegalovirus prophylaxis trial (ACTG 204). *Medicine* 1997; **76**:369–380.

Bernstein DI, Stanberry LR. Herpes simplex virus vaccines. *Vaccine* 1999; **17**:1681–1689.

Beutner KR, Friedman DJ, Forszpaniak C, Andersen PL, Wood MJ. Valaciclovir compared with acyclovir for improved therapy for herpes zoster in immunocompetent adults. *Antimicrob Agents Chemother* 1995; **39**:1546–1553.

Brik D, Dunkel E, Pavan-Langston D. Herpetic keratitis: persistence of viral particles despite topical and systemic antiviral therapy. Report of two cases and review of the literature. *Arch Ophthalmol* 1993; **111**:522–527.

Burns FR, Stack MS, Gray RD, Paterson CA. Inhibition of purified collagenase from alkali-burned rabbit corneas. *Investig Ophthalmol Visual Sci* 1989; **30**:1569–1575.

Coleman VR, Tsu E, Jawetz E. "Treatment-resistance" to idoxuridine in herpetic keratitis. Proceedings of the Society for Experimental Biology and Medicine. *Exp Biol Med* 1968; **129**:761–765.

De Paiva CS, Corrales RM, Villarreal AL, et al. Corticosteroid and doxycycline suppress MMP-9 and inflammatory cytokine expression, MAPK activation in the corneal epithelium in experimental dry eye. *Exp Eye Res* 2006; **83**:526–535.

Federici TJ. The non-antibiotic properties of tetracyclines: clinical potential in ophthalmic disease. *Pharmacol Res* 2011; **6**:1–10.

Garcia DD, Farjo Q, Musch DC, Sugar A. Effect of prophylactic oral acyclovir after penetrating keratoplasty for herpes simplex keratitis. *Cornea* 2007; **26**:930–934.

Gebhardt BM, Wright GE, Xu H, et al. 9-(4-Hydroxybutyl)-N2-phenylguanine (HBPG), a thymidine kinase inhibitor, suppresses herpes virus reactivation in mice. *Antiviral Res* 1996; **30**:87–94.

Gnann JW, Crumpacker CS, Lalezari JP, et al. Sorivudine versus acyclovir for treatment of dermatomal herpes zoster in human immunodeficiency virus-infected patients: results from a randomized, controlled clinical trial. Collaborative Antiviral Study Group/AIDS Clinical Trials Group, Herpes Zoster Study Group. *Antimicrob Agents Chemother* 1998; **42**:1139–1145.

Goodfellow JF, Nabili S, Jones MN, et al. Antiviral treatment following penetrating keratoplasty for herpetic keratitis. *Eye* 2011; **25**:470–474.

Gordon YJ. The evolution of antiviral therapy for external ocular viral infections over twenty-five years. *Cornea* 2000; **19**:673–680. http://www.ncbi.nlm.nih.gov/pubmed/11009319 (Last accessed 18 April 2013.)

Gündüz K, Ozdemir O. Topical cyclosporin as an adjunct to topical acyclovir treatment in herpetic stromal keratitis. *Ophthalmic Res* 1997; **29**:405–408.

Haque RM, Torkildsen GL, Brubaker K, et al. Multicenter open-label study evaluating the efficacy of azithromycin ophthalmic solution 1% on the signs and symptoms of subjects with blepharitis. *Cornea* 2010; **29**:871–877.

Heiligenhaus A, Bauer D, Meller D, Steuhl KP, Tseng SC. Improvement of HSV-1 necrotizing keratitis with amniotic membrane transplantation. *Investig Ophthalmol Visual Sci* 2001; **42**:1969–1974.

Heiligenhaus A, Steuhl KP. Treatment of HSV-1 stromal keratitis with topical cyclosporin A: a pilot study. *Graefe's Arch Clin Exp Ophthalmol (Albrecht von Graefes Archiv für klinische und experimentelle Ophthalmologie)* 1999; **237**:435–438.

Hoh HB, Hurley C, Claoue C, et al. Randomised trial of ganciclovir and acyclovir in the treatment of herpes simplex dendritic keratitis: a multicentre study. *Br J Ophthalmol* 1996; **80**:140–143.

Holbach LM, Font RL, Baehr W, Pittler SJ. HSV antigens and HSV DNA in avascular and vascularized lesions of human herpes simplex keratitis. *Curr Eye Res* 1990a; 10 suppl:63–68.

Holbach LM, Font RL, Naumann GO. Herpes simplex stromal and endothelial keratitis. Granulomatous cell reactions at the level of Descemet's membrane, the stroma, and Bowman's layer. *Ophthalmology* 1990b; **97**:722–728.

Holdiness MR. Contact dermatitis from topical antiviral drugs. *Contact Dermatitis* 2001; **44**:265–269.

Hutnik C, Mohammad-Shahi MH. Bacterial conjunctivitis. *Clin Ophthalmol* 2010; **4**:1451–1457. doi: 10.2147/OPTH.S10162.

Jansen AFG, Rijneveld WJ, Remeijer L, et al. Five-year follow-up on the effect of oral acyclovir after penetrating keratoplasty for herpetic keratitis. *Cornea* 2009; **28**:843–845.

Jun EJ, Won MA, Ahn J, et al. An antiviral small-interfering RNA simultaneously effective against the most prevalent enteroviruses causing acute hemorrhagic conjunctivitis. *Investig Ophthalmol Visual Sci* 2011; **52**:58–63.

Kalkanci A, Ozdek S. Ocular fungal infections. *Curr Eye Res* 2011; **36**:179–189.

Kaufman HE. Treatment of viral diseases of the cornea and external eye. *Prog Retin Eye Res* 2000; **19**:69–85.

Kaufman HE, Varnell ED, Wright GE, et al. Effect of 9-(4-hydroxybutyl)-N2-phenylguanine (HBPG), a thymidine kinase inhibitor, on clinical recurrences of ocular herpetic keratitis in squirrel monkeys. *Antiviral Res* 1996; **33**:65–72.

Krause PR, Straus SE. Herpesvirus vaccines. Development, controversies, and applications. *Infect Dis Clin North Am* 1999; **13**:61–81, vi.

Laibson PR, Arentsen JJ, Mazzanti WD, Eiferman RA. Double controlled comparison of IDU and trifluorothymidine in thirty-three patients with superficial herpetic keratitis. *Trans Am Ophthalmol Soc* 1977; **75**:316–324.

Langford MP, Ball WA, Ganley JP. Inhibition of the enteroviruses that cause acute hemorrhagic conjunctivitis (AHC) by benzimidazoles; enviroxime (LY 122772) and enviradone (LY 127123). *Antiviral Res* 1995; **27**:355–365.

Langford MP, Carr DJ, Yin-Murphy M. Activity of arildone with or without interferon against acute hemorrhagic conjunctivitis viruses in cell culture. *Antimicrob Agents Chemother* 1985; **28**:578–580.

Liesegang TJ. Herpes zoster ophthalmicus natural history, risk factors, clinical presentation, and morbidity. *Ophthalmology* 2008; **115**:S3–S12.

McDonald MB, Protzko EE, Brunner LS, et al. Efficacy and safety of besifloxacin ophthalmic suspension 0.6% compared with moxifloxacin ophthalmic solution 0.5% for treating bacterial conjunctivitis. *Ophthalmology* 2009; **116**:1615.e1-1623.e1.

McKendrick MW, McGill JI, White JE, Wood MJ. Oral acyclovir in acute herpes zoster. *Br Med J* 1986; **293**:1529–1532.

Mencucci R, Paladini I, Menchini U, Gicquel JJ, Dei R. Inhibition of viral replication in vitro by antiviral-treated amniotic membrane. Possible use of amniotic membrane as drug-delivering tool. *Br J Ophthalmol* 2011; **95**:28–31.

Moyes AL, Sugar A, Musch DC, Barnes RD. Antiviral therapy after penetrating keratoplasty for herpes simplex keratitis. *Arch Ophthalmol* 1994: **112**:601–607.

O'Brien TP. Management of bacterial keratitis: beyond exorcism towards consideration of organism and host factors. *Eye* 2003; **17**:957–974.

Pavan-Langston D, Lass J, Campbell R. Antiviral drops: comparative therapy of experimental herpes simplex keratouveitis. *Arch Ophthalmol* 1979; **97**:1132–1135.

Pelletier JS, Stewart K, Trattler W, et al. A combination povidone-iodine 0.4%/dexamethasone 0.1% ophthalmic suspension in the treatment of adenoviral conjunctivitis. *Adv Ther* 2009; **26**:776–783.

Quarterman MJ, Johnson DW, Abele DC, et al. Ocular rosacea. Signs, symptoms, and tear studies before and after treatment with doxycycline. *Arch Dermatol* 1997; **133**:49–54.

Rao SN. Treatment of herpes simplex virus stromal keratitis unresponsive to topical prednisolone 1% with topical cyclosporine 0.05%. *Am J Ophthalmol* 2006; **141**:771–772.

Rietveld RP, ter Riet G, Bindels PJ, et al. The treatment of acute infectious conjunctivitis with fusidic acid: a randomised controlled trial. *Br J Gen Pract* 2005; **55**:924–930.

van Rooij J, Rijneveld WJ, Remeijer L, et al. Effect of oral acyclovir after penetrating keratoplasty for herpetic keratitis: a placebo-controlled multicenter trial. *Ophthalmology* 2003; **110**:1916–1919; discussion 1919.

Rose PW, Harnden A, Brueggemann AB, et al. Chloramphenicol treatment for acute infective conjunctivitis in children in primary care: a randomised double-blind placebo-controlled trial. *Lancet* 2005; **366**:37–43

Sanders ME, Moore QC, Norcross EW, Shafiee A, Marquart ME. Efficacy of besifloxacin in an early treatment model of methicillin-resistant Staphylococcus aureus keratitis. *J Ocul Pharmacol Ther* 2010; **26**:193–198.

Sanders ME, Norcross EW, Moore QC, Shafiee A, Marquart ME. Efficacy of besifloxacin in a rabbit model of methicillin-resistant Staphylococcus aureus keratitis. *Cornea* 2009; **28**:1055–1060.

Seedor JA, Perry HD, McNamara TF, et al. Systemic tetracycline treatment of alkali-induced corneal ulceration in rabbits. *Arch Ophthalmol* 1987; **105**:268–271.

Seitsalo H, Niemelä RK, Marinescu-Gava M, et al. Effectiveness of low-dose doxycycline (LDD) on clinical symptoms of Sjögren's syndrome: a randomized, double-blind, placebo controlled cross-over study. *J Negative Results Biomed* 2007; **6**:11.

Shaw MM, Gürr WK, Watts PA, Littler E, Field HJ. Ganciclovir and penciclovir, but not acyclovir, induce apoptosis in herpes simplex virus thymidine kinase-transformed baby hamster kidney cells. *Antivir Chem Chemother* 2001; **12**:175–186.

Skevaki CL, Galani IE, Pararas MV, Giannopoulou KP, Tsakris A. Treatment of viral conjunctivitis with antiviral drugs. *Drugs* 2011; **71**:331–347.

Tabbara KF, Al Balushi N. Topical ganciclovir in the treatment of acute herpetic keratitis. *Clin Ophthalmol* 2010; **4**:905 912.

Tambasco FP, Cohen EJ, Nguyen LH, Rapuano CJ, Laibson PR. Oral acyclovir after penetrating keratoplasty for herpes simplex keratitis. *Arch Ophthalmol* 1999; **117**:445–449.

Teuchner B, Nagl M, Schidlbauer A, et al. Tolerability and efficacy of N-chlorotaurine in epidemic keratoconjunctivitis—a double-blind, randomized, phase-2 clinical trial. *J Ocul Pharmacol Ther* 2005; **21**:157–165.

The Herpetic Eye Disease Study Group. A controlled trial of oral acyclovir for the prevention of stromal keratitis or iritis in patients with herpes simplex virus epithelial keratitis. The Epithelial Keratitis Trial. *Arch Ophthalmol* 1997; **115**:703–712.

Tyring S, Barbarash RA, Nahlik JE, et al. Famciclovir for the treatment of acute herpes zoster: effects on acute disease and postherpetic neuralgia. A randomized, double-blind, placebo-controlled trial. Collaborative Famciclovir Herpes Zoster Study Group. *Ann Intern Med* 1995; **123**:89–96.

Veldman P, Colby K. Current evidence for topical azithromycin 1 % ophthalmic solution in the treatment of blepharitis and blepharitis-associated ocular dryness. *Int Ophthalmol Clin* 2011; **51**:43–52.

Wilhelmus K. Antiviral treatment and other therapeutic interventions for herpes simplex virus epithelial keratitis. Cochrane Database Syst Rev 2010; CD002898. http://www.update-software.com/BCP/WileyPDF/EN/CD002898.pdf (Last accessed 18 April 2013.)

Wilhelmus KR, Gee L, Hauck WW, et al. Herpetic Eye Disease Study. A controlled trial of topical corticosteroids for herpes simplex stromal keratitis. *Ophthalmology* 1994; **101**:1883–1895; discussion 1895–1896.

Chapter 36 Anti-allergic treatment strategies

Andrea Leonardi

INTRODUCTION

Ocular allergy can involve all the components of the ocular surface including the lid, the lid margin, the conjunctiva, and the lacrimal system. Approximately one third of the world population is affected by some form of allergic disease, and ocular involvement is estimated to be present in 40–60% of this population. Allergic conjunctivitis is a localized allergic condition frequently associated with rhinitis but often observed as the only or prevalent allergic sensitization. The severity of this disease ranges from mild, which can still interfere significantly with quality of life, to severe, which is characterized by potential impairment of visual function. The term 'allergic conjunctivitis' refers to a collection of hypersensitivity disorders that affects the lid and conjunctiva. Various clinical forms are included in the classification of ocular allergy: seasonal allergic conjunctivitis (SAC), perennial allergic conjunctivitis (PAC), vernal keratoconjunctivitis (VKC), atopic keratoconjunctivitis (AKC), giant papillary conjunctivitis (GPC), and contact- or drug-induced dermato-conjunctivitis. Corneal involvement is typically restricted to the two most severe forms of ocular allergy, VKC and AKC, which requires particular care in their management.

TREATMENT OF OCULAR ALLERGY

The most common diseases, SAC and PAC, are classic IgE-mediated disorders, in which the therapeutic focus is mostly confined to the local suppression of mast cells, their degranulation, and the effects of histamine and other mast-cell-derived mediators using topical drugs. Corticosteroids are usually not needed in SAC and PAC, and have potentially important side effects if used for periods longer than occasional short cycles to control severe recurrences, if any. Conversely, severe chronic disorders such as VKC and AKC are both IgE- and T-cell mediated, leading to a chronic inflammation in which eosinophil, lymphocyte, and structural cell activation characterizes the conjunctival allergic reaction. In these cases, stabilization of mast cells and histamine or other mediator receptor antagonists is frequently insufficient for control of conjunctival inflammation and the frequent corneal involvement.

Treatment of ocular allergy includes non-pharmacological management, topical ocular pharmacological treatment, topical ocular non-pharmacological treatments, topical non-ocular pharmacological treatment, systemic pharmacological treatments, and immunotherapy.

Non-pharmacological management

The first treatment of ocular allergy should be avoidance of the offending allergens. This can be usually achieved for indoor, professional, or food allergens. Thus, the identification of allergens by skin or blood testing is necessary to allow for avoidance of precipitating factors. Non-pharmacological treatments include tear substitutes and lid hygiene for the washing out of allergens and mediators from the ocular surface, and cold compresses for decongestion. Patients should be informed of the duration of the disease based on allergen diffusion and exposure.

Topical ocular pharmacological treatment

Currently available topical drugs for allergic conjunctivitis belong to different pharmacological classes (**Table 36.1**): vasoconstrictors, antihistamines, mast cell stabilizers, 'dual-acting' agents (with antihistaminic and mast cell stabilizing properties), non-steroidal anti-inflammatory agents, corticosteroids, and immunosuppressive drugs.

Decongestant or vasoconstrictors are a-adrenergic agonists approved topically for relief of conjunctival redness (Lanier et al. 1983). They have little place in the pharmacological treatment of SAC and PAC except for the immediate removal of injection for cosmetic reasons, but they do have an adverse effect profile locally (glaucoma) and systemically (hypertension). Topical decongestants do not reduce the allergic response because they do not antagonize any of the mediators of allergic inflammation. Prolonged use of topical decongestants as well as the discontinuation of these agents following prolonged use can lead to rebound hyperemia and conjunctivitis medicamentosa (Spector & Raizman 1994). To minimize this potential side effect, topical decongestants should be used as infrequently and for as short a duration as possible (days vs. weeks) (Fraunfelder & Meyer 1987). These are usually associated with topical first-generation antihistamines (H1 receptor [H1R] competitive antagonists) pheniramine and antazoline, available as over-the-counter products.

Mast cell stabilizers

Mast cell stabilizers inhibit degranulation by interrupting the normal chain of intracellular signals resulting from the cross-linking and activation of the high-affinity IgE receptor (FceRI) by the allergen (Cook et al. 2002). They inhibit the release of histamine and other preformed mediators and the arachidonic acid cascade of mediator synthesis. Several mast cell stabilizers are available for use in the eye: sodium cromoglycate 2%, nedocromil sodium 2%, lodoxamide tromethamine 0.1%, spaglumic acid 4%, and pemirolast potassium 0.1%. These drugs are approved for the treatment of allergic conjunctivitis, VKC, and GPC with four times daily dosing regimen. In order to provide this effect, mast cell stabilizers should be used prophylactically (Leonardi 2005), although patients may notice some improvements in SAC signs and symptoms within 24–48 hours if they are used following exposure to the allergen (Bielory 2008, Bielory & Friedlaender 2008, Cook et al. 2002). Topical mast cell stabilizers are generally safe and have minimal ocular side effects, although there may be some tolerability concerns, such as transient burning or stinging upon application.

Sodium cromoglycate (2 and 4% solutions) was the first of these molecules to be developed, and has an enormous body of literature devoted to proving its efficacy in all clinical forms of ocular allergy (Leino et al. 1994, Owen et al. 2004). The recommended dosing schedule is four to six times daily, with a loading period of at least 7 days and an onset of activity after as much as 2 weeks. It is approved for children

Table 36.1 Topical ocular allergy medications

Class	Drug	Indication	Comments
Vasoconstrictor–antihistamine combinations	Naphazoline/pheniramine	Rapid onset of action SAC Episodic allergy	Short duration of action Tachyphylaxis Mydriasis Ocular irritation Hypersensitivity Hypertension Potential for inappropriate patient use
Antihistamines	Levocabastine Emedastine	Rapid onset of action Relief of itching Relief of signs or symptoms SAC, PAC, AKC, VKC, GPC	Short duration of action
Mast cell stabilizers	Cromolyn Nedocromil Lodoxamide NAAGA Pemirolast	Relief of signs and symptoms SAC, PAC, AKC, VKC, GPC	Long-term usage Slow onset of action Prophylactic dosing
Antihistamine or mast cell stabilizers (dual-acting)	Alcaftadine Azelastine Bepotastine Epinastine Ketotifen Olopatadine	Treatment of signs and symptoms of SAC Rapid onset of action Long duration of action Excellent comfort SAC, PAC, AKC, VKC, GPC	Bitter taste (azelastine) No reported serious side effects Olopatadine 0.2% once a day
Corticosteroids	Loteprednol Fluorometholone Desonide Rimexolone Dexamethasone	Treatment of allergic inflammation Use in severe forms of allergies PAC, AKC, VKC	Risk for long-term side effects No mast cell stabilization Potential for inappropriate patient use Requires close monitoring

AKC, atopic keratoconjunctivitis; GPC, giant papillary conjunctivitis; PAC, perennial allergic conjunctivitis; SAC, seasonal allergic conjunctivitis; VKC, vernal keratoconjunctivitis.

3 years and older. The major adverse effect is burning and stinging, which has been reported in 13–77% of patients treated.

Nedocromil sodium 2% appears to be more potent than cromolyn, and is approved for two times daily dosing (Kjellman & Stevens 1995). Nedocromil is a pyranoquinoline that inhibits various activities on the multiple cells involved in allergic inflammation including eosinophils, neutrophils, macrophages, mast cells, monocytes, and platelets. Nedocromil inhibits activation and release of inflammatory mediators such as histamine, prostaglandin D2, and leukotrienes C4 from mast cells (Kjellman & Stevens 1995). The mechanism of action of nedocromil may be due partly to inhibition of axon reflexes and release of sensory neuropeptides, such as substance P, neurokinin A, and calcitonin-gene-related peptides (Benbow et al. 1993). Nedocromil has been shown to improve clinical symptoms in the control of ocular pruritus and irritation in the treatment of SAC (Blumenthal et al. 1992, Melamed et al. 2000). Its safety profile is similar to that of sodium cromoglycate, but is more potent and can be given just twice daily.

Lodoxamide tromethamine 0.1% has been available for the treatment of VKC; however, it has also been shown to be effective against allergic conjunctivitis. Its mechanism of action is thought to be similar to that of cromolyn, since it was shown to prevent tryptase release (Bonini et al. 1997). Inhibition of eosinophil activation and degranulation is the proposed mechanism for its efficacy against corneal signs such as keratitis and shield ulcers in severe allergic disease (Leonardi et al. 1997). Lodoxamide has been shown as superior to placebo (Cerqueti et al. 1994), cromolyn (Leonardi et al. 1997), and N-acetyl-aspartyl glutamic acid (NAAGA) for treatment of VKC (Gunduz et al. 1996). Its recommended dosing is four times daily. Lodoxamide may be used continuously for 3 months in children older than 2 years.

Pemirolast potassium is mast cell stabilizer that has been shown to alleviate the signs of allergic conjunctivitis (Abelson et al. 2002a). Pemirolast is currently approved for a four times daily dosing regimen (Gous & Ropo 2004).

Dipeptide NAAGA 6% has been widely used in Europe as topical eye drops in the treatment of allergic conjunctivitis, VKC (Leonardi et al. 2007), and GPC (Meijer et al. 1993). NAAGA is known to inhibit leukotriene synthesis, histamine release by mast cells, and complement-derived anaphylatoxin production. This anti-allergic compound was also shown to directly inhibit leukocyte adhesion to endothelial cells induced by proinflammatory stimuli, and abrogates tumor necrosis factor-a-induced expression of adhesion molecules on granulocytes and endothelial cells (Lapalus et al. 1986). These pharmacological properties confer a potential anti-inflammatory activity to NAAGA.

■ Antihistamines

Topical antihistamines are the first line of treatment for ocular allergy. Antihistamines act via histamine receptor antagonism to block the inflammatory effects of endogenous histamine and prevent or relieve the signs and symptoms that are associated with histamine. Most antihistamines used in the treatment of allergy are H1R antagonists, although some agents may have affinity for other subtypes (Bielory et al. 2005) H2 receptor (H2R) subtype antagonism has been shown to modulate both cell growth and migration (Bielory et al. 2005). H1 stimulation principally mediates the symptom of conjunctival pruritus whereas the H2R appears to be clinically involved in vasodilation (Abelson & Udell 1981, Bielory et al. 2005).

Drugs with antihistaminic activity may offer therapeutic advantages to patients with allergic conjunctivitis by inhibiting proinflammatory cytokine secretion from human conjunctival epithelial cells (Yanni et al. 1999b).

The first-generation antihistamines, pheniramine and antazoline, have a long safety record, but are known for the burn upon their instillation, the rapid onset and disappearance of their effects, and their limited potency (Yanni et al. 1999a). They may be irritating to the eye, especially with prolonged use, and may be associated with ciliary muscle paralysis, mydriasis, angle-closure glaucoma, and photophobia, especially those that are non-selective and block muscarinic receptors. These are still available in over-the-counter products, particularly in association with vasoconstrictors.

The newer antihistamines are still H1R antagonists, but have a longer duration of action (4–6 hours), and are more tolerable than their predecessors. These include levocabastine hydrochloride 0.5% and emedastine difumarate 0.05%.

Levocabastine hydrochloride 0.05% was shown to be more effective than artificial tears in controlling acute symptoms of allergic conjunctivitis, demonstrating that the selective H1R antagonist action is rapidly effective in a clinical setting (Abelson et al. 1994), is superior to cromolyn in treating allergen-induced conjunctivitis, and has a duration of action of at least 4 hours (Abelson et al. 1995). Levocabastine reduces in vivo inflammatory cell infiltration due to allergen challenge, the adhesion molecule expression on conjunctival epithelium (Buscaglia et al. 1996), and also reduced in the animal model the clinical aspects of the late-phase reaction and the conjunctival expression of a(4)b(1) integrin by reducing infiltrated eosinophils (Qasem et al. 2008).

Emedastine difumarate 0.05% appears to be stronger and more selective than levocabastine (Secchi et al. 2000a, 2000b). In fact, in direct comparison with levocabastine, emedastine proved significantly more effective in alleviating signs of SAC. Both drugs were effective and well tolerated in pediatric subjects with allergic conjunctivitis; however, emedastine was superior for relief of itching, redness, and eyelid swelling in the follow-up visits (Secchi et al. 2000a). Emedastine was found to be economically dominant relative to levocabastine, that is, more effective and less expensive, in Belgium, Germany, Portugal, and Sweden; in France, The Netherlands, and Norway, the incremental cost was low (<€1 per additional symptom-free day) (Pinto et al. 2001). Emedastine was also superior to the non-steroidal anti-inflammatory drug, ketorolac, in controlling itching and redness, the cardinal symptom and sign of allergic conjunctivitis (Discepola et al. 1999). In patients with SAC, olopatadine, ketotifen, epinastine, and emedastine are more efficacious than fluorometholone acetate in preventing itching and redness (Borazan et al. 2009).

In two in vitro studies, emedastine and, to a much lesser degree, levocabastine blocked histamine-stimulated proinflammatory cytokines [interleukin (IL)-8 and IL-6] release from conjunctival epithelial cells (Yanni et al. 1999a) and fibroblasts (Leonardi et al. 2002). Antazoline, emedastine, levocabastine, olopatadine, and pheniramine attenuated histamine-stimulated phosphatidylinositol turnover and IL-6 and IL-8 secretion (Yanni et al. 1999a). Emedastine was the most potent in ligand binding, phosphatidylinositol turnover, and IL-6 secretion, with dissociation constant and 50% inhibitory concentrations of 1–3 nmol/L, while levocabastine (dissociation constant, 52.6 nmol/L) exhibited greater functional activity (50% inhibitory concentration, 8–25 nmol/L) than either antazoline or pheniramine (Yanni et al. 1999b).

Topical antihistamines with multiple anti-inflammatory activities

The antihistamines, alcaftadine, azelastine, bepotastine, epinastine, ketotifen, and olopatadine, which have mast cell stabilizing and additional anti-inflammatory properties (called 'double or multiple action'), are presently available and show evident benefits in treating all forms of ocular allergy. The advantage offered by these molecules is the rapidity of symptomatic relief given by immediate histamine receptor antagonism, which alleviates itching and redness, coupled with the long-term disease-modifying benefit of mast cell stabilization. All these medications are well tolerated and none are associated with significant acute ocular drying effects.

Alcaftadine is the newest of the Food and Drug Administration (FDA)-approved ophthalmic antihistamines with evidence for multiple anti-inflammatory properties in preclinical studies reflecting the expected pharmacological profile of a broad-spectrum antihistamine (Greiner et al. 2011). In the animal model, alcaftadine reduced conjunctival eosinophil recruitment, and had a protective effect on epithelial tight junction protein expression (Ono & Lane 2011). In the conjunctival allergen challenge (CAC) model, alcaftadine showed a statistically and clinically significant effect on the prevention of itching, with a fast onset and prolonged duration of action (Greiner et al. 2011, Torkildsen & Shedden 2011).

Azelastine 0.05% is a second-generation H1R antagonist with additional prophylactic anti-allergic properties downregulating intercellular adhesion molecule 1 (ICAM-1) expression during the early- and late-phase components of ocular allergic response (Ciprandi et al. 2003). Azelastine significantly improved itching and conjunctival redness compared to both cromoglycate and placebo for the treatment of SAC (James et al. 2003). Topical azelastine progressively improved itching and conjunctival redness in patients with moderate to severe PAC (Nazarov et al. 2003). Azelastine has demonstrated in a pediatric SAC study that the response rate to azelastine eye drops group (74%) was significantly higher than that in the placebo group (39%) and comparable with that in the levocabastine group (Giede et al. 2000). It is safe to use in children aged ≥3 years.

Bepotastine besilate 1.5% is one of the new FDA-approved ophthalmic antihistamines with evidence for multiple anti-inflammatory properties. Bepotastine is a non-sedating, highly specific H1R antagonist that acts as an inhibitor of allergic response through multiple mechanisms: H1R antagonism, mast cell stabilization, and inhibition of eosinophil migration to ocular inflammatory sites (Kida et al. 2010).

Bepotastine ophthalmic solutions 1.0 and 1.5% substantially decreased CAC-induced ocular itching for at least 8 hours after dosing; however, the reduction in conjunctival hyperemia after a CAC, although statistically significant, was modest when compared with placebo (Macejko et al. 2010). The 1.5% bepotastine formulation produced statistically significant reductions after a CAC in individual non-ocular symptoms at onset of allergic response and for at least 8 hours after instillation, with the greatest reduction seen for nasal congestion and rhinorrhea (Torkildsen et al. 2010).

Epinastine 0.05% is a topical antihistamine with other anti-inflammatory properties that include H2R antagonism, mast cell stabilization, and inhibition of cytokine production. Pretreatment by epinastine differentially reduced histamine, tumor necrosis factor-a and b, IL-5, IL-8, and IL-10. In vivo, epinastine pretreatment significantly reduced the clinical scores and the numbers of eosinophils and neutrophils (Galatowicz et al. 2007). In an animal model of histamine-induced vascular leakage, epinastine, azelastine, and ketotifen had a shorter duration of effect than olopatadine (Beauregard et al. 2007). In CAC placebo trials, multiple signs and symptoms (ocular itching, eyelid swelling, conjunctival and episcleral hyperemia, and chemosis) of allergic conjunctivitis were significantly reduced by instillation of epinastine compared with vehicle (Abelson et al. 2004a). In a study of patients with SAC, epinastine instillation twice daily clearly reduced ocular itching, but ocular itching and hyperemia scores were similar when compared to levocabastine (Whitcup et al. 2004). One randomized, double-masked, crossover study showed that a single drop of epinastine was more comfortable than azelastine and ketotifen in patients with active allergic conjunctivitis (Torkildsen et al. 2008).

Ketotifen fumarate 0.025% is a benzocycloheptathiophene that has been shown to display several anti-inflammatory properties including strong histamine H1R antagonism, mast cell stabilization, leukotriene formation inhibition, and eosinophil inhibition (helps decrease chemotaxis and activate eosinophils) (Nishimura et al. 1987, Tomioka et al. 1979). Ketotifen has also been shown to have pronounced antihistaminic and antianaphylactic properties that result in moderate to marked symptom improvement in the majority of patients with asthma, atopic dermatitis, seasonal or perennial rhinitis, allergic conjunctivitis, chronic or acute urticaria, and food allergy. Topical ketotifen has a favorable safety and tolerability profile, which may have a positive impact on compliance, an important aspect of effective symptomatic control of allergic conjunctivitis (Abelson et al. 2002b). Ketotifen is safe and effective in reducing ocular itching and hyperemia associated with allergic conjunctivitis (Abelson et al. 2003, Greiner et al. 2003). In a CAC trial in a pediatric population, ketotifen was found to be an effective and safe treatment option for children with allergic conjunctivitis (Abelson et al. 2004b). In the United States, topical ketotifen is now available as an over-the-counter therapy for ocular allergy.

Olopatadine hydrochloride 0.1% possesses antihistaminic activity and mast cell stabilizing effects (Leonardi & Quintieri 2010). Olopatadine pretreatment of conjunctival mast cells inhibited the mediator release associated with eosinophil adhesion to conjunctival epithelial cells and eosinophil degranulation (Cook et al. 2004). In conjunctival epithelial cell cultures, olopatadine inhibited histamine-induced production of IL-1, IL-6, IL-8, and granulocyte-macrophage-colony stimulating factor (GM-CSF) (Yanni et al. 1999b), and was notably more potent than pheniramine and antazoline in inhibiting histamine-induced phosphoinositide turnover (Sharif et al. 1996). In vivo, olopatadine has been shown to be significantly more effective than placebo in relieving itching and redness for up to 8 hours (Abelson 1998). Comparison studies revealed that olopatadine was superior than azelastine (Spangler et al. 2001), epinastine (Lanier et al. 2004, Mah et al. 2007), and ketotifen (Berdy et al. 2000) in preventing ocular itching and redness in the CAC model. In addition, olopatadine caused less ocular discomfort than ketotifen and was preferred by approximately three times as many patients as for ketotifen (Berdy et al. 2000).

Olopatadine 0.2% has an extended duration of action of up to 24 hours and is indicated once daily for the treatment of ocular itching (Abelson & Gomes 2008). It has been shown to be safe in both adults and children as young as 3 years of age, and its once-daily dosing regimen increases convenience and compliance for all ocular allergy patients. Using the CAC model, one drop of olopatadine 0.2% had an efficacy profile comparable to two drops (separated by 8 hours) of olopatadine 0.1% in the prevention of ocular itching (Abelson et al. 2007). Both concentrations showed significant activity at the 24-hour time point and were statistically superior to placebo (Abelson et al. 2007). Olopatadine 0.2% was significantly more effective than placebo in reduction of conjunctival redness, chemosis, and eyelid swelling. Previous users of the 0.1% solution were switched to 0.2%, which showed a significant improvement in all categories of the Rhinoconjunctivitis Quality of Life Questionnaire using the once-a-day preparation (Scoper et al. 2007).

Non-steroidal anti-inflammatory drugs

Non-steroidal anti-inflammatory drugs can be considered in the treatment of ocular allergy for a short period having some efficacy on ocular itching.

Ketorolac tromethamine 0.5% has been approved for the treatment of SAC with a primary mechanism of action on the inhibition of cyclooxygenase, thus blocking the production of prostaglandins but not the formation of leukotrienes. Ketorolac proved to be effective in reducing mast cell degranulation, as indicated by significantly decreased tryptase tear levels, as well as the clinical and cytological allergic reaction (Leonardi et al. 2000). In double-masked clinical studies, ketorolac was found safe and effective in alleviating the signs and symptoms of allergic conjunctivitis when compared to placebo (Ballas et al. 1993, Tinkelman et al. 1993) and equivalent to levocabastine (Donshik et al. 2000), but less effective than emedastine (Discepola et al. 1999) and olopatadine (Deschenes et al. 1999) in the CAC model.

Ketorolac 0.4%, a reformulation of the original 0.5% and indicated for the reduction of ocular pain and burning or stinging following corneal refractive surgery, is effective in the treatment of allergic conjunctivitis when used as either monotherapy or as adjunct therapy to steroids (Schechter 2008).

Non-steroidal anti-inflammatory drugs are classically associated with a low-to-moderate incidence of burning and stinging upon instillation into the eye and should be carefully used, since corneal melting and perforation have been described as occasional side effects (Congdon et al. 2001).

Topical corticosteroids

Corticosteroids relieve the signs and symptoms of SAC by non-specific anti-inflammatory effects. However, they are not recommended in the long-term use because of possible ocular side effects, including increases in intraocular pressure (IOP), induction or exacerbation of glaucoma, formation of cataracts, delay in wound healing, and increase in susceptibility to infections or superinfections. Inappropriate use of topical corticosteroid in the presence of corneal infections also continues to be a cause of ocular morbidity. Other risks of locally administered ophthalmic corticosteroids include tear-film instability, epithelial toxicity, crystalline keratopathy, decreased wound strength, orbital fat atrophy, ptosis, limitation of ocular movement, inadvertent intraocular injection, and reduction in endogenous cortisol (McGhee et al. 2002). These side effects depend, in part, on the structure, dose, duration of treatment, and gender disposition (McGhee et al. 2002). In fact, following daily administration of corticosteroids for 4–6 weeks, approximately one third of the normal population are expected to be 'high or moderate responders,' with an increase in IOP of between 6 and 15 mmHg (McGhee et al. 2002).

Corticosteroid formulations (including the so called 'soft steroids') should be reserved for and carefully used in only the most severe cases that are refractive to other types of medications. Corticosteroids do not directly stabilize immune cell membranes and do not inhibit histamine release; however, they may modulate the mast cell response by inhibiting cytokine production and inflammatory cell recruitment and activation. Thus, they are not the ideal therapy choice for inhibiting the acute allergic reaction; however, clinically, they are the most effective anti-inflammatory agents in active ocular allergy. Fluorometholone 0.1%, loteprednol 0.2%, rimexolone 1%, and desonide, called 'soft' steroids, are the ones considered when a mild, weakly penetrating drug is needed.

Prednisolone 1% and dexamethasone 0.1% are about equipotent and both are suitable, but preservative-free formulations are preferred, especially when frequent dosing of up to hourly application may be required. Their use is recommended as short pulses for acute flare-ups.

Loteprednol etabonate 0.2% is an FDA-approved ophthalmic suspension for the treatment of ocular allergy. It is a site-specific steroid, since the active drug resides at the target tissue long enough to render a therapeutic effect but rarely long enough to cause secondary effects.

Loteprednol 0.2% was more effective than placebo in the treatment of SAC with a safety profile comparable to placebo (Dell et al. 1998, Shulman et al. 1999). The higher dose, loteprednol 0.5%, has been shown to be effective in reducing the signs and symptoms of GPC (Bartlett et al. 1993b), and as an effective prophylactic treatment for the ocular signs and symptoms of SAC administered 6 weeks before the onset of the allergy (Dell et al. 1997). In a retrospective review, loteprednol was shown to be safe when used on a long-term basis for the treatment of both SAC and PAC (Ilyas et al. 2004). The results of analysis in a large population of subjects undergoing long-term therapy and of a previously published controlled, double-masked study in corticosteroid responders suggest that loteprednol has less propensity to cause clinically significant elevations in IOP than prednisolone acetate (Bartlett et al. 1993a). IOP elevation of ≥ 10 mmHg occurred in 1.7% of patients taking long-term loteprednol, 0.5% of those taking vehicle and 6.7% of those taking prednisolone acetate (Novack et al. 1998). However in a recent review, patients treated with loteprednol for dry eye diasease, postoperative therapy, or allergic conjunctivitis required IOP-lowering medications in 24% of cases and surgery in 8% of cases (Rajpal et al. 2011).

Calcineurine inhibitors

Cyclosporin A (CsA) is effective in controlling VKC-associated ocular inflammation by blocking T_H2 lymphocyte proliferation and IL-2 production. It inhibits histamine release from mast cells and basophils through a reduction in IL-5 production, and may reduce eosinophil recruitment and effects on the conjunctiva and cornea. CsA is lipophilic and thus must be dissolved in an alcohol–oil base. Unavailability of a commercial preparation of topical cyclosporine, technical difficulties in dispensing cyclosporine eye drops, and legal restrictions in many countries on its topical use preclude its widespread use in the treatment of VKC.

The 2% formulation has the longest track record, but lower concentrations (e.g. 1%, 0.5%, and 0.05%) have been tried and shown to be effective, although only the 0.05% formulation is commercially available as a treatment for dry eye disease. CsA 1 or 2% emulsion in castor or olive oil can be considered for treatment of severe VKC and can serve as a good alternative to steroids (Pucci et al. 2002, Utine et al. 2010). CsA 1% was reported to be the minimum effective concentration in the treatment of vernal shield ulcer, with recurrence observed at lower concentrations (Cetinkaya et al. 2004). In a randomized,

controlled trial, the effects of 0.05% topical cyclosporine were similar to placebo in the treatment of VKC (Daniell et al. 2006). Conversely, in another study, topical CsA 0.05% decreased the severity of symptoms and clinical signs significantly after 6 months and the need for steroids was reduced, suggesting that CsA at low doses is an effective steroid-sparing agent in severe allergic conjunctivitis (Ozcan et al. 2007). Frequent instillation may be inconvenient, but no significant side effects of topical CsA, except for a burning sensation during administration, have been reported. Thus, topical CsA can control the symptoms of VKC but further trials are required to establish the optimal concentration needed to treat the disease. Recently, a randomized, controlled crossover 2-year study showed the safety and efficacy of topical cyclosporine 0.05% for long-term prevention of VKC relapses (Lambiase et al. 2011). Patients treated with ketotifen had a 2.4 times higher risk of recurrence than patients treated with CsA. In addition, CsA significantly improved itching, photophobia, and conjunctival hyperemia scores with respect to ketotifen. These data are of great importance for the long-term management of pediatric patients at risk of visual impairment, whether due to steroid abuse or to continued recurrences of acute inflammation (Lambiase et al. 2011).

Topical CsA 2% is an effective and safe steroid-sparing agent in AKC and, despite difficulties in patient tolerance, improves symptoms and signs (Hingorani et al. 1998). The lower dose of topical CsA 0.05% seems to be safe and has some effect in alleviating signs and symptoms of severe AKC refractory to topical steroid treatment (Utine et al. 2010). In a multicentered, randomized, controlled trial, CsA 0.05% six times per day followed by four times per day was found to be effective in alleviating the signs and symptoms of AKC (Utine et al. 2010). Although CsA 1% has been shown to be more effective, frequent instillations may compensate for the low concentration of CsA in the currently available commercial preparations in the United States and South America.

Systemic CsA may be an alternative to systemic corticosteroids for treatment of AKC. Atopic dermatitis in patients with and without keratoconus impairs graft prognosis statistically significantly. Systemic CsA improves graft prognosis in atopic dermatitis with keratoconus and the dermatitis itself as long as the drug is used (Reinhard et al. 1999).

In severe cases, systemic treatment with T-lymphocyte signal transduction inhibitors such as CsA or tacrolimus may ameliorate both the dermatological and ocular manifestations in severe patients who are refractory to conventional treatment (Anzaar et al. 2008).

Tacrolimus is a potent drug similar to CsA in its mode of action, but chemically distinct. A skin ointment of tacrolimus is licensed for the treatment of moderate to severe atopic eyelid diseases and may have secondary benefits for AKC (Rikkers et al. 2003, Vichyanond et al. 2004, Virtanen et al. 2006). A recent study reported great efficacy of tacrolimus 0.1% ointment in the treatment of severe VKC patients (Vichyanond et al. 2004). Topical tacrolimus can be used for at least 1 year without apparent adverse reaction in some patients, although possible adverse reaction should be carefully monitored.

Topical non-ocular pharmacological treatment

The efficacy of intranasal corticosteroids in treating allergic nasal symptoms is well established. Recent data show promising effect of intranasal corticosteroids on ocular symptoms of allergic rhinoconjunctivitis (Bielory 2008). In recent retrospective analyses of randomized clinical trials using topical nasal corticosteroids compared with placebo, ocular symptom scores have been reduced (Bielory 2008, Scadding & Keith 2008).

The mechanism by which an intranasal corticosteroid reduces ocular allergic symptoms has been under investigation; some effects on both the reflex neural activity and the local inflammation facilitating the nasolacrimal drainage have been proposed (Baroody et al. 2009).

In SAC and PAC associated with allergic rhinitis, topical nasal steroids (and particularly new molecules with low systemic bioavailability, such as mometasone furoate and fluticasone furoate) have been shown to control the nasal–ocular reflex component of eye symptoms without increasing the risk of cataracts or of an increased ocular pressure (Bielory 2008). In fact, intranasal corticosteroids are considered safe due to their low systemic bioavailability. Analysis of an intranasal corticosteroid on individual ocular symptoms supported the positive impact of mometasone furoate on ocular symptoms (Bielory 2008). Mometasone improved individual symptoms (eye itching, tearing, and redness) and subject-reported total ocular symptom scores compared with placebo, in addition to its established efficacy in reducing nasal symptoms of seasonal allergic rhinitis (Bielory 2008).

Meta-analysis studies showed that there was no significant difference in improvement of eye symptoms between intranasal corticosteroids and oral antihistamines (Weiner et al. 1998), including non-sedating antihistamines. Thus, nasal corticosteroids that have an effect on congestion may also benefit patients with ocular symptoms and may be more beneficial as a single agent to be initiated in allergy treatment.

Systemic pharmacological treatment

Systemic antihistamines should be used in patients with concomitant major non-ocular allergic manifestations. In fact, allergic rhinoconjunctivitis is an equally frequent condition generally treated with systemic antihistamines that have been proven effective in relieving nasal and conjunctival signs and symptoms (Bielory et al. 2005). When allergic symptoms are isolated, focused therapy with topical (ophthalmic) antihistamines is often efficacious and clearly superior to systemic antihistamines, either as monotherapy or in conjunction with an oral or intranasal agent. First-generation H1R antagonists may provide some relief of ocular itching, but are sedating and have anticholinergic effects such as dry mouth, dry eyes, blurred vision, and urinary retention. Second-generation antihistamines offer the same efficacy as their predecessors, but with a low-sedating profile and lack of anticholinergic activity. These drugs include acrivastine, cetirizine, ebastine, fexofenadine, loratadine, and mizolastine. However, even their use has been associated with drying effects, particularly of the ocular surface (Bielory et al. 2005). Desloratadine and levocetirizine are considered a subsequent evolution of these second-generation agents and are preferred over first-generation antihistamines for the treatment of allergic conjunctivitis (Hingorani & Lightman 1995). However, no single agent has been conclusively found to achieve superior overall response rates. Second-generation antihistamines have been shown to reduce individual ocular symptoms following allergen conjunctival challenges or continuous treatment for allergic rhinoconjunctivitis, respectively (Canonica et al. 2008, Torkildsen et al. 2009).

Anti-IgE

Omalizumab is an anti-IgE recombinant, humanized non-anaphylactogenic antibody, directed against the receptor-binding domain of IgE. This binding is specific to free IgE, so that IgE is unable to interact with high-affinity IgE receptors (FceRI) on cells, thereby preventing the antibody from attaching to the mast cell. This molecule was found to improve symptom scores, rescue-medication use, quality-of-life scores, and peak expiratory flows in patients with allergic asthma. In patients with seasonal allergic rhinitis, there was a significant reduction in the nasal and ocular symptoms as well as in the use of rescue medications. Omalizumab also demonstrated a high level of safety in adults, adolescents, and children with a side-effect profile no different from the placebo (Plewako et al. 2002).

In a study on allergic rhinitis patients, blood eosinophils, free IgE in serum, and the number of eosinophils in nasal biopsy specimens were reduced by omalizumab treatment as compared to the placebo (Plewako et al. 2002). Furthermore, the number of IgE(+) staining cells decreased significantly in the omalizumab group during season compared to placebo.

Specific immunotherapy

Allergen-specific immunotherapy (SIT) is indicated only when a clearly defined systemic hypersensitivity to identified allergens exists. The choice of the allergen to be employed for SIT should be made in accordance with the combination of clinical history and results of skin prick test. SIT is one of the cornerstones of allergic rhinoconjunctivitis treatment. Since the development of non-invasive formulations with better safety profiles, there is an increasing tendency to prescribe immunotherapy in youngsters. In these cases, sublingual immunotherapy (SLIT), which is better tolerated in children, can be considered, since it is equally effective as traditional subcutaneous injections. Since the approval of SLIT by the World Health Organization in 1988, the efficacy and safety of SLIT have been confirmed in several new double-blind, placebo-controlled studies for mono-sensitized patients who are allergic to house dust mites, grass pollens, ragweed, and birch pollen. Documented immunological responses to SLIT have included decreased serum eosinophilic cationic protein and IL-13 levels, an elevation in IL-12 levels, a reduction in late-phase responses, and increases in IgG4/IgE ratios. However, successful treatment requires at least 2 years of therapy and adjustment of tolerated doses during the pollen season.

A recent systematic review and meta-analysis of double-blind, placebo-controlled, randomized, controlled trials confirmed that SLIT significantly reduces both the total and individual ocular symptoms scores (redness, itchiness, and watery eyes) in patients with allergic conjunctivitis (AC) with or without rhinitis (Calderon et al. 2011). SLIT is clinically effective, safe, and provides an antigen-specific protective immune effect.

In the same review, it was found that a reduction of eye drops use was not one of the significant effects of SLIT. This lack of effect could be explained by the fact that participants generally are instructed to use intranasal steroids and take systemic antihistamines as rescue medications. These medications are easy to take, and both have been demonstrated to be effective in reducing ocular symptoms in patients with allergic rhinoconjunctivitis.

SLIT and treatment with anti-IgE antibody may be complementary approaches to treating allergic rhinoconjunctivitis, which may be used for single or combined treatment.

REFERENCES

Abelson MB. Evaluation of olopatadine, a new ophthalmic antiallergic agent with dual activity, using the conjunctival allergen challenge model. *Ann Allergy Asthma Immunol* 1998; **81**:211–218.

Abelson MB, Berdy GJ, Mundorf T, Amdahl LD, Graves AL. Pemirolast potassium 0.1% ophthalmic solution is an effective treatment for allergic conjunctivitis: a pooled analysis of two prospective, randomized, double-masked, placebo-controlled, phase III studies. *J Ocul Pharmacol Ther* 2002a; **18**:475–488.

Abelson MB, Chapin MJ, Kapik BM, Shams NB. Ocular tolerability and safety of ketotifen fumarate ophthalmic solution. *Adv Ther* 2002b; **19**:161–169.

Abelson MB, Chapin MJ, Kapik BM, Shams NB. Efficacy of ketotifen fumarate 0.025% ophthalmic solution compared with placebo in the conjunctival allergen challenge model. *Arch Ophthalmol* 2003; **121**:626–630.

Abelson MB, Ferzola NJ, McWhirter CL, Crampton HJ. Efficacy and safety of single- and multiple-dose ketotifen fumarate 0.025% ophthalmic solution in a pediatric population. *Pediatr Allergy Immunol* 2004a; **15**:551–557.

Abelson MB, George MA, Smith LW. Evaluation of the new ophthalmic antihistamine, 0.05% levocabastine, in the clinical allergen challenge model of allergic conjunctivitis. *J Allergy Clin Immunol* 1994; **94**:458–464.

Abelson MB, George MA, Smith LM. Evaluation of 0.05% levocabastine versus 4% sodium cromolyn in the allergen challenge model. *Ophthalmology* 1995; **102**:310–316.

Abelson MB, Gomes PJ. Olopatadine 0.2% ophthalmic solution: the first ophthalmic antiallergy agent with once-daily dosing. *Expert Opin Drug Metab Toxicol* 2008; **4**:453–461.

Abelson MB, Gomes P, Crampton HJ, et al. Efficacy and tolerability of ophthalmic epinastine assessed using the conjunctival antigen challenge model in patients with a history of allergic conjunctivitis. *Clin Ther* 2004b; **26**:35–47.

Abelson MB, Spangler DL, Epstein AB, Mah FS, Crampton HJ. Efficacy of once-daily olopatadine 0.2% ophthalmic solution compared to twice-daily olopatadine 0.1% ophthalmic solution for the treatment of ocular itching induced by conjunctival allergen challenge. *Curr Eye Res* 2007; **32**:1017–1022.

Abelson MB, Udell IJ. H2-receptors in the human ocular surface. *Arch Ophthalmol* 1981; **99**:302–304.

Anzaar F, Gallagher MJ, Bhat P, et al. Use of systemic T-lymphocyte signal transduction inhibitors in the treatment of atopic keratoconjunctivitis. *Cornea* 2008; **27**:884–888.

Ballas Z, Blumenthal M, Tinkelman DG, Krlz R, Rupp G. Clinical evaluation of ketorolac tromethamine 0.5% ophthalmic solution for the treatment of seasonal allergic conjunctivitis. *Surv Ophthalmol* 1993; **38**:141–148.

Baroody FM, Shenaq D, DeTineo M, Wang J, Naclerio RM. Fluticasone furoate nasal spray reduces the nasal-ocular reflex: a mechanism for the efficacy of topical steroids in controlling allergic eye symptoms. *J Allergy Clin Immunol* 2009; **123**:1342–1348.

Bartlett JD, Horwitz B, Laibovitz R, Howes JF. Intraocular pressure response to loteprednol etabonate in known steroid responders. *J Ocul Pharmacol* 1993a; **9**:157–165.

Bartlett JD, Howes JF, Ghormley NR, et al. Safety and efficacy of loteprednol etabonate for treatment of papillae in contact lens-associated giant papillary conjunctivitis. *Curr Eye Res* 1993b; **12**:313–321.

Beauregard C, Stephens D, Roberts L, Gamache D, Yanni J. Duration of action of topical antiallergy drugs in a Guinea pig model of histamine-induced conjunctival vascular permeability. *J Ocul Pharmacol Ther* 2007; **23**:315–320.

Benbow AG, Eady R, Jackson D. The immunopharmacological actions of nedocromil sodium relative to the use of its 2% ophthalmic solution. *Eye* 1993; **7**:26–28.

Berdy GJ, Spangler DL, Bensch G, Berdy SS, Brusatti RC. A comparison of the relative efficacy and clinical performance of olopatadine hydrochloride 0.1% ophthalmic solution and ketotifen fumarate 0.025% ophthalmic solution in the conjunctival antigen challenge model. *Clin Ther* 2000; **22**:826–833.

Bielory L. Ocular symptom reduction in patients with seasonal allergic rhinitis treated with the intranasal corticosteroid mometasone furoate. *Ann Allergy Asthma Immunol* 2008; **100**:272–279.

Bielory L, Friedlaender MH. Allergic conjunctivitis. *Immunol Allergy Clin North Am* 2008; **28**:43–58.

Bielory L, Ghafoor S. Histamine receptors and the conjunctiva. *Curr Opin Allergy Clin Immunol* 2005; **5**:437–440.

Bielory L, Lien KW, Bigelsen S. Efficacy and tolerability of newer antihistamines in the treatment of allergic conjunctivitis. *Drugs* 2005; **65**:215–228.

Blumenthal M, Casale T, Dockhorn R, et al. Efficacy and safety of nedocromil sodium ophthalmic solution in the treatment of seasonal allergic conjunctivitis. *Am J Ophthalmol* 1992; **113**:56–63.

Bonini S, Schiavone M, Bonini S, et al. Efficacy of iodoxamide eye drops on mast cells and eosinophils after allergen challenge in allergic conjunctivitis. *Ophthalmology* 1997; **104**:849–853.

Borazan M, Karalezli A, Akova YA, et al. Efficacy of olopatadine HCl 0.1%, ketotifen fumarate 0.025%, epinastine HCl 0.05%, emedastine 0.05% and fluorometholone acetate 0.1% ophthalmic solutions for seasonal allergic conjunctivitis: a placebo-controlled environmental trial. *Acta Ophthalmol* 2009; **87**:549–554.

Buscaglia S, Paolieri F, Catrullo A, et al. Topical ocular levocabastine reduces ICAM-1 expression on epithelial cells both in vivo and in vitro. *Clin Exp Allergy* 1996; **26**:1188–1196.

Calderon MA, Penagos M, Sheikh A, Canonica GW, Durham SR. Sublingual immunotherapy for allergic conjunctivitis: Cochrane systematic review and meta-analysis. *Clin Exp Allergy* 2011; **41**:1263–1272.

Canonica GW, Fumagalli F, Guerra L, et al. Levocetirizine in persistent allergic rhinitis: continuous or on-demand use? A pilot study. *Curr Med Res Opin* 2008; **24**:2829–2839.

Cerqueti PM, Ricca V, Tosca MA, Buscaglia S, Ciprandi G. Lodoxamide treatment of allergic conjunctivitis. *Int Arch Allergy Immunol* 1994; **105**:185–189.

Cetinkaya A, Akova YA, Dursun D, Pelit A. Topical cyclosporine in the management of shield ulcers. *Cornea* 2004; **23**:194–200.

Ciprandi G, Cosentino C, Milanese M, Tosca MA. Rapid anti-inflammatory action of azelastine eyedrops for ongoing allergic reactions. *Ann Allergy Asthma Immunol* 2003; **90**:434–438.

Congdon NG, Schein OD, von Kulajta P, et al. Corneal complications associated with topical ophthalmic use of nonsteroidal antiinflammatory drugs. *J Cataract Refract Surg* 2001; **27**:622–631.

Cook EB, Stahl JL, Barney NP, Graziano FM. Mechanisms of antihistamines and mast cell stabilizers in ocular allergic inflammation. *Curr Drug Targets Inflamm Allergy* 2002; **1**:167–180.

Cook EB, Stahl JL, Sedgwick JB, Barney NP, Graziano FM. The promotion of eosinophil degranulation and adhesion to conjunctival epithelial cells by IgE-activated conjunctival mast cells. *Ann Allergy Asthma Immunol* 2004; **92**:65–72.

Daniell M, Constantinou M, Vu HT, Taylor HR. Randomised controlled trial of topical ciclosporin A in steroid dependent allergic conjunctivitis. *Br J Ophthalmol* 2006; **90**:461–464.

Dell SJ, Lowry GM, Northcutt JA, et al. A randomized, double-masked, placebo-controlled parallel study of 0.2% loteprednol etabonate in patients with seasonal allergic conjunctivitis. *J Allergy Clin Immunol* 1998; **102**:251–255.

Dell SJ, Shulman DG, Lowry GM, Howes J. A controlled evaluation of the efficacy and safety of loteprednol etabonate in the prophylactic treatment of seasonal allergic conjunctivitis. Loteprednol Allergic Conjunctivitis Study Group. *Am J Ophthalmol* 1997; **123**:791–797.

Deschenes J, Discepola M, Abelson M. Comparative evaluation of olopatadine ophthalmic solution (0.1%) versus ketorolac ophthalmic solution (0.5%) using the provocative antigen challenge model. *Acta Ophthalmol Scand Suppl* 1999; (228):47–52.

Discepola M, Deschenes J, Abelson M. Comparison of the topical ocular antiallergic efficacy of emedastine 0.05% ophthalmic solution to ketorolac 0.5% ophthalmic solution in a clinical model of allergic conjunctivitis. *Acta Ophthalmol Scand Suppl* 1999; (228):43–46.

Donshik PC, Pearlman D, Pinnas J, et al. Efficacy and safety of ketorolac tromethamine 0.5% and levocabastine 0.05%: a multicenter comparison in patients with seasonal allergic conjunctivitis. *Adv Ther* 2000; **17**:94–102.

Fraunfelder FT, Meyer SM. Systemic reactions to ophthalmic drug preparations. *Med Toxicol Adverse Drug Exp* 1987; **2**:287–293.

Galatowicz G, Ajayi Y, Stern ME, Calder VL. Ocular anti-allergic compounds selectively inhibit human mast cell cytokines in vitro and conjunctival cell infiltration in vivo. *Clin Exp Allergy* 2007; **37**:1648–1656.

Giede C, Metzenauer P, Petzold U, Ellers-Lenz B. Comparison of azelastine eye drops with levocabastine eye drops in the treatment of seasonal allergic conjunctivitis. *Curr Med Res Opin* 2000; **16**:153–163.

Gous P, Ropo A. A comparative trial of the safety and efficacy of 0.1 percent pemirolast potassium ophthalmic solution dosed twice or four times a day in patients with seasonal allergic conjunctivitis. *J Ocul Pharmacol Ther* 2004; **20**:139–150.

Greiner JV, Edwards-Swanson K, Ingerman A. Evaluation of alcaftadine 0.25% ophthalmic solution in acute allergic conjunctivitis at 15 minutes and 16 hours after instillation versus placebo and olopatadine 0.1%. *Clin Ophthalmol* 2011; **5**:87–93.

Greiner JV, Mundorf T, Dubiner H, et al. Efficacy and safety of ketotifen fumarate 0.025% in the conjunctival antigen challenge model of ocular allergic conjunctivitis. *Am J Ophthalmol* 2003; **136**:1097–1105.

Gunduz K, Ucakhan O, Budak K, Eryilmaz T, Ozkan M. Efficacy of iodoxamide 0.1% versus N-acetyl aspartyl glutamic acid 6% ophthalmic solutions in patients with vernal keratoconjunctivitis. *Ophthalmic Res* 1996; **28**:80–87.

Hingorani M, Lightman S. Therapeutic options in ocular allergic disease. *Drugs* 1995; **50**:208–221.

Hingorani M, Moodaley L, Calder VL, Buckley RJ, Lightman S. A randomized, placebo-controlled trial of topical cyclosporin A in steroid-dependent atopic keratoconjunctivitis. *Ophthalmology* 1998; **105**:1715–1720.

Ilyas H, Slonim CB, Braswell GR, Favetta JR, Schulman M. Long-term safety of loteprednol etabonate 0.2% in the treatment of seasonal and perennial allergic conjunctivitis. *Eye Contact Lens* 2004; **30**:10–13.

James IG, Campbell LM, Harrison JM, et al. Comparison of the efficacy and tolerability of topically administered azelastine, sodium cromoglycate and placebo in the treatment of seasonal allergic conjunctivitis and rhino-conjunctivitis. *Curr Med Res Opin* 2003; **19**:313–320.

Kida T, Fujii A, Sakai O, et al. Bepotastine besilate, a highly selective histamine H(1) receptor antagonist, suppresses vascular hyperpermeability and eosinophil recruitment in in vitro and in vivo experimental allergic conjunctivitis models. *Exp Eye Res* 2010; **91**:85–91.

Kjellman NI, Stevens MT. Clinical experience with Tilavist: an overview of efficacy and safety. *Allergy* 1995; **50**:14–22; discussion 34–38.

Lambiase A, Leonardi A, Sacchetti M, et al. Topical cyclosporine prevents seasonal recurrences of vernal keratoconjunctivitis in a randomized, double-masked, controlled 2-year study. *J Allergy Clin Immunol* 2011; **128**:896–897.

Lanier BQ, Finegold I, D'Arienzo P, et al. Clinical efficacy of olopatadine vs epinastine ophthalmic solution in the conjunctival allergen challenge model. *Curr Med Res Opin* 2004; **20**:1227–1233.

Lanier BQ, Tremblay N, Smith JP, deFaller JM. A double-masked comparison of ocular decongestants as therapy for allergic conjunctivitis. *Ann Allergy* 1983; **50**:174–177.

Lapalus P, Moulin G, Bayer V, Fredj-Reygrobellet D, Elena PP. Effects of a new anti-allergic agent: the magnesium salt of N-acetyl-aspartyl-glutamic acid on experimental allergic inflammation of the rabbit eye. *Curr Eye Res* 1986; **5**:517–522.

Leino M, Montan P, Njå F. A double-blind group comparative study of ophthalmic sodium cromoglycate, 2% four times daily and 4% twice daily, in the treatment of seasonal allergic conjunctivitis. *Allergy* 1994; **49**:147–151.

Leonardi A. Emerging drugs for ocular allergy. *Expert Opin Emerg Drugs* 2005; **10**:505–520.

Leonardi A, Borghesan F, Avarello A, Plebani M, Secchi A. Effect of lodoxamide and disodium cromoglycate on tear eosinophil cationic protein in vernal keratoconjunctivitis. *Br J Ophthalmol* 1997; **81**:23–26.

Leonardi A, Bremond-Gignac D, Bortolotti M, et al. Clinical and biological efficacy of preservative-free NAAGA eye-drops versus levocabastine eye-drops in vernal keratoconjunctivitis patients. *Br J Ophthalmol* 2007; **91**:1662–1666.

Leonardi A, Busato F, Fregona I, Plebani M, Secchi AG. Anti-inflammatory and antiallergic effects of ketorolac tromethamine in the conjunctival provocation model. *Br J Ophthalmol* 2000; **84**:1228–1232.

Leonardi A, DeFranchis G, De Paoli M, et al. Histamine-induced cytokine production and ICAM-1 expression in human conjunctival fibroblasts. *Curr Eye Res* 2002; **25**:189–196.

Leonardi A, Quintieri L. Olopatadine: a drug for allergic conjunctivitis targeting the mast cell. *Expert Opin Pharmacother* 2010; **11**:969–981.

Macejko TT, Bergmann MT, Williams JI, et al. Multicenter clinical evaluation of bepotastine besilate ophthalmic solutions 1.0% and 1.5% to treat allergic conjunctivitis. *Am J Ophthalmol* 2010; **150**:122–127.e5.

Mah FS, Rosenwasser LJ, Townsend WD, Greiner JV, Bensch G. Efficacy and comfort of olopatadine 0.2% versus epinastine 0.05% ophthalmic solution for treating itching and redness induced by conjunctival allergen challenge. *Curr Med Res Opin* 2007; **23**:1445–1452.

McGhee CN, Dean S, Danesh-Meyer H. Locally administered ocular corticosteroids: benefits and risks. *Drug Saf* 2002; **25**:33–55.

Meijer F, Pogany K, Kok JH, Kijlstra A. N-acetyl-aspartyl glutamic acid (NAAGA) topical eyedrops in the treatment of giant papillary conjunctivitis (GPC). *Doc Ophthalmol* 1993; **85**:5–11.

Melamed J, Schwartz RH, Blumenthal MN, Zeitz HJ. Efficacy and safety of nedocromil sodium 2% ophthalmic solution b.i.d. in the treatment of ragweed seasonal allergic conjunctivitis. *Allergy Asthma Proc* 2000; **21**:235–239.

Nazarov O, Petzold U, Haase H, et al. Azelastine eye drops in the treatment of perennial allergic conjunctivitis. *Arzneimittelforschung* 2003; **53**:167–73.

Nishimura N, Ito K, Tomioka H, Yoshida S. Inhibition of chemical mediator release from human leukocytes and lung in vitro by a novel antiallergic agent, KB-2413. *Immunopharmacol Immunotoxicol* 1987; **9**:511–521.

Novack GD, Howes J, Crockett RS, Sherwood MB. Change in intraocular pressure during long-term use of loteprednol etabonate. *J Glaucoma* 1998; **7**:266–269.

Ono SJ, Lane K. Comparison of effects of alcaftadine and olopatadine on conjunctival epithelium and eosinophil recruitment in a murine model of allergic conjunctivitis. *Drug Des Devel Ther* 2011; **5**:77–84.

Owen CG, Shah A, Henshaw K, Smeeth L, Sheikh A. Topical treatments for seasonal allergic conjunctivitis: systematic review and meta-analysis of efficacy and effectiveness. *Br J Gen Pract* 2004; **54**:451–456.

Ozcan AA, Ersoz TR, Dulger E. Management of severe allergic conjunctivitis with topical cyclosporin a 0.05% eyedrops. *Cornea* 2007; **26**:1035–1038.

Pinto CG, Lafuma A, Fagnani F, Nuijten MJ, Berdeaux G. Cost effectiveness of emedastine versus levocabastine in the treatment of allergic conjunctivitis in 7 European countries. *Pharmacoeconomics* 2001; **19**:255–265.

Plewako H, Arvidsson M, Petruson K, et al. The effect of omalizumab on nasal allergic inflammation. *J Allergy Clin Immunol* 2002; **110**:68–71.

Pucci N, Novembre E, Cianferoni A, et al. Efficacy and safety of cyclosporine eyedrops in vernal keratoconjunctivitis. *Ann Allergy Asthma Immunol* 2002; **89**:298–303.

Qasem AR, Bucolo C, Baiula M, et al. Contribution of alpha4beta1 integrin to the antiallergic effect of levocabastine. *Biochem Pharmacol* 2008; **76**:751–762.

Rajpal RK, Digby D, D'Aversa G, et al. Intraocular pressure elevations with loteprednol etabonate: a retrospective chart review. *J Ocul Pharmacol Ther* 2011; **27**:305–308.

Reinhard T, Moller M, Sundmacher R. Penetrating keratoplasty in patients with atopic dermatitis with and without systemic cyclosporin A. *Cornea* 1999; **18**:645–651.

Rikkers SM, Holland GN, Drayton GE, et al. Topical tacrolimus treatment of atopic eyelid disease. *Am J Ophthalmol* 2003; **135**:297–302.

Scadding GK, Keith PK. Fluticasone furoate nasal spray consistently and significantly improves both the nasal and ocular symptoms of seasonal allergic rhinitis: a review of the clinical data. *Expert Opin Pharmacother* 2008; **9**:2707–2715.

Schechter BA. Ketorolac tromethamine 0.4% as a treatment for allergic conjunctivitis. *Expert Opin Drug Metab Toxicol* 2008; **4**:507–511.

Scoper SV, Berdy GJ, Lichtenstein SJ, et al. Perception and quality of life associated with the use of olopatadine 0.2% (Pataday) in patients with active allergic conjunctivitis. *Adv Ther* 2007; **24**:1221–1232.

Secchi A, Ciprandi G, Leonardi A, Deschenes J, Abelson MB. Safety and efficacy comparison of emedastine 0.05% ophthalmic solution compared to levocabastine 0.05% ophthalmic suspension in pediatric subjects with allergic conjunctivitis. Emadine Study Group. *Acta Ophthalmol Scand Suppl* 2000a; (230):42–47.

Secchi A, Leonardi A, Discepola M, et al. An efficacy and tolerance comparison of emedastine difumarate 0.05% and levocabastine hydrochloride 0.05%: reducing chemosis and eyelid swelling in subjects with seasonal allergic conjunctivitis. *Acta Ophthalmol Scand Suppl* 2000b; **230**:48–51.

Sharif NA, Xu SX, Yanni JM. Olopatadine (AL-4943A): ligand binding and functional studies on a novel, long acting H1-selective histamine antagonist and anti-allergic agent for use in allergic conjunctivitis. *J Ocul Pharmacol Ther* 1996; **12**:401–407.

Shulman DG, Lothringer LL, Rubin JM. A randomized, double-masked, placebo-controlled parallel study of loteprednol etabonate 0.2% in patients with seasonal allergic conjunctivitis. *Ophthalmology* 1999; **106**:362–369.

Spangler DL, Bensch G, Berdy GJ. Evaluation of the efficacy of olopatadine hydrochloride 0.1% ophthalmic solution and azelastine hydrochloride 0.05% ophthalmic solution in the conjunctival allergen challenge model. *Clin Ther* 2001; **23**:1272–1280.

Spector SL, Raizman MB. Conjunctivitis medicamentosa. *J Allergy Clin Immunol* 1994; **94**:134–136.

Tinkelman DG, Rupp G, Kaufman H, Pugely J, Schultz N. Double-masked, paired-comparison clinical study of ketorolac tromethamine 0.5% ophthalmic solution compared with placebo eyedrops in the treatment of seasonal allergic conjunctivitis. *Surv Ophthalmol* 1993; **38**:133–140.

Tomioka H, Yoshida S, Tanaka M, Kumagai A. Inhibition of chemical mediator release from human leukocytes by a new antiasthma drug, HC 20-511 (ketotifen). *Monogr Allergy* 1979; **14**:313–317.

Torkildsen G, Shedden A. The safety and efficacy of alcaftadine 0.25% ophthalmic solution for the prevention of itching associated with allergic conjunctivitis. *Curr Med Res Opin* 2011; **27**:623–631.

Torkildsen GL, Gomes P, Welch D, Gopalan G, Srinivasan S. Evaluation of desloratadine on conjunctival allergen challenge-induced ocular symptoms. *Clin Exp Allergy* 2009; **39**:1052–1059.

Torkildsen GL, Ousler GW 3rd, Gomes P. Ocular comfort and drying effects of three topical antihistamine/mast cell stabilizers in adults with allergic conjunctivitis: a randomized, double-masked crossover study. *Clin Ther* 2008; **30**:1264–1271.

Torkildsen GL, Williams JI, Gow JA, et al. Bepotastine besilate ophthalmic solution for the relief of nonocular symptoms provoked by conjunctival allergen challenge. *Ann Allergy Asthma Immunol* 2010; **105**:57–64.

Utine CA, Stern M, Akpek EK. Clinical review: topical ophthalmic use of cyclosporin A. *Ocul Immunol Inflamm* 2010; **18**:352–361.

Vichyanond P, Tantimongkolsuk C, Dumrongkigchaiporn P, et al. Vernal keratoconjunctivitis: result of a novel therapy with 0.1% topical ophthalmic FK-506 ointment. *J Allergy Clin Immunol* 2004; **113**:355–358.

Virtanen HM, Reitamo S, Kari M, Kari O. Effect of 0.03% tacrolimus ointment on conjunctival cytology in patients with severe atopic blepharoconjunctivitis: a retrospective study. *Acta Ophthalmol Scand* 2006; **84**:693–695.

Weiner JM, Abramson MJ, Puy RM. Intranasal corticosteroids versus oral H1 receptor antagonists in allergic rhinitis: systematic review of randomised controlled trials. *BMJ* 1998; **317**:1624–1629.

Whitcup SM, Bradford R, Lue J, Schiffman RM, Abelson MB. Efficacy and tolerability of ophthalmic epinastine: a randomized, double-masked, parallel-group, active- and vehicle-controlled environmental trial in patients with seasonal allergic conjunctivitis. *Clin Ther* 2004; **26**:29–34.

Yanni JM, Sharif NA, Gamache DA, et al. A current appreciation of sites for pharmacological intervention in allergic conjunctivitis: effects of new topical ocular drugs. *Acta Ophthalmol Scand Suppl* 1999a; (228):33–37.

Yanni JM, Weimer LK, Sharif NA, et al. Inhibition of histamine-induced human conjunctival epithelial cell responses by ocular allergy drugs. *Arch Ophthalmol* 1999b; **117**:643–647.

Chapter 37 Lacrimal punctal occlusion

Stefan Schrader, Frank H. W. Tost, Gerd Geerling

■ INTRODUCTION

Dry eye disease can be due to aqueous tear deficiency and excessive evaporation, both causing damage to the interpalpebral ocular surface and being associated with symptoms of ocular discomfort (Lemp 1998, Pflugfelder et al. 2000). Aqueous tear deficiency can be compensated by improving external conditions to reduce evaporation, applying artificial tears, or reducing lacrimal outflow.

While mild degrees of discomfort resulting from aqueous deficiency can usually be successfully managed with pharmaceutical tear substitutes alone, in moderate-to-severe disease, partial or complete blockage of the lacrimal drainage system is a commonly used modality to treat dry eye disease by increasing the residence time of tear substitutes or natural tears—the fluid with the best lubricant and nutrient capacity for the ocular surface. Occlusion of the lacrimal punctae can be achieved by plugs or surgical methods (Murube & Murube 1996, Tost & Geerling 2008).

However, disadvantages of this approach include signs and symptoms of mechanical irritation such as discomfort, abrasion of the conjunctiva and cornea, epiphora and pyogenic granuloma formation, or loss of the device (Murube & Murube 1996). Yen et al. (2001) found that punctal occlusion can also reduce tear production, clearance, and ocular surface sensation. Also, especially if there is a high inflammatory component of the dry eye disease, punctual occlusion can lead to increased concentrations of proinflammatory cytokines in the tear film, which could promote inflammation resulting in an aggravation of the disease (Pflugfelder et al. 1999, Yen et al. 2001).

This chapter discusses the indications and provides an overview of the methods used for iatrogenic blockage of the lacrimal drainage system.

■ INDICATIONS FOR LACRIMAL PUNCTAL OCCLUSION

Lacrimal punctal occlusion is a non-pharmacological intervention for dry eye disease. It can be used in the management of the disease, if the application of artificial teardrops alone is insufficient to relieve patient's signs or symptoms (Balaram et al. 2001, Willis et al. 1987). The Dry Eye Workshop Report 2007 states that the extensive literature on the use of punctal plugs in the management of dry eye disease has documented their utility. However, as recent reports have suggested that the absorption of tears by the nasolacrimal ducts may provide a feedback mechanism and that punctal occlusion might decrease tear production, this should be carefully considered when deciding about the inclusion of punctal plugs in the management of dry eye disease (Dry Eye Workshop, 2007).

For temporal or semipermanent occlusion, punctum plugs are inserted into the lacrimal puncta or canaliculi, whereas permanent occlusion can be achieved by thermal cautery, argon laser, or different surgical techniques.

Clinical studies have established objective and subjective benefit from punctual occlusion in moderate-to-severe forms of the disease (Nava-Castaneda et al. 2003, Tai et al. 2002). This approach is therefore well established in the stepwise management of dry eye disease (Balaram et al. 2001, Goto & Tseng 2003) where it has been found to improve tear volume, stability, and symptoms. In addition, it decreases hyperosmolarity and improves Rose Bengal positive staining of the ocular surface, although impression cytologic abnormalities tend to persist for at least 6 weeks (Gilbard et al. 1989, Patel & Grierson 1994, Willis et al. 1987). As a general guideline punctal plugs should be considered in patients with symptoms of dry eye disease, a Schirmer's test of ≤5 mm, and positive superficial punctate staining (Tost & Geerling 2008).

Punctal occlusion plugs have also shown to increase the duration of daily contact lens wear in contact lens-induced symptoms of dry eye disease and are beneficial in patients undergoing lid surgery such as ptosis surgery or blepharoplasty, which increases ocular surface exposure (Becker 1991, Virtanen et al. 1996).

Similar advantages of punctual occlusion have been reported for more severe forms of dry eye disease, often induced by an underlying immune disorder directed against mucous membrane or glandular tissue, such as Sjögren's syndrome, Stevens–Johnson syndrome, or ocular mucous membrane pemphigoid (Mansour et al. 2007, Tost & Geerling 2008). Inflammation as well as subsequent scarring of the tissues involved can lead to the aqueous deficient as well as the evaporative form of dry eye disease, due to occlusion of the canaliculi of the lacrimal or meibomian glands. If the lacrimal drainage system is not already blocked as a consequence of the disease, these eyes can benefit from prolonging the residence time of any remaining natural tears or applied substitute medication (Tost & Geerling 2008).

However, extensive surgical manipulation as well as retention of proinflammatory cytokines or potentially cytotoxic medication on the ocular surface can also lead to acute exacerbation or chronic levels of conjunctival inflammation (Dogru & Tsubota 2004, Pflugfelder 2004, Pflugfelder et al. 1999). In this special group of patients, systemic immunosuppression can be necessary to control inflammation, simultaneously avoiding toxicity of topically applied anti-inflammatory medication. It is also important that other contributing factors such as malposition of lid margin and resulting trichiasis are treated adequately.

Refractive corneal surgery, such as photorefractive keratectomy, laser-assisted in situ keratomileusis, or laser-assisted subepithelial keratomileusis, permanently alter corneal morphology including corneal innervation. If the sensitive corneal nerve fibers originating from the trigeminal nerve are severed, the afferent part of the lacrimal reflex loop is impaired and this can result in impaired epithelial wound healing. Huang et al. reported that temporary lacrimal drainage occlusion reduced postoperative symptoms and the need for lubricants. It also improved conjunctival goblet cell density, corneal wound healing, and finally visual acuity (Huang et al. 2004).

Lacrimal plugs can also be used as an adjunctive modality to modulate the effect or minimize potential side effects of other forms of topical treatment. When tumors or neovascular disease of the ocular surface is treated with topical mitomycin C or vascular endothelial growth factor (VEGF) inhibitors, blocking the lacrimal drainage not only expands the retention time and efficacy of the drug but may also reduce nasal mucosal irritation or the risk for serious systemic side effects (Basti & Macsai 2003).

OCCLUSION OF THE LACRIMAL DRAINAGE SYSTEM WITH PLUGS

There are many different types of plugs available on the market that can be differentiated according to their material and their intended location (punctal or canalicular).

Punctal plugs

Punctal plugs usually consist of a flat cap, a cylindrical neck, and a cone-shaped base (**Figure 37.1**). They are placed directly into the punctum, which makes it easy to control their position and, if necessary, to remove the plug. The disadvantages of their superficial location are that they may cause irritation and ocular surface inflammation and can also be lost more easily due to patient manipulation (Tost & Geerling 2008).

At present, most of the punctal plugs dominating the market are made of silicone material (Fayet et al. 2001, Tai et al. 2002). Other materials tested include teflon, hydroxyethylmethacrylate, or polymethylmethacrylate, but none of these showed significant advantages over silicone plugs (Tost & Geerling 2008). In a study by Tai et al. (2002), the mean retention time for silicone plugs was 85.1 ± 7.3 weeks.

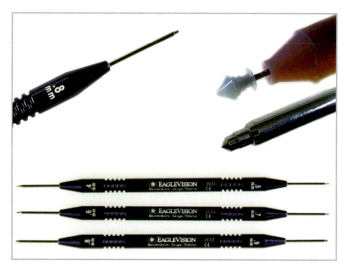

Figure 37.1 Silicone punctum plug applicator and punctum dilators of different diameters. The conical tip of measurement system equipped with two steps. The first step corresponds to diameter of lacrimal punctum; this helps determine individual size of the punctual plug and avoid overstretching the punctual opening.

Intracanalicular plugs

Intracanalicular plugs can be inserted into the ampulla or the horizontal portion of the lacrimal canaliculi and have the advantage of avoiding contact with the ocular surface (**Figure 37.2**). Therefore, mechanical irritation is avoided and discomfort is uncommon. However, these plugs are more difficult to follow up, and if this should become necessary due to complications, this is more difficult compared to punctal plugs (Tost & Geerling 2008).

Non-dissolvable intracanalicular plugs are available in different materials. In clinical practice, silicone plugs (Lee & Flanagan 2001) are used most commonly. Thermodynamic acrylic polymer plugs, which expand in diameter after exposure to body temperature (Burgess et al. 2008), and hydrogel plugs, which also expand after insertion, are supposed to reduce bacterial adhesion and biofilm formation and therefore might be a good future alternative to silicone plugs (Tost & Geerling 2008).

Dissolvable plugs are usually rod-shaped and are made from different materials such as collagen, gelatin, or hydroxypropyl cellulose. They are mainly used for diagnostic purposes and to test whether a patient might develop epiphora following permanent surgical occlusion (Murube & Murube 1996).

However, temporary lacrimal plugs made of collagen have been shown to effectively occlude the canaliculi for only <48 hours, reduce the outflow of tears only by 60–80%, and therefore may be insufficient to mimic full occlusion and simulate a situation caused by permanent occlusion (Tost & Geerling 2008).

Clinical outcome of lacrimal drainage system occlusion with plugs

Among the permanent devices, punctal or intracanalicular plugs show the same degree of objective and subjective improvement, such as reduced need of artificial tear substitute application or punctate surface staining and increased break-up time as goblet cell density in impression cytology (Tost & Geerling 2008).

There is a lack of strong evidence in randomized clinical trials for the long-term efficiency of collagen plugs as a treatment modality for dry eye disease as reviewed in a Cochrane review by Ervin et al. (2010). One study reported no statistically significant effect on either objective or subjective measures of dry eye disease after 5 days of occlusion with collagen plugs (Lowther & Semes 1995) and Tsifetaki et al. (2003) showed oral pilocarpine to be more effective than collagen punctal plugs after 12 weeks of dry eye disease treatment in Sjögren's syndrome patients. However, as pointed out in the Cochrane review by Ervin and colleagues these studies do not report on the use of collagen plugs as a means of predicting the efficiency of permanent plugs, a purpose for which collagen plugs are usually used.

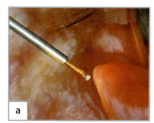
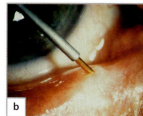
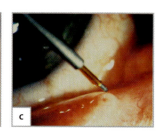

Figure 37.2 Intracanalicular hydrogel plug with the applicator. (a) Before, (b) during, and (c) after insertion, where the plug is completely inserted into the ampulla of proximal canaliculus.

Randomized clinical studies of permanent silicone or combined silicone–collagen punctal occlusion in the treatment of dry eye disease have shown evidence of their clinical efficacy (Burgess et al. 2008, Mansour et al. 2007). The most convincing evidence at present for the efficacy of punctal occlusion comes from a trial by Nava-Castaneda et al. (2003). In that study, a structured therapeutic regimen using temporal collagen plugs followed by silicone plugs was used. Patients with dry eye disease were randomized to either a treatment or a sham group and the outcome was assessed at 1 hour and then 2, 4, and 8 weeks after implantation. The results showed highly significant improvements in moisturizing agent use, fluorescein staining, ocular discomfort, and visual performance in the treatment compared to the sham group. Also, the therapeutic effect of punctal occlusion increased significantly as the duration of the treatment increased.

The most common adverse outcomes in the treatment with punctum plugs are plug loss and epiphora, inhibited tear clearance, and desensitization of the corneal surface (Lemp 1994, Sheppard 2003, Tai et al. 2002). In addition, ocular irritation, foreign body sensation, inflammatory reactions against silicone, corneal melting, and perforation have been reported (Burgess et al. 2008, Mansour et al. 2007, Nava-Castaneda et al. 2003).

Contraindications include allergy to plug materials, punctal ectropion, and preexisting canalicular obstruction. Obvious severe inflammatory changes of the lids and ocular surface should also be treated to reduce the load of proinflammatory cytokines, since reduced tear clearance may otherwise exacerbate chronic surface disease.

In a retrospective study by Tai et al. (2002) on 203 eyes, lacrimal plugs had to be removed in 6.9% of the eyes due to severe itching, a sensation of pressure, and mechanical irritation. These were more commonly reported for punctal plugs than intracanalicular plugs. The high rate of spontaneously lost punctal plugs may also be a consequence of these problems (Balaram et al. 2001, Fayet et al. 2001, Lee & Flanagan 2001).

Spontaneous loss of punctal plugs has been described by various authors to occur in 29–51% and this is more common in patients with horizontal lid laxity and dilated punctae (Willis et al. 1987). In Tai's study, the estimated probability of plug retention was 49%, with a mean survival time of 85.1 ± 7.3 weeks (Tai et al. 2002). Most of the extruded implants (50%) are lost within 4 weeks. Retention is better in the lower than in the upper punctum (Sakamoto et al. 2004). Dislocation into the deeper segments of the lacrimal drainage system is very rare, but can result in more severe consequences (Glatt 1991). If canaliculitis or dacryocystitis evolve, canaliculotomy, external dacryocystorhinostomy, or endoscopic-microsurgical management are required.

If a plug is lost spontaneously, punctal devices can be anchored by placing a non-absorbable suture through its collar and to the lid margin. Alternatively, an intracanalicular plug may be used for more permanent lacrimal drainage occlusion, since 20-MHz ultrasonography has shown that all of 40 implanted thermodynamic acrylic plugs remained in their original position over a period of 2 years (Obata et al. 2006, Tost et al. 2004). However, to reduce patient discomfort and costs in these cases due to repeated device insertion, and if permanent outflow obstruction is required, a surgical blockage of the lacrimal drainage system should be considered.

Surgical occlusion of the lacrimal drainage system

Permanent occlusion of the lacrimal drainage system should only be performed if symptoms (i.e. foreign body sensation, and dryness)

and signs of aqueous deficiency (Schirmer's test repeatedly ≤5 mm in 5 minutes) coincide with signs of severe ocular surface disease and persist despite frequent application of unpreserved lubricants.

Lacrimal punctal occlusion using plugs should be performed and well tolerated without unwanted effects beforehand (Dursun et al. 2003, Kaido et al. 2004).

If surface staining preoperatively is completely negative, other reasons for ocular discomfort have to be evaluated, since the reliability and repeatability of the Schirmer's test are low and patients with a test result of as little as 1 mm can be free of symptoms and signs of disease (Geerling & Tost 2008).

Lacrimal syringing should always be performed prior to opting for permanent iatrogenic outflow occlusion to make sure that the canaliculi are not already occluded (i.e. due to cicatrizing conjunctivitis) and that the epiphora is not absent just due to the reduced tear volume. Also, symptoms of irritation may have been induced by subclinical dacryocystitis due to the backwash of proinflammatory cytokines from the tear sack, which can be treated by a simple dacryocystorhinostomy; also in patients with preexisting nasolacrimal duct stenosis additional occlusion of the canaliculi may cause serious complications such as acute dacryocystitis (Glatt 1991, Marx et al. 1992).

The question regarding which and how many punctae or canaliculi should be occluded remains controversial. In a normal individual, the volume drained via the lower or upper part of the system is approximately the same. Since the lower punctum is more easily accessible, it is frequently occluded first. If signs and symptoms of aqueous deficiency persist, the complementary part of the system is occluded. It has been established that one patent canaliculus is sufficient to prevent epiphora, unless reflex tearing evolves. Although in the dry eye disease situation the occlusion of both punctae gives better results, sequential occlusion (i.e. permanent occlusion in lower punctum and temporary plug in upper punctum) strategies may be preferable in individual patients, especially if permanent occlusion is attempted (Murube & Murube 1996).

Surgical principles

Permanent punctal or canalicular occlusion can be both difficult to achieve as well as—once successfully established—impossible to reverse (Liu & Sadhan 2002). The less destructive the surgical method is, the more frequently the recanalization will occur. Laser punctal occlusion was reported to have a median time to reopening of 22 weeks versus cautery occluded puncta with 28 weeks (Vrabec et al. 1993). On the other hand, an extensive iatrogenic canalicular block will require bypass surgery if epiphora should become a problem. It is therefore advisable to reserve surgical occlusion for severe cases of dry eye disease and to assess the patient's response to punctal or canalicular plugs as a temporary measure first. However, it should be noted that undersized plugs, which produce only an incomplete block, may fail to predict epiphora after permanent punctal occlusion (Glatt 1992). Interventions to block the lacrimal drainage system are not only destructive but also—with the exception of cautery—consume more time and financial resources than the use of plugs.

Irreversible techniques
Heat-induced damage or shrinkage of tissue

Damage or shrinkage of the canalicular and pericanalicular tissues by a hot cautery probe, diathermy, or lasers has been used to occlude the lacrimal outflow. Of these, cauterization is the most simple and frequently practiced method. Variable efficacy has been reported, which seems to depend on the technique used. Superficial cauterization of the lacrimal punctum results in a reopening in 56% cases within 1 month. If the entire vertical portion of the canaliculus is cauterized, this rate is reduced to 7% at 1 month (Knapp et al. 1989). 'Deep cautery' of the vertical plus the horizontal canalicular section of the system is likely to provide an even higher rate of primary and lasting closure.

Alternatively, an argon laser can be used to occlude the punctum. With this technique, 15–500 spots of 100–750 µm diameter and 0.1–2.0 W are applied in the continuous mode for up to 9 seconds (most commonly, 10 burns of 200 µm at 0.4 W) around the punctum. Although this is associated with less postoperative discomfort and a reduced inflammatory reaction, it is also associated with a higher recanalization rate since the laser is not capable of inducing sufficiently deep and extensive tissue necrosis that is required for a long-term effect (Benson et al. 1992, Murube & Murube 1996). Therefore, cautery remains by far the fastest and easiest heat-based method to induce a profound destruction of the canalicular wall.

Occlusion with tissue adhesive (cyanoacrylate)

Occlusion with tissue adhesive is an alternative method of occluding the lacrimal outflow on the level of the ampulla or canaliculus. Patten applied a drop of cyanoacrylate to the punctum, which lasted for a mean of 2.5 weeks (Patten 1976). Diamond et al. used the glue to permanently occlude the entire lacrimal drainage system (Diamond et al. 1995).

Although one would expect that in a biological environment the glue will dissolve in the course of several weeks resulting in recanalization, Diamond could show by means of dacryoscintigraphy that this method was capable of occluding the canaliculi for the full follow-up of a mean of 15 months (11–19 months) in all patients of a case series of eight patients. Patten and Diamond reported only minor complications such as irritation immediately following adhesive application, due to a protrusion of polymer. This was easily managed by trimming the glue. However, with longer follow-up, several cases of canaliculitis or acute dacryocystitis have been reported following glue occlusion of the canalicular part of the drainage system. In these cases, histology showed persistent glue as foreign bodies inducing a severe giant-cell reaction (Koehler 1986). Methods that avoid the use of foreign body material in the nasolacrimal ducts should therefore be preferred for permanent occlusion.

Punctal or canalicular ligature

Charleux described a procedure in which—following local anesthesia—the vertical and horizontal canaliculus is cauterized, the punctum is excised, and the vertical portion is closed with a suture (Charleux & Brun 1978). Liu described the results of a prospective study in which the technique was slightly modified by using a corneal burr (diameter: 0.6 mm) to remove the epithelium from the punctum and the vertical 2 mm of the canaliculus of 26 punctae in 11 patients. A single 6.0 interrupted absorbable suture was placed parallel to the lid margin to approximate and occlude the punctum. This procedure achieved occlusion of punctum or vertical canliculus in 92% cases for a follow-up of 14–34 months and was associated with significant subjective improvement in 64% cases (Liu & Sadhan 2002). No complications were observed. Despite the anatomic success and symptomatic relief, the postoperative signs of surface disease (i.e.

epitheliopathy after Rose Bengal or fluorescein staining) did not improve. Since no quantitative Schirmer's test data were reported, subjective improvement could have been the result of a placebo effect. DeMartelaere et al. reported about 29 patients in whom 59 canaliculi were ligated following vertical trans-section of the horizontal portion of the canaliculus. The procedure resulted in a symptomatic relief in 91% cases. Due to complaints of epiphora, two canaliculi were later reconstructed successfully with repeated vertical trans-section and routine canalicular repair using a silicone intubation. This procedure may therefore be also considered reversible in nature (DeMartelaere et al. 2006).

Canalicular excision

Canalicular excision is a procedure where a Bowman's probe is advanced via the canaliculus into the lacrimal sac. The posterior wall of the canaliculus is incised through the conjunctiva with a D11 surgical blade from the punctum up to the medial canthus, just as in an extensive canaliculotomy. The canaliculus is than grasped with a pair of forceps and the desired length of the canalicular wall is excised with the blade, before the wound is closed with interrupted stitches of a long-acting absorbable 7.0 suture. If the intention is to excise only one individual canaliculus, the opposite canaliculus together with the common canalicular duct should be probed to avoid accidental damage to these structures (Putterman 1991). The only complications of canalicular excision reported include a very mild medial entropion or ectropion. The technique was described to have a 100% success rate, but should be considered irreversible, since tear drainage into the nose can only be re-established by means of a conjunctivodacryocysto(rhino)stomy (Farris 1989).

Dacryocystectomy

Dacryocystectomy is reserved for patients with severe dry eye disease simultaneously suffering from dacryocystitis. As discussed above, nasolacrimal duct obstruction can be associated with signs of ocular surface disease, such as punctate keratopathy (Glatt 1991). This is probably due to the backwash of inflammatory cytokines or pus from the occluded nasolacrimal ducts. Dacryocystectomy is then performed transcutaneously. The medial canthal tendon is detached and the lacrimal sac identified, mobilized, and severed from the common canaliculus and the nasolacrimal duct. The procedure has a 100% rate for success and irreversibility (Geerling & Tost 2008).

■ Potentially reversible surgical techniques

Transfer of the punctum to 'dry dock'

The transfer of the punctum to 'dry dock' was first described by Murube, and it involves transferring the lacrimal punctum toward the external lid margin. Of all surgical methods, this procedure is the least invasive one, and has been shown to be reversible. Migration of the punctum to its original position is rare, but may occur. Although, frequently, primary or secondary atrophy of the lacrimal punctum to a pinpoint size results, this can be dilated and successfully syringed (Murube-del-Castillo & Hernandez-King 1993).

Punctal tarsorrhaphy

Punctal tarsorrhaphy involves the rectangular excision of the superficial 1 mm tissue around the upper and lower punctum. No reports on the long-term success of this procedure exist, but conceptually it should be considered equivalent or superior to a regular tarsorrhaphy. Although this shortens the horizontal length of the palpebral fissure by approximately 5–7 mm, cosmetics is usually acceptable (Murube & Murube 1996).

Punctal patch

The punctal patch was also introduced by Murube and Murube (1996). Under local anesthesia and with the help of an operating microscope, an approximately 2 × 2 mm large piece of superficial rectangular piece of tissue including the punctum is excised. The obtained piece of tissue is used as a template to mark and prepare a graft from the bulbar conjunctiva, which is fixed with 7.0 interrupted absorbable sutures to cover the ampulla. In a study on 40 patients (160 punctae) Shalaby compared punctal patch and cautery. At 1 year, he reported 100% success with the patch method, while a 20% recanalization rate was observed following cautery (Shalaby et al. 2001). However, despite early anatomic success at 1 week, we have observed recanalization due to necrosis of the graft during further follow-up in four out of four puncta within 3 months (Geerling & Tost 2008). The approach has a few conceptual disadvantages, for example, in severe dry eye disease resulting from cicatrizing conjunctival disorders, such as ocular mucous membrane pemphigoid or Stevens–Johnson syndrome. In these, loss of even a small amount of conjunctiva may not be acceptable for functional reasons. Also, progression of the inflammatory component may be triggered by any form of conjunctival trauma, which therefore should be avoided. Additionally, the graft tissue is relatively thin and it is suspended over the lacrimal ampulla without any underlying tissue. Hence, no mechanical support or blood supply is provided to the central, that is, vital part of the graft. A modification of the technique by Geerling et al. provides a biomechanically stronger graft tissue and avoids the need for a conjunctival incision, while simultaneously maintaining the conceptual advantages of a complete and permanent occlusion and reversibility (Geerling & Tost 2008). This procedure was termed 'punctum switch graft'. In short, this involves an eccentric autorotational superficial tarsomarginal graft. The procedure is performed under an operating microscope following local anesthesia with approximately 1.0 mL of lignocaine injected into the medial lid margin. A 4.0 Prolene suture is placed to evert the lid margin with traction over a spatula. A large chalazion clamp helps to evert and stabilize the peripunctal lid margin. With a D11 blade, a 3 × 2 mm superficial area is marked on the lid margin immediately posterior to the lid lashes and including the punctum in the medial half. The marked area is then excised at a depth of approximately 1 mm. Obvious bleeders are cauterized while trying to avoid any excessive thermal damage to the donor or recipient bed. Following this, the graft is rotated 180° and sutured back in place with a continuous 7.0 long-acting absorbable suture. This leaves the excised punctum lateral to the ampulla, which itself is covered by full-thickness lid margin tissue. The surgical approach is usually easier in the lower than in the upper lid. Topical antibiotics are applied for 5 days and the sutures removed, if required, at 2 weeks postoperatively (**Figure 37.3**).

At 3 months postoperatively, 12 out of 18 canaliculi remained occluded and all punctae remained patent until the last follow-up. Six grafts showed necrosis or partial wound dehiscence. This approach largely avoids a surgical trauma to the conjunctiva and covers the drainage system with a biomechanically stronger piece of tissue. Although to date no procedure have had to be reversed, the number of patients treated and our follow-up are still limited and more extensive studies are required. The technique is also certainly more demand-

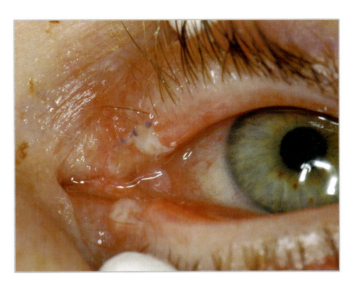

Figure 37.3 Left eye after punctum switch graft procedure.

ing on time and equipment than simple cautery. However, while the punctae may atrophy with postoperative time a 'punctum switch' procedure is potentially reversible.

■ CONCLUSIONS

Occlusion of the lacrimal drainage system with plugs has been shown to preserve natural tears, prolong the retention time of artificial tears on the ocular surface, and substantially improve the quality of life of patients with moderate to severe dry eye disease.

However, before blocking a lacrimal drainage system, a preexisting blepharitis or other forms of ocular surface inflammation must be treated in order to reduce the load of proinflammatory cytokines on the ocular surface. A possible benefit of lacrimal canalicular closure can be simulated with absorbable plugs, although a long-term treatment with dissolvable plugs might not be efficient in relieving patient's symptoms.

Occlusion of the lacrimal drainage system with plugs is usually easier to reverse than surgical approaches; however, discomfort and a high rate of spontaneous loss due to extrusion are a relevant disadvantage. If a punctal plug is sufficient to control signs and symptoms of dry eye disease, but is repeatedly lost, surgical measures to reduce tear drainage should be considered.

Before performing permanent surgical occlusion of the punctae or canaliculi, the lacrimal outflow system should be carefully assessed, since nasolacrimal duct obstruction can also be the cause of symptoms and signs of ocular surface irritation. Additionally, prior to permanent surgical occlusion, the effect of temporarily blocking the lacrimal drainage system should be tested with silicone or other plugs, since it can be difficult to re-establish transcanalicular lacrimal drainage once the system has been successfully occluded.

When permanent occlusion is considered necessary to improve the patient's symptoms, the lower lacrimal canaliculus should be blocked first and the common canaliculus should be spared. Of all methods, cautery is the simplest one; however, the primary thermal damage needs to be substantial in order to achieve long-term occlusion. Canalicular ligature can be considered as a simple and successful alternative. If after the surgery, symptoms or signs of dryness persist or reoccur, the punctae should be probed and syringed, since late recanalization is not uncommon. Epiphora, granuloma formation, suppurative canaliculitis, and acute dacryocystitis have been reported as complications weeks to months after iatrogenic lacrimal outflow occlusion; however, these reported complications are rare and should not prevent the use of this successful therapeutic strategy in the management of severe aqueous deficient dry eyes.

■ REFERENCES

Balaram M, Schaumberg DA, Dana MR. Efficacy and tolerability outcomes after punctal occlusion with silicone plugs in dry eye syndrome. *Am J Ophthalmol* 2001; **131**:30–36.

Basti S, Macsai MS. Ocular surface squamous neoplasia: a review. *Cornea* 2003; **22**:687–704.

Becker BB. Punctal occlusion and blepharoplasty in patients with dry eye syndrome. *Arch Otolaryngol Head Neck Surg* 1991; **117**:789–791.

Benson DR, Hemmady PB, Snyder RW. Efficacy of laser punctal occlusion. *Ophthalmology* 1992; **99**:618–621.

Burgess PI, Koay P, Clark P. SmartPlug versus silicone punctal plug therapy for dry eye: a prospective randomized trial. *Cornea* 2008; **27**:391–394.

Charleux J, Brun P. Traitement chirurgical des syndromes secs oculaires. *Bull Mém Soc Fr Ophthalmol* 1978; **89**:177–185.

Diamond JP, Morgan JE, Virjee J, Easty DL. Cannalicular occlusion with cyanoacrylate adhesive: a new treatment for the dry eye. *Eye* 1995; **9**:126–129.

DeMartelaere SL, Blaydon SM, Tovilla-Canales JL, Shore JW. A permanent and reversible procedure to block tear drainage for the treatment of dry eye. *Ophthal Plast Reconstr Surg* 2006; **22**:352–355.

Dogru M, Tsubota K. New insights into the diagnosis and treatment of dry eye. *Ocular Surf* 2004; **2**:59–75.

Dry Eye Workshop. Management and therapy of dry eye disease: report of the Management and Therapy Subcommittee of the International Dry Eye WorkShop (2007). *Ocular Surf* 2007; **5**:163–178.

Dursun D, Ertan A, Bilezikçi B, Akova YA, Pelit A. Ocular surface changes in keratoconjunctivitis sicca with silicone punctum plug occlusion. *Curr Eye Res* 2003; **26**:263–269.

Ervin AM, Wojciechowski R, Schein O. Punctal occlusion for dry eye syndrome. *Cochrane Database Syst Rev* 2010; CD006775.

Farris RL. The Sjögren's syndrome handbook. Sjögren's Syndrome Foundation Inc., Bethesda, MD; 1989:29–42.

Fayet B, Assouline M, Hanush S, et al. Silicone punctal plug extrusion resulting from spontaneous dissection of canalicular mucosa: a clinical and histopathologic report. *Ophthalmology* 2001; **108**:405–409.

Geerling G, Tost FH. Surgical occlusion of the lacrimal drainage system. *Dev Ophthalmol* 2008; **41**:213–229.

Gilbard JP, Rossi SR, Azar DT, Gray KL. Effect of punctal occlusion by Freeman silicone plug insertion on tear osmolarity in dry eye disorders. *CLAO J* 1989; **15**:216–218.

Glatt HJ. Acute dacryocystitis after punctal occlusion of keratoconjunctivitis sicca. *Am J Ophthalmol* 1991; **111**:769–770.

Glatt HJ. Failure of collagen plugs to predict epiphora after permanent punctal occlusion. *Ophthalmic Surg* 1992; **23**:292–293.

Goto E, Tseng SC. Kinetic analysis of tear interference images in aqueous tear deficiency dry eye before and after punctal occlusion. *Invest Ophthalmol Vis Sci* 2003; **44**:1897–1905.

Huang B, Mirza MA, Qazi MA, Pepose JS. The effect of punctal occlusion on wavefront aberrations in dry eye patients after laser in situ keratomileusis. *Am J Ophthalmol* 2004; **137**:52–61.

Kaido M, Goto E, Dogru M, Tsubota K. Punctal occlusion in the management of chronic Stevens-Johnson syndrome. *Ophthalmology* 2004; **111**:895–900.

Knapp ME, Frueh BR, Nelson CC, Musch DC. A comparison of two methods of punctal occlusion. *Am J Ophthalmol* 1989; **108**:315–318.

Koehler U. Kompliaktionen nach vorübergehendem Tränennasenwegsverschluß mit Gewebekleber (Histoacryl). *Klin Mbl Augenheilk* 1986; **189**:486–490.

Lee J, Flanagan JC. Complications associated with silicone intracanalicular plugs. *Ophthalmic Plastic Reconstructive Surg* 2001; **17**:465–469.

Lemp MA. Management of the dry-eye patient. *Int Ophthalmol Clin* 1994; **34**:101–113.

Lemp MA, Epidemiology and classification of dry eye. *Adv Exp Med Biol* 1998; **438**:791–803.

Liu D, Sadhan Y. Surgical punctal occlusion: a prospective study. *Br J Ophthalmol* 2002; **86**:1031–1034.

Lowther GE, Semes L. Effect of absorbable intracanalicular collagen implants in hydrogel contact lens patients with symptoms of dryness. *International Contact Lens Clinic* 1995; **22**:238–243.

Mansour K, Leonhardt CJ, Kalk WW, et al. Lacrimal punctum occlusion in the treatment of severe keratoconjunctivitis sicca caused by Sjogren syndrome: a uniocular evaluation. *Cornea* 2007; **26**:147–150.

Marx JL, Hillman DS, Hinshaw KD, et al. Bilateral dacryocystitis after punctal occlusion with thermal cautery. *Ophthalmic Surg* 1992; **23**:560–561.

Murube-del-Castillo J, Hernandez-King J. Treatment of dry eye by moving the lacrimal punctum to dry dock. *Ophthalmic Surg* 1993; **24**:53–58.

Murube J, Murube, E. Treatment of dry eye by blocking the lacrimal canaliculi. *Surv Ophthalmol* 1996; **40**:463–480.

Nava-Castaneda A, Tovilla-Canales JL, Rodriguez L, Tovilla Y, Pomar JL. Effects of lacrimal occlusion with collagen and silicone plugs on patients with conjunctivitis associated with dry eye. *Cornea* 2003; **22**:10–14.

Obata H, Ibaraki N, Tsuru T. A technique for preventing spontaneous loss of lacrimal punctal plugs. *Am J Ophthalmol* 2006; **141**:567–569.

Patel S, Grierson D. Effect of collagen punctal occlusion on tear stability and volume. *Adv Exp Med Biol* 1994; **350**:605–608.

Patten JT. Punctal occlusion with n-butyl cyanoacrylate tissue adhesive. *Ophthalmic Surg* 1976; **7**:24–26.

Pflugfelder SC. Antiinflammatory therapy for dry eye. *Am J Ophthalmol* 2004; **137**:337–342.

Pflugfelder SC, Jones D, Ji Z, Afonso A, Monroy D. Altered cytokine balance in the tear fluid and conjunctiva of patients with Sjögren's syndrome keratoconjunctivitis sicca. *Curr Eye Res* 1999; **19**:201–211.

Pflugfelder SC, Solomon A, Stern ME. The diagnosis and management of dry eye: a twenty-five-year review. *Cornea* 2000; **19**:644–649.

Putterman AM. Canaliculectomy in the treatment of keratitis sicca. *Ophthalmic Surg* 1991; **22**:478–480.

Sakamoto A, Kitagawa K, Tatami A. Efficacy and retention rate of two types of silicone punctal plugs in patients with and without Sjogren syndrome. *Cornea* 2004; **23**:249–254.

Shalaby O, Rivas L, Rivas AI, Oroza MA, Murube J. Comparison of 2 lacrimal punctal occlusion methods. *Arch Soc Esp Oftalmolo* 2001; **76**:533–536.

Sheppard JD. Dry eye moves beyond palliative therapy. *Managed Care* 2003; **12**:6–8.

Tai MC, Cosar CB, Cohen EJ, Rapuano CJ, Laibson PR. The clinical efficacy of silicone punctal plug therapy. *Cornea* 2002; **21**:135–139.

Tost FH, Darman J, Clemens S. 20-MHz ultrasound and its value in imaging of lacrimal plugs. *Ophthalmologica* 2004; **218**:14–19.

Tost FH, Geerling, G. Plugs for occlusion of the lacrimal drainage system. *Dev Ophthalmol* 2008; **41**:193–212.

Tsifetaki N, Kitsos G, Paschides CA, et al. Oral pilocarpine for the treatment of ocular symptoms in patients with Sjögren's syndrome: a randomised 12 week controlled study. *Ann Rheumatic Dis* 2003; **62**:1204–1207.

Virtanen T, Huotari K, Härkönen M, Tervo T.Lacrimal plugs as a therapy for contact lens intolerance. *Eye* 1996; **10**:727–731.

Vrabec MP, Elsing SH, Aitken PA. A prospective, randomized comparison of thermal cautery and argon laser for permanent punctal occlusion. *Am J Ophthalmol* 1993; **116**:469–471.

Willis RM, Folberg R, Krachmer JH, Holland EJ. The treatment of aqueous-deficient dry eye with removable punctal plugs. A clinical and impression-cytologic study. *Ophthalmology* 1987; **94**:514–518.

Yen MT. Pflugfelder SC, Feuer WJ. The effect of punctal occlusion on tear production, tear clearance, and ocular surface sensation in normal subjects. *Am J Ophthalmol* 2001; **131**:314–323.

Chapter 38 Bioadhesives

Jorge L. Alio, M. Emilia Mulet

■ INTRODUCTION

Bioadhesives are surgical devices with a major potential for application in conjunctiva and corneal surgery. Due to the relative simplicity of their use, and the evidence that this use may consistently save surgical time, this topic has recently attracted the attention of a number of industries interested in the development of ophthalmic surgery products. In general, the adequate closure of the different surgical planes is an essential step following any surgical procedure in order to achieve an adequate anatomical and functional result. The method used for the replacement of the tissue planes must be effective enough to join the reconstructed tissues, well tolerated by the biology of the reconstructed tissues, deprived of toxicity for all the tissues affected by the closure and the other neighboring ones, resistant to bacterial contamination, and easily absorbable or biodegradable. Additionally, it should not constitute a barrier for the normal healing process, which would follow the surgical reconstruction. The accessibility of the ocular surface has made the cornea, sclera, and conjunctiva the ocular tissues in which bioadhesives have been more extensively tested and used.

Corneal ulcer lacerations or perforations may be caused by trauma, infection, and inflammation and represent a common ophthalmic emergency with potentially blinding sequelae due to corneal scarring, astigmatism, and intraocular potential for complications, including lens damage and endophthalmitis. Sutures are used to repair corneal wounds and the pattern and extent of the injury will determine the number and type of sutures required to restore the integrity of the cornea. The process of suturing further causes additional trauma to the corneal tissue and increases the risk of infection, inflammation, and vascularization. Sutures require postoperative removal, in addition to the risk of loosening or breaking, and commonly induce astigmatism.

For all these reasons, the use of tissue adhesives has become a standard treatment for the temporary occlusion of perforations of the cornea since it was first described by Webster in 1968 (Webster et al. 1968). Interest in tissue adhesives has increased and numerous studies on many different types have been reported. Additionally, the use of bioadhesives in scleral and conjunctival surgery has received the attention of different investigators, both for the management of emergencies and also as a coadjuvant in the management of routine surgical procedures. Examples of indications for the application of bioadhesives include corneal perforations (Refojo et al. 1968), descematoceles (Arentsen et al. 1985), leaking filtering blebs (Kajiwara 1990), retinal holes (Seelenfreund et al. 1970), scleral thinning, stromal thinning, wound leaks, exposure keratopathy (Leahey et al. 1993), amniotic membrane transplantation, lamellar transplant (Cardarelli & Basu 1969, Kaufman et al. 2003), limbal wounds (Ellis & Levine 1963), corneal transplantation, strabismus surgery (Mulet et al. 2006, Ricci et al. 2000), tarsorrhaphy, punctal occlusion (Patten 1976), pterygium or conjunctive surgery (Alio et al. 2003), and cataract surgery or refractive surgery (Alió et al. 1996, Mulet et al. 1997).

However, in spite of the obvious reported advantages of ocular bioadhesives in the management of these conditions, its use has still not gained popularity due to different reasons, which include accessibility, irregular tolerance, cost, and potential biological hazards. In this chapter, we shall review the progress that this interesting and newly emerging topic has undergone during recent years.

■ TYPES OF TISSUE ADHESIVES USED IN OPHTHALMIC SURGERY

Figure 38.1 shows the classification of adhesives used in ophthalmic practice.

■ Cyanoacrylates

The use of cyanoacrylates has perhaps received the most attention as they have been widely used and many different acrylate substances have been proposed and investigated for the purpose of corneal,

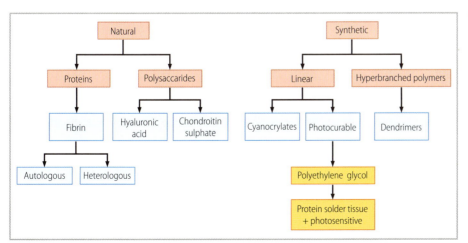

Figure 38.1 Adhesives types.

scleral, and conjunctival reconstruction, jointly with a wide range of polymerization promoters, inhibitors, or stabilizers.

The most extensively used cyanoacrylates include N-heptyl (6),2-octyl (Dermabond, Ethicon Inc, USA), isobutyl (Histacryl, Germany) (Cardarelli & Basu 1969), methyl-2 (Eastman 910, Eastman Kodak, USA), carbohexoxymethyl-2, N-butyl, isobutyl-2 (Tisuacryl, Cuba), N-butyl-2 (Histacryl-N-Blue, Braun, Germany), hexyl (Adal-2, Alicante University, Spain), ethyl, alkyl (Adal-1, Alicante University, Spain), and decyl-2 (Leahey et al. 1993). They differ in the length of the carbon side chains (**Figure 38.2**). These adhesives have limitations, which include their well-known capability for immediate polymerization upon contact with wet surfaces, generation of heat, as with all exothermic reactions, and their capability to degrade, generating toxic degradation products that include formaldehyde. The polymerization of the cyanoacrylate adhesive is inversely proportional to the length of the string. The shorter string will produce a faster cure, higher exothermic reaction, and more toxicity to tissues. Cyanoacrylates and derivatives have a good tensile strength and are efficient in joining tissues. However, their rigidity, hardness, limited effect in the presence of water or highly hydrated tissues, and their exothermicity have been their main drawbacks for their use in ophthalmic surgery.

Use of cyanoacrylates in ophthalmic surgery

Once cyanoacrylates are applied onto the ocular surface, the bond formed is rigid and, therefore, fragile. The longer range decreases the rate of polymerization, the adhesive is more flexible, and the exothermic reaction is lower, with less toxicity to tissues.

These derivatives have some limitations, which consist of a moist substrate reactivity with heat (exothermic reaction) such as cross-linking opaque spicules and cured product (**Figure 38.3**).

The degree of exothermicity depends on the speed that elapses from the polymerization reaction, the amount of adhesive applied, and the degree of wetting of the biological substrates (Refojo et al. 1968, Weiss et al. 1983). The release of energy as heat is likely to cause cell necrosis, which is a major limitation in the use of such adhesives in surgical practice. The opacity with which these cyanoacrylate bioadhesives polymerize makes their use limited to corneal injury or surgery. Rigid cross-linking makes these adhesives fragile and may cause ulcers in those tissues of the eye that are subjected to repeated friction (**Figure 38.4a–b**).

Another limitation of N-butyl adhesive is the amount of time it takes to be eliminated from biological tissues, which in some cases can go up to 3 or 4 months from the time of being instilled, inhibiting the healing process (Henderson & Stephenson 1992, Moschos et al. 1997). El isobutyl-2-cyanoacrylate is effective and better tolerated, and is the glue of choice for eye surgery (Alió et al. 1996).

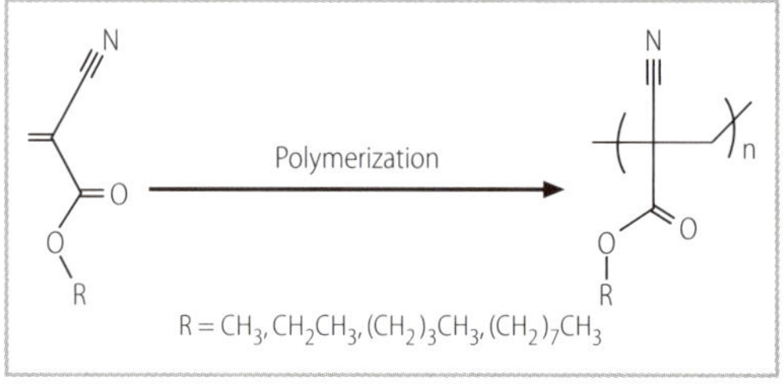

Modifying the molecular chain structure of cyanoacrylate produces a mixture of ethyl cyanoacrylate and 6-hydroxihexile (Adal-2). Cross-linked adhesive has a transparent appearance and consistency is supple to touch, such that the tissues surrounding the bond experience no ulcerative type lesion (**Figure 38.5**).

Depending on the tissues to be joined by the bioadhesive, a feature to be considered is the tensile strength of the joint, as it is not the same for the closure of conjunctival or corneal planes to attach muscle to sclera in strabismus surgery. The bond must be strong enough to withstand the eye movements. The hardness of the cured sealant produced by very rigid polymers can cause ulcers (Leahey et al. 1993, Moschos et al. 1997). The final hardness of the adhesive can delay the polymerization without losing the final efficiency producing a strong adhesive mix for this type of surgery. Adal-1 is an adhesive mixture of an alkyl and a new semisynthetic acrylic derivative. The results in rabbits and humans (Mulet et al. 2006) showed comparable efficacy in the sutures. The muscles were kept in the default site, with ocular movements in the adhesives group in comparison to the muscle control group, and no cases of ulceration of the surrounding tissue, blanching, or retinal necrosis were observed (**Figure 38.6a** and **38.6b**).

Another limitation in using the tissue adhesive has been the size of the perforations and the condition of the surrounding tissue. These factors influence glue adherence.

Existing options such as sutures or cyanoacrylate glues have been used to aid corneal wound healing for many years, but most surgeons agree that they are not ideal. Cyanoacrylate adhesives have been an effective therapeutic option in certain ophthalmic situations, such as sealing small perforations (1–3 mm) and pre-emptive treatment of corneal thinning disorders; however, the limitations of this method include difficult application techniques, limited effectiveness, discomfort, toxicity, and lack of biodegradation. Complications with cyanoacrylates that have been reported include cataract formation, corneal infiltration, granulomatous keratitis, glaucoma, and even retinal toxicity (Hida et al. 1988, Seelenfreund et al. 1970).

Cyanoacrylates and their derivatives, in spite of being proven as useful, are less used today for the purpose of tissue gluing than tissue sealants, due to their complications and limitations. For these reasons, a number of new alternatives for corneal repair are now being proposed.

Figure 38.2 Cyanoacrylate monomers used as surgical adhesives.

Polymerization

$R = CH_3, CH_2CH_3, (CH_2)_3CH_3, (CH_2)_7CH_3$

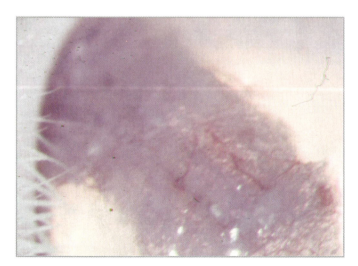

Figure 38.3 Experimental corneal laceration sealed by cyanoacrylate adhesive after the polymerization process.

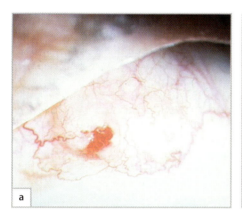

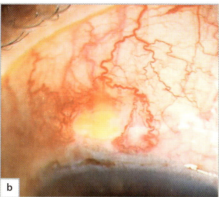

Figure 38.4 (a) Conjunctival ulcer produced by cyanoacrylate spicules. The adhesive was used to seal a conjunctival surgical incision for strabismus surgery. (b) Rigid spicules produced by cured cyanoacrylate. The adhesive was used for the purpose of sealing a conjunctival incision.

Fibrin adhesives

Fibrin sealant is a complex, plasma-derived product that is increasingly used as a biodegradable tissue adhesive or sealant, to stop or control bleeding or to provide a barrier to air and fluid during many surgical procedures. This product mimics the last step of the blood coagulation cascade, through the proteolysis of fibrinogen by thrombin, and factor XIII, which leads to the formation of a semirigid fibrin clot (**Figure 38.7**). The fibrin sealant can be applied in the following ways: sequential application, simultaneous application, and spray applica-

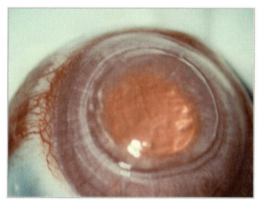

Figure 38.5 Experimental corneal flap sealed by Adal-2 bioadhesive.

tion (Kaetsu et al. 2000). Fibrin has a low tensile strength that limits its application for the purpose of joining tissues, especially if they are elastic or if the joining process needs to be forced by approximation. As the commercial presentations are all of animal origin, they are affected by a biological hazard that has further limited their registration and use, jointly to the high cost in many parts of the globe.

Use of fibrin glues in ophthalmic surgery

Tisseel adhesive, a fibrin glue (Tisseel, Baxter, USA), is a product frequently used with LASIK surgery flaps to prevent epithelial ingrowth because sutures do not create a continuous seal and can cause astigmatism (Kaufman et al. 2003). It is also used for conjunctiva and pterygia repair and amniotic membrane grafts. The fibrin glue is a biocompatible and totally biodegradable compound that induces minimal stromal inflammation and foreign body reaction and does not cause tissue necrosis. Some authors reported a 93% success rate in corneal perforations (Lagoutte et al. 1989) and comparable with N-butyl-2 cyanoacrylate in the closure of corneal perforations of up to 3 mm (Ashok et al. 2003), although the fibrin produces a faster scar response and a lower degree of corneal vascularization. The limitations of this type of adhesives are a low-protein cohesive force that results in low-strength adhesive bonds and the relatively short lifespan of fibrin adhesives (<2 weeks), which requires repeated application. In addition, there is an associated risk of viral contamination (Chan & Boisjoly 2004), to be extracted from blood plasma, and of allergic

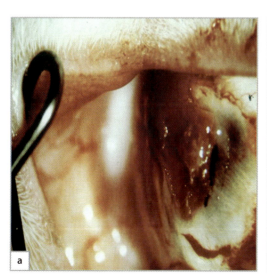

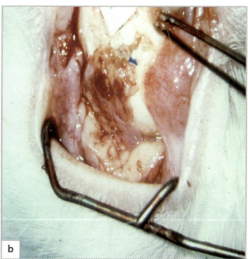

Figure 38.6 (a) Muscle joint sealed to sclera by Adal-1 (appearance immediately after sealing muscle to sclera). (b) One week after application. The muscle remains at the blue mark without suffering displacements caused by eye movements.

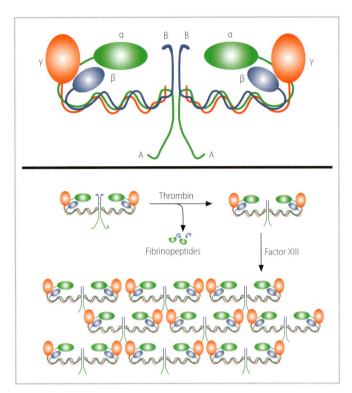

Figure 38.7 Blood coagulation cascade: proteolysis of fibrinogen by thrombin. Reproduced by permission of The Royal Society of Chemistry.

reaction (to bovin products). It is autologous in form and has a lengthy preparation time, complex application, and a high cost (Bathia 2006). However, recently, we have described a new approach for the use of autologous fibrin in sealing ulcers or perforations of the cornea with excellent results as a tectonic element and promoter of the wound healing process when associated to solid platelet-rich plasma (Alió et al. 2007, 2012) (**Figure 38.8**).

Protein tissue solder adhesives

Laser-induced tissue soldering and welding has been used as surgical adhesives since the 1960s (Bass & Treat 1995). Tissue welding occurs by heating the tissues of opposing wound edges until they flow together and entangle. Tissue welding is disadvantageous due to low repair strength and thermal damage to surrounding tissue.

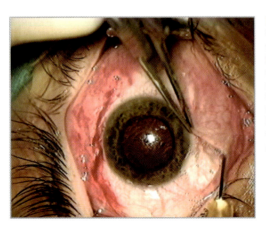

Figure 38.8 Conjunctive sealed with fibrin adhesive showing the gelatinous texture of the residual bioadhesive, which is easily eliminated.

Although conventional adhesives such as cyanoacrylates and fibrin have the potential to effectively close wounds, these adhesives suffer from some disadvantages. Many of the drawbacks of fibrin and cyanoacrylate adhesives have been overcome by the development of ophthalmic adhesives composed of protein tissue solders as well as natural and synthetic polymer hydrogels, which are soft, flexible, and hydrophilic materials. Protein-based tissue solders have been prepared from fibrinogen, albumin, and gelatine and have been mixed with linear polymers and polymer films for increased adhesion strength. The protein tissue solder and natural polymer hydrogel adhesives are advantageous due to their biocompatibility, but the cost, purity, and large-scale production are of concern due to the necessity of isolating adhesive components from human or animal sources. Hydrogel adhesives composed of synthetic polymers such as polyethyleneglycol (PEG) have attracted recent interest due to their ease of synthesis and purification, low costs, tunable molecular weight, choice of the monomer, and functional groups. The physical properties of a protein tissue solder can be modified by changes in the concentration of the original protein solution, as well as in the concentration of the absorbing chromophore. The cure time of these solders was ≤2 minutes and with little preparation time, only requiring simple mixing of components.

There are two general cross-linking strategies used to prepare hydrogel adhesives: photo-activated free radical cross-linking and nucleophilic substitution cross-linking. In both cases, new covalent bonds are being formed between the various cross-linkable polymers or monomers. In the nucleophilic substitution cross-linking approach, chemical reactions occur under physiological conditions of pH and temperature. The hydrogel formation time can be tuned from seconds to minutes in order to address the specific challenges of different wound models. Hydrogel adhesives are also formed by photolysis of a cross-linkable polymer in the presence of a photo-initiator system. Polymers are typically modified with methacrylate or acrylate groups. An advantage of using photo-induced cross-linking is that it allows for precise real-time control of cross-linking over the wound space by selective use of handheld laser optics. An important difference between hydrogels prepared by photo-induced free radicals and by nucleophilic substitution cross-linking is that, depending on the specific chemistry used, the latter type of hydrogel can bond chemically to the protein of the ocular surface (Oelker & Grinstaff 2008).

Use of protein solder adhesives in ophthalmic surgery

Several experimental models have been used to investigate the efficacy of tissue solders in the management of corneal wounds, including central corneal incisions, full-thickness corneal transplants, scleral incisions, and ocular muscle reattachment. In an animal in vivo model, protein solders have been tested for efficacy in the repair of corneal incisions (Khadem et al. 2004). Various mixtures have been tested, including albumin, hyaluronic acid, chondroitin sulfate, and indocyanine green dye cross-linked with an 808 mm diode laser for closing 8 mm scleral incisions in an in vitro porcine model (Oelker & Grinstaff 2008). All experiments have been conducted ex vivo. The enucleated eyes were then pressurized and the intraocular pressure was evaluated for observing the leakage presence in the wound site. Protein solders made of fibrinogen and riboflavin-5-phospate were applied to 5 mm central corneal incisions in enucleated human eyes and cured with an argon ion laser for 2 minutes at 600 mW. The leakage pressure of adhesive-treated wounds was within normal ranges, and no tissue distortion around the wound site was observed (Khadem et al. 2004). A similar mixture of fibrinogen and riboflavine-4-phosphate was used in an in vitro model of full-thickness 7 mm transplants and showed a higher leakage pressure obtained with adhesive plus 4 sutures than the control wounds sealed with 16 sutures.

An important step forward in the use of tissue solders to seal corneal wounds is the application of polymer film patches soaked with solder that are cross-linked onto the eye to provide additional structural support. The film–solder adhesive strength was dependent upon solder concentration, porosity of the polymer films, and wound type.

Dendritic polymers

Dendritic polymers are composed of glycerol and succinic acid. Polymers can be synthesized with specific chemical, physical, and medicinal properties that suit a diverse set of applications. Dendrimers are monodisperse, hyperbranched polymers possessing three main structural zones—a central core, internal branching layers, and peripheral end groups (**Figure 38.9**). The monomer units are assembled in a controlled step-growth polymerization process and are organized in layered 'generations.' The branched structure of dendrimers allows a globular, three-dimensional macromolecular shape and generally confers an important series of positive characteristics when compared to the other sealants, such as high solubility, low viscosity, adhesivity, and glass-transition temperatures that differ from the corresponding linear analogue. Medical applications of dendritic polymers vary owing to their size, ease of functionalization, large number of surface end groups, and well-defined structure (Luman et al. 2004). Dendrimers have been investigated as magnetic resonance imaging contrast agent carriers, gene transfection vehicles, drug delivery systems, and tissue sealants (Oelker & Grinstaff 2008).

A degradable, photo-curable biodendrimer sealant was prepared by reacting the (G1-PGLSA-OH)2-PEG dendritic linear polymer (Carnahan et al. 2002) with methacrylic anhydride to allow the methacrylated derivative. The resulting polymer can be subsequently photo-cross-linked to form a hydrogel using visible light in conjunction with a photo-initiating system (eosin, triethanolamine, and N-vinyl pyrrolidone). This system is capable of closing a wound or filling a defect. The adhesive was applied onto the inner borders of the laceration as well as to the surface of the corneal laceration. An argon ion laser (200 mW; 1-second pulse duration) was used to polymerize the biodendrimer and form a clear cross-linked gel that subsequently

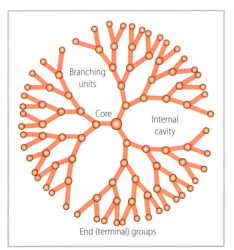

Figure 38.9 Dendrimer polymer.

closed the wound. The wounds that received the biodendrimer sealant were histologically superior and possessed more uniform corneal structure than the suture-treated wounds (Hovanesian 2009).

Use of dendritic polymers in ophthalmic surgery

A synthetic dendritic hydrogel has been used as an ocular bandage to seal corneal incisions (Vivagel, Dendritic Nanotechnologies, USA; and Starpharma, Australia) (Luman et al. 2004), and this ocular bandage can protect against mechanical stress and irritation in postsurgical, post-traumatic, and non-traumatic conditions (Hovanesian 2009). Although endopthalmitis is rare (0.2%) (Barry et al. 2006), the clear corneal incision increases the risk for endophthalmitis following a cataract surgery.

The synthetic, dendritic hydrogel is activated by mixing two separate components, and is easily applied with a special applicator onto the ocular surface as a liquid and after 30 seconds forms a low-profile, smooth, soft, and transparent protective barrier film on the ocular surface. The ultrastructure of the ocular bandage may provide insight into the microbial barrier. Scanning electron microscopy has revealed the pore size in the polymer network of this ocular sealant to be very small (1–3 µm). No discomfort, complications, or adverse events have been reported. The liquid ocular bandage has proved to be safe, well tolerated, and effective in human patients (Meskin et al. 2005).

On the other hand, linear lacerations require minimal or no suturing; shelved linear lacerations may self-seal with only a bandage contact lens placed over it. The laceration with a jagged edge can cause irregular, stellate wound and may require surgical intervention. When it is difficult to close, it requires multiple passes of sutures and causes a leak in another area to open up. Contrary to the use of cyanoacrylate, which becomes stiff and opaque and can cause patient discomfort, the biodendrimer hydrogel polymer polymerizes into a hydrogel that posesses the ideal properties for this use. It is transparent and flexible, so there is some give to it; it has a very smooth, silicone-like texture, so you should not need a bandage contact lens on top of it; and it can be applied in a very thin profile, to minimize the chance of dislodgement and patient discomfort. The limitation of this polymer is the time it remains on the eye, but this is somewhat modulated by various factors, such as the type of tissue and wound, the status of the surface epithelium, and perhaps other local environmental factors.

Biologically derived hydrogels

Recent developments in the area of ophthalmic adhesives have in part focused on biologically derived polysaccharides such as hyaluronic acid and chondroitin sulfate. Hyaluronic acid, composed of repeating disaccharide units (D-glucuronate and N-acetyl-D-glucosamine), is an important component of extracellular matrices, synovial fluid, and the vitreous humor in the eye. The main sources of commercial hyaluronic acid are chicken combs and bovine vitreous. These types of bioadhesives have a minimal tensile strength and a very fast degradation process and have not been found useful for the purpose of ocular surface reconstruction, either at the cornea, sclera, or conjunctiva. They may offer some advantages as intraocular sealants, but that does not come within the scope of this chapter.

Chondroitin sulfate

Chondroitin sulfate is a linear polysaccharide found in the extracellular matrix of tissue (**Figure 38.10**). Chondroitin sulfate is a major

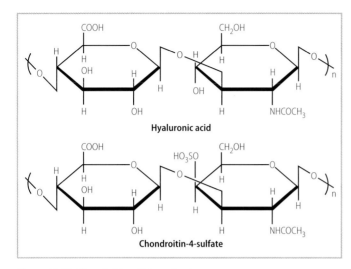

Figure 38.10 Chondroitin sulfate molecule.

component of most of the tissue of the body, including the cornea. When aldehyde of chondroitin sulfate modification is combined with polyvinyl alcohol covinylamine (CS-ald/PVA-A), adhesive properties are activated and polymerization occurs in 30 seconds. A thin layer is applied that coats the incision and the external third of the corneal tunnel in from the wound edge. The mixture becomes gelatinous and very soft, like corneal tissue. This hydrogel induces epithelial regeneration and serves as a repository for cytokines and growth factors that promote wound healing. The adhesive is biodegradable, and does not interfere with the wound healing. It acts as a matrix for regrowth of tissue and collagen. Intraocular pressure resistance of this glue is comparable to single and triple sutures (Reyes et al. 2005).

In order to chemically obtain cross-linked hydrogels, these polysacharides have been modified with a variety of functional groups. Chondroitin sulfate has been modified with adipic dihydrazide, methacrylate, and aldehyde groups.

Use of chondroitin sulfate adhesives in ophthalmic surgery

These adhesives have been evaluated for use as ophthalmic sealants and tested in two different wound models in an experimental study: 3 mm clear corneal incisions and flaps from 6.5 mm trephinations for microkeratome-assisted posterior lamellar keratoplasty. No leakage was observed in adhesive-treated eyes at the maximum intraocular pressure, and the eyes treated with CS-ald/PVA-A exhibited lower astigmatism but lower leakage pressures as well than sutured eyes (Reyes et al. 2005). However, the tensile strength of these adhesives limits their potential application for ocular surface reconstruction.

Gelatine

Tissue adhesives based on collagen or gelatine (denatured collagen), the most abundant protein in the extracellular matrix of animal tissue, are insoluble and form large fibrils through intramolecular hydrogen bonding. Upon heating collagen fibrils to 39°C, the hydrogen bonding is disrupted and the collagen loses the tertiary structure to form gelatine. The gelatine-based hydrogel formulation used as an ophthalmology adhesive was cross-linked by the reaction of gelatine with calcium-independent microbial transglutaminase. This form of cross-linking is quite similar to that of fibrin during blood coagulation.

Transglutaminase cross-linked gelatine hydrogels exhibited gelation times ranging from 5 to 30 minutes at different concentrations.

Use of gelatine adhesives in ophthalmic surgery

These adhesives have been evaluated for use as ophthalmic sealants, with potential for use in retinal reattachment surgery, bonded choroids, and scleral tissue. The adhesive was able to bond retinal tissue in vitro under wet conditions. Analysis of retinal tissue sections showed no evidence of retinal damage such as necrosis, cellular dropout, nuclear loss, or retinal edema (Chen et al. 2006).

◼ Synthetic polymer hydrogels

Hydrogels made from synthetic linear polymers have been explored for use as ophthalmic adhesives. They predominately include derivates of PEG. PEG hydrogel polymers used in many biomaterials have a long track record of being safe and tolerable, made mostly of water that can be placed on the eye for extended periods. This type of adhesives offer a good potential for the reconstruction of the tissues of the ocular surface, especially in the form of macromolecules, and have received recent attention by a number of investigators.

◼ Polyethylenglycol biomacromolecules

Multiple thiazolidines as the chemical ligation between macromolecules render a cross-linked hydrogel for the repair of acute corneal wounds (Oelker & Grinstaff 2008, Wathier et al. 2004). PEG biomacromolecules are useful in applications where hydrogel adhesives are required for longer periods, such as in a corneal transplant. The use of pseudoproline ligations between a dendron and PEG possessing N-terminal cysteines and aldehyde esters has been investigated.

Pseudoproline formation is one type of chemoselective and orthogonal peptide ligation method that has been successfully applied to the synthesis of a variety of proteins (Degoricija et al. 2007). A peptide possessing a C-terminal glycol aldehyde ester is reacted with another peptide possessing an N-terminal cysteine. The hydrogel formed between the dendron and PEG diester aldehyde is stable and retains its shape and size over time. This pseudoproline-cross-linked hydrogel remains intact for >6 months with a <10% change in weight when placed in a humidity chamber. This hydrogel is a contrast to a hydrogel formed between the dendron and PEG dialdehyde. In this latter reaction, a hydrogel is formed via formation of multiple thiazolidines. This thiazolidine formation is reversible and the hydrogel is intact for relatively short periods. When placed in a humidity chamber, the thiazolidine-cross-linked hydrogel loses its original cylindrical shape and is an unstructured gelatinous mass at approximately 1 week.

Use of polyethylenglycol biomacromolecules in ophthalmic surgery

When applied on a corneal ulcer, corneal re-epithelization occurs in humans in about 3 days; however, for the repair of large corneal wounds such as corneal transplants, a sealant is desired that can remain longer at the wound site (Wathier et al. 2006).

PEG bioadhesives have been used in corneal grafting surgery but with limited success. The disadvantages found were related to delayed visual recovery, suprachoroidal hemorrhage, neovascularization, microbial keratitis, postoperative suture removal, and surgically induced astigmatism. A corneal sutureless transplant procedure would significantly improve the multiple intraoperative and postoperative complications. These sealants cannot totally replace sutures, but preliminary information indicates that these hydrogels would reduce the number of sutures necessary to secure the incision between the host and graft corneal tissue (Wathier et al. 2006).

The PEG polymer requires mixing of components immediately before application and a surgical technique is used to apply the desired quantity on the eye. Visualization of the mixed hydrogel on the eye is aided by a blue dye that is included in the material. The blue color assists in the determination of coverage and thickness and then diffuses from the polymer within 1–2 hours, leaving an optically clear, untinted hydrogel bandage that has a smooth surface and is not visible without magnification (I-ZIP Ocular Bandage, I-Therapeutix, USA).

The PEG polymer was studied with an in vitro model and the watertight barrier properties of the adhesive were evaluated during transient fluctuations of intraocular pressure and mechanical manipulation when applied to a uniplanar clear corneal small cataract incision in human cadaver eyes and in rabbit eyes. Previous laboratory studies established the safety characteristics of this ocular bandage in the extraocular environment non-cytotoxic, non-sensitizing, and non-irritating, with no systemic toxicity. No heat is released during the polymerization of this material. In rabbits, no intraocular toxicity was noted after intentional injection of the material into the anterior chamber. In addition, clear corneal incisions closed with this ocular bandage did not experience inflammation, swelling, discharge, flare, corneal opacity, or pannus. Histopathology found that the healing of rabbit eyes treated with this hydrogel polymer was at least equivalent to, and potentially faster than, untreated corneal incisions. The liquid bandage did not penetrate into wounds. In a pilot study of human eyes with cataract surgery, the hydrogel bandage spontaneously sloughed from the ocular surface 3–5 days after application and did not cause giant papillary conjunctivitis, nor act as a nidus for infection or interfere in any detectable way with postoperative eye drop medications. Tissue-adherent hydrogel polymer ocular bandages may provide more secure closure of clear corneal cataract wounds than the current standard of care, which is to leave non-leaking wounds uncovered and unsutured (Hovanesian 2009).

Another new hydrogel polymer developed by HyperBranch is OcuSeal (Hyperbranch Technology, USA); it is a liquid when applied, but within 30 seconds to 1 minute it polymerizes into a hydrogel that possesses the ideal properties for this use. It is transparent, flexible, so there is some give to it; it has a very smooth, silicone-like texture, so a bandage contact lens is usually not needed on top of it; and it can be applied in a very thin profile, to minimize the chance of dislodgement and patient discomfort. This synthetic dendritic hydrogel has been used in rabbits and human patients (**Figure 38.11**). The average duration of the bandage varied depending on the type of wound, lasting 1 day in normal eyes, 1.5 days in abraded eyes, and 6.3 days in eyes that received a linear partial-thickness incision. There was no evidence of any inflammation or other abnormal findings, and fluorescein staining of the surface helped to identify and confirm the presence of the ocular bandage.

This synthetic adhesive has also been proposed as a surgical coadjuvant for the protection of ocular incisions caused by procedures such as parsplana vitrectomy and treating complications related to LASIK surgery and glaucoma filtering blebs.

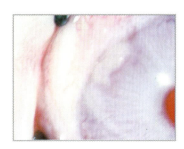

Figure 38.11 Corneal incision sealed by hydrogel adhesive.

Table 38.1 Commercially available adhesives

Adhesive type	Mixture	Registered name	Company
Cyanoacrylate	Methyl-2	Eastman 910	Eastman Kodak, USA
	N-Butyl-2	Histoacryl-N-Blue	Braun, Germany
	Isobutyl	Histoacryl	Braun, Germany
	2-Octyl	Dermabond	Ethicon, USA
	2-Octyl + paranbens	Liquid bandage	Johnson & Johnson, USA
	Isobutyl-2	Tissuacryl	Habana University, Cuba
		Adal-1	Alicante University, Cuba
	Hexyl	Adal-2	Alicante University, Spain
Fibrine		Tisseel	Baxter, USA
		TachoSeal	Baxter, USA
Hydrogel	Polyethylenglycol	I-ZIP	I-Therapeutix, USA
		OcuSeal	Hyperbranch Technology, USA
Gelatine	Gelatine + poly (L-glutamic acid)	Bolheal	Chemo-Sero-Therapeutic Research Institute, Japan.
	Transglutaminase cross-linked gelatine adhesive		Payne
Biodendrimer	Polyglycerol + succinic acid	Vivagel	Dendritic Nanotechnologies, USA Starpharma, Australia

Future of ocular surface bioadhesives

Bioadhesives offer an excellent opportunity today both for the ophthalmic industry and for clinical researches. The evidence accumulated during the last 10 years clearly proves the practicality and advantages of their use compared to the conventional suturing technique. The 'perfect' ocular surface bioadhesive will be totally biocompatible, with adequate tensile strength to fix the cornea, sclera, and conjunctiva, biodegradable in a maximum of few weeks to months depending on the tissue and surgery involved in the closure. It will also be easy and fast to use, with adequate plasticity and crystallization process to allow the different surgical steps involved in the surgery and cheap enough to be cost effective.

Ocular bioadhesives fit well in the concept of minimal invasiveness that is being promoted in modern ophthalmic surgery today. Their main applications in the future will be conjunctival reconstruction following strabismus, vitreoretinal, pterygium, pinguecula, tumors and trauma surgery. Corneal surgery indications will be the different types of modern corneal graft surgery, especially deep anterior lamellar surgery, refractive surgery, trauma, and different varieties of chronic ulcers. Scleral surgery, especially glaucoma and strabismus surgery, will be also an indication, jointly with all types of surgery of the ocular adnexa, including oculoplastic surgery. Cataract surgery will also use bioadhesive sealants to close leaky incisions following cataract removal or doubtfully stable incisions. In **Table 38.1**, we show the ocular bioadhesives that are currently commercially available in the different parts of the world or will appear in the global market in the coming 5 years. We also display the companies currently involved in their development. These bioadhesives, and probably others, still unknown today to the authors will make the longstanding dream of ophthalmic suture substitution possible, promoting a faster recovery by a more perfect reconstruction of the ocular tissues, with less closure-related complications. A very exciting future is awaiting this topic.

■ REFERENCES

Alió JL, Abad M, Artola A, et al. Use of autologous platelet rich-plasma in the treatment of dormant corneal ulcers. *Ophthalmology* 2007; **114**:1286–1293.

Alió JL, Arnalich-Montiel F, Rodriguez AE. The role of "eye platelet rich-plasma" (E-PRP) for wound sealing in ophthalmology. *Curr Pharm Biotechnol* 2012; **13**:1257–1265.

Alió JL, Gomez J, Mulet ME, et al. A new acrylic tissue for conjunctival surgery: experimental study. *Ophthalmic Res* 2003; **85**:306–312.

Alió JL, Mulet ME, Garcia JC. Use of cyanocrylate tissue adhesive in small incision cataract surgery. *Ophthalmic Surg Lasers* 1996; **27**:270–274.

Arentsen JJ, Laibson PR, Cohen EJ. Management of corneal descemetocel and perforations. *Opthalmic Surg* 1985; **16**:29–33.

Ashok S, Ravinder K, Sudarshan K, et al. Fibrin glue versus N-butyl-2-cyanocrylate in corneal perforations. *Ophthalmology* 2003; **110**:291–298.

Barry P, Seal DV, Gettinby G, et al. ESCRS study of prophylaxis of postoperative endophthalmitis after cataract surgery. Preliminary report of principle results from a European multicenter study. *J Cataract Refract Surg* 2006; **32**:407–410.

Bass LS, Treat MR. Laser tissue welding a comprehensive review of current and future clinical applications. *Lasers Surg Med* 1995; **17**:315–349.

Bathia SS. Ocular Surface sealants and adhesives. *Ocular Surf* 2006; 4146–4154.

Cardarelli J, Basu PK. Lamellar corneal transplantation in rabbits using isobutyl cyanocrilate. *Can J Ophthalmol* 1969; **4**:179–182.

Carnahan MA, Middleton C, Kim J, et al. Hybrid dendritic-linear polyester-ethers for in situ photopolymerization. *J Am Chem Soc* 2002; **124**:5291–5293.

Chan SM, Boisjoly H. Advances in the use of adhesives in ophthalmology. *Curr Opin Ophthalmol* 2004; **15**:305–310.

Chen T, Janjua R, McDermont MK, et al. Gelatin-based biometric tissue adhesive potential for retinal reattachment. *J Biomed Mater Res* 2006; 77B:416–422.

Degoricija L, Starck C, Wathier M, et al. Photo cross-linkable biodendrimers as ophthalmic adhesives for central lacerations and penetrating keratoplasties. *Invest Ophthalmol Vis Sci* 2007; **48**:2037–2042.

Ellis RA, Levine A. Experimental sutureless ocular surgery. *Am J Ophthalmol* 1963; **55**:733–741.

Henderson AM, Stephenson M. 3-methoxybutylcyanocrylate: evaluation of biocompatibility and bioresorption. *Biomaterials* 1992; **13**:1077–1084.

Hida T, Sheta SM, Proia AD et al. Retinal toxicity of cyanocrylate tissue adhesive in the rabbit. *Retina* 1988; **8**:148–153.

Hovanesian JA. Cataract wound closure with a polymerizing liquid hydrogel ocular bandage. *J Cataract Refract Surg* 2009; **35**:912–916.

Kaetsu H, Uchida T, Shinya N. Increased effectiveness of fibrin-sealant with a higher fibrin concentration. *Int J Adhesion & Adhesives* 2000; **20**:27–31.

Kajiwara K. Repair of a leaking bleb with fibrin glue. *Am J Ophthalmol* 1990; **109**:599–601.

Kaufman HE, Insler MS, Ibrahim-Elzembely HA, et al. Human fibrin tissue adhesive for sutureless lamellar keratoplasty and scleral patch adhesion: a pilot study. *Ophthalmology* 2003; **110**:2168–2172.

Khadem J, Martino M, Anatelli F, et al. Healing of perforating rat corneal incisions closed with photodynamic laser-activated tissue glue. *Lasers Surg Med* 2004; **35**:304–311.

Lagoutte FM, Gauthier L, Comte PRM. A fibrin sealant for perforated and preperforated corneal ulcers. *Br J Ophthalmol* 1989; **73**:757–761.

Leahey BA, Gottsch DJ, Start JW. Clinical experience with N-butyl cyanocrylate (Nexactyl) tissue adhesives. *Ophthalmology* 1993; **100**:173–180.

Luman NR, Kim T, Grinstaff MW. Dendritic polymers composed of glycerol and succinic acid: synthetic methodologies and medical applications. *Pure Appl Chem* 2004; **76**:1375–1385.

Meskin SW, Ritterband DC, Shapiro DE, et al. Liquid bandage a (2-octyl cyanocrylate) as a temporary wound barrier in clear corneal cataract surgery. *Ophthalmology* 2005; **112**:2015–2021.

Moschos M, Droutsas D, Boussalis P, et al. Clinical experience with cyanocrylate tissue adhesive. *Doc Ophthalmol* 1997; **93**:237–245.

Mulet ME, Alió JL, Gobby F. Efficacy of fibrinogen as bioadhesive in cataract surgery through scleral tunnel. *Arch Soc Esp Oftalmologia* 1997; **72**:427–430.

Mulet ME, Alió JL, Mahiques MM, et al. Adal-1® bioadhesive for sutureless resecction muscle surgery: a clinical trial. *Br J Ophthalmol* 2006; **90**:208–212.

Oelker AM, Grinstaff MW. Ophthalmic adhesives: a materials chemistry perspective. *J Mater Chem* 2008; **18**:2509–2616.

Patten JT. Punctal occlusion with n-butyl cyanocrylate tissue adhesive. *Ophthalmic Surg* 1976; **7**:24–26.

Refojo MF, Dohlman CH, Ahmad B, et al. Evaluation of adhesives for corneal surgery. *Arch Ophthalmol* 1968; **80**:645–656.

Reyes JM, Herretes S, Pirouzmanesh A, et al. A modified chondroitin sulphate aldehyde adhesive for sealing corneal incisions. *Invest Ophthalmol Vis Sci* 2005; **46**:1247–1250.

Ricci B, Ricci F, Bianchi PE. Octyl-cyanocrylate in sutureless surgery of extraocular muscles: an experimental study in the rabbit model. *Graefes Arch Clin Exp Ophtalmol* 2000; **238**:454–458.

Seelenfreund MH, Refojo MF, Schepens CL. Sealing choroidal perforations with cyanocrylate adhesives. *Arch Ophthalmol* 1970; **83**:619–625.

Wathier M, Jung PJ, Carnaham MA, et al. Dendritic macromers as in situ polymerizing biomaterials for securing cataract incisions. *J Am Chem Soc* 2004; **126**:12744–12745.

Wathier M, Starck C, Kim T, et al. Hydrogels formed by multiple peptide ligation reactions to fasten corneal transplants. *Bioconjugate Chem* 2006; **17**:873–876.

Webster RG Jr, Slansky HH, Refojo M, et al. The use of adhesive for the closure of corneal perforations. Report of two cases. *Arch Ophthalmol* 1968; **80**:705–709.

Weiss JL, Williams P, Lindstrom RL, et al. The use of tissue adhesive in corneal perforations. *Ophthalmology* 1983; **90**:610–615.

Chapter 39

The role of amniotic membrane for managing dry eye disease

Hosam Sheha, Scheffer C. G. Tseng

INTRODUCTION

Dry eye disease (DED) refers to a spectrum of ocular surface diseases with diverse and multiple etiologies. A common feature of DED is an abnormal tear film that adversely affects its ability to perform essential functions such as providing a clear optical interface, supporting the ocular surface epithelium, and preventing microbial invasion. Tear film abnormalities are caused by either compositional tear deficiency, owing to insufficient supply or excessive loss of lipid, aqueous fluid, and mucin components, or hydrodynamic tear deficiency owing to ineffective tear spread or clearance or excessive evaporation or exposure. Despite different underlying pathogenic processes, DED is also characterized by a common denominator, ocular surface inflammation, which in turn causes cell damage, resulting in a self-perpetuating cycle of deterioration. Progress has been made in our understanding of the etiology and pathogenesis of DED as well as other ocular surface diseases that mimic or aggravate DED. These advances have led us to adopt a practical algorithm for clinicians to restore the integrity of the ocular surface with an attempt to maintain a stable tear film. In this chapter, we focus on how transplantation of cryopreserved amniotic membrane (AM) can be an important surgical modality to achieve this goal.

FUNDAMENTAL MECHANISMS OF DRY EYE DISEASE

Tear film instability

The integrity of the tear film is achieved by both compositional and hydrodynamic elements. The compositional elements comprise the lacrimal glands, the ocular surface, and the meibomian glands, while the hydrodynamic elements comprise tear evaporation, spread, and drainage or clearance, which are controlled by eyelid blinking and closure. These two elements are integrated as one unit controlled by two reflexes via the first branch of trigeminal nerve as the sensory input, the parasympathetic branch as secretory and the motor branch of the facial nerve (**Figure 39.1**). A sound neuroanatomic integration of the above two elements ensures a stable tear film that dictates ocular surface integrity when the eye is open (Tseng & Tsubota 1997).

Dysfunction of any components in either compositional or the hydrodynamic elements in the aforementioned neuroanatomic integration destabilizes the preocular tear film, leading to DED. Among these dysfunctional elements that may lead to DED, the four common causes include aqueous tear deficiency (ATD) due to lacrimal gland dysfunction, lipid tear deficiency (LTD) due to meibomian gland dysfunction, delayed tear clearance (DTC) due to ineffective tear spread, and neurotrophic and exposure keratopathy (Tseng 2011).

Delayed tear clearance

DTC commonly occurs when there is a mechanical or functional obstruction in the lacrimal drainage system (**Figure 39.2**). It can also develop in severe ATD in which the tear meniscus is too low to reach the punctum, or when there is mucosal swelling or irregularity of the ocular surface that interrupts the tear meniscus or drainage. DTC is commonly associated with chronic ocular surface inflammation. One common cause is conjunctivochalasis (CCh), which has been reported to cause DTC by interfering with tear drainage via punctae (Di Pascuale et al. 2004a). It aggravates ocular irritation by prolonging the contact of the irritative stimuli to the ocular surface that may lead to inflammation and epithelial damage (Prabhasawat & Tseng 1998). CCh also interferes with the formation of the tear meniscus leading

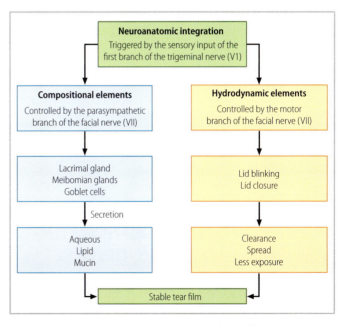

Figure 39.1 Neuroanatomic integration stabilizes the tear film. Two neuronal reflexes are involved in integrating the compositional and hydrodynamic elements to form an integral unit to maintain a stable tear film. Both reflexes are triggered by the sensory input of the first branch of the trigeminal nerve (V1), the compositional one is mediated by the parasympathetic branch of the facial nerve (VII), and the hydrodynamic one is mediated by the motor branch of the facial nerve. Modified with permission from Tseng and Tsubota (1997).

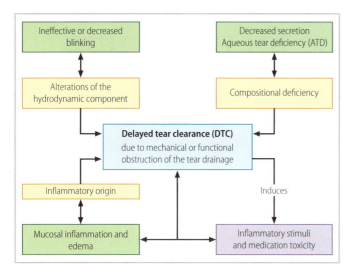

Figure 39.2 Pathophysiology of delayed tear clearance (DTC). Functional and/or mechanical obstruction of tear drainage leads to DTC, which induces ocular irritation or inflammation. Modified with permission from Prabhasawat and Tseng (1998).

to DED by inducing poor tear spread over the ocular surface during blinking (see below) (Gumus et al. 2011).

Exposure and neurotrophic keratopathy

Another common but often overlooked cause of DED is exposure keratopathy, which leads to excessive tear evaporation and increases the difficulty in tear spread. It has been suggested that excessive evaporation increases tear osmolarity, which in turn induces damage to the surface epithelium by activating a cascade of inflammatory events (Lemp 2008).

For patients with normal corneal sensation, exposure keratopathy can be caused by incomplete blinking or closure because of disparity between the eyelid and the globe or anatomic abnormality of eyelids (i.e. ectropion) or fornix (i.e. symblepharon). For patients with poor ocular sensation (i.e. neurotrophic state), exposure keratopathy is a common sequel. Although both types of patients may present ocular surface morbidity, for example, punctate keratopathy or epithelial defects, the former is relatively milder and more symptomatic, while the latter tends to have disproportionally fewer symptoms and the ocular surface damage usually falls outside of radar detection. As stated above, once epithelial damage ensues, the tear film stability is further threatened, thereby creating a vicious cycle.

A PRACTICAL ALGORITHM FOR MANAGING DRY EYE DISEASE

To formulate a practical algorithm, first, it is important to identify all dysfunctional elements needed for sound neuroanatomic integration. Although an unstable tear film is the hallmark of DED, simple detection of tear break-up time or pattern is not sufficient. Before any testing, simple observation of patient's blinking frequency and amplitude can raise the concern of possible neurotrophic exposure issues. One useful clinical test is the fluorescein clearance test, which simultaneously detects basic and reflex aqueous tear secretion and aqueous tear clearance (Afonso et al. 1999, Macri & Pflugfelder 2000, Prabhasawat

& Tseng 1998, Xu & Tsubota 1995). Besides detecting epithelial abnormalities, fluorescein staining is useful in evaluating the status of tear meniscus, i.e. height and uniformity, and hence for assessing CCh. Rose Bengal staining further highlights ocular surface epithelial cells that exhibit a mucin-deficient state (Feenstra & Tseng 1992a, 1992b). The interpalpebral pattern suggests dryness due to ATD or exposure, while a linear pattern of the eyelid in contact with the ocular surface suggests DTC and CCh. Kinetic analysis of tear interference images is effective in detecting the precorneal lipid film, and the resultant pattern can further differentiate ATD from LTD (Goto & Tseng 2003a, 2003b). Once the dysfunctional elements are delineated, a clinical treatment plan can be formulated according to the following steps.

Step 1: elimination of intrinsic irritative stimuli especially in the presence of delayed tear clearance

Elimination of intrinsic irritative stimuli such as infection, allergy, and inflammatory causes is the first step to restore ocular comfort. One overlooked intrinsic irritative stimulus is the toxic effect derived from topical medications including preservatives. Ocular irritation is exacerbated by DTC, which gives rise to a vicious cycle by perpetuating the concentration of intrinsic inflammatory cytokines or toxic substances. Hence, detection of DTC by fluorescein clearance test further strengthens one's suspicion of the aforementioned pathogenic process. We have proposed to use preservative-free steroids to resolve ocular irritation by suppressing inflammation while eliminating DTC at the same time in eyes with or without ATD (Marsh & Pflugfelder 1999, Prabhasawat & Tseng 1998). Future studies are needed to determine whether other preservative-free formulations containing cyclosporin A (Utine et al. 2010), doxycyclines (Dursun et al. 2001), or glucocorticoid receptor antagonist (Cavet et al. 2010) may also better resolve DTC in DED patients.

Step 2: correction of tear spread deficiency caused by conjunctivochalasis

Ocular surface irregularities that may induce ineffective tear spread have been well recognized. One classical example is dellen formation adjacent to elevated areas such as pinguecula, pterygium, Salzmann's nodular degeneration, or filtering bleb. Nonetheless, the most common but unrecognized cause of ineffective tear spread is CCh, which may also interfere with the normal tear distribution by interrupting the tear meniscus (**Figure 39.3**). CCh manifests an array of dysfunctional elements according to its severity; in mild-to-moderate cases, DTC may occur, resulting in ocular surface inflammation. In severe cases, DED usually arises along with dellen and exposure (Meller & Tseng 1998). In addition, CCh depletes the tear reservoir in the fornix (**Figure 39.3**), further depleting the overall tear holding capacity of an eye. This aggravates the DED symptoms and renders topical artificial tears ineffective. Therefore, one needs to consider treating CCh first before addressing compositional tear deficiency.

The exact pathogenesis of CCh remains unclear; however, recent studies suggest that degradation of the Tenon capsule may result in the lack of adherence of the conjunctiva to the underlying ocular tissue (Kheirkhah et al. 2007, Li et al. 2000, Meller et al. 2000a, 2000b). Simple excision of the redundant conjunctival might not be effective if the fornix is not deepened. Excision of residual mobile Tenon together with replacement of the Tenon and the conjunctival tissue by cryopreserved AM has been reported to relieve ocular irritation in DED by deepening the fornix while reducing the scar formation for both inferior (Meller et al. 2000b) and superior (Kheirkhah et al. 2007) CCh, of which the latter has also been found to be associated with superior limbic keratoconjunctivitis (Gris et al. 2010). Now knowing that the primary abnormality of CCh resides in dissolution of the Tenon capsule, it is logical to consider using AM to replace this missing tissue (**Figure 39.4**). Consequently, the overlying conjunctiva can be better adhering to the sclera without scarring in between, so that the conjunctival tissue can be spared.

Step 3: treating aqueous tear deficiency dry eye disease before lipid tear deficiency dry eye disease

The conventional treatment of ATD DED starts with topical application of artificial tears. To avoid toxicity to the ocular surface from prolonged uses of artificial tears, preservative-free tear substitutes are preferred. Nonetheless, it soon becomes impractical when the application of artificial tears reaches a certain daily frequency. Punctal occlusion remains the mainstay of managing ATD DED. If plugs are not available or are repeatedly lost, cauterization is preferred to achieve permanent closure. Punctal occlusion invariably creates DTC, which can potentially precipitate the concomitant ocular surface inflammation, which is why we advise eliminating all intrinsic irritative stimuli in step 1. Because CCh might cause DTC confounding the complexity, surgical correction of CCh is advised in step 2 before punctal occlusion is contemplated. In cases with DED primarily caused by the neurotrophic state, punctal occlusion should be the first measure to take before using autologous serum drops and bandage contact lens, which can be more practically instituted later to resolve corneal epithelial breakdown and improve the visual acuity.

In the presence of ATD, the spread of meibum lipids is also retarded (Goto & Tseng 2003b), because spread of polar lipids into a thin film depends on the presence of sufficient water (Khamene et al. 2000). Therefore, it is more effective to manage LTD DED after ATD is adequately managed. Common treatments for LTD caused by meibomian gland dysfunction include lid hygiene, warm compress, and mechanical expression. The accompanied inflammation or infection can be managed similarly. Instillation of artificial tears with components that may stabilize the lipid film has been attempted (Di Pascuale et al. 2004b). One way of maintaining a stable tear film without replacing the missing meibum might be to wear a bandage contact lens or a sclera lens. Additional studies are needed to investigate the efficacy of such new approaches, such as canalization of meibomian gland orifices in managing LTD (Maskin 2010), as well as new devices to warm and massage the meibomian glands.

Step 4: treat underlying ocular surface deficits

Ocular surface irregularities that interfere with the normal distribution of the tear film can aggravate the DED and cause cell damage. Therefore, ocular surface deficits or complications of DED should be treated at the same time or should follow the three steps mentioned previously. For example, exposure keratopathy usually develops epithelial irregularities that induce blurry vision and can be detected under the slit lamp (**Figure 39.5a**). AM can be used as a temporary biological bandage to restore a healthy and smooth corneal epithelium. AM can be secured by sutures to cover the cornea or by a self-retaining device (ProKera, Bio-Tissue, USA) without sutures (**Figure 39.5b**). Upon healing (**Figure 39.5c** and **39.5d**) AM usually dissolves or is removed.

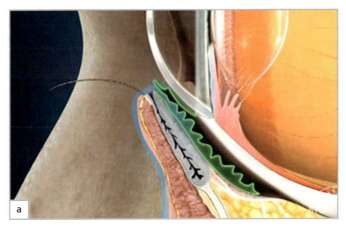
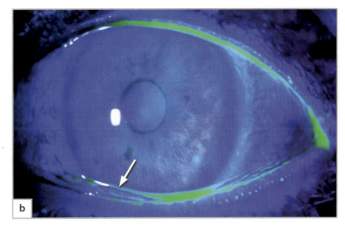

Figure 39.3 Conjunctivochalasis. The wrinkled conjunctiva [green in (a)] observed at the lid margin is only the 'tip of the iceberg' [arrow in (b)]. The bulk occupies the fornix depleting the tear reservoir.

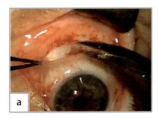
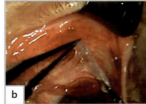
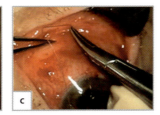

Figure 39.4 Tenon's replacement with amniotic membrane (AM) graft. (a) Under topical anesthesia, limbal-based conjunctival flap is made. (b) AM is secured to the episclera using fibrin glue (arrow). (c) The conjunctiva is secured over the AM using 8-0 Vicryl sutures.

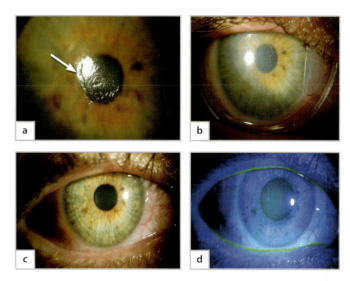

Figure 39.5 Exposure keratopathy. (a) Irregular corneal epithelium (arrow). (b) Treated with ProKera. (c) and (d) Healthy and smooth ocular surface restored.

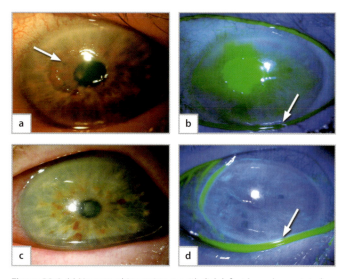

Figure 39.6 (a) Neurotrophic persistent epithelial defect (arrow), associated with (b) low tear meniscus (arrow). ProKera was placed to promote scarless healing immediately after lower punctal occlusion. (c) Complete healing occurred within 7 days without scarring. (d) The patient maintained a good tear meniscus (arrow).

In cases of persistent epithelial defect due to neurotrophic keratopathy, AM with or without tarsorrhaphy can also be considered following punctal occlusion (Solomon et al. 2000) (**Figure 39.6**).

In eyes with cicatricial complications, other ocular deficits ensue. One major deficit is 'blink-related microtrauma' caused by lid margin pathologies such as keratinization, scarring, and misdirected lashes. Correction of these pathologies is important because they are significantly correlated with corneal blindness in diseases such as Stevens–Johnson syndrome (Di Pascuale et al. 2005). In this scenario, the hydrodynamic reflex, which is normally in concert with the compositional reflex to help stabilize the tear film, becomes pathogenic by causing progressive ocular surface failure due to the presence of these lid margin pathologies. Recently, we reported our experience in using oral mucosal graft (OMG) to correct lid margin pathological features in cicatricial ocular surface diseases (Fu et al. 2011).

The other major deficit that is frequently caused by cicatricial complications is 'exposure' due to infrequent blinking and incomplete closure as a result of entropion, symblepharon/fornix foreshortening, and lid skin contracture. Recently, we have reported that infrequent blinking, lagophthalmos, and pathogenic symblepharon are additional risk factors contributing to corneal epithelial breakdown (Liang et al. 2009). This deficit can be corrected by symblepharon lysis, fornix reconstruction, AMT, OMG, and skin graft.

Kheirkhah et al. (2008) proposed a new surgical strategy for conjunctival surface reconstruction after symblepharon lysis by selectively using AMT, mitomycin C, anchoring sutures, and OMG according to the severity of symblepharon. For mild cases, the recessed conjunctiva is large enough to cover the entire palpebral area where it is secured using fibrin glue. The bare sclera is covered with AM, with the stromal side down, using fibrin glue or sutures (**Figure 39.7a** and **39.7b**). For moderate cases, the recessed conjunctiva is just enough to cover the tarsal area. A double-armed 4-0 black silk suture, secured to the skin with a bolster, is needed to keep it in place. One such anchoring suture is needed per quadrant. The remaining bare sclera, fornix, and palpebral area are covered by AM using fibrin glue (**Figure 39.7c** and **39.7d**). For severe cases, there is not enough of the recessed conjunctiva to cover the tarsal area. Therefore, OMG is used to substitute the tarsal conjunctiva. OMG is secured to the tarsal plate with fibrin glue, sutured to the posterior lid margin using 8-0 vicryl sutures, and then anchored to the skin with a bolster as previously described. The remaining bare sclera, fornix, and palpebral area are covered with AM in the same manner (**Figure 39.7e** and **39.7f**).

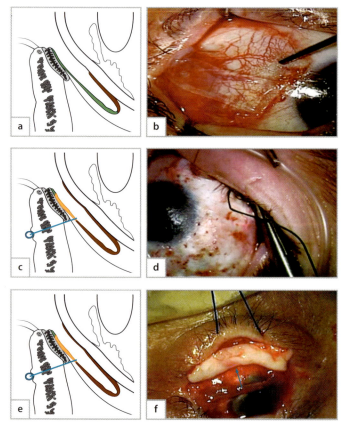

Figure 39.7 Surgical strategy for fornix reconstruction after symblepharon lysis. Modified with permission from Kheirkhah et al. (2008).

CONCLUSION

By understanding the pathogenesis of DED within the context of neuroanatomic integration and taking the logical algorithm in resolving dysfunctional elements, we have developed a practical approach for managing DED. These measures span to cover common causes as well as relatively uncommon ones with a common goal to eliminate ongoing insults and to restore a stable tear film. The sooner this goal is attained, the better the outcome in relieving patient's irritative symptoms and maintaining ocular surface health.

REFERENCES

Afonso AA, Monroy D, Stern ME, et al. Correlation of tear fluorescein clearance and Schirmer test scores with ocular irritation symptoms. *Ophthalmology* 1999; **106**: 803–810.

Cavet ME, Harrington KL, Ward KW, Zhang JZ. Mapracorat, a novel selective glucocorticoid receptor agonist, inhibits hyperosmolar-induced cytokine release and MAPK pathways in human corneal epithelial cells. *Mol Vis* 2010; **16**:1791–1800.

Di Pascuale MA, Espana EM, Liu DT, et al. Correlation of corneal complications with eyelid cicatricial pathologies in patients with Steven Johnson syndrome and toxic epidermal necrolysis syndrome. *Ophthalmology* 2005; **112**:904–912.

Di Pascuale MA, Espana EM, Tseng SCG. Clinical importance of conjunctivochalasis in dry eye management. EyeNet 2004a.

Di Pascuale MA, Goto E, Tseng SCG. Changes of lipid tear film in dry eye patients and normal subjects following one drop of a new emulsion eye drop using kinetic analysis of tear interference images. *Ophthalmology* 2004b; **111**:783–791.

Dursun D, Kim MC, Solomon A, Pflugfelder SC. Treatment of recalcitrant recurrent corneal erosions with inhibitors of matrix metalloproteinase-9, doxycycline and corticosteroids. *Am J Ophthalmol* 2001; **132**:8–13.

Feenstra RPG, Tseng SCG. Comparison of fluorescein and rose bengal staining. *Ophthalmology* 1992a; **99**:605–617.

Feenstra RPG, Tseng SCG. What is actually stained by rose bengal? *Arch Ophthalmol* 1992b; **110**:984–993.

Fu Y, Liu J, Tseng SC. Oral mucosal graft to correct lid margin pathologic features in cicatricial ocular surface diseases. *Am J Ophthalmol* 2011; **152**:600–608.

Goto E, Tseng SC. Differentiation of lipid tear deficiency dry eye by kinetic analysis of tear interference images. *Arch Ophthalmol* 2003a; **121**:173–180.

Goto E, Tseng SC. Kinetic analysis of tear interference images in aqueous tear deficiency dry eye before and after punctal occlusion. *Invest Ophthalmol Vis Sci* 2003b; **44**:1897–1905.

Gris O, Plazas A, Lerma E, et al. Conjunctival resection with and without amniotic membrane graft for the treatment of superior limbic keratoconjunctivitis. *Cornea* 2010; **29**:1025–1030.

Gumus K, Crockett CH, Rao K, et al. Non invasive assessment of the tear film stability in patients with tear dysfunction using the Tear Film Stability Analysis System (TSAS). *Invest Ophthalmol Vis Sci* 2011; **52**:456–461.

Khamene A, Negahdaripour S, Tseng SC. A spectral-discrimination method for tear-film lipid-layer thickness estimation from fringe pattern images. *IEEE Trans Biomed Eng* 2000; **47**:249–258.

Kheirkhah A, Blanco G, Casas V, et al. Surgical strategies for fornix reconstruction based on symblepharon severity. *Am J Ophthalmol* 2008; **146**:266–275.

Kheirkhah A, Casas V, Blanco G, et al. Amniotic membrane transplantation with fibrin glue for conjunctivochalasis. *Am J Ophthalmol* 2007; **144**:311–313.

Lemp MA. Advances in understanding and managing dry eye disease. *Am J Ophthalmol* 2008; **146**:350–356.

Li D-Q, Meller D, Tseng SCG. Overexpression of collagenase (MMP-1) and stromelysin (MMP-3) by cultured conjunctivochalasis fibroblasts. *Invest Ophthalmol Vis Sci* 2000; **41**:404–410.

Liang L, Sheha H, Tseng SC. Long-term outcomes of keratolimbal allograft for total limbal stem cell deficiency using combined immunosuppressive agents and correction of ocular surface deficits. *Arch Ophthalmol* 2009; **127**:1428–1434.

Macri A, Pflugfelder SC. Correlation of the Schirmer 1 and fluorescein clearance tests with the severity of corneal epithelial and eyelid disease. *Arch Ophthalmol* 2000; **118**:1632–1638.

Marsh P, Pflugfelder SC. Topical nonpreserved methylprednisolone therapy for keratoconjunctivitis sicca in Sjogren syndrome. *Ophthalmology* 1999; **106**:811–816.

Maskin SL. Intraductal meibomian gland probing relieves symptoms of obstructive meibomian gland dysfunction. *Cornea* 2010; **29**:1145–1152.

Meller D, Li D-Q, Tseng SCG. Regulation of collagenase, stromelysin, and gelatinase B in human conjunctival and conjunctivochalasis fibroblasts by interleukin-1b and tumor necrosis factor-a. *Invest Ophthalmol Vis Sci* 2000a; **41**:2922–2929.

Meller D, Maskin SL, Pires RTF, Tseng SCG. Amniotic membrane transplantation for symptomatic conjunctivochalasis refractory to medical treatments. *Cornea* 2000b; **19**:796–803.

Meller D, Tseng SC. Conjunctivochalasis: literature review and possible pathophysiology. *Surv Ophthalmol* 1998; **43**:225–232.

Prabhasawat P, Tseng SCG. Frequent association of delayed tear clearance in ocular irritation. *Br J Ophthalmol* 1998; **82**:666–675.

Solomon A, Touhami A, Sandoval H, Tseng SCG. Neurotrophic keratopathy: basic concepts and therapeutic strategies. *Comp Ophthalmol Update* 2000; **3**:165–174.

Tseng SC. A practical treatment algorithm for managing ocular surface and tear disorders. *Cornea* 2011; **30**:S8–S14.

Tseng SC, Tsubota K. Important concepts for treating ocular surface and tear disorders: *Am J Ophthalmol* 1997; **124**:825–835.

Utine CA, Stern M, Akpek EK. Clinical review: topical ophthalmic use of cyclosporin A. *Ocul Immunol Inflamm* 2010; **18**:352–361.

Xu KP, Tsubota K. Correlation of tear clearance rate and fluorophotometric assessment of tear turnover. *Br J Ophthalmol* 1995; **79**:1042–1045.

Chapter 40

Sequential sectorial conjunctival epitheliectomy and superficial keratectomy

Jose Güell, Oscar Gris, Diego Aristizabal, Daniel Elies, Felicidad Manero, Merce Morral

INTRODUCTION

Corneal epithelial wound healing in normal and pathological states: corneal epithelial stem cells

The maintenance of a healthy functional corneal epithelium depends on a unique subpopulation of stem cells (SC) located in the limbus at the limbal palisades of Vogt (Cotsarelis et al. 1989, Schermer et al. 1986). Limbal epithelial crypts (LEC) are solid cords of epithelial SCs that extend from the peripheral end of some limbal palisades of Vogt into the underlying stroma, deeper into the substantia propia, and constitute SC niches (Dua & Azuara-Blanco 2000, Dua & Forrester 1990, Dua et al. 2005, 2010, Shanmuganathan et al. 2007). As the location of the LEC is predominantly in the mid- or distal limbus, toward the conjunctival end of the limbus, preservation of the conjunctiva in any procedure to transplant limbus is essential. A 3 mm rim of conjunctiva measured from the visible edge of the cornea (start of the limbus) would include almost all LECs (Shanmuganathan et al. 2007). Apart from containing the SCs, the limbal epithelium acts as a barrier that prevents the migration of conjunctival epithelial cells onto the cornea (Dua 1998).

Thoft and Friend proposed an 'X, Y, Z hypothesis of corneal epithelial maintenance' in which desquamated cells (Z component) are continuously replaced by basal cells (X) that divide, and by cells that migrate from the periphery (Y). Such daughter cells are called 'transient amplifying cells' (TACs) and are distributed in the corneal basal cell layer. The TACs migrate centripetally, and after a number of mitoses, they further differentiate into 'postmitotic cells,' which do not divide any further. These postmitotic cells differentiate into terminally differentiated corneal epithelial cells, which die after a certain time. Thus, in presence of healthy limbal epithelium, SCs divide and differentiate, acquiring features of corneal epithelium. Migration occurs centripetally and circumferentially from the limbus and vertically from the basal layer (Thoft & Friend 1983).

When limbal epithelial SCs are destroyed and/or their supporting stromal environment becomes dysfunctional, limbal stem cell deficiency (LSCD) develops, and the healthy ocular surface status and regeneration capacity is affected (Lavker et al. 2004). In such cases, healing occurs by (1) centripetal migration of epithelial cells from the remaining intact corneal and conjunctival epithelium, and (2) circumferential migration of limbal epithelial cells along the limbus from the two ends of the remaining intact limbal epithelium (Dua et al. 2010).

Moreover, as the barrier function is lost, conjunctival epithelium often migrates across the denuded limbus to cover the corneal surface, which is known as conjunctivalization. Conjunctival epithelium covering the cornea was believed to undergo a slow transformation to corneal epithelium, a process referred to as conjunctival transdifferentiation. However, later studies showed that there is little clinical evidence to support the occurrence of conjunctival transdifferentiation in humans (Dua 1998). The pathophysiology and etiology of LSCD are discussed in more detail in Chapter 24.

Limbal stem cell deficiency: diagnosis and management

Diagnosis of LSCD is essentially clinical. Symptoms of LSCD include decreased vision, redness, watering, photophobia, and recurrent pain due to epithelial breakdown. Conjunctivalization of the cornea is the main feature of LSCD, and results in thickened, irregular, unstable epithelium. When it covers the pupillary area, vision can be significantly affected. This conjunctival epithelium covering the corneal surface presents as columns, whorls, or sheets with late fluorescein staining, as it is more permeable than corneal epithelium (**Figure 40.1a**). In partial LSCD, a clear demarcation line is often visible between corneal and conjunctival phenotype of cells. At the line of contact between the two phenotypes, tiny bud-like projections of normal corneal epithelium can be seen extending into the conjunctivalized area. Other signs include superficial and deep vascularization, fibrovascular pannus, persistent epithelial defects, and scarring. Slit-lamp exam is generally sufficient to determine the extent of LSCD, and is confirmed by the presence of conjunctival epithelial and goblet cells on the cornea, demonstrated by in vivo confocal microscopy, impression cytology, or biopsy (Donisi et al. 2003, Dua & Azuara-Blanco 2000, Puangsricharern & Tseng 1995). Other findings on biopsy specimens are destruction of the basement membrane, superficial neovascularization, chronic inflammation, scarring, and poor epithelial integrity (Dua et al. 2000).

The treatment of choice depends on the extent of LSCD, which is defined as unilateral or bilateral and partial (visual axis affected or spared) or total. Preoperative ophthalmological examination should include: visual acuity evaluation and prognosis, slit-lamp examination with evaluation of the extent of LSCD and thickness and clarity of the corneal stroma underlying the fibrovascular pannus, intraocular pressure, and fundus examination. Some cases of total LSCD may require determination of the visual potential by electrophysiological tests. Finally, for allolimbal transplantation techniques, HLA typing of the patient and potential living related donors and a thorough work-up of the patient for immunosuppression are mandatory.

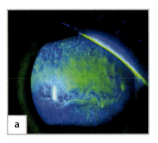 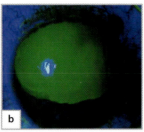 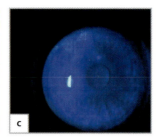

Figure 40.1 Sequential sectorial conjunctival epitheliectomy (SSCE) for partial limbal stem cell deficiency. (a) Preoperative clinical photograph showing the pattern of fluorescein staining. A clear demarcation between corneal and conjunctival epithelial phenotypes can be seen. The conjunctival epithelium appears irregular, with areas of fluorescein pooling, and fine neovessels. The pupillary area is entirely covered by conjunctival epithelium. Tiny 'buds' of corneal epithelium can be seen along the line of contact between corneal and conjunctival epithelium. Visual acuity was <20/400. (b) Immediate postoperative period after removal of all conjunctival epithelium from the corneal surface (SSCE). An epithelial defect affecting two thirds of the cornea is seen. Note that the removal of epithelium was not extended across the limbus. Autologous serum drops were prescribed. (c) Three weeks after SSCE. The pupillary area is covered by corneal healthy epithelium, which appears much smoother. Visual acuity improved to 20/30.

Table 40.1 summarizes the main treatment strategies. Surgical treatment is only required when the visual axis is affected, or in cases of recurrent or persistent corneal epithelial defects. For eyes with total LSCD, corneal surface reconstruction resorts to transplantation of limbal epithelial SCs (Dua et al. 2010, Kheirkhah et al. 2008). Limbal transplantation techniques are further discussed in Chapter 43. However, for eyes with partial LSCD and visual axis affected, the corneal surface can be reconstructed by debridement of conjunctival epithelium with or without transplantation of amniotic membrane (AM), or by anterior keratectomy. The repeated removal of conjunctival epithelium covering the cornea is known as sequential sectorial conjunctival epitheliectomy (SSCE), and was first described by Harminder Dua in 1998 (Dua 1998, 2002).

Sequential sectorial conjunctival epitheliectomy

SSCE consists of staged or repeated removal of conjunctival epithelium covering a sector of the cornea and limbus, or adjacent bulbar conjunctiva, until the denuded surface is covered by corneal epithelium-derived cells. The aim of SSCE is to encourage conjunctival epithelium cover for conjunctiva and corneal epithelium cover for cornea. As the conjunctival epithelium migrates faster than the limbal sheets, mechanical scrape of the advancing conjunctival epithelial sheet may have to be repeated two or three times. This procedure is usually followed by rapid re-epithelization of the cornea with corneal epithelium. Interestingly, in Dua's study, it was the corneal epithelial sheet that rapidly advanced to cover the defect rather than conjunctival epithelium from the limbus (Dua 1998, Dua et al. 1994).

Indications and contraindications for sequential sectorial conjunctival epitheliectomy

Table 40.2 summarizes the main indications and contraindications of SSCE. As a general rule, SSCE is indicated in cases of partial LSCD with conjunctivalization affecting the visual axis, and vision consequently affected. SSCE is not required when the visual axis is not involved. For total LSCD, a limbal SC replacement technique is required to restore a normal phenotypical corneal epithelium, but SSCE may be required in the postoperative period of limbal SC transplantation. Care should be taken in eyes with thin underlying stroma, and SSCE is not effective when fibrovascular pannus is present. Finally, SSCE should not be performed in case of severe dry eyes or anesthetic corneas, as the potential for re-epithelialization is hampered.

Surgical technique

SSCE is usually performed under topical anesthesia at the slit lamp or under the operating microscope. The abnormal epithelium is scraped with a crescent blade or a dry spear. To avoid any contact inhibition mechanisms by the conjunctival epithelium that would delay or stop corneal epithelial proliferation and migration, the abnormal epithelium in contact with the corneal epithelium should be completely removed. Finally, a bandage contact lens is placed, and topical antibiotics and steroids, and artificial tears should be prescribed, avoiding or minimizing toxic drops and preservatives. When more than 50% of the corneal surface is de-epithelialized, autologous serum drops have been reported to be an effective adjunct for the postoperative

Table 40.1 Treatment of limbal stem cell deficiencies

| Visual axis spared (partial or total) | Visual axis affected | | | |
| | Partial | | Total | |
	No fibrovascular pannus	Fibrovascular pannus	Unilateral	Bilateral
Conservative measures (lubricants, autologous serum, bandage contact lens, etc.)	SSCE or anterior keratectomy ± AMT	SSCE or anterior keratectomy ± AMT and/or SLT	Autolimbal transplant or ex vivo expansion of stem cells	Allolimbal transplant (living related, or cadaver donor) or ex vivo expansion of stem cells

Taken from Dua et al. (2010).
AMT, amniotic membrane transplantation; SLT, sector limbal transplant; SSCE, sequential sectorial conjunctival epitheliectomy.
Treatment depends on the extent of limbal abnormality. All associated abnormalities (e.g. lids, conjunctiva, and intraocular pressure) should be treated before limbal deficiency management.

Table 40.2 Indications and contraindications of sequential sectorial conjunctival epitheliectomy

Indications	Contraindications
Acute ocular surface defects involving the cornea and limbus (i.e. acute chemical burns)	Partial LSCD and visual axis not involved
Partial LSCD with established conjunctivalization of the cornea	Total LSCD
	Dense fibrovascular pannus
Postoperatively, in patients undergoing limbal auto- or allografts in total LSCD	Thin underlying stroma
	Severe dry eye disease
After excision of sectorial limbal lesions	Anesthetic cornea

LSCD, limbal stem cell deficiency.

management of patients undergoing ocular surface reconstruction (**Figure 40.1**) (Tsubota et al. 1999). Patients should be closely monitored on a daily basis until re-epithelialization is complete. As denuded area is covered by corneal epithelium cells derived from the intact limbus, the conjunctival epithelium also grows over the corneal surface in the areas of limbal deficiency. Therefore, repeated brushing or scraping of this conjunctival epithelium is usually required every 24–48 hours, and should be performed as many times as required until the corneal surface is covered by corneal epithelium cells. If the conjunctival epithelium is thick or in presence of fibrovascular pannus, Vannas scissors may be used (Dua et al. 1994, 2010).

Partial limbal stem cell deficiencies

SSCE is performed as described above. In partial LSCD, with fibrovascular pannus involving the stroma, an abnormal epithelium may remain on the corneal surface, preventing the corneal epithelium to regenerate through contact inhibition. In such cases, a sector limbal transplant (SLT) may be required (Dua 2002). Moreover, SSCE does not remove superficial neovascularization, whereas SLT may remove neovascularization, recover the normal corneal architecture, and decrease inflammation (Huang et al. 2001).

SSCE can be employed to improve visual function and reduce symptoms even when as little as two clock hours of normal limbus and peripheral cornea remain. The aim should be to achieve normal corneal epithelial cover over the visual axis. An attempt to achieve normal epithelial cover for the entire cornea, when only two clock hours or less of limbus are surviving, may stretch the capacity of the remaining limbus and could eventually lead to epithelial breakdown (Dua et al. 2000).

Amniotic membrane and partial limbal stem cell deficiencies

AM may be used individually, or be associated to both SSCE and anterior keratectomy to enhance corneal re-epithelialization and reduce inflammation and neovascularization. In partial limbal deficiencies, AM re-establishes the SC environment in the stroma of the sclerocorneal limbus, reduces inflammation, and stimulates proliferation of limbal SCs, avoiding limbal transplant. Although in some cases, AM may be used as a graft, AM is generally used as a patch to provide a proper environment for the cells to grow underneath. Moreover, AM presents anti-inflammatory properties, which are especially useful in the acute phase of chemical burns (Dua et al. 2004, Gomes et al. 2003, Guell et al. 2011, Sangwan et al. 2004).

Dua suggested that partial LSCD with <90° of intact limbus could not be treated with simple epithelial debridement without AM transplantation (Dua 2002). In contrast, AM as a permanent graft after pannus resection has been shown to restore the entire corneal surface in eyes with partial LSCD with as little as 30–60° of intact limbus left (Anderson et al. 2001a, Dua et al. 2004, Guell et al. 2011).

Postoperative care of limbal auto- or allografts in total limbal stem cell deficiencies

Following SLT for total LSCD, generally in autografts, conjunctival epithelium often reaches the limbus and grows over the corneal surface despite peritomy and conjunctival recession. SSCE is performed to prevent conjunctival epithelium from reaching the limbus, until repopulation of the limbus from surviving or donor limbal cells is completed, and to remove conjunctivalization over the cornea (Dua 2002).

Amniotic membrane and total limbal stem cell deficiencies

In total limbal deficiencies, as AM is devoid of SC, a limbal transplant is essential to re-establish the population of limbal SC. Amniotic membrane transplantation (AMT) associated with a limbal transplant constitutes a substrate for SC proliferation and epithelial migration that may accelerate re-epithelization following surgery (Dua et al. 2004, Gomes et al. 2003). AMT may also be performed as a prior procedure to restore the microenvironment of the sclerocorneal limbal stroma. Both AMT and the use of systemic immunosuppressors have reduced the incidence of limbal allograft rejection (Dua et al. 2004, Meallet et al. 2003).

Acute chemical and thermal ocular injuries

Immediately after acute ocular burns, a large or total corneal epithelial defect may be present. The ability of the eye to heal the defect depends on the extent of limbal SC injury. The amount of limbal damage can be estimated by evaluating perilimbal ischemia. However, in most cases of chemical injury, the extent of LSCD cannot be determined in the acute phase. Only time would tell if enough limbus survived to regenerate the cornea with normal corneal epithelium (Schwartz & Holland 2011).

In the acute phase of chemical and thermal burns with partial limbal deficiency, conjunctival epithelium should be prevented from crossing the limbus and covering the corneal surface when possible until the circumferentially migrating sheets of limbal epithelium meet each other, and the limbal barrier is re-established. However, in severe ocular surface diseases involving the entire or a very extensive area limbus, it may be preferred to allow the conjunctival epithelium to cover the cornea until the inflammation settles; since, according to Dua's advice, conjunctival epithelium is better than no epithelium. Conjunctival epithelium may be removed or limbal transplantation techniques may be attempted at a later date.

Amniotic membrane in the acute phase of chemical or thermal burns

AMT may also be used as an adjuvant to restore corneal and conjunctival surfaces, as it enhances epithelial regeneration, reduces inflammation and limbal stromal infiltration, and limits symblepharon formation, especially when applied immediately after the burn (**Figure 40.2**) (Dua et al. 2004, Guell et al. 2011, Meller et al. 2000).

ANTERIOR OR SUPERFICIAL KERATECTOMY

Indications

Anterior or superficial keratectomy consists of removal of corneal lesions affecting the epithelium, subepithelium, and anterior stroma. It may be useful to treat any corneal opacity involving the surface of the cornea [i.e. Salzmann's nodular degeneration and band keratopathy (BK)]. Additionally, de-epìthelialization may be required to enhance corneal healing in neurotrophic corneal ulcers with rolled edges.

Surgical technique

Superficial keratectomy may be performed mechanically (using a surgical blade and/or Vannas scissors, or with a mechanical microkeratome) or with excimer or femtosecond laser.

Under topical anesthesia, a crescent blade is used to remove the corneal lesions. In presence of thick fibrovascular pannus, or thick lesions, Vannas scissors may be used to remove the lesions. A dissection plane free of disease is frequently reached. Care should be taken to avoid creating irregularities in the corneal stroma, which could lead to irregular astigmatism and delayed epithelial healing. Finally, a bandage contact lens is placed, and topical antibiotics and steroids, and artificial tears should be prescribed. Patients should be closely monitored until re-epithelialization is complete.

In some eyes, subsequent phototherapeutic keratectomy may be necessary to smooth the surface, especially in eyes with lesions involving the Bowman's layer and superficial stroma, or with major peripheral neovascularization. In presence of deep defects in Bowman's layer and superficial stroma after difficult mechanical removal of corneal superficial lesions, multiple masking or laser ablation procedures may be required to acquire a homogenous surface. Alternatively, anterior lamellar keratoplasty (ALK) may be performed. Phototherapeutic keratectomy is discussed in more detail in Chapter 42.

Salzmann's degeneration

Salzmann's nodular degeneration consists of single or multiple, yellowish-white to grayish-blue, elevated nodular lesions that are often annular in location and in the mid-periphery of the cornea. Nodules are often seen adjacent to corneal scarring or pannus, with an iron line at the edge (Farjoo et al. 2006). Lesions experience slow progression, and they may be unilateral or bilateral. It predominantly affects women in the sixth decade of their life (Graue-Hernández et al. 2010, Severin & Kirchhof 1990, Vannas et al. 1975).

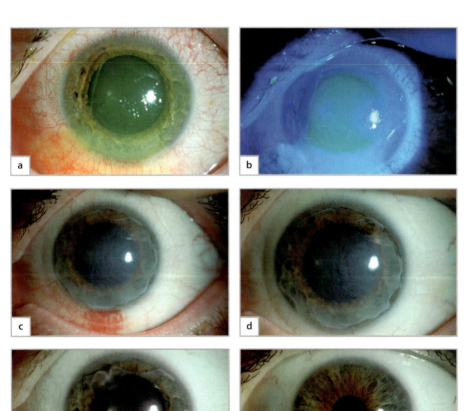

Figure 40.2 Amniotic membrane transplantation (AMT) in a patient with an acute chemical burn because of an alkali (sodium hydroxide). (a) and (b) Clinical photographs showing an extensive epithelial defect affecting three fourths of the cornea. Mild corneal edema, and perilimbal ischemia affecting the inferior half of the cornea are seen. Visual acuity was counting fingers. (c) One week and (d) three weeks after AMT, visual acuity had improved to 20/100. Partial reabsortion of the amniotic membrane (AM) is seen. (e) Five weeks and (f) two months after AMT visual acuity had improved to 20/60 and 20/20, respectively. The epithelial defect had healed with normal corneal epithelium phenotype, and the AM was completely reabsorbed.

Salzmann's nodular degeneration may occur following episodes of keratitis (i.e. phlyctenulosis, trachoma, vernal keratoconjunctivitis, measles, scarlet fever, interstitial keratitis, and other viral diseases). It is rarely associated with anterior basement membrane dystrophy and corneal surgery, such as LASIK (Lim & Chan 2009, Werner et al. 2000). Currently, most cases are idiopathic or in association with any corneal inflammatory disease. In a series of 180 eyes, meibomian gland dysfunction was the most common coexistent condition, identified in 41.7% of the cases (Graue-Hernández et al. 2010). It has also been associated with contact lens wear (**Figure 40.3**) (Farjoo et al. 2006).

Histopathologically, it is composed of dense collagen plaques with hyalinization between epithelium and Bowman's layer or beyond. The corneal epithelium presents degenerative changes, and it may be atrophic or absent in nodular areas. There is excessive secretion of a basement-membrane-like material, and Bowman's membrane is absent. Causative factors include external irritation because of poor epithelial protection and other tissue repair mechanisms (Das et al. 2005).

Salzmann's degeneration is generally asymptomatic. Decreased visual acuity, occurring in 30.6% of patients, is the most common symptom and the main indication for surgical treatment. Salzmann's nodules induce a central corneal flattening with high hyperopic refractive error and significant increment of corneal aberrations. Lacrimation, photophobia, and irritation may occur if the epithelium over the nodules breaks down (Graue-Hernández et al. 2010).

Manual removal, phototherapeutic keratectomy with or without the use of topical mitomycin C 0.02%, and lamellar or penetrating keratoplasty have been used (Khaireddin et al. 2011). Under topical anesthesia, lamellar dissection of Salzmann's nodules with Bowman's membrane as 'guiding' structure is performed by grasping of nodules with Colibri forceps and careful planar dissection with a hockey knife. Roszkowska et al. used 25% ethanol as an adjuvant to mechanically remove the nodules and showed that manual alcohol-assisted removal of Salzmann's was effective in improving visual acuity and refractive change, as well as normalizing corneal topography and aberrometry in a case where the underlying corneal stroma appeared smooth (Roszkowska et al. 2009). AM as a patch may also be used to enhance corneal re-epithelialization (**Figure 40.3** and **40.4**) (Gris et al. 1999, Yoon & Park 2003).

However, even when a cleavage plane is easily detected and tissue can be separated easily from the corneal surface leaving Bowman's layer almost untouched, some cases require phototherapeutic keratectomy to further smooth the corneal surface. On the other hand, eyes with deep defects in Bowman's layer and superficial stroma after difficult mechanical removal of nodules may require multiple phototherapuetic keratectomies homogenizing procedures, and will be more prone to recurrences. In a series of 35 eyes documented to have Salzmann's nodular degeneration, 22 needed phototherapeutic keratectomies (Das et al. 2005). As a routine, laser ablation should be combined with previous conventional removal of nodules and excessive pannus tissue. By doing so, lamellar and penetrating keratoplasty techniques may only be required for lesions extending to the mid-stroma (Das et al. 2005, Khaireddin et al. 2011). Recurrences have been reported to be of 21.9% (Graue-Hernández et al. 2010).

Band keratopathy

BK consists of calcium deposits in the form of hydroxyapatite, a phosphate salt, at the level of Bowman's membrane, epithelial basement membrane, and anterior stroma related to excess of calcium, and/or a change of corneal metabolism that causes increased tissue pH and precipitation of calcium. Although there are noncalcific forms as well, such as in advanced spheroidal degeneration, chronic use of topical medications with mercurial compounds, or urate keratopathy, typically the term BK refers to the calcific forms most frequently related to chronic uveitis and other inflammatory diseases, or hypercalcemic states (i.e. chronic renal failure or sarcoidosis). The incidence of BK in juvenile idiopathic arthritis and juvenile rheumatoid arthritis has been reported to be as high as 46 and 60%, respectively (Kump et al. 2006, Ozdal et al. 2005). The use of topical medications containing phosphates has also been associated to BK (Taravella et al. 1994). In those patients with BK of unknown origin, possible systemic causes

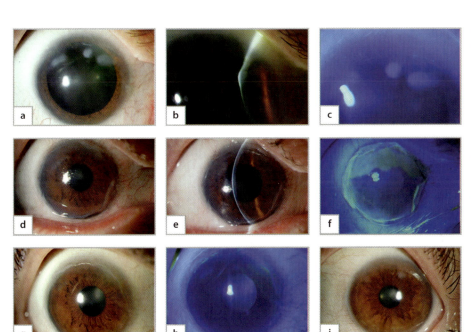

Figure 40.3 Salzmann's nodular degeneration in the right eye of a 51-year-old male, contact lens wearer. (a) and (b) Preoperative clinical photographs show grayish, raised nodules on the superior peripheral cornea with clear margins. (c) Fluorescein staining shows negative staining of the Salzmann's nodules and partial limbal stem cell deficiency. (d)–(f) One day after superficial keratectomy and amniotic membrane (AM) transplantation. (g) and (h) One month postoperatively, visual acuity was 20/25. Slit-lamp examination showed partial reabsortion of the AM, and smooth cornea. Faint superficial leucomas can be seen in the areas previously affected by the nodules. (i) Left eye of the same patient showing mild, asymptomatic Salzmann's nodules superiorly that did not require treatment.

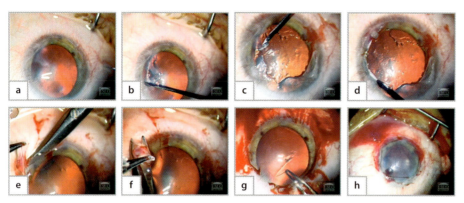

Figure 40.4 Superficial keratectomy and amniotic membrane (AM) transplantation for Salzmann's nodular degeneration: surgical technique. This patient underwent phacoemulsification and intraocular lens implantation during the same procedure. (a) Preoperative clinical photograph shows grayish, raised nodules on the temporal half of the cornea. (b)–(d) The corneal epithelium and the nodules are removed using a beaver blade with Bowman's membrane as the 'guiding' layer. Careful planar dissection is mandatory to avoid inducing irregularities on the corneal stroma. (e) and (f) Vannas scissors are used to smoothly cut the thicker tissue at the periphery of the cornea. (g) Phacoemulsification: methylcellulose is applied onto the cornea, which allows perfect visualization during phacoemulsification. Capsulorhexis is shown. (h) AM is sutured as a patch (epithelial side down) using a running 10-0 Nylon suture with the knot buried at 11 o'clock position.

should be investigated as recurrences are high or guaranteed if the cause persists. A medical work-up should include serum calcium, phosphorus, uric acid, and renal function values, and parathyroid hormone and angiotensin-converting enzyme levels (elevated in sarcoid disease).

Clinically, BK appears as a grayish opacity of the cornea, which begins in the corneal periphery in the horizontal meridian, and is separated from the limbus by a narrow clear zone. As the degeneration develops, BK gradually progresses centrally as an interpalpebral band dotted with holes, giving it a 'Swiss cheese' appearance (**Figure 40.5**). These holes are thought to be the sites where the opacity is perforated by corneal nerves. The lesions are subepithelial but may break through the epithelium in advanced stages, forming a continuous band from limbus to limbus.

Histopathologically, calcium deposits are intracellular when associated with hypercalcemia, and extracellular when associated with local disease or renal failure. They are first encountered at the level of Bowman's layer, but later invade the superficial stroma. Hyaline-like material is deposited around the calcific depositions, and a fibrous

pannus separates the epithelium and Bowman's layer. The overlying epithelium may be atrophic (Cursino & Fine 1976).

Early stages of BK are usually asymptomatic, and do not require treatment. BK can cause discomfort, foreign body sensation, and recurrent episodes of sharp pain as a result of epithelial breakdown. Visual acuity is affected when BK covers the central cornea. The treatment of BK should be directed toward both relieving or solving the symptoms (decrease in visual acuity, and resolution of pain) and treating the cause to decrease the likelihood of recurrences. The mainstay of treatment is the application of disodium ethylenediamine-tetraacetic acid (EDTA) in 0.05 M concentration, after an adequate scrape of the epithelium to expose the calcium deposits. Chelation with EDTA has shown a recurrence rate of about 18%, with a higher recurrence rate of about 60% in patients with chronic uveitis (**Figure 40.5**) (Najjar et al. 2004). EDTA chelation may be associated with other treatment strategies including mechanical superficial keratectomy, phototherapeutic keratectomy, laser-assisted subepithelial keratectomy, or ALK or penetrating keratoplasty (Biser et al. 2004, O'Brart et al. 1993, de Ortueta et al. 2006, Saini et al. 2003, Sharma et al. 2011). A diamond burr or

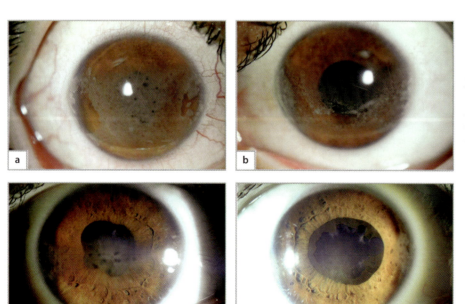

Figure 40.5 Band keratopathy secondary to chronic uveitis in patients with juvenile idiopathic arthritis (a) and (b), and juvenile rheumatoid arthritis (c) and (d). (a) and (c) Preoperative clinical photographs show a grayish band of calcium deposits dotted with holes, giving it a 'Swiss cheese' appearance. (b) and (d) Three months after mechanical corneal de-epithelialization, and chelation with 0.05 M disodium ethylenediaminetetraacetic acid. Significant improvement is observed.

No.15 blade may be used to smooth the corneal surface (Bokosky et al. 1985). A combination of treatment strategies is often used, such as EDTA + superficial keratectomy and/or phototherapeutic keratectomy + AMT (**Figures 40.6–40.8**) (Im et al. 2010, Kwon et al. 2004). AM has been used after chelation with EDTA to improve re-epithelialization and reduce postoperative pain (Anderson et al. 2001b).

Neurotrophic ulcers

The spectrum of dry eye disease ranges from mild irritation with minimal ocular surface disease to severe and disabling irritation with persistent epithelial defects and stromal ulcerations related to neurotrophic keratopathy. This entity is a degenerative disease of the corneal epithelium characterized by impaired healing. Absence of corneal sensitivity is the hallmark of the condition, which may end in corneal stromal melting and perforation. The causes of decreased corneal sensation are multiple and may affect sensory nerve supply from the trigeminal nucleus to the corneal nerve endings (Kruse et al. 1999). Neurotrophic keratopathy is discussed in more detail in Chapter 26.

Currently, dry eye disease is considered a multifactorial disease and, therefore, treatment strategies are focused on improving the different factors involved in an individual case, which include increasing and stabilizing the tear film, controlling inflammation, and treating meibomian gland dysfunction. Conservative treatments include (1) intense lubrication of the ocular surface, specially with preservative-free artificial tears or ointments to prevent preservative-induced epithelial toxicity; (2) therapeutic soft contact lenses (Lemp 1986);

(3) punctal plugs of the lower and/or upper puncta (Tai et al. 2002); (4) and autologous serum drops in concentrations ranging from 20 to 100%. Autologous serum is believed to inhibit apoptosis in the conjunctival and corneal epithelium due to the effect of growth factors, fibronectin, vitamins, and immunoglobulins contained in the serum (Fox et al. 1984, Poon et al. 2001). Medical treatment is sufficient in the vast majority of patients with mild-to-moderate forms of dry eye disease. However, patients with very severe forms of dry eye disease with complicated neurotrophic ulcers may need surgical interventions.

The procedure of choice is desepithelialization and/or superficial keratectomy. Under topical anesthesia, the epithelium near the edge of the ulcer, which is usually reduplicated and thick, is removed with a beaver blade. An AM patch generally enhances postoperative re-epithelialization. The AM patch covers the whole cornea, and is sutured to the episclera near the limbus, epithelial side down, using a 10/0 Nylon running suture with the knot buried at 11 o'clock. In cases with stromal loss, a monolayer or multilayer AM graft may be also sutured underneath to fill the stromal defect. Finally, a therapeutic contact lens is placed, and topical antibiotic and anti-inflammatory drops are prescribed until complete re-epithelialization is achieved. The AM graft gets embedded in the area of stromal defects, whereas the AM patch may be removed, reabsorbed, or it falls off. The AM protects the ocular surface from external insults and provides substances that reduce inflammation and promote epithelialization beneath the membrane by facilitating migration of epithelial cells, reinforcing adhesion of basal epithelial cells, and preventing apoptosis (Dua et al. 2004, Gris et al. 2002, Guell et al. 2011).

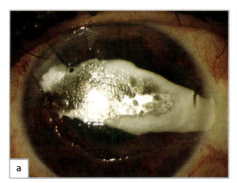
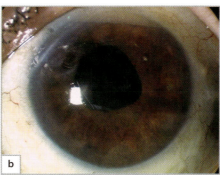

Figure 40.6 Dense band keratopathy in a patient who had undergone multiple vitreoretinal surgeries and temporary silicone oil tamponade. (a) Preoperative clinical photograph showing a dense plaque of calcium deposits extending from limbus to limbus, and an extense epithelial defect. (b) Three months after chelation with 0.05 M disodium ethylenediaminetetraacetic acid, mechanical superficial keratectomy, and amniotic membrane transplantation. Autologous serum eyedrops were also prescribed. A clear cornea with no calcium deposits or epithelial defect is seen.

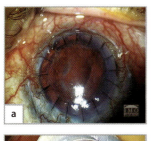
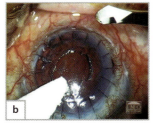
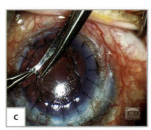
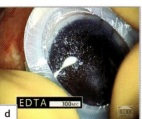
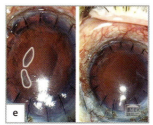
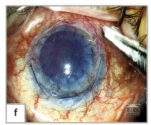

Figure 40.7 Band keratopathy after penetrating keratoplasty. (a) Preoperative clinical photograph showing two plaques of calcium deposits in the temporal cornea (b) The corneal epithelium is removed to expose the calcium deposits using a beaver blade and a microsponge. (c) Vannas scissors are used to ensure clean margins of the epithelial defect. (d) Chelation with 0.05 M disodium ethylenediaminetetraacetic acid (EDTA). (e) Before (left) and immediately after (right) EDTA chelation, showing complete removal of the calcium deposits. (f) Finally, amniotic membrane is sutured as a patch (epithelial side down) using a running 10-0 Nylon suture with the knot buried at 11 o'clock position.

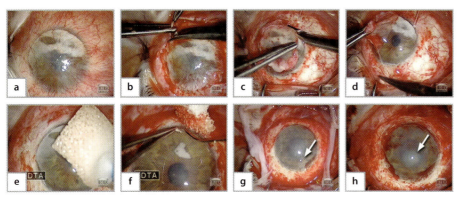

Figure 40.8 Total limbal stem cell deficiency with dense band keratopathy after ocular chemical burn. (a) Preoperative clinical photograph showing 360° conjunctivalization of the cornea, and a dense plaque of calcium deposits extending from limbus to limbus superiorly. (b) 360° conjunctival peritomy. (c) and (d) The conjunctival epithelium covering the cornea is easily removed using forceps and Vannas scissors. The corneal stroma underneath appears clear. (e) Calcium deposits are removed by mechanical friction and chelation using a microsponge soaked with 0.05 M disodium ethylenediaminetetraacetic acid. (f) Small remnants of calcium are removed using forceps and a blunt blade. (g) and (h) Ex vivo expanded corneal stem cells on amniotic membrane are finally implanted. The amniotic membrane is sutured as a patch (epithelial side down) using a running 10-0 Nylon suture with the knot buried at 11 o'clock position. The biopsy specimen (yellow arrow) is placed on the center of the cornea, as the highest density of expanded cells is expected surrounding the area.

ANTERIOR LAMELLAR KERATOPLASTY IN OCULAR SURFACE DISEASE

Indications

ALK is rarely indicated in patients with severe dry eye disease or severe ocular surface diseases because it carries a poor prognosis. However, ALK may be considered the procedure of choice in cases of persistent superficial stromal scarring, neurotrophic corneal ulcers with impending perforation, or corneal perforations. In such cases, the integrity of the globe is the primary aim. Anterior lamellar corneal transplantation techniques are preferred to full-thickness grafts because they present important advantages, which include extraocular surgery, absence of risk of endothelial graft rejection as the host endothelium is preserved, faster wound healing, and shorter topical corticosteroid regimes (Reinhart et al. 2011).

Surgical technique

Whenever possible, the procedure of choice is a deep ALK, as it presents better optical results than other ALK techniques. The big bubble technique, first described by Anwar and Teichmann in 2002, with several modifications published and presented later, provides a clean pre-Descemet's plane lamellar dissection that reduces the incidence and severity of interface-related complications (Anwar & Teichmann 2002).

Under retrobulbar anesthesia, a partial-thickness trephination is performed with a Hessburg-Barron suction trephine (Katena, New Jersey, USA). The Barron trephine cuts 0.250 mm downward per turn. Partial trephination should aim for 75% corneal thickness, which is preoperatively determined by ultrasonic pachymetry or optical coherence tomography pachymetry maps. A portion of the anterior stroma is dissected with a crescent knife for a better judgment of the needle depth for the air injection. Alternatively, a femtosecond laser may be used to remove an anterior cap of the host cornea.

A 30-gauge disposable needle attached to a syringe filled with air is inserted, deeply and bevel down, into the paracentral corneal stroma. Air is injected to form a large air bubble that separates the endothelium–Descemet's membrane from the rest of the corneal stroma. This same maneuver may be performed directly with an ophthalmic viscosurgical device (OVD). Then, a small opening is made in the air bubble by a stromal cut, using a sharp tip of a blade, and a viscosurgical device is injected in the interface to protect the Descemet's membrane from being damaged. Special care should be taken not to cut the Descemet's membrane. The remaining stromal layers are lifted with an iris spatula, severed with a blade, and excised with curved scissors. We use the Katzin left-right keratoplasty scissors to create a more vertical cut. Usually, a side port incision is made to lower the intraocular pressure and check the formation of the air bubble by injecting air in the anterior chamber and visualizing its shape in the peripheral cornea. Finally, the corneal donor button is stripped of Descemet's membrane and endothelium (which can conceptually be used for a Descemet's membrane endothelial keratoplasty), and sutured with 16 interrupted 10-0 Nylon sutures in the recipient's corneal bed after the OVD is profusely washed out. An AM patch is used in those cases where troublesome epithelialization is expected (i.e. postherpetic keratitis, neurotrophic keratitis, and severe dry eye disease states).

CONCLUSIONS

SSCE is effective in restoring the corneal surface with healthy corneal epithelium in cases of partial LSCD. AM may be associated to enhance corneal re-epithelialization, especially in cases with <90° of intact limbus. However, SSCE cannot be performed if AM is used. Anterior or superficial keratectomy is an alternative when dense fibrovascular pannus has developed. However, for eyes with total LSCD, corneal surface reconstruction requires transplantation of limbal epithelial SCs.

Desepithelialization of the rolled edges of neurotrophic corneal ulcers is sometimes required to allow appropriate corneal healing response. AMT is often required in such cases. Manual superficial keratectomy is an effective surgical approach for lesions affecting the corneal epithelium, Bowman's membrane, and anterior stroma. However, lesions deeper in the stroma or cases with impending corneal perforation may require lamellar keratoplasty both to improve visual acuity and preserve the integrity of the globe.

REFERENCES

Anderson DF, Ellies P, Pires RT, et al. Amniotic membrane transplantation for partial limbal stem cell deficiency. Br J Ophthalmol 2001a; 85:567–575.

Anderson DF, Prabhasawat P, Alfonso E, Tseng SCG. Amniotic membrane transplantation after the primary surgical management of band keratopathy. Cornea 2001b; 20:354–361.

Anwar M, Teichmann KD. Big-bubble technique to bare Descemet's membrane in anterior lamellar keratoplasty. J Cataract Refract Surg 2002; 28:398–403.

Biser SA, Donnenfeld ED, Doshi SJ, et al. Lamellar keratectomy using an automated microkeratome. Eye Contact Lens 2004; 30:69–73.

Bokosky JE, Meyer RF, Sugar A. Surgical treatment of calcific band keratopathy. Ophthalmic Surg 1985; 16:645–647.

Cotsarelis G, Cheng SZ, Dong G, et al. Existence of slow-cycling limbal epithelial basal cells that can be preferentially stimulated to proliferate: implications on epithelial stem cells. Cell 1989; 57:201–209.

Cursino JW, Fine BS. A histologic study of calcific and noncalcific band keratopathies. Am J Ophthalmol 1976; 82:395–404.

Das S, Link B, Seitz B. Salzmann's nodular degeneration of the cornea: a review and case series. Cornea 2005; 24:772–777.

Donisi PM, Rama P, Fasolo A, Ponzin D. Analysis of limbal stem cell deficiency by corneal impression cytology. Cornea 2003; 22:533–538.

Dua H. Sequential sector conjunctival epitheliectomy. In: Holland EJ, Mannis M (eds), Ocular surface disease, medical and surgical management. New York: Springer, 2002: 168–174.

Dua HS. The conjunctiva in corneal epithelial wound healing. Br J Ophthalmol 1998; 82:1407–1411.

Dua HS, Azuara-Blanco A. Limbal stem cells of the corneal epithelium. Surv Ophthalmol 2000; 44:415–425.

Dua HS, Forrester JV. The corneoscleral limbus in human corneal epithelial wound healing. Am J Ophthalmol 1990; 110:646–656.

Dua HS, Gomes JA, King AJ, Maharajan VS. The amniotic membrane in ophthalmology. Surv Ophthalmol 2004; 49:51–77.

Dua HS, Gomes JAP, Singh A. Corneal epithelial wound healing. Br J Ophthalmol 1994; 78:401–408.

Dua HS, Miri A, Said DG. Contemporary limbal stem cell transplantation—a review. Clin Experiment Ophthalmol 2010; 38:104–117.

Dua HS, Saini JS, Azuara-Blanco A, Gupta P. Limbal stem cell deficiency: concept, aetiology, clinical presentation, diagnosis and management. Indian J Ophthalmol 2000b; 48:83–92.

Dua HS, Shanmuganathan VA, Powell-Richards AO, et al. Limbal epithelial crypts: a novel anatomical structure and a putative limbal stem cell niche. Br J Ophthalmol 2005; 89:529–532.

Farjoo AA, Halperin GI, Syed N, et al. Salzmann's nodular corneal degeneration clinical characteristics and surgical outcomes. Cornea 2006; 25:11–15.

Fox RI, Chan R, Michelson JB, et al. Beneficial effect of artificial tears made with autologous serum in patients with keratoconjunctivitis sicca. Arthritis Rheum 1984; 27:459–461.

Gomes JA, dos Santos MS, Cunha MC, et al. Amniotic membrane transplantation for partial and total limbal stem cell deficiency secondary to chemical burn. Ophthalmology 2003; 110:466–473.

Graue-Hernández EO, Mannis MJ, Eliasieh K, et al. Salzmann nodular degeneration. Cornea 2010; 29:283–289.

Gris O, del Campo Z, Wooley-Dod C, et al. Amniotic membrane implantation as a therapeutic contact lens for the treatment of epithelial disorders. Cornea 2002; 21:22–27.

Gris O, Güell JL, Lopez-Navidad A, et al. Application of the amniotic membrane in ocular surface pathology. Ann Transplant 1999; 4:82–84.

Guell JL, Gris O, Morral M. Indications for and uses of amniotic membrane. In: Krachmer JH, Mannis MJ, Holland EJ (eds), Cornea, chapter 146. Mosby/Saunders: Elsevier, 2011: 1647–1654.

Huang T, Wang Y, Zhang H, et al. Limbal allografting from living-related donors to treat partial limbal deficiency secondary to ocular chemical burns. Arch Ophthalmol 2001; 129:1267–1273.

Im SK, Lee KH, Yoon KC. Combined ethylenediaminetetraacetic acid chelation, phototherapeutic keratectomy and amniotic membrane transplantation for treatment of band keratopathy. Korean J Ophthalmol 2010; 24:73–77.

Khaireddin R, Katz T, Baile RB, et al. Superficial keratectomy, PTK, and mitomycin C as a combined treatment option for Salzmann's nodular degeneration: a follow-up of eight eyes. Graefes Arch Clin Exp Ophthalmol 2011; 249:1211–1215.

Kheirkhah A, Raju VK, Tseng SCG. Minimal conjunctival limbal autograft for total limbal stem cell deficiency. Cornea 2008; 27:730–733.

Kruse FE, Rohrschneider K, Völcker H. Multilayer amniotic membrane transplantation for reconstruction of deep corneal ulcers. Ophthalmology 1999; 106:1504–1510.

Kump LI, Castañeda RA, Androudi SN, et al. Visual outcomes in children with juvenile idiopathic arthritis-associated uveitis. Ophthalmology 2006; 113:1874–1877.

Kwon YS, Song YS, Kim JC. New treatment for band keratopathy: superficial lamellar keratectomy, EDTA chelation and amniotic membrane transplantation. J Korean Med Sci 2004; 19:611–615.

Lavker RM, Tseng SC, Sun TT. Corneal epithelial stem cells at the limbus: looking at some old problems from a new angle. Exp Eye Res 2004; 78:433–446.

Lemp MA. Contact lenses and the dry-eye patient. Int Ophthalmol Clin 1986; 26:63–71.

Lim MC, Chan WK. Salzmann nodular degeneration after laser in situ keratomileusis. Cornea 2009; 28:577–578.

Meallet MA, Espana EM, Grueterich M, et al. Amniotic membrane transplantation with conjunctival limbal autograft for total limbal stem cell deficiency. Ophthalmology 2003; 110:1585–1592.

Meller D, Pires RTF, Mack RJS, et al. Amniotic membrane transplantation for acute chemical or thermal burns. Ophthalmology 2000; 107:980–990.

Najjar DM, Cohen EJ, Rapuano CJ, Laibson PR. EDTA chelation for calcific band keratopathy: results and long-term follow-up. Am J Ophthalmol 2004; 137:1056–1064.

O'Brart DP, Gartry DS, Lohmann CP, et al. Treatment of band keratopathy by excimer laser phototherapeutic keratectomy: surgical techniques and long term follow up. Br J Ophthalmol 1993; 77:702–708.

de Ortueta D, Schreyger F, Baatz H. Band keratopathy: a modified treatment. Eur J Ophthalmol 2006; 16:618–620.

Ozdal PC, Vianna RN, Deschênes J. Visual outcome of juvenile rheumatoid arthritis-associated uveitis in adults. Ocul Immunol Inflamm 2005; 13:33–38.

Poon AC, Geerling G, Dart JK, et al. Autologous serum eyedrops and epithelial defects: clinical and in vitro toxicity studies. Br J Ophthalmol 2001; 85:1188–1197.

Puangsricharern V, Tseng SCG. Cytologic evidence of corneal diseases with limbal stem cell deficiency. Ophthalmology 1995; 102:1476–1485.

Reinhart WJ, Musch DC, Jacobs DS, et al. Deep anterior lamellar keratoplasty as an alternative to penetrating keratoplasty a report by the American Academy of Ophthalmology. Ophthalmology 2011; 118:209–218.

Roszkowska AM, Colosi P, De Grazia L, et al. One year outcome of manual alcohol-assisted removal of Salzmann's nodular degeneration. Graefes Arch Clin Exp Ophthalmol 2009; 247:1431–1434.

Saini JS, Jain AK, Sukhija J, Saroha V. Indications and outcome of optical partial thickness lamellar keratoplasty. Cornea 2003; 22:111–113.

Sangwan VS, Matalia HP, Vemuganti GK, et al. Amniotic membrane transplantation for reconstruction of corneal epithelial surface in cases of partial limbal stem cell deficiency. Indian J Ophthalmol 2004; 52:281–285.

Schermer A, Galvin S, Sun T-T. Differentiation-related expression of a major 64K corneal keratin in vivo and in culture suggests limbal location of corneal epithelial stem cells. J Cell Biol 1986; 103:49–62.

Schwartz GS, Holland EJ. Classification and staging of ocular surface disease. In: Krachmer JH, Mannis MJ, Holland EJ (eds), Cornea, chapter 154. Mosby/Saunders, Elsevier 2011: 1713–1725.

Severin M, Kirchhof B. Recurrent Salzmann's corneal degeneration. Graefes Arch Clin Exp Ophthalmol 1990; 228:101–104.

Shanmuganathan VA, Foster T, Kulkarni BB, et al. Morphological characteristics of the limbal epithelial crypt. Br J Ophthalmol 2007; 91:514–519.

Sharma N, Mannan R, Sinha R, et al. Excimer laser phototherapeutic keratectomy for the treatment of silicone oil-induced band-shaped keratopathy. Eye Contact Lens 2011; 37:282–285.

Tai MC, Cosar CB, Cohen EJ, et al. The clinical efficacy of silicone punctal plug therapy. Cornea 2002; 21:135–139.

Taravella MJ, Stulting RD, Mader TH, et al. Calcific band keratopathy associated with the use of topical steroid-phosphate preparations. *Arch Ophthalmol* 1994; **112**:608–613.

Thoft RA, Friend J. The X, Y, Z hypothesis of corneal epithelial maintenance. *Invest Ophthalmol Vis Sci* 1983; **24**:1442–1443.

Tsubota K, Satake Y, Kaido M, et al. Treatment of severe ocular-surface disorders with corneal epithelial stem-cell transplantation. *N Engl J Med* 1999; **340**:1697–1703.

Vannas A, Hogan MJ, Wood I. Salzmann's nodular degeneration of the cornea. *Am J Ophthalmol* 1975; **79**:211–219.

Werner LP, Issid K, Werner LP, et al. Salzmann's corneal degeneration associated with epithelial basement membrane dystrophy. *Cornea* 2000; **19**:121–123.

Yoon KC, Park YG. Recurrent Salzmann's nodular degeneration. *Jpn J Ophthalmol* 2003; **47**:401–404.

Chapter 41 Phototherapeutic keratectomy

Miguel J. Maldonado

INTRODUCTION

The acronym 'PTK' is derived from the term 'phototherapeutic keratectomy,' which specifically refers to keratectomy (the removal of corneal tissue) through the application of an excimer laser ('photo'), with primarily therapeutic rather than refractive purposes, thus, the difference between PTK and PRK (photorefractive keratectomy). Since PTK pioneers began working with this technique in the late 1980s and PTK received FDA approval in 1995, its evolution has added other more complex objectives to the primary aim of removing altered corneal tissue, such as obtaining a more optically regular surface and improving the health of the ocular surface (Rapuano 2010).

OBJECTIVES OF PHOTOTHERAPEUTIC KERATECTOMY

In addition to the objectives of manual superficial keratectomy, PTK seeks to add the advantages of diminishing the amount of tissue removed and minimizing surgical trauma to the cornea (Ayres & Rapuano 2006). When the appropriate technique for PTK application is used in a way that takes advantage of the submicrometric precision in the excimer laser ablation, the end result of the procedure should be an improved corneal surface regularity that does not generate an excessive scarring reaction and acts as an adequate substrate to promote the correct adherence of the epithelium. Therefore, the cornea will have improved in optical surface quality, in transparency, in being less reactive to scarring and in displaying a more adherent epithelium (Seitz & Lisch 2011) (**Table 41.1**). Thanks to all of the above, it is often possible to delay, or even avoid, keratoplasty, which is a more invasive surgery that poses the added risk of immunological failure in the penetrating technique (Ayres & Rapuano 2006, Fagerholm 2003).

PHOTOTHERAPEUTIC KERATECTOMY PRESURGICAL EVALUATION

First of all, we must take into account that PTK is not the sole therapeutic option, as manual keratectomy still plays a role, and also that PTK is not the first choice of treatment for all anterior corneal disorders (Hersh et al. 1996). From this perspective, which states that PTK should not be used in an indiscriminate manner, we must bear in mind four

Table 41.1 Goals and indications for phototherapeutic keratectomy

Primary goals*	Secondary goals*	Examples of indication
Corneal opacity removal (from anterior 10–20% of the cornea)		Shallow corneal scar, central leukoma
Decreasing irregular surface and astigmatism		Salzmann's nodular degeneration
Increasing epithelial adherence		Anterior basement membrane epithelial dystrophy or recurrent corneal erosion syndrome from trauma
	Increasing contact lens tolerance	Keratoconus nodule
	Microbial debulking and increased drug penetration	Uncontrolled keratitis (bacterial, fungal, or amebic)
	Pain relief	Bullous keratopathy
	Promoting re-epithelialization	Shield ulcer
	Amblyopia prevention	Corneal opacities in children
	More accurate intraocular lens power calculation and increased intraoperative visualization	Coexisting band keratopathy and cataract
	Improving results after refractive surgery complications	Buttonholed flap, corneal haze, corneal higher order aberrations
	Deferral of primary or repeat keratoplasty	Granular corneal dystrophy
	Cosmetic and symptomatic improvement in eyes with low visual potential for keratoplasty	Silicone oil keratopathy
	Enhancement of ocular surface status	Avellino corneal dystrophy

*Various primary and secondary goals often coincide in the same phototherapeutic keratectomy treatment.
IOL, intraocular lens.

general aspects: (1) the localization and nature of the corneal disease, (2) the associated subjective symptoms, (3) the accompanying refractive error, and (4) the previously established goals and expectations.

Anatomical localization of the corneal pathology

To begin with, it is necessary to study the topographical location of the lesion, its distribution pattern, and the depth the keratectomy must reach. Generally, the more extensive and central the lesion is, the more homogeneously it is distributed, and only occasionally, the deeper the lesion is, the greater the advantages that excimer laser keratectomy will have over manual keratectomy (Hersh et al. 1996). On the other hand, the deeper the corneal pathology, the more amenable to keratoplasty is in most instances.

Location of the disorder on the cornea

The localization may be central, paracentral, or peripheral (**Figure 41.1**). Central localization, which is within the central 3–4 mm, implies that the lesion is over the pupil entrance, and therefore vision is affected either directly due to lack of transparency or due to induced irregular astigmatism. The paracentral area comprises the midperipheral cornea, situated within a diameter of 4 mm and 7–8 mm. Pathology in this localization will normally affect vision indirectly, causing irregular astigmatism or glare in situations with low luminosity. In the peripheral area, existing pathology will cause symptoms, but will rarely affect vision, and in such cases PTK will exceptionally be advantageous (Wagoner 1996).

Distribution pattern

According to the regularity and extension of the lesions in the optical zone, their distribution can be classified into nodular, segmental, diffuse, or complete (**Figure 41.2**). Nodular lesions are well-circumscribed alterations, surrounded by healthy cornea, which are isolated or present in low numbers. Segmental lesions are similar to nodular but occupy a larger extension of the cornea, therefore involving the pupillary aperture. Diffuse pathology refers to the presence of various lesions regularly distributed throughout the cornea, without occupying a major part of its extension. Complete distribution comprises lesions that occupy the entire central cornea (Wagoner 1996).

Depth

The depth is not measured by the localization of the lesion, but by the depth, the keratectomy must reach in order to obtain the desired therapeutic results (Rapuano 2003). In order to be able to determine the deepest level of the keratectomy and to classify the accessibility of the lesion, it is important to be able to objectively determine the anteroposterior extension of the lesion (Stark et al. 1990). In addition to a detailed slit-lamp examination, invaluable imaging techniques can be used for this purpose, such as an optical pachymeter, confocal microscopy, Scheimpflug photography, or optical coherence tomography (OCT) (**Figure 41.3**). When considering the pachymetry of the cornea to be treated, it is important to bear in mind that some scanning-slit topography and tomography systems underestimate true corneal thickness proportional to the density of an existing corneal opacity.

The considered levels according to depth are pre-Bowman's, Bowman's, anterior stromal, and profound stromal. Pre-Bowman's localized lesions include lesions incorporated in the epithelium and basement membrane. The pathology in the Bowman's membrane localization also includes concomitant alterations in the epithelium and basement membrane. Anterior stroma lesions include pathologies that are mainly located in the superficial 100–150 μm of the cornea. Profound stroma pathology is localized deeper than 150 μm (**Figure 41.3**).

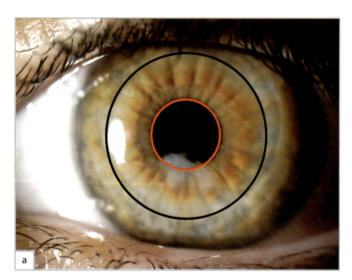

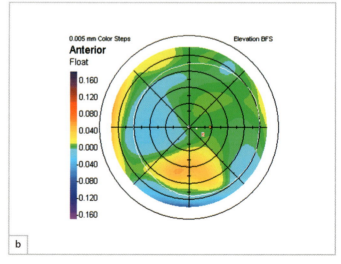

Figure 41.1 Surface location of corneal pathology, which may be performed at the slit lamp or, when the lesion is protruding, based on corneal topographical elevation maps. (a) In this eye, the pathology is predominantly located in the central cornea, but does not encroach the visual axis, as seen at the slit lamp. The red circle depicts a 3 mm-diameter area for a central location. The black circle delineates the 7 mm-diameter area, which outlines the paracentral region in between this and the red circle, and the peripheral area outside it. (b) The elevation topographical map shows the location by the bulging (as coded in yellow and orange) of the same lesion as in 'a', but at an earlier stage. In this map, the first inner circle delineates 3 mm in diameter central area and each circle delineates increments of 2 mm in diameter. In this case, the lesion has grown and migrated centripetally during the 2-year span in between (a) and (b). Centrally located pathology may be a good indication for PTK alone or in combination with manual keratectomy, particularly if the visual axis is involved. Paracentral lesions should be treated with PTK cautiously because the visual axis is not affected initially and the laser ablation should not alter the clarity and regularity over the pupil entrance. In peripherally located corneal disorders, while there is not a contraindication for PTK, excimer laser ablation offers little advantage over manual keratectomy. PTK, phototherapeutic keratectomy.

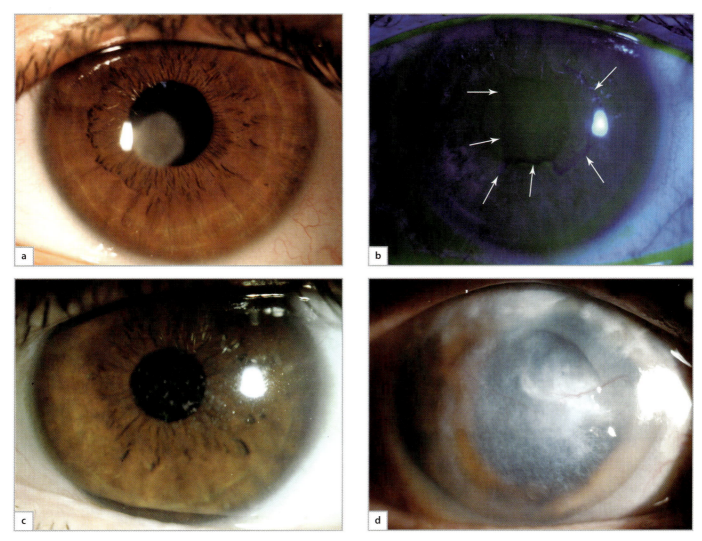

Figure 41.2 Pattern of distribution of corneal pathology, which largely determines the strategy of the best PTK technique. (a) A pseudomonas corneal ulcer scar presents as nodular pathology. (b) Basement membrane epithelial corneal dystrophy with segmental pattern is delineated by negative fluorescein staining. (c) Granular corneal dystrophy displays a diffuse pattern of scattered opacities in the central and paracentral cornea. (d) Longstanding bullous keratopathy presents as a complete corneal disorder. PTK, phototherapeutic keratectomy. Parts a and b: courtesy of Dr M. Calonge.

■ Symptomatology

In addition to the requirements of visual acuity, both with and without optical correction, it is common for the patient to present photophobia, eye watering, pain, or significant discomfort, or visual disturbances such as halos, glare, monocular diplopia, or clouding, either fluctuating during the day or constantly.

Refractive error

Central PTK induces hyperopia proportional to the ablation depth, which is not so likely to happen after manual keratectomy (Hersh et al. 1996). Conversely, a paracentral ablation can cause myopic shifts or induce variable amounts of astigmatism, both regular and irregular. Thus, for instance, a patient with Reis–Bücklers dystrophy and myopia will tolerate PTK much better than a patient with emmetropia or hyperopia will. In the latter, the level of satisfaction will be expected to be higher when treated with manual keratectomy instead, unless a combined PTK–hyperopic PRK procedure is performed.

The refractive status of the fellow eye should also be considered in unilateral conditions to avoid severe anisometropia. When the pathology is anterior, it might be worth considering combining manual de-epithelialization or a shallow transepithelial PTK with a laser refractive keratectomy to correct the preexisting ametropia (Stasi & Chuck 2009).

Goals and expectations of the surgery

The patient's expectations for good visual acuity, either with or without optical correction, must be always considered and discussed. The expected PTK-induced refractive shifts and their compensation are an integral part of this dialogue.

■ TREATMENT PLANNING

When making a decision as to the most adequate keratectomy, the first factor to consider is the localization of the lesion. From there, we can proceed to consider the pathology distribution, depth and

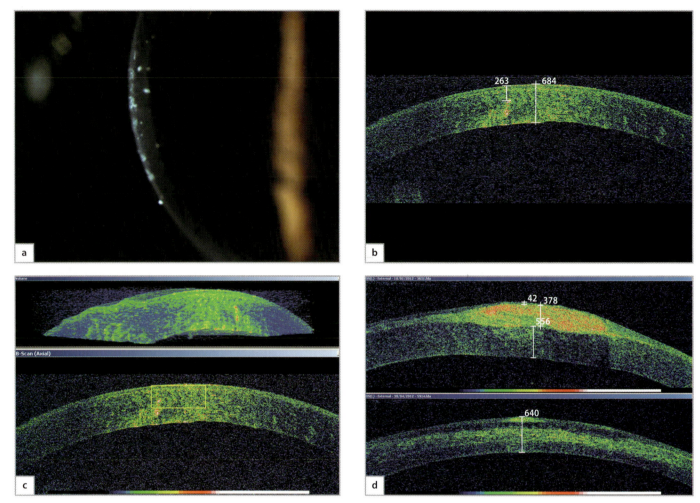

Figure 41.3 Assessment of ablation depth. Usually, the goal of PTK is not to ablate down completely to the deepest aspect of the corneal disturbance but to a depth that favorably balances the expected improvement in clarity, with the risk of excessive corneal thinning, scarring or inducing unwanted large refractive defects or irregular astigmatism. For this reason, it is so important to evaluate the bottom allocation of the corneal pathology. (a) A careful slit-lamp examination discloses that in this case of granular dystrophy most of the opacities lie in the anterior cornea, making PTK a feasible and worthwhile treatment option. (b) OCT allows for quantitative assessment of corneal pathology depth. In this case of polymorphic amyloid degeneration, the caliper function of the OCT permits accurate measurement of the opacities depth, showing that the optically densest deposits are located deeper (263 μm) than 20% of total pachymetry (684 μm × 20% = 137 μm). (c) Modern OCT technology also offers three-dimensional reconstruction of the scans (top) so that a better overview of the distribution of corneal pathology than in two-dimensional scans (bottom) can be achieved. (d) Salzmann's nodular degeneration shows how OCT technology discloses preoperatively (top) not only the diseased tissue but also the epithelium, which gets thinner at the apex of the nodule and exhibits compensatory hyperplasia on both sides of the prominence. This allows accurate planning of the surgery that comprised a manual keratectomy to debulk the nodule followed by a PTK with a masking agent to regularize the surface. Postoperatively (bottom), OCT confirms that the above-mentioned goals were achieved. OCT, optical coherence tomography; PTK, phototherapeutic keratectomy.

associated symptoms, as well as the patient's refraction and requirements (Wagoner 1996).

■ Central corneal lesions
Nodular or segmental distribution

In lesions situated within the optical zone where the alteration is nodular or segmental, the procedure should aim to remove the lesion without altering the surrounding healthy cornea. This is often adequately achieved with manual keratectomy. In this situation, the advantages offered by a primary PTK procedure are few; perhaps the removal of the lesion would be somewhat more thorough; however, this would only be an advantage if the disorder was situated in the intersection of the visual axis. On the other hand, it is important to take

into account that photoablation of a dense focal scar is difficult due to the lower ablation rate of the scar tissue in comparison with the surrounding healthy tissue. Furthermore, ablating adjacent areas of the healthy cornea could induce irregular astigmatism, which would be visually significant due to the central location. A good strategy consists of combining a manual keratectomy to debulk the lesion with a PTK to regularize the surface at the end of the procedure (Rapuano 2010).

Diffuse or complete distribution

When the disorder presents a diffuse or complete distribution, the selective removal of diseased tissue is usually unviable; therefore, keratectomy of the entire affected corneal layer is often considered. Thus, other factors such as the depth of the keratectomy must be considered in order to make the most appropriate decision.

Lesions that only affect the pre-Bowman's level can be manually eliminated without much difficulty or risk of inducing an intense scarring reaction. The application of the excimer laser could be justified when there is also the aim to minimally treat Bowman's membrane, as is the case in recurrent corneal erosion syndrome. In cases where a refractive error is also present, it is possible to proceed with a PRK.

Disorders that affect the Bowman's membrane level are more susceptible to benefiting specifically from PTK, even though manual keratectomy plays a relevant role in many cases. In those cases, other aspects such as refraction or corneal thickness will be the deciding factors when choosing one technique over another. Reis–Bücklers dystrophy is a classical example, as it can primarily be treated manually (especially in foresight of recurrence and scant corneal thickness for successive photoablations), but in a patient with myopia, the application of the excimer laser (with PTK in very mild myopia or PRK if the myopia is medium to high) would be the more pertinent therapeutic decision (McDonnell & Seiler 1992). When the disorder is not easily removed by manual keratectomy, as is the case in postinfectious scarring or in climatic keratopathy, the role of PTK is unquestionable.

When disorders affect the anterior stromal level, the complexity of carrying out a good manual keratectomy is greatly increased, as is the risk of inducing a significant postoperative scar (Hersh et al. 1996). In these cases, PTK must be applied with the most appropriate surgical strategy, making it possible to delay, or even avoid, performing keratoplasty.

Disorders that affect the profound stromal level can only be partially treated with PTK and are usually managed with grafting techniques. However, in cases such as bullous keratopathy or macular dystrophy, the excimer laser may alleviate the waiting period for a patient until keratoplasty is performed, particularly by diminishing ocular pain (Rathi et al. 2012).

Paracentral corneal lesions

Those disorders that do not affect the pupil entrance must be primarily treated by manual keratectomy. In these cases (such as paracentral Salzmann's nodular degeneration), the fundamental objectives are to diminish the irritating symptoms, the recurrence of erosions, and the probability that the disorder will extend centrally; improving visual acuity is not the primary objective. Therefore, it is not usually necessary to remove the entire lesion in order to obtain the required therapeutic benefit. Incidentally, a primary PTK does not offer clear advantages in such cases, and, furthermore, may induce further irregular astigmatism by ablating the adjacent healthy cornea if the latter is not thoroughly masked (Hersh et al. 1996).

Peripheral corneal lesions

When the alteration is located in the peripheral areas of the cornea, the indications are mostly symptomatic, as the probability of inducing visually significant irregular astigmatism is very low due to the distance from the visual axes. Therefore, keratectomy may be either manual or laser, or even combined.

PHOTOTHERAPEUTIC KERATECTOMY TECHNIQUES

What needs to be known about the excimer laser?

Nature of the excimer laser and its interaction with the corneal stroma and epithelium

The excimer laser utilizes 193 nm wavelength ultraviolet C light to break molecular bonds in the cornea to remove tiny amounts of tissue. It eliminates tissue from the surface of the cornea (0.25 μm per pulse) over an area identical to the diameter of the beam it projects through a process called ablative photodecomposition (Rapuano 2003).

The ablation rate of the corneal epithelium per pulse is greater than for stromal tissue, and in turn, greater for stromal tissue than for Bowman's membrane (Seiler et al. 1990). Also, when the epithelium is ablated, it emits a characteristic blue fluorescence that can be seen when the lights in the room are turned off (Phillips & McDonnell 1997). The autofluorescence disappears when the ablation reaches the stromal tissue. This phenomenon is due to its low water content. Dark areas will appear then and are the result of the interaction with the collagen present in Bowman's membrane.

Excimer laser liberation systems

There are three basic types of liberation systems:
1. Wide beam: this type of laser projects a large circular beam over the cornea that has an adjustable diameter
2. Scanner slit beam: in this system, a slit-shaped beam acts by continually scanning from right to left and from left to right so that a diaphragm with an adjustable aperture can determine which area of the cornea is exposed to the laser
3. Flying spot: this system utilizes a laser diameter of between <1 and 2 mm and sends pulses to changing spots in the area of the cornea to be treated. The latter requires a good eye tracker system to achieve precise ablations, but it is thought to induce less refractive change in PTK (Rathi et al. 2012)

Photogerapeutic keratectomy ablation profile

PTK ablates corneal tissue with a flat profile; the same amount of tissue removal is intended from the center than from the outer edges of the selected optical zone (**Figure 41.4**). This is unlike excimer laser application for the correction of myopia, which ablates more tissue from the center of the cornea than from the peripheral area with the purpose of flattening the central cornea. However, in practice, even if no refractive change is intended during a PTK stromal ablation, the healing corneal epithelium creates a peripheral meniscus that leads to a hyperopic shift in centrally located ablations and a myopic change in paracentral ones (Hersh et al. 1996, Rapuano 2003). Due to this, many lasers in their PTK operation mode provide an ablation transition

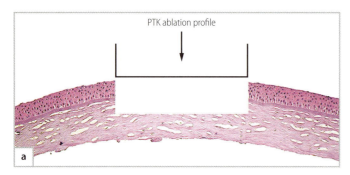
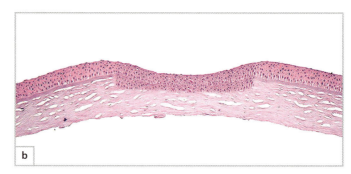

Figure 41.4 PTK ablation profile, corneal healing, and refractive shifts. (a) A typical PTK ablation profile is flat by intending to etch as much tissue in the center as in the periphery of the optical zone, for which the ablation would be expected to be neutral from a refractive perspective. (b) However, the epithelial healing and remodeling with constant blinking tend to smooth out the surface postoperatively, creating a negative meniscus effect that is more pronounced; the smaller the diameter of the optical zone, the deeper the intended ablation or the drying of the surface (increased ablation rate), and the more abrupt the transition between the optical zone and the untreated cornea is (less peripheral blending). Thus, when a central PTK is performed, there is a tendency toward a hyperopic shift due to central flattening of the anterior corneal contour that should be counterbalanced by antihyperopia strategies (minimizing ablation depth, increasing optical zone and peripheral transition zone, or adding a hyperopic PRK). When the PTK is paracentral or peripheral, there is a tendency toward induction of myopic shift because the central corneal contour steepens whereas the peripheral flattens. With any PTK location, great care should be taken not to induce or aggravate regular and irregular astigmatism. PRK, photorefractive keratectomy; PTK, phototherapeutic keratectomy.

zone outside the selected optical zone, creating a progression of the ablated stromal tissue in order to minimize tendency of the corneal epithelium to create a peripheral meniscus. Also, the retraction of the corneal lamellae in the cornea adjacent to the ablation crater seems to play a role in the hyperopic refraction switch following a central PTK (Dupps & Roberts 2001). In general, the risk of inducing hyperopia as a consequence of PTK is lower; the shallower the ablation depth, the less the drying of the cornea during the procedure, the larger the optical zone to be treated, and the more progressive the peripheral transition (Rathi et al. 2012). Some surgeons who work with wide beam lasers, unable to create programmed PTK peripheral transition zones, and no eye tracker, usually apply a gentle rotating movement to the patient's head during the ablation in order to achieve a similar effect and thus lower the hyperopic shift (known as 'polishing maneuver').

Finally, only some lasers allow the choice of PTK ablation mode through 'joystick' control; the beam can be directed by a stick that is operated by the surgeon, with movement along an 'x' and 'y' axis. This is a useful procedure when trying to focally ablate a lesion that is surrounded by healthy tissue (Rapuano 2010).

Patient preparation

Before carrying out any type of keratectomy, it is important to ensure that there is no inflammatory activity on the ocular surface. If there is an infection, it should be treated and controlled before the procedure, the exception being certain keratitis in which the excimer laser is used to directly debulk the microbial load and increase drug penetration (Rathi et al. 2012). Blepharitis must also be checked for, as treating it beforehand is a prerequisite for the eye to be in the best possible condition for surgery. Intraocular inflammation must also be treated, or it may become worse due to the tissue liberation of inflammatory mediators. Last, care should be taken to avoid patients with uncontrolled diabetes or collagen vascular disease.

Antiviral prophylaxis should be provided in all cases of PTK not only for herpetic scar, but also with a history of herpes simplex virus keratitis and in all patients with a corneal scar of unknown origin because exposure to the excimer laser (ultraviolet C light) can induce the reactivation of latent herpes simplex virus (Asbell 2000). Useful regimens include systemic acyclovir 800 mg thrice a day or

systemic valacyclovir 500 mg twice a day (de Rojas Silva et al. 2007). As to timing, while no protocol has been demonstrated superior to other, it seems wise to prescribe oral prophylaxis beginning at least 2 weeks prior to surgery and to continue oral prophylaxis for weeks or months, depending on the duration of topical steroid administration. The role of topical antiviral drugs is uncertain but may be limited by the unwanted potential local toxicity in the healing cornea. In addition to the use of systemic antiviral prophylaxis, prudence would dictate selecting patients in whom the herpes has been inactive for a minimum of 1 year before surgery and corneal sensitivity levels are not severely decreased.

Treatment strategies

PTK comprises a spectrum of techniques that range from the all-laser excimer ablation procedure to the one in which the excimer laser contributes to, or completes, a manual keratectomy (Hersh et al. 1996). This section begins with its predecessor, manual keratectomy, and a discussion of its current treatment options.

Manual keratectomy

In the manual technique, the altered epithelium or the one overlying lesion is usually gently scraped using a dry surgical spear, a #15 blade scalpel, or a blunt spatula (Wagoner 1996). Extreme care must be taken so as not to damage healthy underlying tissue or the limbal epithelium, to ensure a good epithelial closure. If the lesion is situated under the epithelium, the cleavage plane must be identified, drying it with the tip of the spear (**Figure 41.5**). Once identified, its border will then be lifted using the tip of the spear, a blunt spatula, or the blunt side of a scalpel. After this, it might help to use forceps to pull the diseased tissue perpendicularly, while the other hand continues to dissect the lesion, keeping the right cleavage plane. When the adhesion is large, the blade of the scalpel may be used carefully. Finally, if there is residue left from the lesion or the surface is not very homogeneous, it can be gently scraped with a lancet or the blunt edge of the scalpel.

In case of band keratopathy, 0.35% ethylenediaminetetraacetic acid (EDTA) should be applied. After the complete removal of the epithelium, the EDTA solution is applied to the cornea as a corneal bath, by continuous irrigation, or by a solution-soaked pledget or sponge for

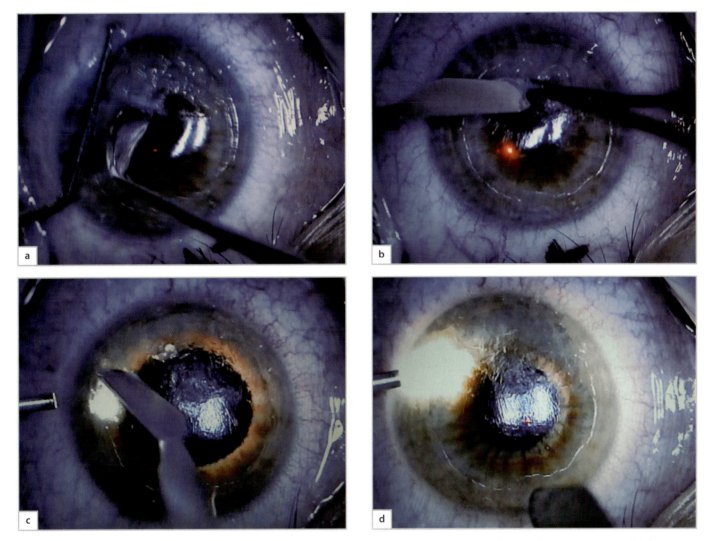

Figure 41.5 Manual keratectomy technique frequently combined with subsequent PTK, as was performed in this Salzmann's degeneration patient. (a) To begin surgery, the epithelium is scraped gently over and around the nodule until normal, smooth Bowman's layer is reached in order to decrease the chance of a future recurrent nodule due to a wider base than expected. (b) With the aid of forceps, the cleavage plane of the lesion is found and a blade is used to debulk the elevated lesion. (c) Visualization of the more residual lesion is enhanced by the use of a light probe tangential to the limbus. (d) The manual keratectomy ends when the elevated lesion has been removed completely. Following, the remaining, irregular base is smoothed out with PTK as explained in the next figures. PTK, phototherapeutic keratectomy.

15–20 minutes. The eye is irrigated after the procedure with a balanced salt solution. Since EDTA does not remove embedded calcium salts well, treatment is often combined with mechanical scraping and/or PTK (Jhanji et al. 2011).

Large-diameter phototherapeutic keratectomy

In this type of application, the diameter of the PTK optical zone will typically vary between 5.5 mm and 7 mm, in addition to the transition zones. This technique, which is the most straightforward form of PTK, is applied over lesions with diffuse or complete distribution, as is the case in Reis–Bücklers dystrophy and reticular dystrophy among others. If the epithelium shows an irregular surface, it must be scraped using a dry surgical spear in the same manner explained previously. This stops the laser from transferring the above-mentioned irregularity to the corneal stroma. On the other hand, if the epithelium

seems to homogeneously cover more abrupt underlying irregularities, the laser can be applied directly over it, benefiting from the role of the epithelium as a 'masking agent' (Rapuano 2010) (**Figure 41.6**). When treating recurrent corneal erosion syndrome due to basement membrane dystrophy, the overlying epithelium is eliminated with a surgical spear so that the laser can be superficially applied (PTK of typically 5–6 μm deep).

When treating corneal scars, only those that are truly superficial (<100 μm) should be treated and corneas that are excessively thin should be avoided, so as not to induce iatrogenic ectasia.

On occasions it is necessary to homogenize the surface of the ablated cornea (**Figure 41.6**). Masking agents must be used for this, such as 0.1% Dextran 70, 1% methylcellulose, or 0.25% sodium hyaluronate (Kornmehl et al. 1991, Alió et al. 2001). They can be dyed with fluorescein to obtain more precise control fluorescence during the application of PTK (**Figure 41.7**). Concentrations of methylcellulose >1% fill in not only the 'valleys' of the irregular profile, but also the

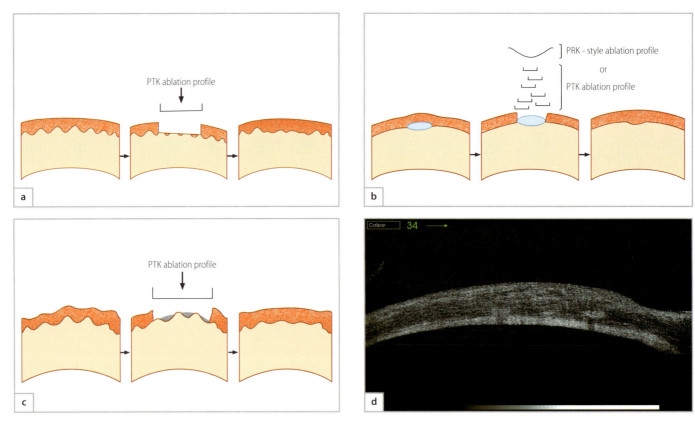

Figure 41.6 Masking and smoothing agents. The understanding of the role of masking and smoothing agents in PTK is crucial for a good surgical outcome. (a) The foremost important 'smoothing agent' to begin considering is the corneal epithelium. If the anterior corneal contour is more even than the expected denuded Bowman's layer or stroma, a transepithelial approach of the PTK ablation is preferred because the surface smoothness is translated and imprinted into the anterior stroma. If the operating room lights are dimmed, it is possible to suspect when the epithelial ablation has ended because the characteristic bluish fluorescence the epithelium emits when the excimer laser interacts with it disappears. Then, the underlying tissue begins to be ablated and the bluish emission turns into dark areas. (b) Also, when a nodular, protruding lesion is surrounded by normal cornea, the epithelium lying over healthy tissue acts as a masking agent. In this situation, two approaches are possible: either a myopic PRK profile centered on the nodule is planned with an optical zone, equaling the size of the lesion, and the ablation depth is calculated according to the preoperative nodule thickness assessment or, if the laser allows for joystick control of the procedure, a spot size about half the diameter of the lesion is selected and centrally overlapping spots are applied so that the apex of the nodule is ablated more than the sides. (c) If the anterior corneal contour is not even and a transepithelial approach is not advisable or if PTK completes a manual keratectomy, smoothing agents (e.g. dextran and methyl cellulose – represented in gray) are then used as indicated. Intermittent spread of the smoothing agent is performed with the aid of a spatula or a soaked surgical spear to ascertain its even distribution. (d) Sitting the patient up and examining the eye at the slit lamp is a must for any PTK procedure aiming deeper than 20 μm of stromal tissue. Otherwise, under the surgical microscope it is easy that overprotected areas along with overtreated areas causing focal thinning and severe irregular astigmatism are overlooked. This OCT image shows an example of pronounced paracentral, segmental corneal thinning, and irregular astigmatism induction due to lack of periodical checking during the PTK procedure despite the use of a masking agent. OCT, optical coherence tomography; PRK, photorefractive keratectomy; PTK, phototherapeutic keratectomy.

peaks, making homogenization largely ineffective. When the amount of methylcellulose is excessive, the typical clicking sound of the laser interacting with the cornea becomes markedly muffled or dull. On the other hand, lower concentrations do not set well over the 'valleys' of the desired area.

Methylcellulose can also be used to mask healthy areas of the cornea adjacent to the lesion that needs to be treated. In this situation, a higher concentration, approximately 2.5%, is very useful because methylcellulose tends to remain compact in the area where it is instilled.

When the area to be treated is very extensive, or when the wide beam laser does not offer a pre-established transition zone, the 'polish' technique, as explained earlier, PTK ablation profile, may be used to avoid a deep crater of perpendicular walls that has a great potential for inducing hyperopia. With the current laser platforms, this would be better achieved through applying hyperopic ablation at the end of PTK (Fagerholm 2003).

In order to carry out an adequate excision, which is not excessively deep or too superficial, it is useful to regularly examine the patient at a slit lamp to check on the state of the ablation depth of both the diseased and the healthy corneal tissue. When the roughness of the stroma prevents the correct identification of the deeper corneal tissue in the slit, it is usually practical to instill a drop of methylcellulose to homogenize the optic surface of the cornea. Additionally, the use of a light probe to produce indirect limbus retroillumination allows for the observation under the surgical microscope of opacities, including residuals (Hayashi et al. 2003), as shown in **Figures 41.5** and **41.7**.

We should remember that for many disorders, the objective of PTK is not the complete removal of all the existing opacity, but its significant reduction, since exhaustive elimination often involves creating a large crater in the cornea with resulting scarring and large refractive shifts (Hersh et al. 1996). At the end of the procedure, the corneal stroma typically looks like 'unpolished crystal,' which will disappear when the epithelium completely heals over it.

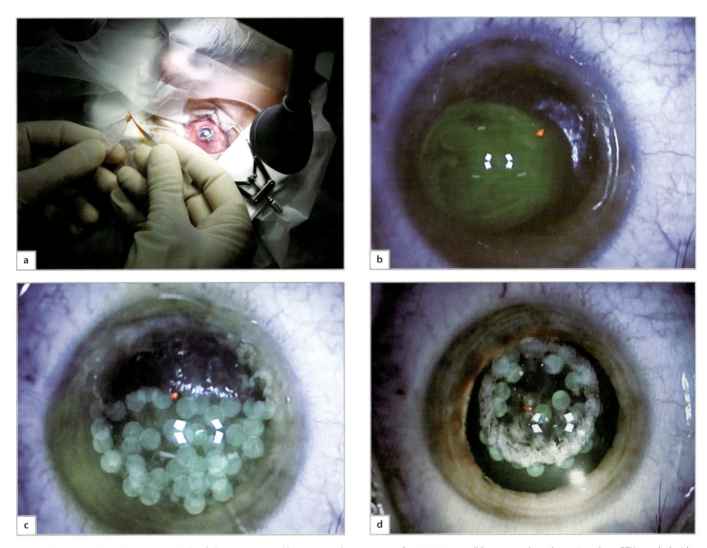

Figure 41.7 PTK with masking agents. Either following a manual keratectomy beginning or after initiating an all-laser procedure, the excimer laser PTK coupled with masking agents is used to further smooth the corneal surface. Here, we continue on the same case shown in Figure 41.5. *Contd...*

Phototherapeutic keratectomy and manual keratectomy combined

A careful manual de-epithelialization and excision of the lesions followed by and application of PTK with methylcellulose masking afterwards gives superior results compared to just using PTK for the entire procedure in disorders where there is a great difference between the consistency of the lesion and the normal surrounding cornea. Indications such as band keratopathy, where calcium is more highly concentrated in some areas than in others, or corneal lesions with vascularization, which partially block the effects of the laser upon bleeding, are good examples. If these cases are treated with different ablation rates for each area from the start of the procedure, the PTK would yield a rather irregular corneal surface (Hersh et al. 1996).

Focal application (smoothing)

The excimer laser can be applied focally over Salzmann's nodular degeneration or keratoconus nodules, for example, to allow for a more comfortable contact lens fit. This 'smoothing' effect can also

be achieved by manual keratectomy or combined manual and laser. Preoperative evaluation of the lesion's elevation is important in these cases, as the laser requirement would be at least four pulses for each micrometer of tissue ablation. The surgery begins by manually removing the overlying epithelium by blunt dissection, while leaving the epithelium that covers the normal cornea intact. In this way, the epithelium masks the healthy areas of the cornea. Additionally, methylcellulose may be used for protecting adjacent healthy areas. The PTK diameter is adjusted not to exceed the frontal area of the lesion, can be half its size, the apex of the nodule being treated more than the sides. Laser application is interrupted to control at the slit lamp so that the lesion has evened out with the normal tissue, without causing a crater due to overtreatment (Rapuano 2010).

■ Postoperative regimen

Once the surgery has finished, a bandage contact lens—silicone hydrogel lens—is applied or the eye is occluded until complete epithelialization. A topical antibiotic must be administered

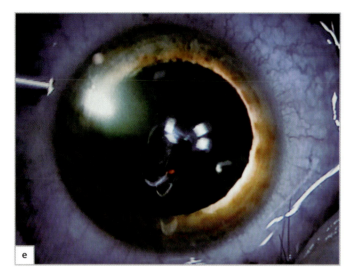
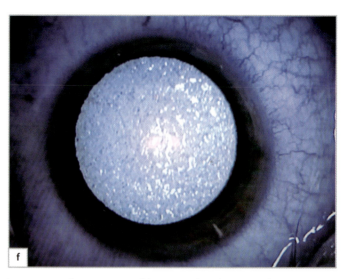

Figure 41.7 *Contd.* PTK with masking agents. Either following a manual keratectomy beginning or after initiating an all-laser procedure, the excimer laser PTK coupled with masking agents is used to further smooth the corneal surface. Here, we continue on the same case shown in Figure 41.5. (a) The masking agent can be stained with fluorescein dye using a soaked strip, as shown. This allows better visualization and control of the ablated and protected areas under the laser microscope with dim light conditions, as illustrated next. (b) The masking agent, in this case 0.5% hydroxyethyl cellulose, an analogue of methyl cellulose, is placed over the corneal surface and spread with a spatula. (c) When the laser spots interact with the fluorescein-stained masking agent, a characteristic bright radiance is seen, which contrasts with the darker areas corresponding to interaction between the excimer laser and the corneal tissue. This way, a better command of the protected and ablated areas is achieved during the procedure for a more regular cornea as an end result. (d) When ablating a layer of methylcellulose or hydroxyethyl cellulose, it is common to see whitening of the surface and the appearance of fine bubbles. When the masking agent is instilled in excess, an audible sign can also be noticed; the typical clicking sound of the laser interacting with the cornea becomes markedly muffled or dull. (e) The scattering sclerocorneal illumination of a light probe can be used to utter existing remnants of diseased and irregular tissue. When the corneal surface has been adequately smoothed out, the ablation process should be halted. (f) An 8 mm-diameter sponge soaked in 0.02% mitomycin C is placed at the end of the procedure for 1 minute, if deemed appropriate. This off-label treatment is a useful adjuvant to prevent postoperative corneal haze. Copious balanced salt solution is passed before the application of the sponge to eliminate the film of masking agents, thus allowing for direct contact between mitomycin and corneal tissue, and at the end of the application, in order to remove any residual antimitotic trace from the ocular surface. PTK, phototherapeutic keratectomy.

(every 3 or 4 hours). If the eye is patched, antibiotic ointment may be preferred. The instillation of a non-steroidal anti-inflammatory drug is usually beneficial in controlling postoperative pain, for which patients sometimes request oral analgesics. However, topical nepafenac should be used with caution because corneal melt has been described after PRK (Rathi et al. 2012). Instilling cycloplegic eye drops every 8 hours also helps to control discomfort until epithelial closure. Once epithelialization is complete, the bandage contact lens is usually removed and the antibiotic and cycloplegic eye drops are discontinued. Artificial tears can begin to be applied frequently as well as fluorometholone at 0.1% four times per day, reducing at the rate by one per day for each elapsed month. In eyes with previous laser-assisted in situ keratomileusis (LASIK), topical steroids are mandatory to avoid the development of diffuse lamellar keratitis. Prednisolone acetate at 1% should only be used when a greater scarring response is expected. When treatment has been minimal, for example a 5 μm ablation for basement membrane dystrophy, steroids may not be necessary. When treating opacity due to herpes virus or of unknown origin, the aforementioned antiviral regimen should be followed.

Tissular response to phototherapeutic keratectomy

There are three distinguishable phases in the response of the cornea to PTK. The first stage is re-epithelialization, which lasts from 3 days up to 2–4 weeks—when it is delayed. Within the next weeks and months, this is followed by the remodeling of the corneal stroma, which tends to replace a small part of the ablated tissue with apparently healthy tissue. When the organization of the anterior stromal cellular matrix is altered, along with the appearance of myofibroblast cells, corneal opacity (haze) may appear (Shah & Wilson 2010). Finally, after the first few months have elapsed, a topographic and refractive stabilization is reached that basically derives from the hyperplasic contribution of the epithelium and, to a lesser extent, from stromal remodeling. Therefore, the postoperative objectives include achieving epithelialization as early as possible, minimizing stromal scarring reaction, and optimizing refractive and topographic results. There is evidence that intraoperative 0.02% mitomycin C for 1 minute (**Figure 41.7**), thiotepa, or the application of amniotic membrane tends to attenuate scarring response following PTK (Rathi et al. 2012).

SPECIFIC INDICATIONS AND RESULTS

Recurrent corneal erosion syndrome

Recurrent corneal erosion syndrome currently constitutes the most frequent indication for PTK (Fagerholm 2003). This syndrome spans as many presentations of undetermined etiology as post-traumatic cases, as well as those associated to several corneal dystrophies that are discussed later.

Faced with a patient with recurring corneal erosion syndrome, the first step is to rule out dry eye disease and/or blepharitis. If it is confirmed that it is not a consequence of either factor, the standard PTK treatment is indicated and includes careful mechanical de-epithelialization over the diseased area, followed by a 5- to 6 µm deep ablation of the Bowman's layer (Rapuano 2010). The epithelial removal over the entrance pupil should be complete to avoid inducing irregularities in the Bowman's membrane. It is also important to apply the laser in an area equal to or greater than the area of the de-epithelialization. Otherwise, the surgeon may induce damage to the basement membrane that cannot be repaired by the excimer laser, with the possibility of creating new areas within the paracentral and peripheral cornea that are prone to future recurrent erosion.

The primary success rate of PTK in recurrent epithelial erosion ranges between 74% and 100%, with higher rates after trauma than in corneal dystrophies (Stasi & Chuck 2009). The outcome of combined manual and PTK laser treatment is superior to the conventional manual treatment (Fagerholm 2003). PTK also seems to be superior to other therapeutic alternatives that have a reported success rate around 40–50% for de-epithelialization followed by micropuncture with Nd: YAG laser, or 60% for mechanical micropuncture. However, epithelial debridement and polishing of Bowman's membrane using a diamond burr seem to have advantages over PTK in the treatment of recurrent corneal erosions (Sridhar et al. 2002). If the syndrome relapses after the first PTK, retreatment with a second PTK seems to significantly reduce recurrence.

Corneal dystrophies

Given that keratoplasty is only a temporary solution in many dystrophies, as many of them recur years after grafting, and since regrafting increases the risk of immunological rejection with respect to the first transplant, any therapy that postpones the need for a corneal transplant should be appropriate and beneficial (Rapuano 2001). In this sense, PTK's partial success is assured, as in the worst-case scenario, a corneal transplant is not hindered by a previous PTK. Furthermore, PTK has achieved very long periods without relapse in primary treatments and has even restored sufficient corneal transparency in grafts where the dystrophy had relapsed (Lee & Kim 2003). However, recurrence can also occur after PTK, and some dystrophies are more prone to relapse than others. Moreover, it should be distinguished between relapses that are solely biomicroscopic as opposed to those that are clinically significant (Rapuano 2001).

In the twenty-first century, the suitability of a corneal dystrophy for a predictable result after PTK can be determined not only by the clinical presentation—phenotype—but also possibly by the chromosomal findings—genotype (Lee & Kim 2003, Stasi & Chuck 2009).

Phototherapeutic keratectomy according to the corneal dystrophy phenotype

Meesmann's dystrophy

In Meesmann's dystrophy, experiences using PTK to eliminate the central epithelium are limited and vary between good (good vision and no signs of ocular irritation) and negative (permanence of symptoms and corneal opacity), to the extent that not even the results in the first eye are predictive of the results in the other eye (Lee & Kim 2003).

Theoretically, eliminating part of the diseased epithelium when it is going to be replaced with equally dystrophic adjacent tissue seems impractical. However, there has been speculation that PTK surgery could partly suppress the expression of the gene responsible for dystrophy (Fagerholm 2003).

Map-dot-fingerprint dystrophy

Map-dot-fingerprint dystrophy constitutes the second most frequent indication of PTK (Fagerholm 2003). PTK can be transepithelial (flat ablation of 7 µm in diameter and ~5 µm deep) only when the biomicroscopic appearance of the epithelium is regular. In any case, and particularly when the epithelial surface is clearly irregular, the best option is to mechanically debride the epithelium using a spatula. Once inside the Bowman's membrane, the aim is to remove about 6 µm of tissue by means of a flat ablation. Postoperative recovery is relatively fast, with refractive stability and a reduction in symptoms achieved approximately 2 months postoperatively. It also allows the combination PTK with PRK (also called 'transepithelial PRK') for the correction of refractive errors in patients with basement membrane dystrophy (Stasi & Chuck 2009).

Results of PTK for epithelial basement membrane dystrophy (EBMD) in general are very satisfactory and, typically, the refraction quickly stabilizes, corrected visual acuity improves (76%), and erosions cease (95%). Nevertheless, a certain change in refraction may occur despite the superficiality of the ablation on the Bowman's membrane (Fagerholm 2003). When the symptoms of this dystrophy relapse, they tend to recur within the first 6–9 months (Lee & Kim 2003).

Reis–Bücklers dystrophy

In Reis–Bücklers dystrophy, the epithelium usually presents sufficient homogeneity to carry out a transepithelial PTK. In this way, the epithelium acts as a masking agent that facilitates the regular ablation of 'peaks' in the projections of the stroma toward the surface, while protecting the 'valleys.' Therefore, it would be unadvisable to carry out manual de-epithelialization in this situation. Only when the epithelium insinuates an already irregular corneal contour, is it worthwhile to use a masking fluid. Results are generally good and any significant recurrences are rare, slow, and deferred (McDonnell & Seiler 1992). Biomicroscopic recurrences have been detected in 59% of cases after an average follow-up of 12.3 months, and significant recurrences were detected after 21.6 months (Dinh et al. 1999).

Thiel–Behnke dystrophy

PTK appears to be useful in treating both primary Thiel–Behnke dystrophy and graft recurrences (Lee & Kim 2003).

Granular dystrophy

The patient usually requests to be treated for photophobia and a reduction in visual acuity. Even though epithelial erosions are observed in some cases, they are infrequent. Results of PTK in granular dystrophy are considered to be good. Although the majority of opacities are located in the anterior stroma, some can be located deeper. Since ablating down to the deepest ones would induce considerable hyperopia and corneal scarring, in this situation, it is best to leave the deeper ones without complete ablation, as they have limited impact on vision. During the postoperative period, some may grow in size in the same way crystallized salt does in saturated water (Fagerholm 2003). Average recurrence time is 32 months, and 40 months on average for a clinically significant relapse (Dinh et al. 1999). It is rare for recurrence to appear before 2 years. The result of PTK on recurrences in eyes with penetrating keratoplasty seems to be good (one recurrence for each seven cases) (Maclean et al. 1996).

Avellino dystrophy

In Avellino dystrophy, PTK has proven useful in the improvement of the ocular surface conditions (in parameters such as corneal sensitivity, tear film break-up time in relation to the lipid layer, and conjunctival squamous metaplasia) (Drogu et al. 2000). Nevertheless, when the disorder recurs, there is accompanying deterioration of the ocular surface status (Drogu et al. 2000). In dystrophies such as this, in which the production of transforming growth factor (TGF)-β is involved, LASIK surgery is contraindicated as it exacerbates the disorder due to the existence of incitement by surgical trauma and the creation of a new space, the interface, where deposits may accumulate (Lee & Kim 2003).

Reticular dystrophy

The ablation of the anterior corneal stroma can remove the diffuse opacity and part of the ramified filaments typical of reticular dystrophy. Because spontaneous erosions are also relatively frequent, the application of transepithelial PTK may be justified in these cases. Even though there are few PTK clinical studies that include this dystrophy, it is known that visual improvement is perceptible but it is usually not very marked (Fagerholm 2003). This is partly due to the difficulty in eliminating the deepest opacities. The rate of recurrence is moderate and its apparition is slow. In a corneal graft, the recurrence of reticular dystrophy presents diffuse superficial opacity that eventually interferes with vision (Dinh et al. 1999). Nevertheless, PTK can eliminate the above-mentioned opacity, achieving better vision for at least a few years. Reticular dystrophy may, on occasions, appear in childhood, causing marked amblyopia. The slow visual rehabilitation associated with keratoplasty makes it an almost ineffective alternative at such early ages. PTK, however, may eliminate much of the opacity with a comparatively quicker and more bearable recuperation for the child. In this way, amblyopia at such a critical age may be prevented (Fagerholm 2003, Stasi & Chuck 2009).

Reticular dystrophy type 2 (Meretoja's syndrome)

Reticular dystrophy type 2 is characterized by presenting fine filaments of more anterior localization than in reticular type 1. Initial results following PTK are satisfactory; however, recurrence may appear after 2 years (Fagerholm 2003). In these cases, complications stem from a reduction in corneal sensitivity, associated with dry eye disease, on occasions resulting in exposure keratopathy, as described in the systemic context of a generalized amyloidosis.

Macular dystrophy

As the localization of the opacities in the stroma is usually quite anterior, especially in the initial stages of presentation, treatment with PTK seems effective and has a long time to recurrence (Wagoner 1999). However, long-term follow-up indicates that recurrences are heavy, so keratoplasty is preferred by some surgeons (Rathi et al. 2012).

Schnyder's dystrophy

In Schnyder's dystrophy, there is an appearance of diffuse opacity in the stroma and crystals of subepithelial localization that cause a light dispersion phenomenon that considerably degrades vision. Treatment with PTK, in the few cases in which it has been applied, has been effective in the elimination of the superficial central crystals. The diffuse opacity tends to persist, limiting vision to the order of 20/40. The relapse speed in these cases seems to be quite slow (Fagerholm 2003).

Fuchs' dystrophy and bullous keratopathy

In Fuchs' endothelial dystrophy, vision is limited due to corneal stromal and epithelial edema and subepithelial fibrosis. Also, many patients present ocular pain due to the rupture of the epithelial bullae on the corneal surface. PTK in this dystrophy benefits through a number of mechanisms: stromal edema tends to diminish when a considerable amount of stromal tissue is removed (25% of the central pachymetry), as the compromised endothelium is more efficient in maintaining deturgescence on a smaller stromal volume, partial sensory denervation of the cornea occurs, and the subepithelial scarring is ablated by the laser (Maini et al. 2001). All of this results in a postoperative cornea that is thinner, less cloudy, less painful, and has a healthier ocular surface, once the epithelial bullae have diminished. Even so, the possibility of an abnormal scarring response exists, for which reason PTK must be judiciously indicated. In practice, PTK has prevented penetrating or endothelial keratoplasty in patients whose eyes presented low visual potential due to other causes and in those who did not wish to undergo the slow visual rehabilitation associated with corneal transplant. Moreover, PTK can provide relief from painful symptoms to patients who are awaiting a corneal transplant.

Phototherapeutic keratectomy according to the corneal dystrophy genotype

Several corneal dystrophies (granular, lattice, Avellino, Reis–Bücklers, and a minority of cases of EBMD) have been linked to a mutation in the transforming growth factor beta 1 (*TGFβI*) gene (also called the *BIGH3* gene). This gene, located on chromosome 5q31, codes for the keratoepithelin protein, which is secreted by the corneal epithelium, and diffuses through the corneal tissues, thus being a normal component of the stroma. However, when mutation of the *BIGH3* gene occurs, the keratoepithelin molecule is abnormal, transforms into an insoluble protein, and accumulates in the cornea (Lee & Kim 2003).

There is evidence to suggest that patients with autosomal dominant TGFβI-linked corneal dystrophies show different results after PTK according to their specific genotype. The Gly623Arg mutation of the *BIGH3* gene has been correlated with a better outcome with PTK (Stasi & Chuck 2009). Moreover, in patients with Avellino corneal dystrophy, the recurrence of corneal deposits after PTK with heterozygous R124 mutation of the *BIGH3* gene is milder and more centrally located than in patients with homozygous mutation, who develop a more severe pattern of recurrence with a diffuse layout and more peripheral involvement. Recurrent-free intervals are also reportedly different for the heterozygous patients (38.4 months) than for the homozygous patients (9.5 months). Therefore, DNA sequencing can guide ophthalmologists as to the adequacy of PTK for an individual patient (Lee & Kim 2003, Stasi & Chuck 2009).

The above-mentioned data also give rise to the use of topical anti-TGFβ therapy (i.e. antibodies or peptides) to suppress recurrence of corneal opacities after PTK in these patients (Lee & Kim 2003).

■ Pseudophakic bullous keratopathy

In non-dystrophic corneas where corneal edema with symptomatology related to ruptured epithelial bullae has developed due to intraocular surgical trauma (**Figure 41.8**), a deep PTK (~120 μm) not only alleviates the painful symptomatology but may also provide a discreet vision improvement. This benefits the comfort of the patient who is on a waiting list for penetrating or endothelial keratoplasty, without interfering with the grafting technique. Also, PTK can represent an alternative to keratoplasty in high-risk eyes for failure and in those with concomitant untreatable visually limiting conditions (Maini et al. 2001, Rathi et al. 2012).

Post-traumatic and postsurgical scars

PTK can ablate superficial scars or superficial aspects of these scars, occurring as a consequence of either eye trauma or surgery, as might happen after refractive procedures (Rathi et al. 2012). In all of these indications, it is usually wise to wait a few months (at least 3–6 months) to obtain not just a more transparent cornea, but more importantly, a more regular cornea due to the compensatory role of the epithelium.

Pterygium

In case of central extension of the pterygium, a bed of scar tissue usually appears in the superficial stroma following manual excision. Applying PTK over this bed may reduce the residual refractive defect following pterygium surgery and can smooth the corneal contour using masking agents. Nevertheless, the smoothing of the bed does not

reduce the rate of pterygium recurrence (Fagerholm 2003). A typical technique consists in a 15 μm deep, 6 mm diameter central ablation of Bowman's membrane followed by the local application of PTK to regularize the remaining scar tissue. Refraction after PTK is not very predictable, and some scarring response may appear postoperatively requiring then retreatments.

Phototherapeutic keratectomy as an adjuvant in conventional corneal surface surgery

PTK may also be used in association with other mechanical or chemical procedures in the treatment of the ocular surface. In the elimination of corneal calcifications, the excimer laser has been a good complement to the application of topical EDTA and mechanical keratectomy

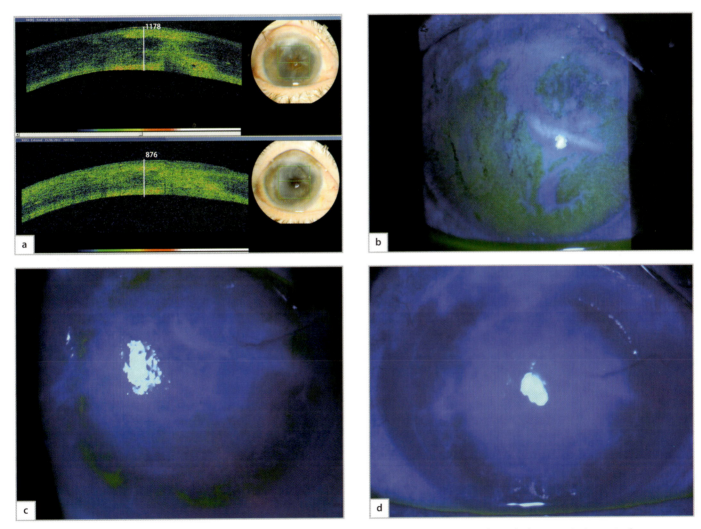

Figure 41.8 PTK in bullous keratopathy. (a) Thickened cornea (1178 μm) in a highly symptomatic red eye is seen after multiple vitreoretinal surgeries for severe ocular trauma complications (top). The cornea is 302 μm thinner and the eye shows notably less hyperemia after PKT (bottom). (b) Preoperative fluorescein staining of the multiple bullae in this long-standing bullous keratopathy. Some central subepithelial fibrosis and neovascular growth are also present. (c) One month after PTK, the number of blisters has decreased significantly. (d) Three months after PTK, scarce bullae are present and the cornea shows subepithelial haze because of the deep ablation. Vision potential was vastly poor due to vitreoretinal complications of the previous ocular trauma, rendering the eye unable to benefit from keratoplasty. However, the patient is satisfied because of the pain relief without the need of wearing bandage contact lenses as a consequence of PTK. By discontinuing the bandage contact lens wear, the risk of infectious keratitis decreases too. PTK, phototherapeutic keratectomy.

to achieve a more uniform and transparent ocular surface. When this combined treatment is applied over irritated and painful eyes, the symptoms are notably alleviated. Various bulky formations of the corneal surface, such as keloids (in Lowe's syndrome) or some dense scarring, can prove too slow to be completely ablated by the excimer laser. In such cases, manual keratectomy can be followed by a smoothing of the surface with PTK. A more uniform surface usually contributes to a reduction of the irritant symptoms and produces a more favorable cosmetic result, or at least, a more uniform corneal contour to allow the adaptation of a contact lens or prosthesis (Fagerholm 2003).

Salzmann's nodular degeneration

These nodules, which are usually located in the midperipheral cornea, induce refractive changes and irregular astigmatism with the aggravating factor of impeding the adequate adaptation of a contact lens. The ablation of the nodules up to the level of the rest of the cornea may be an alternative to their manual excision (Rapuano 2010). The adequate technique has already been explained. PTK treatment provides the patient with a situation where vision may be improved in respect to the preoperative situation, whether with glasses or contact lenses, which can now be adapted (**Figure 41.9**). The rate of recurrence is close to 4% at 2 years (Rapuano 2001). Nevertheless, and even though the disorder tends to be a continuous process, PTK can allow for keratoplasty deferral for almost a decade. Intraoperative application of mitomycin C has proven effective in preventing future relapses (Rapuano 2010).

Keratoconus

When an apical opacity appears, typically following an episode of corneal hydrops, not only loss of corneal transparency but also a protrusion that impedes the adaptation of a contact lens without irritation appears. In this context, the patient, who may be on a waiting list for keratoplasty, can benefit temporarily from PTK by reducing blur, symptoms, and contact lens intolerance. Nevertheless, keratolysis and the formation of descemetoceles have been described in a patient with keratoconus as a complication of PTK associated with a lack of epithelial closure (Fagerholm 2003).

Scars following infectious keratitis

Bacterial keratitis

Opacities following bacterial keratitis are usually dense and are occasionally associated with significant focal thinning. The latter may impede these cases from being considered appropriate for PTK. Otherwise, it is possible that these eyes may benefit from topography-guided surface ablations. In trachoma-induced opacities, PTK has proven useful in cases where the condition of the rest of the ocular surface was sufficiently acceptable (Rathi et al. 2012).

Viral keratitis

Corneal opacities within this group of disorders that allow treatment with PTK are herpes simplex, herpes zoster, and epidemic keratoconjunctivitis. Determination of the thinnest corneal point is crucial to plan the adequate ablation depth, especially in herpes simplex cases. Generally, the presence of significant thinning jeopardizes the achievement of good clinical results.

Preoperative prophylactic antiviral therapy should be administered, as explained earlier. As both herpes simplex and zoster reduce corneal sensitivity, the closure of the epithelium and the scarring process must be closely monitored. Reportedly, cases of herpes simplex or zoster in children younger than 7 years may benefit from PTK to prevent amblyopia, which could otherwise be very severe (Fagerholm 2003).

Subepithelial opacities following adenoviral keratoconjunctivitis may be treated with PTK; however, the rates of recurrence are not exactly known, and relapse of opacities with a deeper localization has been described as a potential complication (Starr 1999).

Thygeson's superficial punctate keratitis

Usefulness of PTK associated with PRK in treating Thygeson's keratitis with multiple relapses associated with the cessation of topical corticoid therapy has been reported in a myopic patient (Goldstein et al. 2002).

Epithelial defects

PTK has been successfully used to promote healing of chronic epithelial defects that would not close after applying other medical or surgical treatment methods. The application of the excimer laser was carried out in trials using PTK mode with a 1 mm diameter and a range of pulses between 150 and 200, and it was directed at elevated epithelial borders surrounding the defect. Complete epithelialization occurred in the majority of eyes within 7 days and only two cases had to wait for 12 days. Although evidence is only experimental, it appears that applying PTK over a caustic corneal ulcer promotes faster epithelialization (Fagerholm 2003).

Allergic ulcers

In vernal keratoconjunctivitis, the ulcers may appear covered by protein precipitates, eosinophilic protein, and major basic protein. As these proteins are toxic to the epithelium, the ulcer tends to remain open. Also, because the immune system of these patients predisposes to a greater risk of microbial keratitis, infected ulcers are frequent complications in patients with atopic dermatitis. Ablation of the superficial proteins by PTK and the subsequent induction of the epithelial closure have been suggested as an adjuvant therapy to conventional treatments for allergic ulcers (Cameron et al. 1995).

Band keratopathy

Band keratopathy constituted one of the earliest indications for PTK. Nevertheless, experience has shown that many cases recurred during the first 2 years. Therefore, many surgeons prefer manual de-epithelialization and direct application of EDTA, with the long-term advantage of not excessively ablating tissue (Fagerholm 2003). However, many of these eyes present poor visual prognosis, and the objective is to smooth the corneal contour to achieve an alleviation of the irritant symptomatology. In these cases, the combined treatments of manual keratectomy for macroirregularities, EDTA, and PTK for surface smoothing have been successfully used. Thus, 85% of patients with band keratopathy and irregular surface should improve their symptoms postoperatively (Rapuano 2001). In the experience of this author and others (Jhanji et al. 2011), functional and anatomical surface rehabilitation is optimal using PTK and amniotic membrane to immediately cover the epithelial defect.

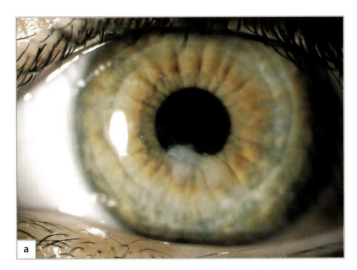

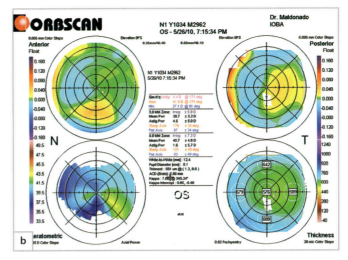

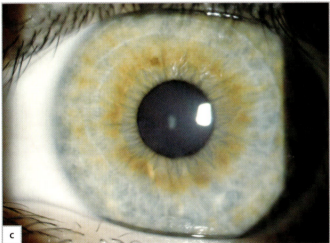

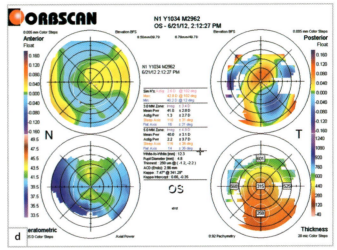

Figure 41.9 PTK for Salzmann's nodular degeneration. Preoperatively, the cornea shows (a) a prominent nodule encroaching the central and paracentral cornea inferiorly, and (b) an irregular topographic map with a 4.5-diopter against-the-rule astigmatism in the central cornea (typical Orbscan II quad map printout is depicted showing from left to right and top to bottom: an elevation map of the anterior corneal surface, an elevation map of the posterior corneal surface, a tangential anterior curvature map and a corneal thickness map). The patient had become contact lens intolerant. Postoperatively, (c) the cornea shows no significant opacification and, (d) the topography is more regular, with a 1.3-diopter with-the-rule central astigmatism. Posterior elevation and pachymetric maps show the artifact from the subepithelial corneal haze peaking 3 months postoperatively. The eye has gained two visual acuity lines, best spectacle-corrected and unaided, and is able to wear contact lenses after combined manual keratectomy and PTK with smoothing agents. PTK, phototherapeutic keratectomy.

Climatic keratopathy

Little is known about the application of PTK in this infrequent keratopathy, but it seems there is a favorable response. PTK before cataract surgery in eyes seems to provide improved intraoperative visualization and patient satisfaction (Rathi et al. 2012).

Ectodermic dysplasia

There is only one reported case of the application of successive PTKs to obtain a significant reduction in the visual limitations caused by an ectodermic dysplasia in a child who otherwise would have probably suffered from profound amblyopia (Stasi & Chuck 2009).

Corneal intraepithelial dysplasia and carcinoma

PTK has been successfully used in the treatment of both intraepithelial dysplasia and recurrent corneal intraepithelial carcinoma, according to anecdotal cases compiled in relevant literature (Dausch et al. 1994). However, when a suspicious lesion is completely ablated, it is not possible to obtain histological confirmation of its nature or its extension. Therefore, a biopsy of the lesion's border prior to applying PTK would be most appropriate.

Topographical irregularities

When the adequate therapeutic strategy is chosen, PTK may help regularize the corneal contour in various ocular surface disorders

(Maloney et al. 1996). Topographical regularity was reportedly improved in 60–70% of cases; it remained basically unaltered in 25–35%, and deteriorated in 2–4%.

Complications of previous refractive surgery

The main indications of PTK in these cases embrace both the topographical alterations (irregular astigmatism causing higher order aberrations) and corneal opacity (haze) (Stasi & Chuck 2009).

PHOTOTHERAPEUTIC KERATECTOMY COMPLICATIONS

Unlike other surgeries with the excimer laser, in PTK, surgery is applied on diseased corneas. Additionally, PTK can easily induce topographical changes, which, in turn, may result in secondary unwanted refractive shifts.

Delayed epithelialization

Various degrees of limbal stem cell deficiency are commonly seen in eyes requiring PTK, possibly leading to delayed epithelial closure. While complete epithelization usually occurs during the first postoperative week, a delayed healing, generally taking 2–4 weeks, occurs with an incidence of around 12% (Hersh et al. 1996, Rapuano 2001). As a consequence, secondary complications, such as the appearance of sterile infiltrates, infectious keratitis, or stromal scarring with opacity, may appear. Therefore, patients with caustications, cicatricial pemphigoid, atopic keratoconjunctivitis, and severe dry eye disease must be carefully selected and specifically treated to improve the ocular surface status before PTK. Similarly, patients who present eyelid position alterations, either static or dynamic, or blepharitis must have these conditions controlled (e.g. eyelid cleaning and oral tetracyclines) as required. Frequent lubrication without preservatives and the aid of therapeutic contact lenses, especially during the early postoperative period, must be prescribed. The addition of topical autologous blood derivatives (serum or others) may be particularly useful in eyes with limbal stem cell deficiency.

Bacterial keratitis

Bacterial keratitis constitutes one of the most frequent serious complications, even though the risk of appearance is less than in keratoplasty. In the longest case series published, the incidence has been 1.2% (Rathi et al. 2012). Aside from some exceptions, it presents during the early postoperative period (1 week, up to 2 months), always while the epithelium is still healing. It is mainly caused by Gram-positive bacteria. For that, a prophylaxis with a topical antibiotic with a low toxicity profile (i.e. fluoroquinolones) is mandatory and should be prolonged until complete epithelial closure and/or therapeutic contact lens removal.

Subepithelial opacities

Although in most instances the haze after PTK is transient and relatively faint, occasionally, a significant fibrotic plaque can develop. This aggressive type of scarring response can be seen more often in treating central pterygium, keratoplasty cases, when delayed epithelialization occurs, and generally when the ablation is deep (Fagerholm 2003). Therefore, all possible measures must be adopted to promote fast and complete epithelialization and control the postoperative response with judicious use of topical corticoids and intraocular pressure monitoring. Rarely an anterior lamellar keratectomy is needed, particularly since the concomitant administration of intraoperative mitomycin C or postoperative topical thiotepa has been included in the PTK protocols (Rapuano 2010).

Disease recurrence

Following PTK, some disorders such as reticular dystrophy, basement membrane dystrophy, and Salzmann's degeneration tend to relapse slowly with time. It must be taken into account that keratectomy eliminates part of the diseased tissue and attempts to regularize the corneal contour, but it does not eliminate all diseased tissues. It is therefore important to inform preoperatively this possibility, tendency in some conditions, so that patients understand the temporary benefit between successive treatments (Dinh et al. 1999).

Graft rejection

In anecdotal cases, it has been possible to confirm the coincidence between the time of a PTK treatment and the triggering of an immune response against the keratoplasty button. Upon appearance it should be conventionally treated. On the other hand, there is no evidence to suggest that keratoplasty is technically more complex in an eye that has undergone PTK previously (Rathi et al. 2012).

Limbal stem cell deficiency

The development of secondary limbal deficiency has been described in a PTK case sustaining extensive epithelial debridement in a patient with general risk factors such as diabetes mellitus and rosacea (Nghiem-Buffet et al. 2003).

Recurrence of herpetic keratitis

Excimer laser radiation, which is ultraviolet C, surgical trauma, and the use of steroids may provoke the reactivation of herpes simplex (Asbell 2000). Therefore, PTK must never be applied to an active herpetic keratitis, and a quiescent period of nearly 1 year is recommended. It is also important to administer the antiviral prophylaxis, as mentioned earlier. In this way, the probability of herpetic reactivation related to PTK is very low (Fagerholm 2003).

Keratectasia

Even though the appearance of keratectasia is very rare, iatrogenic ectasia following PTK has been described in a similar way to its presentation following LASIK (Maldonado et al. 2008). Therefore, extreme care must be taken with primary treatments, and above all in retreatments on thin corneas. Although intraoperative pachymetry is useful, sitting the patient at the slit lamp several times during the procedure discloses areas of possible excessive thinning and provides better control on the amount of opacity ablated (Rapuano 2010).

Recurrent erosions

When manual de-epithelialization involves touching areas of the exposed Bowman's layer that are not ablated by the excimer laser during the procedure, it is possible that recurrent erosions of the epithelium develop in such areas. Although its incidence is very low, it may be seen during the first postoperative year (Fagerholm 2003).

Endothelial alterations

Endothelial alterations are very rarely encountered since endothelial changes occur if the ablation reaches within 90 μm of the posterior cornea.

Diminished corneal sensitivity and dry eye disease

A reduction in corneal sensitivity occurs following excimer laser surgery. However, sensitivity tends to be restored through nerve regeneration within the treated area. During this period, it is normal to experience varying degrees of dry eye disease that must be quickly and appropriately treated. Also, in many disorders requiring PTK, reduced corneal sensitivity and dry eye disease already exist. However, in these cases PTK usually improves the ocular surface eventually. Reportedly PTK improves corneal sensitivity, tear break-up time, tear film lipid layer, and the degree of conjunctival squamous metaplasia in Avellino, granular and reticular dystrophies, band keratopathy, and eyes with corneal scars (Drogu et al. 2000). It appears that in addition to improving corneal regularity and clarity, the end result of a typical PTK is a more stable tear film and a better mucin production in a healthier epithelium (Ayres & Rapuano 2006).

Induced refractive changes

In general, leaving the patient with hyperopia, marked anisometropia, high astigmatism, or a large bilateral refractive error is perceived as a refractive complication (Rathi et al. 2012). The considerations made in the previous sections (**The refractive error; PTK ablation profile**) should always be kept in mind.

FUTURE DEVELOPMENTS IN PHOTOTHERAPEUTIC KERATECTOMY

It is expected that the corneal response to PTK in many of the dystrophic disorders will be characterized by the type of chromosomal mutation causing it so that a genotypic analysis will indicate a priori individual suitability of this treatment (Stasi & Chuck 2009). The excimer laser is very effective in the removal of corneal tissue, but with the refinement of the masking agents and combined surface ablation wavefront-guided treatments, PTK might eventually achieve a totally regular corneal surface, something that is far from reality to date. The generalization of real-time non-invasive intraoperative pachymetry monitoring through OCT or other technologies will enhance the treatment precision and prevent excessive corneal thinning (Maldonado et al. 2008). Advances in pharmacomodulation for scarring will bring us nearer to our desired result. In addition to mitomycin C, which seems particularly useful in corneal dystrophies related to TGF-β, and thiotepa, new anti-TGF-β therapies may possibly help avoid relapses in corneal opacities following PTK. Also combining ocular surface reconstruction techniques such as amniotic membrane surgery and cultured limbal stem cells should provide better control on the healing response of the cornea to PTK (Stasi & Chuck 2009). Furthermore, with the refinement of laser ablation techniques (Maldonado et al. 2008), flying spot systems guided by accurate corneal topography diagnostics will be able to treat corneal surface disorders more precisely, providing the patient with better unaided vision, while bringing the patient closer to emmetropia, as well as achieving at the same time a more optically perfect cornea and clinically healthier ocular surface.

ACKNOWLEDGMENT

The author thanks Margarita Calonge, MD, PhD, for her contribution with the figures of this chapter, and to Cecilio Jesús Muzquiz Buron, OD, MSc, for his assistance in the acquisition of the intraoperative images and figure editing.

FURTHER READING

Azar DT, Steinert RF, Stark WJ. Excimer laser phototherapeutic keratectomy, 1st edn. Baltimore: Williams & Willkins, 1997.

Hersh PS, Wagoner MD. Excimer laser surgery for corneal disorders, 1st edn. New York: Thieme, 1998.

REFERENCES

Alió JL, Belda JI, Shalaby AM. Correction of irregular astigmatism with excimer laser assisted by sodium hyaluronate. *Ophthalmology* 2001; **108**:1246–1260.

Asbell PA. Valacyclovir for the prevention of recurrent herpes simplex virus eye disease after excimer laser photokeratectomy. *Trans Am Ophthalmol Soc* 2000; **98**:285–303.

Ayres BD, Rapuano CJ. Excimer laser phototherapeutic keratectomy. *Ocul Surf* 2006; **4**:196–206.

Cameron JA, Antonios SR, Badr IA. Excimer laser phototherapeutic keratectomy for shield ulcers and corneal plaques in vernal keratoconjunctivitis. *J Refract Surg* 1995; **11**:31–35.

Dausch D, Landesz M, Schroder E. Phototherapeutic keratectomy in recurrent corneal intraepithelial dysplasia. *Arch Ophthalmol* 1994; **112**:22–23.

de Rojas Silva V, Rodríguez-Conde R, Cobo-Soriano R, et al. Laser in situ keratomileusis in patients with a history of ocular herpes. *J Cataract Refract Surg* 2007; **33**:1855–1859.

Dinh R, Rapuano CJ, Cohen EJ, Laibson PR. Recurrence of corneal dystrophy after excimer laser phototherapeutic keratectomy. *Ophthalmology* 1999; **106**:1490–1497.

Drogu M, Katakami C, Miyashita M. Ocular surface changes after excimer laser phototherapeutic keratectomy. *Ophthalmology* 2000; **107**:1142–1152.

Dupps WJ, Roberts C. Effect of acute biomechanical changes on corneal curvature after photokeratectomy. *J Refract Surg* 2001; **17**:658–669.

Fagerholm P. Phototherapeutic keratectomy: 12 years of experience. *Acta Ophthalmol Scand* 2003; **81**:19–32.

Goldstein MH, Feistmann JA, Bhatti MT. PRK-PTK as a treatment for a patient with Thygeson's superficial punctate keratopathy. *CLAO J* 2002; **28**:172–173.

Hayashi H, Maeda N, Ikeda Y, et al. Sclerotic scattering illumination during phototherapeutic keratectomy for better visualization of corneal opacities. *Am J Ophthalmol* 2003; **135**:559–561.

Hersh PS, Burnstein Y, Carr J, et al. Phototherapeutic keratectomy: surgical strategies and clinical outcomes. *Ophthalmology* 1996; **103**:1210–1222.

Jhanji V, Rapuano CJ, Vajpayee RB. Corneal calcific band keratopathy. *Curr Opin Ophthalmol* 2011; **22**:283–289.

Kornmehl EW, Steinert RF, Puliafito CA. A comparative study of masking fluids for excimer laser phototherapeutic keratectomy. *Arch Ophthalmol* 1991; **109**:860–863.

Lee ES, Kim EK. Surgical do's and don'ts of corneal dystrophies. *Curr Opin Ophthalmol* 2003; **14**:186–191.

Maclean H, Robinson LP, Wechsler AW, Goh A. Excimer phototherapeutic keratectomy for recurrent granular dystrophy. *Aust N Z J Ophthalmol* 1996; **24**:127–130.

Maini R, Sullivan L, Snibson GT, et al. A comparison of different depth ablations in the treatment of painful bullous keratopathy with phototherapeutic keratectomy. *Br J Ophthalmol* 2001; **85**:912–915.

Maldonado MJ, Nieto JC, Piñero DP. Advances in technologies for laser-assisted in situ keratomileusis (LASIK) surgery. *Expert Rev Med Devices* 2008; **5**:209–229.

Maloney RK, Thompson V, Ghiselli G, et al. A prospective multicenter trial of excimer laser phototherapeutic keratectomy for corneal vision loss. The Summit Phototherapeutic Keratectomy Study Group. *Am J Ophthalmol* 1996; **122**:149–160.

McDonnell PJ, Seiler T. Phototherapeutic keratectomy with excimer laser for Reis–Bücklers corneal dystrophy. *Refract Corneal Surg* 1992; **8**:306–310.

Nghiem-Buffet MH, Gatinel D, Jacquot F, et al. Limbal stem cell deficiency following phototherapeutic keratectomy. *Cornea* 2003; **22**:482–484.

Phillips AF, McDonnell PJ. Laser-induced fluorescence during photorefractive keratectomy; a method for controlling epithelial removal. *Am J Ophthalmol* 1997; **123**:42–47.

Rapuano CJ. Excimer laser phototherapeutic keratectomy. *Curr Opin Ophthalmol* 2001; **12**:288–293.

Rapuano CJ. Excimer laser phototherapeutic keratectomy in eyes with anterior corneal dystrophies: preoperative and postoperative ultrasound biomicroscopic examination and short-term clinical outcomes with and without an antihyperopia treatment. *Trans Am Ophthalmol Soc* 2003; **101**:371–399.

Rapuano CJ. Phototherapeutic keratectomy: who are the best candidates and how do you treat them? *Curr Opin Ophthalmol* 2010; **21**:280–282.

Rathi VM, Vyas SP, Sangwan VS. Phototherapeutic keratectomy. *Indian J Ophthalmol* 2012; **60**:5–14.

Shah RA, Wilson SE. Use of mitomycin-C for phototherapeutic keratectomy and photorefractive keratectomy surgery. *Curr Opin Ophthalmol* 2010; **21**:269–273.

Seiler T, Kriegerowski M, Schnoy N, Bende T. Ablation rate of human corneal epithelium and Bowman's layer with the excimer laser (193 nm). *Refract Corneal Surg* 1990; **6**:99–102.

Seitz B, Lisch W. Stage-related therapy of corneal dystrophies. *Dev Ophthalmol* 2011; **48**:116–153.

Sridhar MS, Rapuano CJ, Cosar CB, et al. Phototherapeutic keratectomy versus diamond burr polishing of Bowman's membrane in the treatment of recurrent corneal erosions associated with anterior basement membrane dystrophy. *Ophthalmology* 2002; **109**:674–679.

Stark WJ, Gilbert ML, Gottsch JD, Munnerlyn C. Optical pachometry in the measurement of anterior corneal disease: an evaluative tool for phototherapeutic keratectomy. *Arch Ophthalmol* 1990; **108**:12–13.

Starr MB. Recurrent subepithelial corneal opacities after excimer laser phototherapeutic keratectomy. *Cornea* 1999; **18**:117–120.

Stasi K, Chuck RS. Update on phototherapeutic keratectomy. *Curr Opin Ophthalmol* 2009; **20**:272–275.

Wagoner MD. Decision making in superficial keratectomy: manual vs. phototherapeutic techniques. *Middle Eastern J Ophthalmol* 1996; **3**:181–193.

Wagoner MD, Badr IA. Phototherapeutic keratectomy for macular corneal dystrophy. *J Refract Surg* 1999; **15**:481–484.

Chapter 42

Autologous limbal transplant and allogenic limbal transplant

Tetsuya Kawakita, Kazuo Tsubota

■ INTRODUCTION

To maintain good quality of vision, the cornea should be transparent with a smooth surface epithelium providing a barrier against environmental stress. The most superficial corneal epithelial cells are regularly shed from the surface of the eye and replaced by new cells that are ultimately provided by corneal epithelial basal cells migrated from limbal location. This concept was proposed as the XYZ theory (Thoft & Friend 1983), which was based on the hypothesis that corneal epithelial stem cells reside in the limbal basal location. This hypothesis (Cotsarelis et al. 1989) has been substantiated by many clinical reports (Tsubota et al. 1995, 1999) (**Figure 42.1**).

Under physiological conditions, corneal epithelial stem cells are not depleted during the human life span. When corneal epithelial homeostasis could not be maintained by pathological conditions, limbal stem cell deficiency (LSCD) occurs. The common cause of LSCD is limbal epithelial depletion by severe inflammation in Stevens–Johnson syndrome, ocular mucous membrane pemphigoid (OcMMP), and corneal alkali burn. The loss of stem cells from the corneal epithelium leads to the invasion of vascularized conjunctival epithelium over the cornea (Kenyon 1989), which may induce functional blindness that cannot be treated by standard penetrating keratoplasty because of the lack of corneal epithelial stem cells in the donor corneal button. If penetrating keratoplasty is performed on the eye without the care of LSCD, corneal allograft fails to maintain transparency. Therefore,

total LSCD has been identified as the exclusion criteria for simple penetrating keratoplasty. When the cornea is totally covered with non-corneal epithelial cells it is defined as total stem cell deficiency, whereas when the corneal surface is invaded by non-corneal epithelium through limbus, it is defined as partial (sectoral) limbal stem cell deficiency. In this case, conjunctival epithelial cells and/or keratinized epithelial cells coexist with the corneal epithelial cells on the corneal surface. If the conjunctival stem cells are further depleted after corneal epithelial depletion, the ocular surface is eventually totally covered with the keratinized epithelium, which may be seen at the end stage of OcMMP or Steven–Johnson syndrome and recognized as the most difficult case to recover.

After the report about successful limbal autograft transplantation in the treatment of severe unilateral ocular surface disease (Kenyon & Tseng 1989), significant advances in surgical technique have been developed. For patients with bilateral disease, allografts obtained from cadaver donor tissue have been used in LSCD. In cases of LSCD combined with severe ocular surface inflammation, amniotic membrane has been applied as a substrate of corneal stem cells, and/or as a tentative overlay on the cornea to reduce inflammation. Finally, the cultivated epithelial sheet has been used for clinical application to cover the entire cornea during surgery, especially in cases of total LSCD with persistent inflammation. Recently different cell sources, including oral mucosal epithelial cells, have been applied as a donor cell source for the cultivated epithelial sheet.

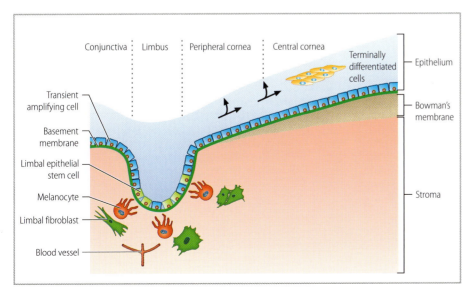

Conjunctiva | Limbus | Peripheral cornea | Central cornea

Terminally differentiated cells

Transient amplifying cell

Basement membrane

Limbal epithelial stem cell

Melanocyte

Limbal fibroblast

Blood vessel

Epithelium

Bowman's membrane

Stroma

Figure 42.1 Structure of limbus: limbal epithelial stem cells and their niche. Limbal epithelial stem cells are located at the limbal basal layer. This epithelial layer has transient amplifying cells, melanocytes, which might work as stem cell niche. Transient amplifying cells proliferate and migrate into the central side of the corneal basal layer, and finally into terminally differentiated superficial cells. The limbal basement membrane, subjacent limbal mesenchymal cells may also serve as niche cells, surrounded by nerves and blood vessels.

TOTAL LIMBAL STEM CELL DEFICIENCY

The symptoms of LSCD include decreased vision, photophobia, tearing, pain, and chronic inflammation with redness. The findings at slit-lamp examination may include a dull and irregular reflex of the corneal epithelium, which varies in thickness and transparency. Severe cases may have an ingrowth of thickened fibrovascular pannus, chronic keratitis, scarring, and calcification. Conjunctivalized areas on the corneal surfaces are frequently stained abnormally by fluorescein dye because conjunctival epithelium is more permeable than corneal epithelium.

Although accurate diagnosis is important for the surgical strategy for LSCD, it is difficult to diagnose LSCD only by signs of the loss of limbal palisades of Vogt, fluorescein staining pattern of the cornea (irregular and abnormal epithelium), persistent epithelial defect, and superficial neovascularization. The most reliable marker might be the existence of goblet cells, which could be confirmed by impression cytology (Kenyon & Tseng 1989). Under healthy conditions, the goblet cells exist only on conjunctivae, and when the limbal stem cells and niche are destroyed, goblet cells migrate with conjunctival epithelial cells from the conjunctiva into the cornea. Therefore, this specifically proves the existence of conjunctival cells on the cornea. However, if goblet cells on the ocular surface are destroyed, including severe keratinization in cicatricial ocular pemphigoid, or Stevens–Johnson syndrome, impression cytology cannot be used for the diagnosis of LSCD. In such cases, the absence of cornea-specific markers (such as the absence of keratin CK3/CK12) could prove loss of corneal epithelial cells on the cornea. In addition, in vivo confocal microscopy could be a candidate to show the existence of goblet cells on the cornea, and a world standard diagnosis criterion for LSCD needs to be determined to compare reported surgical data of LSCD accurately.

Patients with LSCD do not require surgical intervention because there are many asymptomatic patients with partial LSCD. Corneal and conjunctival epithelial cells can coexist stably on the cornea for long periods (Dua et al. 1994). Pseudopterygium has been sometimes misdiagnosed as partial or total LSCD. Surgical intervention should be performed only when most of the corneal surface is covered with conjunctival or keratinized epithelium accompanied by other signs of LSCD and poor vision. In partial LSCD with the capacity of functional epithelial stem cells, only mechanical debridement of the abnormal epithelium induces resurfacing of corneal epithelial cells on the denuded area. Therefore the criteria for surgical intervention are very important (**Figure 42.2**). LSCD is discussed in more detail in Chapter 24.

PARTIAL LIMBAL STEM CELL DEFICIENCY

In partial stem cell deficiency, a clear line of demarcation is often visible between the corneal and conjunctival phenotypes of cells. At the line of contact of the two phenotypes, fluorescein dye tends to pool on the conjunctivalized side of the line of contact because it is relatively thin. Partial LSCD may be subclinical in some patients at the time of the insult, and may eventually progress to total LSCD as the stem cell population depletes completely. When they maintain good vision, asymptomatic patients with partial and peripheral conjunctivalization of the corneal surface may not require intervention. Corneal

and conjunctival epithelial cell phenotypes have coexisted on the corneal surface for prolonged periods without significant extension of the conjunctivalized area (Dua et al. 1994). If the central area or most of the corneal surface is covered with conjunctival epithelium, mechanical debridement of conjunctival epithelium may improve adequate corneal epithelial healing from the remaining intact limbal epithelium (Coster et al. 1995). Mechanical debridement of conjunctival epithelium and encouraging the denuded area to be resurfaced with corneal epithelial cells is a valid, simple, and effective alternative to limbal transplantation in partial LSCD. This procedure can improve visual function and reduce symptoms even when normal limbus and peripheral cornea remain little. It may be better to consider it before ocular surface reconstruction (discussed in more detail in Chapter 41). Mechanical debridement may have a role to prevent migration of conjunctival epithelium onto the corneal surface in partial LSCD. Amniotic membrane transplantation might be performed with the mechanical debridement to treat partial LSCD.

AUTOLOGOUS LIMBAL TRANSPLANT

Concept of surgery

Autologous conjunctival transplant was first described in 1977 (Thoft 1977), and was shown to be clinically applicable for monocular chemical burn: successful re-epithelialization with increasing vision was achieved in 18% (3/17 eyes). After this report, several clinical studies proved the effectiveness of autologous conjunctival transplant in LSCD (Holland & Schwartz 1996, Thoft 1982, Vastine et al. 1982). However, this concept was based on the hypothesis that conjunctival epithelial

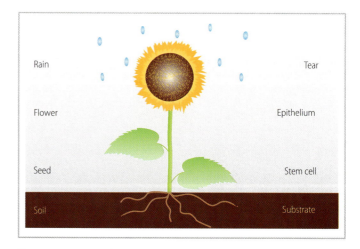

Figure 42.2 Strategy for stem cell transplantation. Ocular surface health is ensured by a close relationship between ocular surface epithelia and the preocular tear film, and supported by stromal fibroblasts and matrix. Therefore, for reconstruction of limbus, adequate substrate and tears were necessary to maintain healthy epithelial homeostasis including stem cells. This analogy describes the similarity in maintaining ocular surface health and growing a flowering plant. Firstly, it is important to have good seeds (equivalent to the stem cells). The seeds grow into healthy plants only when provided with sufficient water (equivalent to the tear fluid). In addition to water, the seeds and roots also need to be nourished by other nutrients from the soil (equivalent to the stromal fibroblasts and matrix). Redrawn with permission from Tseng and Tsubota (1997).

cells differentiate into corneal epithelial cells. In a rabbit model of LSCD, the comparison between autologous limbal transplant and autologous conjunctival transplant was performed. The results showed that only limbal transplant could recover the corneal epithelial phenotype (Tsai et al. 1990). Therefore, autologous conjunctival transplant was modified into autologous limbal transplant; the concept was based on the hypothesis that corneal epithelial stem cells exist in the limbus (Kenyon & Tseng 1989). This surgical concept and procedure improves the results of autologous limbal transplant and is widely performed in unilateral LSCD all over the world.

Indications for surgery

The surgical procedure is indicated for LSCD when the corneal surface is covered with conjunctival epithelium. However, the most severe case of LSCD with total invasion of keratinocyte (skin) with no conjunctival epithelium is contraindication. Limbal autologous transplantation is a useful surgery to treat LSCD; however, this surgical procedure could be only performed when the contralateral eye remains in a healthy condition. Small pieces of limbal tissue are removed from the upper and lower parts of the limbus in the contralateral eye, possibly resulting in reduced numbers of stem cells in that eye. Therefore, even if the cornea in the contralateral eye remains transparent with no inflammatory signs, the limbal tissue should not be removed in cases of Stevens–Johnson syndrome, OcMMP, and/or any conditions that may predispose it to later development of LSCD. Even long-term contact lens wear had been reported to be the risk of LSCD, which affected the result of autologous limbal transplant (Jenkins et al. 1993).

Preoperative considerations

In the preoperative surgical procedure, the primary advantage is no immunological rejection of the transplanted tissue. Furthermore, autograft is used just after removal from the contralateral eye, so the tissue is very fresh and supported by their niche cells/components. However, the biggest problem is the source of epithelial stem cells, which is sometimes too small to recover the whole surface of the cornea. Because it might take time to expand epithelial cells from the small autograft into the recipient corneal surface, sustained inflammation might attack and destroy the transplanted epithelial cells before starting to expand the epithelium from the autograft. The poor clinical outcomes after autograft in LSCD have been reported, especially in LSCD with underlying immunologically mediated diseases, such as Stevens–Johnson syndrome, toxic epidermal necrolysis, or OcMMP. Lower success rates have reported to be related to inflammatory ocular surface diseases (Samson et al. 2002). Anterior segment structure, the shape of eye lid, keratinization of lid margin, palpebral conjunctival scaring, and aqueous tear production need to be carefully examined before surgery, which may affect re-epithelialization of corneal surface. After surgery, it is important to keep wetness on ocular surface, and when lagopthalmos or poor lid closure exists, punctual occlusion and/or lateral tarsorrhaphy improve the wetness on ocular surface. These risk factors should be considered before all the ocular surface surgeries.

Surgical procedure

The fellow eye is marked with a 12-blade radial keratotomy marker. Two clock hours of limbal conjunctival tissue at the 12 o'clock and 6 o'clock positions are resected. A conjunctival incision is made 3–4 mm posterior to the limbus. The donor sites are left open to heal. A 360° limbal peritomy is performed, and subepithelial fibrotic tissue is removed from ocular surface by scissors or knife. To prevent re-invasion of the active fibrovascular tissue, mitomycin C treatment (0.02–0.04% for 2–5 minutes) may be performed. Subsequently the limbal autografts are transplanted in the same positions (the corresponding 12 o'clock and 6 o'clock positions) sutured by 10-0 nylon. Because autograft will be taken before the start of the recipient eye, epithelial side of autograft needs to maintain wetness until use by the viscoelastic device in a moist chamber. To reduce inflammation and improve epithelialization, amniotic membrane is sometimes used as covering the whole corneal surface after limbal autograft transplantation. This amniotic membrane is removed after 1 week and epithelial surface is checked. Sometimes amniotic membrane is melted by inflammation before removing (**Figure 42.3**).

Postoperative management

After autograft surgery, how to maintain the ocular surface until complete epithelialization is the key issue to achieve a healthy ocular surface. Using autologous serum drops and maintaining tear volume to avoid desiccation stress should be considered (Tsubota 1999). Amniotic membrane at the same time of surgery should also considered in autograft with signs of inflammation to inhibit neovascularization, support epithelial growth, and prevent microtraumatic stress by blepharoconjunctiva. In severe alkali burn cases, amniotic membrane transplantation is necessary to improve the prognosis of very severe corneal surface disorders (Muraine et al. 2000). Limbal autograft transplantation is a reliable and effective procedure in LSCD, after careful patient selection and considering the therapeutic strategy after surgery.

Collectively, autograft is a useful and safe surgical procedure for LSCD; this procedure should be used in patients with unilateral stem cell deficiency with normal conjunctival surface and minimal ocular

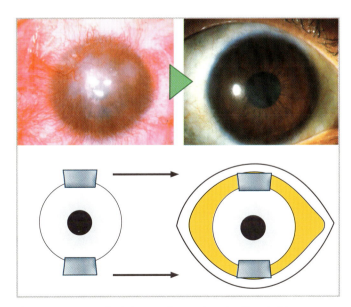

Figure 42.3 A case of limbal autograft transplantation. Two clock hours of limbal conjunctival tissue at the 12 o'clock and 6 o'clock positions were resected. A conjunctival incision was made 3–4 mm posterior to the limbus. The donor sites were left open to heal (illustration). Using this procedure, total limbal stem cell deficiency with severe fibrovascular tissue after chemical burn was treated.

surface inflammation. If the surgical criteria are applied, the clinical outcome after limbal autograft may be better.

Allogenic limbal transplant

In bilateral or unilateral total LSCD, transplantation of allogeneic limbal graft is the remaining alternative therapeutic option where the limbal allograft will be prepared from cadaveric donors (Tsubota et al. 1995) (**Figures 42.4** and **42.5**) or from living-related donors (Daya & Ilari 2001). From cadaveric donors, 360° entire limbus could be used for transplantation, but from living-related donors, small portions of the limbal tissue can be transplanted, same as autograft.

LIVING-RELATED LIMBAL ALLOGRAFT

Concept of surgery, indication, and clinical outcome

When autologous limbal transplant cannot be considered mainly by bilateral ocular surface disease, allograft will be considered. Limbus location is highly vascularized, and it is difficult to manage the risk of graft rejection. Therefore, to reduce the risk, living-related limbal allograft may be considered. Although this surgical procedure has limitations on the amount of tissue for transplantation, just as for

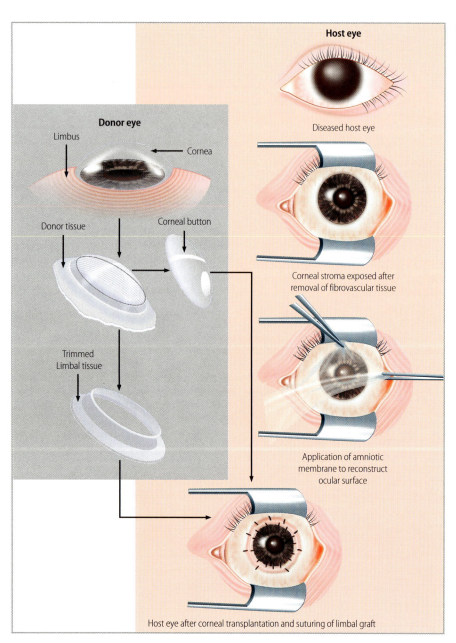

Figure 42.4 The limbal allograft transplantation. Reprinted with permission by Massachusetts Medical Society from Tsubota et al. (1999).

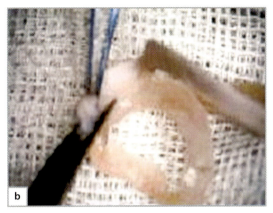

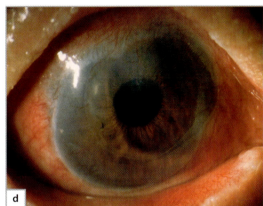

Figure 42.5 Allogeneic limbal transplantation. (a) Total limbal stem cell deficiency after chemical burn with severe symblepharon is shown. (b) Superficial lamellar dissection was carried out in donor limbal tissue after removed corneoscleral buttons. (c) The keratolimbal allograft was transplanted on epithelial-denuded surface of the recipient after removing all fibrovascular tissue, invading the ocular surface. (d) Corneal transparency and healthy ocular surface was maintained at 6 months after transplantation.

autograft, some degree of immune histocompatibility could be provided (Daya & Ilari 2001). The advantage of this procedure is similar to that autograft of fresh limbal tissue (maintains cell viability) and reduced systemic immunosuppression (avoids severe systemic side effect). The best human leukocyte antigen (HLA)-matched relative is the ideal donor. Donor eyes are evaluated not to have any history of ocular surface diseases and/or surgeries.

Preoperative considerations

In the preoperative surgical procedure, the primary advantage is less immunological rejection of the transplanted tissue similar to autograft. Graft rejection has been reported after living-related allograft transplantation, and the influence of HLA and ABO compatibility is unclear and difficult to establish in a small cohort in which there are numerous other variables to take into consideration. A good HLA match in which two or more class I antigens are matched has been shown by some studies to provide long-term benefit in corneal transplantation (Sanfilippo et al. 1986). Blood ABO matching is also considered an influential factor because epithelial cell expression of blood group antigens has been demonstrated (Dua et al. 1998). Most of rejection episodes occurred in eyes that had previously had Stevens–Johnson syndrome, toxic epidermal necrolysis, or chemical injuries (Kwitko et al. 1995, Rao et al. 1999). Living-related allograft also has cell source problem, which is sometimes too small to recover the whole surface of the cornea under inflammation.

Surgical procedure

Surgical procedures are similar to autograft surgery. Procedures on both the donor and the recipient are performed. The recipient follows

the donor immediately on the operating list. The donor eye is marked with a 12-blade radial keratotomy marker. Two clock hours of limbal conjunctival tissue at the 12 o'clock and 6 o'clock positions are resected. A conjunctival incision is made 3–4 mm posterior to the limbus. Careful attention to the limbal conjunctiva should be taken to ensure maximal resection. This is accomplished by dissecting conjunctival tissue, including palisades of Vogt anteriorly onto the corneal surface. The epithelial sides of the two donor tissues are covered by the viscoelastic device in a moist chamber and transferred for transplantation. Surgery on the recipient is also similar to autograft. A conjunctival peritomy is performed at the 12 o'clock and 6 o'clock positions, and limbal conjunctiva is undermined and allowed to retract posteriorly. The corneal pannus is carefully dissected, and the conjunctival grafts are secured using 10-0 nylon suture. To prevent reinvasion of the active fibrovascular tissue, mitomycin C treatment (0.02–0.04% for 2–5 minutes) may be performed before transplantation. The limbal portion of the graft is sutured to the bare corneal limbus, and the posterior side is sutured to the episcleral tissue and host conjunctiva. To reduce inflammation by the contact of lid and improve epithelialization, amniotic membrane is sometimes used to cover the entire corneal surface after limbal allograft transplantation. This amniotic membrane is removed after 1 week and epithelial surface is checked.

Postoperative management

After allograft surgery, the key issue to achieve a healthy ocular surface is same as autograft. It is necessary to maintain the wet ocular surface with less inflammation until complete epithelialization. The use of autologous serum drops (Tsubota 1999) and amniotic membrane at the same time of surgery should also be considered, if signs of inflammation are present, to inhibit neovascularization, support epithelial growth, and prevent microtraumatic stress by blepharoconjunctiva. With postoperative systemic immunosuppression (steroids and/or cyclosporine), the clinical outcome might be better in living-related allograft. Using systemic immunosuppression, a high ratio of allograft survival up to 80% was reported (Daya & Ilari 2001).

LIMBAL ALLOGRAFT FROM CADAVER DONOR

Concept of surgery and indication

After the achievement of autologous limbal transplant, limbal tissue from the cadaver donor has been applied for limbal transplantation (Tan et al. 1996). For patients with bilateral disease, first Tsai and Tseng (1994) reported the transplantation of limbal allografts obtained from cadaver donor tissue, and the modification of the technique by the use of amniotic membrane as a substrate replacement (Kim & Tseng 1995) has permitted new approaches to the treatment of even endstage of total LSCD. Such severe diseases had been considered contraindications to surgery because of the extremely poor prognosis of patients treated with corneal transplantation. In this surgical procedure, the primary advantage is cell source, which could be the whole limbus of the cadaver donor eye. However after surgery, immunological rejection of the transplanted tissue needs to be considered. Compared with autograft, freshness of the tissue and damage by air exposure vary among donors.

Surgical procedure

The surgical procedure is designed to remove all abnormal tissue invading the ocular surface and to provide corneal stem cells by transplantation of limbal allografts from cadaver donors. Conjunctival or keratinized epithelium covering the cornea and then dissected fibrous tissue and any existing symblepharon that might have interfered with eye movement are removed. A 360° cadaveric donor corneolimbal ring graft, obtained from the donor corneoscleral button, is used in this surgery. After the central corneal button is removed with an 8 mm trephine, the remaining corneoscleral ring is trimmed of excessive sclera and flattened with the epithelial surface, facing down on a protective layer of the viscoelastic device. The posterior half of the stroma, including the endothelium, is removed by a pair of sharp scissors or knife. Additional tapering of the corneal and limboscleral edges is performed with scissors so that their contact with the recipient surface would be smooth. The amniotic membrane is transplanted on the scleral surface as a niche of stem cells before allograft transplant. The donor corneolimbal ring is secured to the surrounding conjunctival edge with 10-0 interrupted nylon sutures, each with episcleral anchorage and corneal surface.

Preoperative considerations

Although the success rate for short follow-up was good, the success rate of limbal allograft for LSCD dramatically dropped to <60% for long-time follow-up of >2 years (Solomon et al. 2002, Tsubota et al. 1999), which was explained mainly by immunological rejection. Allograft rejection sometimes could not be managed under continuous systemic cyclosporin A with steroid, and the long-term results for limbal allograft remained unsatisfactory. All of the recipient limbal location (360°) was covered by allograft, and the drainage system of the aqueous humor might be destroyed, resulting in a possible increase of intraocular pressure. Furthermore, maintaining wetness on the ocular surface is important to reduce inflammation before and after surgery (Shimazaki et al. 2000). For that purpose, bandage contact lens, tarsorrhaphy, punctal occlusion, autologous serum eye drops, fornix reconstruction, amniotic membrane transplantation, and lid reconstruction might be considered to be combined with the allograft surgery.

Just as limbal autograft, the poor clinical outcomes after allograft in LSCD have been reported, especially in LSCD with underlying immunologically mediated diseases, such as Stevens–Johnson syndrome. The existence of preoperative conjunctival keratinization has also been shown to have a poor prognosis (Holland 1996). Preoperatively anterior segment structure, the shape of eye lid, keratinization of lid margin, palpebral conjunctival scaring, and aqueous tear production need to be carefully examined, which may affect re-epithelialization of the corneal surface.

Postoperative management

After allograft surgery, how to maintain the ocular surface until complete epithelialization is the key issue to achieve a healthy ocular surface just as for autograft surgery. The use of autologous serum drops (Tsubota 1999) and amniotic membrane covering might be also considered. Amniotic membrane transplantation may be necessary to improve the prognosis of very severe corneal surface disorders.

Intraocular pressure is also controlled by glaucoma drainage/implant surgery or by medications. In the cases with corneal stromal opacity, penetrating keratoplasty is performed for visual rehabilitation after a stable epithelium has been achieved. Collectively, allograft surgery should be considered due to the higher rate of complications than autograft, including rejection and glaucoma, and following the strategy for maintaining a healthy ocular surface is necessary. More effective therapies for rejection, reversing keratinization, and suppressing persistent ocular surface inflammation improve the surgical outcome of allograft.

Limbal allograft transplantation can be adversely affected by several risk factors, threatening ocular surface health and transplanted stem cell survival. Current consensus is that autologous limbal grafts have a better prognosis than allografts, and the most significant advantage is the absence of immunological rejection. However, persistent inflammation of the ocular surface resulting from the original disease, infection, or abnormal eyelids can also cause loss of donor limbal tissue (Shimmura & Tsubota 2008). Although limbal allograft rejection is considered the major cause of failure, other risk factors, such as keratinization, symblepharon, inflammation, and dry eye disease, have been implicated. Stevens–Johnson syndrome has been shown to have the worst prognosis after limbal allograft in terms of ambulatory vision and success of penetrating keratoplasty. They are also found in younger patients when performing penetrating keratoplasty simultaneously with limbal allograft, which resulted in poor prognosis and poor ambulatory vision (Solomon et al. 2002).

CONCLUSIONS

Transplantation of corneal epithelial auto/allografts is efficacious for the treatment of LSCD. Severe inflammation and/or abnormal ocular surface epithelium (i.e. keratinization and symblepharon) are risk factors for poor prognosis. The control of persistent epithelial defects, ocular hypertension, dry eye disease, and graft rejection may further increase the efficacy of this method of transplantation.

■ REFERENCES

Coster DJ, Aggarwal RK, Williams KA. Surgical management of ocular surface disorders using conjunctival and stem cell allografts. *Br J Ophthalmol* 1995; **79**:977–982.

Cotsarelis G, Cheng SZ, Dong G, et al. Existence of slow-cycling limbal epithelial basal cells that can be preferentially stimulated to proliferate: implications on epithelial stem cells. *Cell* 1989; **57**:201–209.

Daya SM, Ilari FA. Living related conjunctival limbal allograft for the treatment of stem cell deficiency. *Ophthalmology* 2001; **108**:126–133; discussion 133–134.

Dua HS, Chan J, Gomes JA, Azuara-Blanco A. Adverse effect of blood group ABO mismatching on corneal epithelial cells. *Lancet* 1998; **352**:1677–1678.

Dua HS, Gomes JA, Singh A. Corneal epithelial wound healing. *Br J Ophthalmol* 1994; **78**:401–408.

Holland EJ. Epithelial transplantation for the management of severe ocular surface disease. *Trans Am Ophthalmol Soc* 1996; **94**:677–743.

Holland EJ, Schwartz GS. The evolution of epithelial transplantation for severe ocular surface disease and a proposed classification system. *Cornea* 1996; **6**:549–556.

Jenkins C, Tuft S, Liu C, Buckley R. Limbal transplantation in the management of chronic contact-lens-associated epitheliopathy. *Eye (Lond)* 1993; **7**:629–633.

Kenyon, KR. Limbal autograft transplantation for chemical and thermal burns. *Dev Ophthalmol* 1989; **18**:53–58.

Kenyon KR, Tseng SC. Limbal autograft transplantation for ocular surface disorders. *Ophthalmology* 1989; **96**:709–722; discussion 722–723.

Kim JC, Tseng SC. Transplantation of preserved human amniotic membrane for surface reconstruction in severely damaged rabbit corneas. *Cornea* 1995; **14**:473–484.

Kwitko S, Marinho D, Barcaro S, et al. Allograft conjunctival transplantation for bilateral ocular surface disorders. *Ophthalmology* 1995; **102**:1020–1025.

Muraine M, Salessy P, Watt L, et al. Limbal autograft transplantation, eight consecutive cases. *J Fr Ophtalmol* 2000; **23**:141–150.

Rao SK, Rajagopal R, Sitalakshmi G, Padmanabhan P. Limbal allografting from related live donors for corneal surface reconstruction. *Ophthalmology* 1999; **106**:822–828.

Samson CM, Nduaguba C, Baltatzis S, Foster CS. Limbal stem cell transplantation in chronic inflammatory eye disease. *Ophthalmology* 2002; **109**:862–868.

Shimazaki J, Shimmura S, Fujishima H, Tsubota K. Association of preoperative tear function with surgical outcome in severe Stevens-Johnson syndrome. *Ophthalmology* 2000; **107**:1518–1523.

Sanfilippo F, MacQueen JM, Vaughn WK, Foulks G. Reduced graft rejection with good HLA-A and B matching in high-risk corneal transplantation. *N Engl J Med* 1986; **315**:29–35.

Shimmura S, Tsubota K. Surgical treatment of limbal stem cell deficiency: are we really transplanting stem cells? *Am J Ophthalmol* 2008; **146**:154–155.

Solomon A, Ellies P, Anderson DF, et al. Long-term outcome of keratolimbal allograft with or without penetrating keratoplasty for total limbal stem cell deficiency. *Ophthalmology* 2002; **109**:1159–1166.

Tan DT, Ficker LA, Buckley RJ. Limbal transplantation. *Ophthalmology* 1996; **103**:29–36.

Thoft RA. Conjunctival transplantation. *Arch Ophthalmol* 1977; **95**:1425–1427.

Thoft RA. Indications for conjunctival transplantation. *Ophthalmology* 1982; **89**:335–339.

Thoft RA, Friend J. The X, Y, Z hypothesis of corneal epithelial maintenance. *Investig Ophthalmol Visual Sci* 1983; **24**:1442–1443.

Tsubota K. Ocular surface management in corneal transplantation, a review. *Jpn J Ophthalmol* 1999; **43**:502–508.

Tsubota K, Satake Y, Kaido M, et al. Treatment of severe ocular-surface disorders with corneal epithelial stem-cell transplantation. *N Engl J Med* 1999; **340**:1697–1703.

Tsubota K, Toda I, Saito H, et al. Reconstruction of the corneal epithelium by limbal allograft transplantation for severe ocular surface disorders. *Ophthalmology* 1995; **102**:1486–1496.

Tsai RJ, Sun TT, Tseng SC. Comparison of limbal and conjunctival autograft transplantation in corneal surface reconstruction in rabbits. *Ophthalmology* 1990; **97**:446–455.

Tsai RJ, Tseng SC. Human allograft limbal transplantation for corneal surface reconstruction. *Cornea* 1994; **13**:389–400.

Tseng SC, Tsubota K. Important concepts for treating ocular surface and tear disorders. *Am J Ophthalmol* 1997; **124**:825–835.

Vastine DW, Stewart WB, Schwab IR. Reconstruction of the periocular mucous membrane by autologous conjunctival transplantation. *Ophthalmology* 1982; **89**:1072–1081.

Chapter 43 | Keratoprosthesis

Borja Salvador Culla, Claes H. Dohlman

INTRODUCTION

Due to the scarcity of donor corneas for standard transplantation in parts of the world, the cost of processing, and the often mediocre long-term keratoplasty outcomes, there is a great need for a well-functioning artificial cornea (keratoprosthesis or KPro) with long-term safety. The concept of an artificial cornea is an obvious one—as obvious as placing a window on a house to be able to see out—and this possibility occurred to French surgeons by the time of the Revolution (Mannis & Dohlman 1999). However, at a time of no anesthesia, no asepsis, no antibiotics, no steroids, etc., the outcomes of these early attempts were predictably disastrous. During the following nineteenth century, there were scattered attempts at KPro implantation, but very often these efforts still resulted in endophthalmitis, extrusion, and loss of the eye. It was not until the early 1950s, with the introduction of transparent non-toxic plastics (Franceschetti 1949, Györffy 1951, Stone & Herbert 1953, Wünsche 1947), antibiotics, and steroids, that some measure of success began to be reported. This trend has gradually continued with a moderate number of surgeons worldwide developing new devices and, more importantly, introducing techniques to preserve the health of the surrounding corneal tissue. Complications such as glaucoma and retinal detachment still pose substantial problems, resulting in unfavorable prognostic categories; however, tissue melt and infection have been brought under reasonable control. Detailed history of KPro developments over the last two centuries is not covered in this chapter; the reader is instead referred to a recent review (Mannis & Dohlman 1999).

Presently, only a small number of groups of physicians and scientists worldwide—perhaps two dozen—are actively involved in the development and testing of new KPro devices and new postoperative management. An even smaller number of researchers, past and present, have succeeded in bringing their results to market to any great extent. The number of patients who have had a KPro implanted during the last 60 years is unknown, but is probably still small—not >15,000. The number of such patients who have truly benefited visually for a long period must be far less. The types of KPro that have been implanted in the largest number have been the Cardona–De Voe devices (Cardona & DeVoe 1977), the osteo-odonto KPro (OOKP) by Strampelli (1963), initially modified by Falcinelli et al. (2005) and Temprano (Michael et al. 2008), and later further modified by Liu et al. (1999), and Hille et al. (2005), those by Worst and Van Andel (2001), Pintucci et al. (1995), Fyodorov et al. (1970), the AlphaCor (Hicks et al. 2006), and the Boston KPro (Zerbe et al. 2006). These are briefly described here, together with outlines of their complications. Space does not allow covering several important smaller series from the past (i.e. Barraquer 1960, Legeais et al. 1995) or newer designs that are under development but have not yet been subjected to the market in large numbers.

TYPES OF KERATOPROSTHESIS

Cardona

One of the first keratoprostheses implanted in humans was developed by Cardona, DeVoe, and Castroviejo in 1962 (**Figure 43.1**). Cardona's initial 'through-and-through' design was made of pure poly(methyl

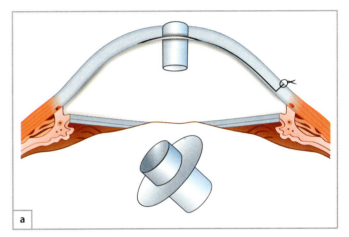

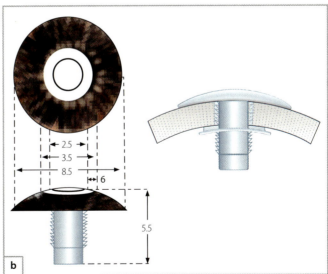

Figure 43.1 Cardona keratoprosthesis: (a) 'through-and-through' and (b) 'nut and bolt' devices. Reproduced from Castroviejo et al. (1969), with permission from the American Ophthalmological Society.

methacrylate) (PMMA), with an optical cylinder of 2 mm in diameter, and an intralamellar plate of 4 mm in diameter (Cardona 1962). He also designed a second 'nut and bolt' model that consisted of an optical cylinder attached to a colored front plate of 9 mm in diameter, and a posterior 'nut' screwed onto the stem from the back. The device was originally designed to be implanted in the patient's own cornea. But in the cases where the cornea was too thin or vascularized, Cardona modified the surgical technique by removing the anterior two thirds of the patient's cornea, and replacing the tissue with a full-thickness graft (Castroviejo et al. 1969). Although short-term results were positive, the long-term extrusion rate remained a problem. Cardona's work also became an inspiration to the field and to subsequent surgeons, such as Pintucci et al. (1995) and Girard (1993), who modified the device by using other materials (such as Dacron) for the intralamellar haptic.

Osteo-odonto keratoprosthesis

Strampelli (1963) introduced a novel concept by using a slice of the patient's own tooth as an anchor for a PMMA rod. The cylinder has a posterior portion 4.1 mm in diameter, and an anterior portion 3.65 mm in diameter. This difference in size creates a step that prevents spontaneous extrusion. The implantation requires two surgical stages over a 3-month period (**Figure 43.2**). Although extrusion rate is lower than Cardona's, other complications are still present, including glaucoma, retroprosthetic membranes (RPM), retinal detachment, and endophthalmitis. In an attempt to reduce these complications, Falcinelli made modifications to Strampelli's original technique (including the use of a relative's tooth, cryoextraction of the lens, anterior vitrectomy, the use of buccal instead of labial mucosa, and iris removal) (Falcinelli et al. 2005). In 1975 Temprano substituted the tooth for a piece of tibia in patients who lacked useful teeth. This technique has been called tibia-KPro (Michael et al. 2008). Further substantial modifications have been made by Liu et al. (2005) and Marchi et al. (1994).

Russian keratoprosthesis

The Russian KPro surgeons include Fyodorov, Zuev, Moroz, Glazko (Fyodorov et al. 1970), and Kalinnikov et al. (2001), as well as Yakimenko (1993) from Ukraine, among others. Their primary device, Moscow Eye Microsurgery Complex, is composed of a PMMA optical stem (2.5 mm diameter, 2.2–2.4 mm length) and an intrastromal butterfly-shaped titanium frame as haptic. The range of dioptric power is +55.00 to +62.00 diopters. The surgical procedure is carried out in two stages (**Figure 43.3**). First, the titanium frame is inserted into a two-third depth lamellar pocket (6 mm × 8 mm). After 3 months, an anterior vitrectomy with removal of iris and lens is performed; 2.5 mm × 2.2 mm holes are trephined in the anterior and posterior central cornea respectively, and the optical cylinder is screwed in. This device has also been used in China for a decade, particularly in chemical burns, with good results reported (Huang et al. 2011). Lately, Ghaffariyeh et al. (2011) have adopted the technique for implanting the device into a carrier corneal graft, analogous to the standard technique for the Boston KPro.

Boston keratoprosthesis

Developed at the Massachusetts Eye and Ear Infirmary in the 1960s, and approved by the FDA in 1992, the Boston KPro type I is made of pure PMMA and designed to be implanted into a carrier corneal graft, like a collar button (Dohlman et al. 1970, 2006). Thus, it has a front plate (5.5 mm diameter) with a central optical cylinder of 3.35 mm diameter (but only 2.3 mm inner optical aperture), and a snap-on back plate

(7.0–8.5 mm diameter) with 8–16 holes (1.3 mm diameter each). A donor cornea is sandwiched between the plates, and the complex is then sutured into the patient's cornea like a standard graft (**Figure 43.4**). The holes in the back plate allow access of aqueous humor to the corneal graft for better nutrition (Harissi-Dagher et al. 2007). Thus, in this device, the haptic (back plate) ends up on the back surface of the cornea, rather than being placed intrastromally. For more severe cases with end-stage dryness, a modified design (type II) exists, with an anterior nub extension that emerges between the lids or through the upper lid (Pujari et al. 2001). As of October 2011, >6000 Boston KPro devices have been implanted worldwide—the vast majority composed of type I.

AlphaCor

Formerly known as the Chirila KPro, AlphaCor is a soft hydrogel disc made of poly(2-hydroxyethyl methacrylate), or PHEMA. The disc (7 mm diameter, 0.6 mm thickness) comprises a central optically clear region fused to a porous skirt, which allows cellular colonization and collagen deposition for a better biointegration (**Figure 43.5**). Its implantation requires two stages separated by a period of about 12 weeks. In stage 1, the device is placed within a lamellar pocket, with a 3.5 mm hole in the posterior lamella. In stage 2, the central 3 mm of the anterior stroma is removed to expose the optical area, while the skirt remains integrated within the corneal stroma (Hicks et al. 2006).

Worst

In 1988, Worst et al. introduced a new design. This prosthesis, resembling a champagne cork, provides a wider visual field to the patients. The device consists of a KF-9 glass core molded into a platinum coating of 3.5 mm length. The glass core has a frontal flange of 6 mm in diameter. The flange has four holes (0.1 mm diameter), through each is placed a 70 μm stainless steel wire (**Figure 43.6**). In order to fixate the prosthesis, the four steel wires are wrapped around the eyeball and knotted two to two. The optical cylinder is placed through a central opening of the cornea, with the frontal flange inserted intrastromally (Worst & Van Andel 2001).

Pintucci

In 1995, the Italian surgeon Pintucci presented his device in which a PMMA optical cylinder (5.4 mm long and 3.5 mm wide) is fused to a filamentous Dacron skirt, the latter to be positioned in the stroma (Pintucci et al. 1995) (**Figure 43.7**). As in the OOKP, the surgical technique consists of two stages. In the first stage, the surface of the eye is covered with buccal mucosa, and the KPro is kept separately in a skin pocket created under the lower lid for tissue colonization. Two months later, the buccal mucosa is folded back and the cornea is partially exposed. Prior to its trephination, three partial-thickness radial incisions are performed. Once the trephination is completed, the radial cuts are completed, the iris and the lens removed, the optical cylinder is positioned, and the Dacron skirt and the radial incisions are sutured. The oral mucosa is then folded back to cover the device, and a hole is made over the optical stem. In severely dry eyes, a tarsorrhaphy is required to keep the integrity of the oral mucosa (Pintucci et al. 1996).

SURGICAL PROCEDURES

Implantation techniques of the described keratoprostheses have been outlined previously. More-detailed descriptions are beyond the scope of this chapter, and the reader is referred to pertinent publications.

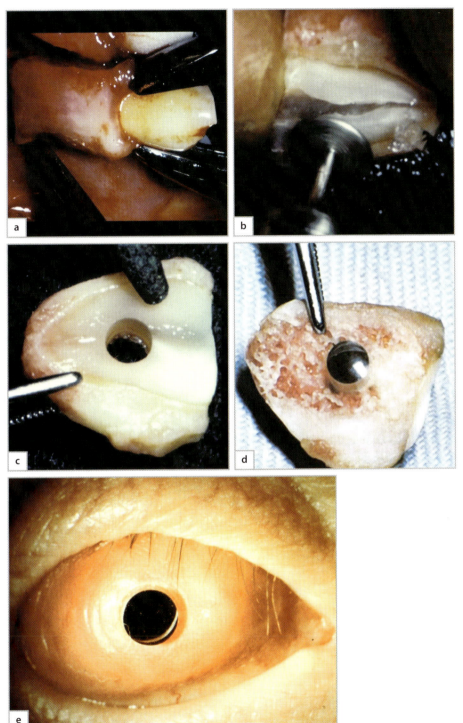

Figure 43.2 Osteo-odonto keratoprosthesis (OOKP). (a-d) The first steps in the surgical technique for the implantation of OOKP, and (e) appearance of the OOKP in a patient 2 years post-surgery. The eye is completely covered with buccal mucosa. Courtesy of Dr Temprano J, Centro de Oftalmología Barraquer, Barcelona.

COMPLICATIONS

The types of complications after KPro surgery can be expected to be similar with all KPro devices, although the rates may vary. A list of the most clinically relevant ones is provided in **Table 43.1**.

Desiccation of the ocular surface

Desiccation of the ocular surface is a process that can lead to substantial chronic surface damage. This is a phenomenon probably caused not so much by the rate of tear secretion, but rather by blink rate and blink completeness. This occurs particularly in bilateral abnormalities, thus with corneal pathology also in the opposite eye. Here, the corneal sensation is diminished because of nerve damage, and therefore blinking is not sufficiently triggered. As a measure to prevent dryness, a soft contact lens should be worn around the clock whenever possible. A lateral tarsorrhaphy can be considered in cases where contact lens retention might be difficult. In fact, in the Boston type I, the use of a soft contact lens is mandatory. In cases where dryness promotes protein deposition over the soft lens, hybrid contact lenses that have a

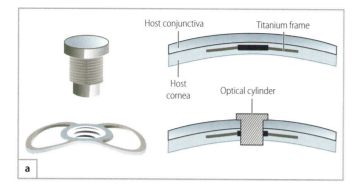

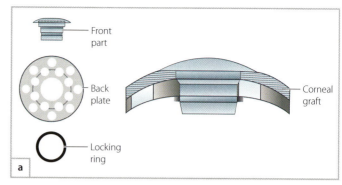

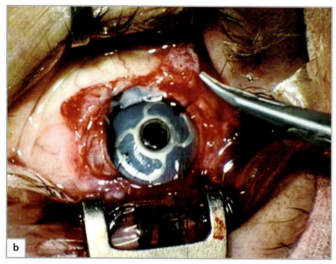

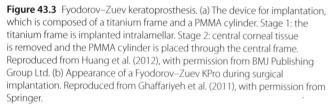

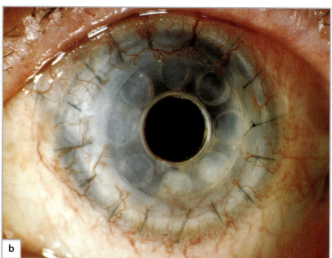

Figure 43.3 Fyodorov–Zuev keratoprosthesis. (a) The device for implantation, which is composed of a titanium frame and a PMMA cylinder. Stage 1: the titanium frame is implanted intralamellar. Stage 2: central corneal tissue is removed and the PMMA cylinder is placed through the central frame. Reproduced from Huang et al. (2012), with permission from BMJ Publishing Group Ltd. (b) Appearance of a Fyodorov–Zuev KPro during surgical implantation. Reproduced from Ghaffariyeh et al. (2011), with permission from Springer.

Figure 43.4 Boston keratoprosthesis: (a) the assembly of the Boston KPro type I and (b) appearance of a patient's eye with a Boston KPro 3 years after implantation.

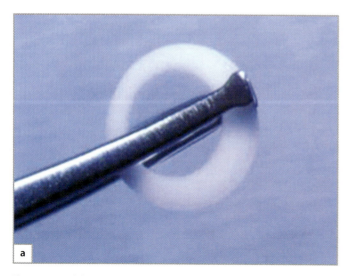

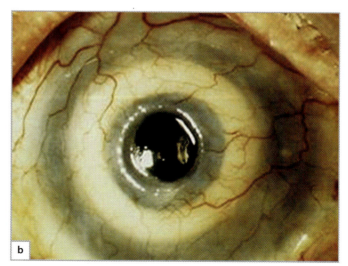

Figure 43.5 AlphaCor KPro: (a) a close-up of the device and (b) appearance of the prosthesis in a patient after removing the central 3 mm of the anterior stroma to expose the optical area (stage 2). Courtesy of Dr Crawford GJ, Lions Eye Institute Nedlands Western Australia, Australia.

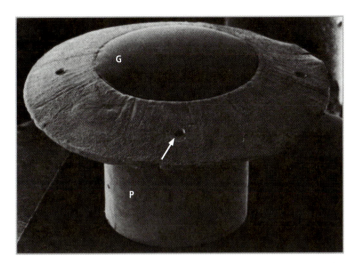

Figure 43.6 Worst keratoprosthesis. Scanning electron microscopy image of the Worst keratoprosthesis (platinum–glass). P, platinum; G, glass; arrow, hole for traction thread. Reproduced from Cuperus et al. (1989), with permission from Kluwer Academic Publishers.

Table 43.1 Most common complications after KPro implantation

Complications	Clinical manifestations
Desiccation of the ocular surface	Persistent epithelial defects
Tissue necrosis	Melt of surrounding tissue Aqueous leak Extrusion
Infection	Keratitis (bacterial and fungal) Endophthalmitis
Inflammation	Retroprosthetic membrane Postoperative uveitis Sudden sterile vitritis Epiretinal membrane Cystoid macular edema Retinal detachment Phthisis
Glaucoma	Preoperative condition Postoperative worsening

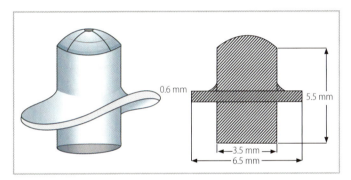

Figure 43.7 Pintucci keratoprosthesis: the Pintucci's PMMA-Dacron KPro. Reproduced from Pintucci et al. (1995), with permission from BMJ Publishing Group Ltd.

hard central core and a soft peripheral skirt usually solve the problem (Beyer et al. 2011, Dohlman et al. 2002).

Tissue necrosis

Being more common in some KPro varieties than in others, tissue necrosis (melt) and even extrusion can still occur with any device. Clinically, it presents as a persistent epithelial defect (PED) that can lead to infectious keratitis, stromal necrosis, and perforation, which in turn can result in aqueous leak, hypotony, choroidal detachment, and even retinal detachment.

Preventing PED formation can be usually achieved with a bandage contact lens wear, except in very dry eyes. Pathologies with increased chronic surface inflammation, limbal stem cell deficiency (LSCD), or autoimmune disease have a higher risk of tissue necrosis after KPro implantation (Sejpal et al. 2011). The chronic inflammatory environment in these situations, with an exacerbated collagenolytic activity, has been suggested to be the main cause of stromal necrosis and tissue melting (Dohlman et al. 2009). It is strongly suspected that collagenase inhibitors such as 0.1% doxycycline and 1.0% medroxyprogesterone drops, two to four times daily, can be helpful. Use of corticosteroids

in tissue necrosis is controversial, since they can inhibit connective tissue repair too much, and can even cause melt and extrusion of the KPro. Should severe tissue melt occur, complete reoperation is often indicated.

Infection

Although the incidence of infection has decreased significantly in the past decade, endophthalmitis remains the most catastrophic complication after KPro implantation. Virulent organisms can cause loss of vision in 24 hours. It can occur at any time after surgery, even years, although it is rare during the first postoperative months. Clinically, if a soft contact lens is in place, infection starts with the colonization of the lens and, if left untreated, progresses to keratitis, which often appears as whiteness around the stem. Penetration into the anterior chamber and the vitreous cavity can then follow (Nouri et al. 2001).

If endophthalmitis is suspected because of tenderness, pain, redness, cells or fibrin in the anterior chamber, etc., immediate aqueous tap (for smear and culture) and intrachamber injection of antibiotics are mandatory. Standard treatment is 1.0 mg vancomycin, 0.4 mg amikacin, and 0.4 mg dexamethasone. The patient should be then admitted to the hospital for further intensive treatment with topical antibiotics (e.g. fortified vancomycin 25 mg/mL and tobramycin 14 mg/mL). An additional systemic intravenous antibiotic regimen (including vancomycin and ceftazidime, or tobramycin, or ciprofloxacin) is also recommended, until the result of the culture allows a more targeted therapy. Vitrectomy is sometimes advocated.

The eventual outcome depends not only on rapid treatment but also on the virulence of the organism. In the worst situation, vision can be lost in a day or two—even with rapid treatment. Therefore, prophylaxis is of overwhelming importance. It is very important to impress upon the patients that a meticulous compliance with a regimen of daily drops of antibiotics is necessary for life. In Boston, our standard regimen consists of one drop of polymyxin B/trimethoprim once daily in standard cases. In autoimmune patients and in only eyes, we add vancomycin (14 mg/mL) once or twice daily (Durand & Dohlman 2009). Prophylaxis against fungal infection in KPro patients is not well defined; however, based on our experience (unpublished), it may include a 'burst' of amphotericin B twice daily for 1 or 2 weeks, repeated every 2–3 months in endemic areas. In addition, use of povidone iodine 2–5% at every visit may also be beneficial. In our experience, the bacterial endophthalmitis rate during the first 5 postoperative years has dropped to about 1%.

Inflammation

In some patients, sudden massive vitritis (uveitis) with temporary severe vision loss has been observed after KPro implantation (Nouri et al. 2005). This vitritis can mimic bacterial endophthalmitis, but the lack of pain, tenderness, or redness should lead us to suspect sterile vitritis. There is no need for a tap or injection but rather increased steroid treatment (including subtenon injection of 40 mg triamcinolone), and increased topical antibiotics. Rarely, sterile vitritis can lead to other complications such as RPM, and vision is regained within a few weeks in the vast majority of patients.

The degree of postoperative inflammation correlates closely with preoperative inflammation. In non-autoimmune diseases, the postoperative inflammatory reaction is short-lived and can be held in check with topical steroids. In severely damaged eyes and in autoimmune diseases—such as Stevens–Johnson syndrome, ocular mucous membrane pemphigoid (OcMMP), and graft-versus-host disease—a low-grade hard-to-detect chronic inflammation may be present for a long time, predisposing these patients to increased risk of tissue melt, RPM, vitreous opacities, and even retinal detachment.

Treatment usually consists of steroids, but due to their effect on repair processes, as well as on the intraocular pressure (IOP), dosage often has to be kept low. RPMs are fairly common, but they can usually be opened with Nd:YAG-laser. If the RPM is very dense or vascularized, it is often safest to repeat the whole KPro graft procedure and completely excise the membrane open sky. Retinal detachments are difficult to repair, and vision is rarely restored.

The incidence rates of these complications are not discussed here. They vary between groups, with much depending on severity of preexisting disease; thus, they are hard to compare. The reader is referred to the publications currently available.

Glaucoma

The incidence of infection has drastically decreased after KPro implantation during the last few decades, leaving glaucoma as the most destructive complication after KPro (Netland et al. 1998). Although glaucoma often has a multifactorial pathogenesis, the most likely cause seems to be gradual closure of the anterior chamber angle from low-grade inflammation.

Often the incidence of preexisting glaucoma is very high in eyes that need a KPro; several studies have shown a preoperative rate of 60–75%. Subsequent KPro surgery, or any surgery, often aggravates the situation. The complicating situation is the difficulty in measuring the IOP after KPro implantation. The rigid back plate precludes accurate readings with tonometers. This leaves finger palpation of the globe, a very crude assessment, the only practical alternative. Evaluations of the optic disc at every visit, as well as periodic visual fields, are mandatory.

In patients with a history or high suspicion of preoperative glaucoma, aggressive treatment must be administered with no delay. In spite of the back plate in some KPros, antiglaucoma medications still penetrate into the eye well, and then have the usual effect in controlling IOP. Carbonic anhydrase inhibitors also have the expected effect. When profound medical control of IOP is insufficient, implantation of aqueous shunts, either at the same time or following the implantation

of a KPro, is often indicated. Endoscopic/trans-scleral photocoagulation has also shown to be effective, but it should be reserved for patients with refractory glaucoma since the results can be unpredictable (Rivier et al. 2009).

INDICATIONS

The severity and the frequency of complications dictate the indications for any KPro. However, over the years a certain consensus on indications has developed, regardless of the type of KPro. A gross categorization is shown in **Table 43.2**.

Wet, blinking eye

In patients with normal blinking and tear secretion, KPro implantation has a low risk of postoperative complications and a good long-term prognosis, with visual recovery being faster compared to that after standard keratoplasty (Yaghouti et al. 2001). In this category we include stromal scarring from multiple graft failure, failed keratoconus surgery, non-inflammatory corneal edema (e.g. Fuchs' dystrophy and postsurgical bullous keratopathy) with stromal opacity, LSCD and aniridia, infectious keratitis (e.g. herpes simplex virus, bacteria, and fungi) in a quiet stage after a period of treatment, severe corneal neovascularization, and corneal dystrophies (Greiner et al. 2011).

Chemical burns

The rate of chemical accidents has decreased in the last few decades, partly due to better protective measures in the working environment and fewer assaults. However, chemical burns still remain a challenge for corneal specialists since standard keratoplasty has poor results. Corneal stem cell transplantation (autograft) is a successful alternative in unilateral cases, but in bilateral injuries a KPro can provide better long-term visual acuity than a keratolimbal allograft (Cade et al. 2011). Acid burns can have relatively good outcomes, but alkali burns are usually much worse. Severe glaucoma is often present preoperatively, and it may progress despite the implantation of a glaucoma shunt or cyclophotocoagulation therapy.

Autoimmune disease

A number of autoimmune diseases (including rheumatoid arthritis and atopy) can adversely affect eye surgery, but Stevens–Johnson syndrome, OcMMP, and graft-versus-host disease are the most dif-

Table 43.2 Indications for KPro

Wet, blinking eye—non-autoimmune (low risk)	Multiple failed grafts Non-inflammatory corneal edema, scarring Corneal dystrophies and degenerations Limbal stem cell deficiency, aniridia Infectious keratitis (herpes simplex virus, Herpes Varicella Zoster (HVZ), bacterial, and fungal)—quiet stage Corneal neovascularization
Chemical burns (moderate risk)	Alkali and acid
Autoimmune disease (high risk)	Stevens–Johnson syndrome Ocular mucous membrane pemphigoid Atopy, graft-versus-host disease, etc. Uveitis

ficult. These entities often have end-stage dry eye disease when first encountered, and their prognosis for KPro is poor. Melt, chronic inflammation, glaucoma, retinal detachment, and infection occur much more often than in non-autoimmune cases (Ciralski et al. 2010, Yaghouti et al. 2001). KPro is presently inadvisable in these conditions; great vision can sometimes be achieved for a year or two, but then severe complications can set in.

RESULTS

In reports on the existing KPros, outcomes in terms of vision and complications are often well detailed. Still, it is often hard to compare the outcomes due to short follow-ups and insufficient details on the composition of the patient cohorts. In addition, the prevalence of autoimmune diseases is not always listed with precision. For further information, the reader is referred to the numerous outcome publications on the separate KPros.

CONCLUSION

For almost a quarter of a millennium, it has been a goal in ophthalmology to develop an artificial cornea with long-term safety. Good optics, simplicity of surgery and management, and low cost would be of additional benefit, particularly in the developing world. As described earlier, past and present scientists and surgeons have made great strides in the field. Although there is still much more development needed for safe mass application, several principles have already been identified, which may serve as a foundation for future work.

Over the years a number of different materials have been employed to constitute KPros. However, after >65 years on the scene, PMMA is still the preferred material for the optical portion in the vast majority of KPros (Franceschetti 1949, Györffy 1951, Stone & Herbert 1953, Wünsche 1947). For the bearing structure (haptic) a wider range of substances have been tried. In terms of tissue compatibility, PMMA, titanium, and hydroxyapatite, as well as autologous tissue (e.g. tooth), have emerged as the most favorable at present, whereas Dacron, fluorocarbons, hydrogels, silicone, etc., have been more problematic. The search for the ideal biocompatible material continues.

In terms of implantation, the haptic has been placed intrastromally or, more rarely, as a back plate. It seems that the latter position better protects against extrusion. Holes in the back plate facilitate nutrition to the overlying cornea (Harissi-Dagher et al. 2007). It has also become clear that implanting the KPro into a carrier corneal graft (or using the patient's own cornea) is advantageous for postoperative retention (Dohlman et al. 1970). Moreover, placement of a soft contact lens for constant wear, after surgery in the wet eye, is very protective (Dohlman et al. 2002).

In terms of tissue response to the KPro, it has become increasingly clear that systemic autoimmune diseases (e.g. Stevens–Johnson syndrome, OcMMP, uveitis, and atopy) constitute a high risk for postoperative complications, including chronic inflammation, corneal tissue melt, leak, vitreous opacities, retinal detachment, and endophthalmitis. This goes for any type of KPro. The mediators that trigger these events in autoimmunity are still largely unknown; however, there are still possibilities to make the surgery safer. Such approaches include not only modifications of design, material, and surgical technique but also employment of immunosuppression and biological anti-inflammatories. Granted that the autoimmune category will probably be the last to be rescued by KPro surgery, rapid progress is presently being made.

Patients without autoimmune disease, on the other hand, with good blink rate and reasonable tear production, often do very well for a long time with several KPro types, as cumulative experience has shown. This category is by far the largest in numbers. In these patients (mostly penetrating keratoplasty failure from microbial keratitis, dystrophies, trauma, etc.), glaucoma control and compliance with prophylactic antibiotics can still remain problematic.

As mentioned previously, the addition of soft or hybrid contact lenses, worn around the clock in eyes that have normal tear production, has a dramatic protective effect in diffusing evaporative forces and preventing localized desiccation of the ocular surface—reducing surface inflammation and tissue melt. Increasing retention rate of the lenses is needed, however. A vaulting hard lens (PROSE—prosthetic replacement of the ocular surface ecosystem) can lead to astonishing improvement in sight and comfort in patients with severe dry disease, and it has also been applied to KPro eyes.

A reduced rate of microbial keratitis/endophthalmitis following KPro surgery has also been a triumph of recent years. The success of using prophylactic low-dose topical antibiotics over many years has been surprising and counterintuitive, but well documented in the United States (Durand & Dohlman 2009). Abroad, especially in developing countries, the statistics are still less favorable; however, this warrants further work on 'biointegration' between the graft and the device to retard or prevent microbial entry into the eye. Antimicrobial coatings are also under investigation. Less expensive antibiotics or antiseptics are desirable, as well as further work on drug-eluting soft contact lenses (Ciolino et al. 2009). Lack of compliance by the patient is often a problem, and one that is only partly amenable to education since meager health resources in many countries contribute to the difficulties in maintaining tight prophylaxis for life.

Necrosis (melt) of the corneal tissue around the KPro, occasionally leading to aqueous leak and disastrous consequences, used to be a substantial problem in the past. However, adding holes or openings in intrastromal or retrocorneal haptics (supporting membranes) has drastically reduced the melting problem (see previously). These openings improve nutrition of corneal keratocytes by allowing better access of aqueous humor. Presently it is mainly in the autoimmune situations where leaks occur, and for this category, anti-inflammation research seems to be the key. Also, since such tissue melt is likely to be mediated by matrix metalloproteinases and other enzymes, better use of inhibitors to such enzymes is presently being investigated.

Chronic intraocular inflammation can ruin many well-positioned KPros in severely diseased eyes. Low-level, clinically invisible inflammation can lead to troublesome consequences such as RPMs, glaucoma, vitreous opacities, or the ultimate disaster—retinal detachment. Prophylactic vitrectomy, immunosuppression, and biological anti-inflammatory treatment (i.e. infliximab) are presently topics of vigorous research. As mentioned previously, autoimmune conditions are the main contributors to these inflammation-based complications.

Postoperative glaucoma is now the most formidable barrier to long-term benefit from KPro implantation. Most patients (60–75%) have glaucoma diagnosed already before surgery, and worsening often follows postoperatively (Netland et al. 1998). Compounding the problem is the difficulty of measuring the IOP accurately (finger palpation only). However, well-tolerated implantable pressure transducers, read from the outside by radiowave telemetry, are presently being tested and will probably be routinely used in KPro eyes within a few years (Todani et al. 2011). Improved valve shunts are also being developed, which promise to bring the IOP to low levels without risking hypotony. A stable pressure of 5–10 mmHg is an important goal for many of these severely damaged eyes.

Thus, compared to a decade or two ago, KPro research worldwide is now flowering at a much greater rate. New designs and materials are steadily emerging from several groups. Investigations are also sharply focused on issues such as optics, glare, light damage to retina, glaucoma and inflammation problems, development of alternative tissues to serve as KPro carriers, chemical burn aspects, and field trials in developing countries. The future of KPros to help restore vision in millions of people with corneal blindness is very bright indeed.

■ REFERENCES

Barraquer J. Inclusión de prótesis ópticas corneanas, córneas acrílicas o queratoprótesis. An Inst Barraquer (Barc.) 1960; 1/2:243–247.

Beyer J, Todani A, Dohlman CH. Prevention of visually debilitating deposits on soft contact lenses in keratoprosthesis patients. *Cornea* 2011; **30**:1419–1422.

Cade F, Grosskreutz CL, Tauber A, Dohlman CH. Glaucoma in eyes with severe chemical burns before and after keratoprosthesis. *Cornea* 2011; **30**:613–614.

Cardona H. Keratoprosthesis: acrylic optical cylinder with supporting interlamellar plate. *Am. J. Ophth* 1962; **54**:284–94.

Cardona H, DeVoe AG. Prosthokeratoplasty. *Trans Am Acad Ophthalmol Otolaryngol* 1977; **83**:271.

Castroviejo R, Cardona H, de Voe AG. The present status of prosthokeratoplasty. *Trans Am Ophthal Soc* 1969; **67**:207–234.

Ciolino JB, Hoare TR, Iwata NG, et al. A drug-eluting contact lens. *IOVS* 2009; **50**:3346–3352.

Ciralski J, Papaliodis GN, Dohlman CH, Chodosh J. Keratoprosthesis in autoimmune disease. *Ocul Immunol Inflamm* 2010; **18**:275–280.

Cuperus PL, Jongebloed WL, Van Andel P, Worst JF. Glass-metal keratoprosthesis: light and electron microscopical evaluation of experimental surgery on rabbit eyes. *Documenta Ophthalmologica* 1989; **71**:29–47.

Dohlman CH, Dudenhoefer E, Khan BF, Morneault S. Protection of the ocular surface after keratoprosthesis surgery. The role of soft contact lenses. *CLAO J* 2002; **28**:72–74.

Dohlman CH, Harissi-Dagher M, Khan BF, et al. Introduction to the use of the Boston Keratoprosthesis. *Expert Rev Ophthalmol* 2006; **1**:41–48.

Dohlman CH, Webster RG, Biswas SK, et al. In: Polack F.M. (ed.), Collar-button prosthesis glued to a corneal graft: cornea and external diseases of the eye. First Inter-American Symposium 1970. Springfield: Charles C Thomas, 189.

Dohlman JG, Foster CS, Dohlman CH. Boston keratoprosthesis in Stevens-Johnson syndrome: a case of using infliximab to prevent tissue necrosis. *Digital J Ophthalmol* 2009; 15.

Durand ML, Dohlman CH. Successful prevention of bacterial endophthalmitis in eyes with the Boston keratoprosthesis. *Cornea* 2009; **28**:896–901.

Falcinelli G, Falsini B, Taloni M, et al. Modified osteo-odonto-keratoprosthesis for treatment of corneal blindness: long-term anatomical and functional outcomes in 181 cases. *Arch Ophthalmol* 2005; **123**:1319–1329.

Franceschetti A. Corneal grafting. *Trans Ophthalmol Soc United Kingdom* 1949; **69**:17–35.

Fyodorov SN, Kivaev AA, Bagrov SN. Keratoprosthesis in the case of serious leukomas and the endothelial epithelial dystrophy of the cornea clinical and experimental researches. *Oftalmologicheskil Zhurnal* 1970; **4**:253–255.

Ghaffariyeh A, Honarpisheh N, Karkhaneh A, et al. Fyodorov-Zuev keratoprosthesis implantation: long-term results in patients with multiple failed corneal grafts. *Graefes Arch Clin Exp Ophthalmol* 2011; **249**:93–101.

Girard LJ. Girard keratoprosthesis with flexible skirt: 28 years experience. *Refract Corneal Surg* 1993; **9**:194–195.

Greiner MA, Li JY, Mannis MJ. Longer-term vision outcomes and complications with the Boston type 1 keratoprosthesis at the University of California, Davis. *Ophthalmology* 2011; **118**:1543–1550.

Györffy I. Acrylic corneal implant in keratoplasty. *Am J Ophthalmol* 1951; **34**:757–758.

Harissi-Dagher M, Khan BF, Schaumberg DA, Dohlman CH. Importance of nutrition to corneal grafts when used as a carrier of Boston keratoprosthesis. *Cornea* 2007; **26**:564–568.

Hicks CR, Crawford GJ, Dart JKG, et al. AlphaCor: Clinical outcomes. *Cornea* 2006; **25**:1034–1042.

Hille K, Grabner G, Liu C, et al. Standards for modified osteoodontokeratoprosthesis (OOKP) surgery according to Strampelli and Falcinelli: the Rome-Vienna Protocol. *Cornea* 2005; **24**:895–908.

Huang Y, Dong Y, Wang L, et al. Long-term outcomes of MICOF keratoprosthesis in the end stage of autoimmune dry eyes: an experience in China. *Br J Ophthal* 2012; **96**:28–33.

Huang Y, Yu J, Liu L, et al. Moscow eye microsurgery complex in Russia keratoprosthesis in Beijing. *Ophthalmology* 2011; **118**:41–46.

Kalinnikov YY, Moroz ZI, Leontieva GD, et al. Clinical results of biokeratoprosthesis for leukomas. *An Inst Barraquer (Barc.)* 2001; **30**: 77–81.

Legeais JM, Renard G, Parel JM, et al. Keratoprosthesis with biocolonizable microporous fluorocarbon haptic. Preliminary results in a 24-patient study. *Arch Ophthalmol* 1995; **113**:757–763.

Liu C, Herold J, Sciscio A, et al. Osteo-odonto-keratoprosthesis surgery. *Br J Ophthalmol* 1999; **83**:127.

Liu C, Paul B, Tandon R, et al. The osteo-odonto-keratoprosthesis (OOKP). *Semin Ophthalmol* 2005; **20**:113–128.

Mannis MJ, Dohlman CH. The artificial cornea: a brief history. In: Mannis MJ, Mannis AA, eds. Corneal transplantation: a History in profiles. *Hirschberg History Ophthalmol* 1999; **6**:321–335.

Marchi V, Ricci R, Pecorella I, et al. Osteo-odonto-keratoprosthesis. Description of surgical technique with results in 85 patients. *Cornea* 1994; **13**:125–130.

Michael R, Charoenrook V, de la Paz MF, et al. Long-term functional and anatomical results of osteo- and osteoodonto-keratoprosthesis. *Graefes Arch Clin Exp Ophthalmol* 2008; **246**:1133–1137.

Netland P, Terada H, Dohlman CH. Glaucoma associated with keratoprosthesis. *Ophthalmol* 1998; **105**:751–757.

Nouri M, Durand ML, Dohlman CH. Sudden reversible vitritis after keratoprosthesis. An immune phenomenon? *Cornea* 2005; **24**:915–919.

Nouri M, Terada H, Alfonso EC, et al. Endophthalmitis after keratoprosthesis: incidence, bacterial etiologies and risk factors. *Arch Ophthalmol* 2001; **119**:484–489.

Pintucci S, Pintucci F, Caiazza S, Cecconi M. The Dacron felt colonizable keratoprosthesis: after 15 years. *Eur J Ophthalmol* 1996; **6**:125–130.

Pintucci S, Pintucci F, Cecconi M, Caiazza S. New Dacron tissue colonisable keratoprosthesis: clinical experience. *Br J Ophthalmol* 1995; **79**:825–829.

Pujari S, Siddique S, Dohlman CH, Chodosh J. Boston keratoprosthesis type II: The Massachusetts Eye and Ear Infirmary experience. *Cornea* 2001; **30**:1298–1303.

Rivier D, Paula JS, Kim E, et al. Glaucoma and keratoprosthesis surgery: role of adjunctive cyclophotocoagulation. *J Glaucoma* 2009; **18**:321–324.

Sejpal K, Yu F, Aldave AJ. The Boston Keratoprosthesis in the managment of corneal limbal stem cell deficiency. *Cornea* 2011; **30**:1187–1194.

Stone Jr W, Herbert E. Experimental study of plastic material and replacement of the cornea. Preliminary report. *Am J Ophthalmol* 1953; **36**:168.

Strampelli B. Osteo-odontocheratoprotesi. *Ann Ottalmol Clin Ocul* 1963; **89**:1039–1044.

Worst JGF, Van Andel MV. The worst keratoprosthesis. *An Inst Barraquer (Barc.)* 2001; **30**:85–86.

Todani A, Behlau I, Fava M, et al. Intraocular pressure measurement by radiowave telemetry. *Invest Ophthalmol Vis Sci* 2011; **52**:9573–9580.

Wünsche G. Versuche zur totalen Keratoplastie und zur cornea artificialis. *Arztliche Forschung* 1947; **1**:345.

Yaghouti F, Nouri M, Abad JC, et al. Keratoprosthesis: preoperative prognosis categories. *Cornea* 2001; **20**:19–23.

Yakimenko S. Results of a PMMA/titanium keratoprosthesis in 502 eyes. *Refract Corneal Surg* 1993; **9**:197–198.

Zerbe BL, Belin MW, Ciolino JB. Boston Type 1 Keratoprosthesis Study Group. Results from the multicenter Boston Type 1 Keratoprosthesis Study. *Ophthalmology* 2006; **113**:1779–1784.

Chapter 44

Future prospects and trends in the diagnosis and treatment of dry eye disease

Jose M. Benitez-del-Castillo, Rocío Herrero-Vanrell, Michael A. Lemp

INTRODUCTION

Dry eye disease (DED) is the most common ocular disease. It is a common practice to use the terms 'ocular surface disease (OSD)' and 'DED' interchangeably because DED is the most common OSD and most other OSD entities lead to the production of DED indirectly. Therefore, the research on DED is growing, and in the near future, we expect significant new advances in diagnosis and treatment.

DIAGNOSIS

From a diagnostic point of view, biomarkers that could help in defining new cases and differentiating the type of DED are being investigated. Compositional analysis of the tear film has been hampered in the past due to the complex nature of the fluid and small sample sizes. With the advent of nanoscale detection and analysis methods, it has become possible to identify specific tear components and properties. Application of these techniques will help to identify biomarkers for specific OSDs, such as blepharitis and DED, and these have already yielded new approaches for high clinical utility. Efforts to explore the human tear proteome, lipidome, and genome to develop new biomarkers of disease continue (Zhou et al. 2012).

Inflammatory markers, such as matrix metalloproteinase 9 (MMP-9), interleukin 6, and interferon-γ, ocular surface health, such as epidermal growth factor, nerve growth factor (NGF), mucins, and tear osmolarity have been reported. A recently commercialized device can rapidly detect in-office elevated levels of MMP-9 in tear fluid. Although not specific for DED, it has the potential to identify patients with significant inflammation who may be responsive to anti-inflammatory treatment. Decreased tear levels of calcitonin gene-related peptide (CGRP) and neuropeptide Y (NPY) in DED are related to impaired lacrimal function, and tear levels of NGF are closely related to corneal epithelial damage, suggesting that NPY, CGRP, and NGF could become useful markers of dry eye severity (Lambiase et al. 2011). The expression levels of mucin 1 (MUC1) may be used as a diagnostic test in DED (Corrales et al. 2011). A novel biomarker panel of five proteins for the diagnosis and monitoring of DED in tears has recently been described by a Spanish company (Bioftalmik), including S100A6, annexin A1 (ANXA1), annexin A11 (ANXA11), cystatin-S (CST4), and phospholipase A2-activating protein. These markers were identified through in gel-based comparative proteomic analyses, and widely validated in tears of control individuals, and patients with DED and blepharitis (Soria et al. 2013). This panel is able to discriminate DED from the control group with a high diagnostic power. All proteins were found to be upregulated in DED, except CST4, which was found downregulated in the pathological condition. These protein biomarkers are mainly involved in inflammatory processes, antimicrobial protection, and apoptosis events.

Osmolarity is, at present, the best approach as a biomarker. There is an extensive literature on the use of tear osmolarity as a diagnostic entity for DED (Suzuki et al. 2010). Recent studies using an in vitro diagnostic technology (TearLab) that collects a 50 nL sample have demonstrated that tear osmolarity is the single most accurate objective test for diagnosing DED (Lemp et al. 2011, Sullivan et al. 2010), parallels disease severity and responds to effective treatment (Sullivan et al. 2012a, 2012b). Reductions in osmolarity preceded changes in symptoms during therapy. This biomarker may serve as a clinically useful objective endpoint in clinical trials of therapeutic products for DED.

THERAPEUTICS

New therapeutic approaches are being developed for DED. They are not based on the replacement of a new tear film similar to the natural one, but instead work by acting against some of the physiopathological events of the disease. In this chapter, current research therapies are presented. Nevertheless, the rapid pace of research suggests that even newer modes of disease management may be apparent by the time of publication of this book.

TEAR SUBSTITUTES

Artificial tears are still the mainstay of DED treatment. In healthy eyes, the lipid and aqueous components of the preocular tear film are capable of maintaining a continuous 10 mm layer, which is regularly respread with the blink of the lids. Alterations of the tear film result in discomfort and visual disturbance with potential damage to the ocular surface of patients. Because the preocular tear film is altered with independence of the subtype of DED, a popular idea for the future will be to develop formulations that resemble the natural film and can remain in contact with the ocular surface for as long as possible.

In this context it would seem logical to provide artificial tears with different components (lipid and aqueous) able to build a multilayer after their instillation. Essentially, ocular lubricants must include lipids, polymers in aqueous solvents (resembling the mucin layer), and amphiphilic substances to help link the lipid and aqueous layers. Moreover, the components included in formulations must be directed to increase tear film break-up time, improving the stability of the tear film. Several pharmaceutical excipients could accomplish the idea of simulating the unique properties of the lacrimal film and are proposed in this chapter.

Table 44.1 New dry eye disease therapeutic options in study

Calcineurin inhibitors	NOVA22007, AL38583 ST603-007 (Zyclorin) Tacrolimus Pimecrolimus LX214
Steroids and NSAIDs	EGP-437 AL-2178 Mapracorat (BOL-303242-X) ISV-101
Other anti-inflammatory drugs	Tofacitinib (CP-690,550) SAR 1118 Cilomilast (AL43546) IL-1Ra ESBA105 CF101 Epigallocatechin gallate PES103 AIN457 (secukinumab) ACZ885 (canakinumab) RX-10005 Oral lactoferrin
Secretagogues	Lacovutide (Moli 1901) 1(S)-HETE Ecabet Rebamipide (OPC12759) OPC-12759 DA-6034 (7-carboxymethyloxy-3′,4′,5-trimethoxy flavone monohydrate)′
Hormones	ARG101, 102, and 103 Testosterone
Ocular surface healing promoters	RGN-259 KCT-0809 NGF MIM-D3
Alternative therapies	Calorie restriction Acupuncture Chinese herbal medicine Ayurveda
Pain treatment	Civamide SYL1001

NSAIDs, non-steroidal anti-inflammatory drugs.

Lipophilic excipients

For several years, oily substances have been included in artificial tears to simulate the lipid layer. Ophthalmic formulations resembling the lipid layer of the preocular tear film must contain non-polar (air–tear interface) and polar (aqueous–lipid interface) lipids. Among the non-polar lipids used in ophthalmic formulations, the most commonly employed have been lanolin alcohol, light liquid paraffin, microcrystalline wax, mineral oil, and white petrolatum. Generally, lipid concentration determines whether the ophthalmic formulation has the consistency of an ointment or a drop.

The polar phase of the preocular tear film serves as an interface between the aqueous and lipid layers. Moreover, the organization and integrity of the non-polar layer depends on the underlying polar phase. Polar lipids include molecules with a polar head group capable of being attached to ionic substances and the non-polar chain that confers solubility in lipophilic solvents. Their amphiphilic properties lead to their use as surfactants and solubilizing agents.

Lanolin, stearic acid, propylene glycol (PG), polyethylene glycol (PEG), polysorbates, and lecithin (phosphatidylcholine) are amphiphilic substances, which have functions as surfactants, emulsifiers, and humectants. The most similar component to the polar lipid components is phosphatidylcholine because it is present in the natural tear film.

One of the advantages of amphiphilic substances included in the artificial tears is that they are able to decrease the surface tension, improving the spreading of the formulation on the ocular surface. Furthermore, the substances mentioned have other advantages as they can help to incorporate and solubilize lipophilic substances such as vitamin A derivatives (retinyl palmitate), cholesterol (a natural component of the lipid layer of the lacrimal film), or other hydrophobic substances. Dendrimers are new polymers with hyperbranched molecules that are modifiable in both size and structure. They can possess both hydrophilic and hydrophobic properties and are under investigation for use in ophthalmic formulations.

The benefit of non-polar and polar lipids combined in the same formulation is that once applied, the non-polar lipids will be present at the tear–air interface.

Artificial tears prepared with lipophilic substances similar to the ones present in the tear film—wax esters and cholesterol for non-polar lipids and phospholipids for polar lipids—will be preferred. Recent results suggest that the lipid layer of the tear film forms a gel in vivo (Leiske et al. 2010). According to this, the combination of several lipids able to form a gel upon instillation may aid in mechanical stabilization of the tear film.

Excipients resembling the aqueous–mucin layer

The main components of the aqueous–mucin layer of the lacrimal film are proteins, electrolytes, and other aqueous soluble components. Among the proteins, mucins have spreading properties, having an important role at the superficial lipid–aqueous tear interface of the preocular tear film. Gel-forming mucins are responsible for the viscoelastic properties and are able to spread across the ocular surface during blinking (Tiffany 2008).

Mucins are high-molecular-weight proteins characterized by their extensive O-glycosylation (Argüeso & Gipson 2001). The rheology of natural tears is believed to be similar to mucins. Solutions of mucins show non-Newtonian behavior. Between two consecutive blinks, mucins form a network of entangled linear polymers. They separate when the movement of lids produces a shearing of their chains, influencing the tear film break-up time. Because mucins affect both tear formation and stability, manufacturers formulate artificial tears with demulcents or viscosity agents to resemble the behavior of ocular mucins. Moreover, new evidence indicates that gel-forming and cell surface-associated mucins make a contribution in the protection of the ocular surface.

Among the viscosity agents employed in artificial tear formulations, cellulose derivatives and the glycosaminoglycan agent (hyaluronic acid) are the most used. They present high ocular biocompatibility and are capable of producing gel formulations, simulating the mucin layer of the preocular tear film. Hyaluronic acid (hyaluronan) increases viscosity and lubricity, as it has a viscoelastic behavior, improving lubrication. Furthermore, it has been shown to improve epithelial repair. Cellulose derivative polymers such as hydroxypropyl methylcellulose, methylcellulose, and carboxymethylcellulose (CMC) are widely used in eye lubricants. Gel formulations of CMC are thought to protect damaged corneal epithelial cells. Some of these polymers are capable of interacting with mucosal membranes, increasing the ocular contact time.

Aqueous solutions of those polymers well tolerated by the ocular surface and included in topical ophthalmic formulations with a poor tolerable active substance (timolol maleate) have been shown to increase cell viability (Andrés-Guerrero et al. 2011).

Another strategy to simulate the mucin layer is to use a combination of polymers able to form a gel upon instillation. This is the case of a derivative of guar gum (hydroxypropyl-guar, HP-guar) which, when mixed with liquid PG and PEG 400 and the ionic buffer borate, is able to form a gel after its instillation.

Different excipients can be added to improve the benefits of artificial tears. Normal tears have a pH of about 7.4, and this is the optimal value of most ophthalmic topical formulations. The pH of solutions must be compatible with the ocular surface and the rest of the excipients present in the ophthalmic formulations. Several buffers offer additional advantages for patients with DED. For example, bicarbonate buffer may help regulate the production of some ocular mucins, borates have preservative properties, and potassium helps maintain corneal thickness.

Lacrimal fluid is isotonic with blood, with an isotonicity value corresponding to that of a 0.9% sodium chloride solution. Ideally, topical ophthalmic solutions should have this tonicity value (natural tears have an osmotic pressure of ~290–305 mOsm/L). However, the eye can tolerate tonicity values ranging from 0.6 to 2% sodium chloride solution without marked discomfort to the patient.

In terms of osmolarity, artificial tears can be isotonic or hypotonic. Because the tonicity of tears increases in patients with DED, the use of hypotonic solutions is considered an additional benefit in the formulations, although any effects of hypotonic solutions are very short-lived. The clinical utility of this approach is in doubt.

The surface tension of the ophthalmic solution must be close to the natural tears. Proteins or lubricants can be included in formulations to improve the extensibility of the lipid layer over the aqueous mucin–gel. For example, inclusion of proteins resembling the lipid-binding lipocalin may provide stability to the tear film. Additional lubricants such as Dextran 70 and povidone or polyvinyl alcohol (water-soluble synthetic polymers with excellent film-forming properties) can be included to help spread the formulation on the ocular surface. Attention to naturally occurring expression of surface agents promoting lubricity, such as occur in the joints, has been lacking. A protein, lubricin, has been found to be expressed on the ocular surface and may represent a promising approach to mitigating the deleterious effects of frictional damage to the ocular surface (Sullivan BD, personal communication).

Antimicrobial properties can be provided by the addition of proteins such as lysozyme, lactoferrin, and cationic peptides (defensins). Peptides belonging to the defensin family have been reported to take part in wound healing.

Growth factors, neuropeptides, and other substances similar to albumin, transferrin, immunoglobulin A (IgA), immunoglobulin M (IgM9), and immunoglobulin G (IgG) could be also present.

Despite the advantages of including proteins in formulations for dry eye treatment, their poor stability makes it difficult to develop ophthalmic products including these components.

A disaccharide, trehalose, has been shown to prevent epithelial cell desiccation. This agent has demonstrated this ability in vitro and has also shown efficacy in treating moderate-to-severe DED in humans compared with hyaluronan- or cellulose-based eye drops and in a mouse dry eye model. Mannitol (polyol) or glucose (monosaccharide) can be used in artificial tears instead of sodium chloride or other salts.

Supplementation with oral antioxidants has already been demonstrated to improve tear stability. Addition of antioxidants such as ascorbate derivatives, lactoferrin or vitamin E, and other compounds such as polyphenolic and terpenoid substances in formulations resembling the preocular film could promote an additional benefit on the ocular surface.

Essential polyunsaturated fatty acids of omega-3 and omega-6 series are promising natural anti-inflammatory agents. Their topical application should result in an improvement of DED.

Preservatives

Preservatives are used in many multidose eye drop dispensers to maintain sterility throughout their shelf life. In the special case of dry eye treatments, these agents can increase the severity of a damaged epithelium. Moreover, preservatives are associated with allergic reactions when the ocular surface is hypersensitized by repeated administrations in long-term therapies (Baudouin et al. 2010).

In vitro, in vivo, and clinical data suggest that preservatives can have a detrimental effect in patients with DED. Furthermore, they can provoke an inflammatory response in predisposed patients, with local activation of immune cells. The most frequently used preservative is the benzalkonium chloride, BAK, a quaternary ammonium derivative with fast-acting activity against many microorganisms. However, BAK causes deleterious effects that have been demonstrated in laboratory, experimental, and human clinical trials (e.g. reductions in tear film break-up time, reduced goblet cell densities, increased tear osmolarity, and a greater amount of epithelial cell squamous metaplasia).

Although milder chemical preservatives have shown higher tolerance than BAK, results from antibacterial efficacy and long-term tolerance studies in patients with DED are necessary if they are to be used in artificial tears. Polyquaternarium-1 is a polycationic preservative that induces considerably less toxicity than BAK. A preservation system based on an ionic buffer that contains borate, sorbitol, PG, and zinc has not shown a significant effect on cellular viability and membrane integrity when tested in the conjunctival cell line. Oxidative preservatives such as sodium perborate or stabilized oxychloro complex have been incorporated in some formulations because of their lower corneal toxicity. In any case, care should be taken to avoid the long-term use of preservatives.

Preservative-free solutions avoid the risk of adverse effects and are preferred over preserved formulations. Multidose bottles that distribute their contents through a filter membrane (0.2 µm) are commercially available as well as unit doses. Both manufactured products minimize the associated risks of long-term exposure to preservatives for all levels of dry eye conditions. Although both strategies lead to higher product cost to the consumer, the risk of surface damage is significantly reduced.

Pharmaceutical systems

Heterogeneous pharmaceutical systems include lipid and aqueous components in the same formulation. Within this group of pharmaceutical products are emulsions, microemulsions, or liposomes. Emulsions are formed of two non-miscible liquid phases (oily and aqueous) in which the inner phase is dispersed in the external phase. Depending on the external phase of the emulsion, they are named as oil-in-water (O/W) if the external phase is an aqueous solvent or water-in-oil (W/O) for lipophilic external phases. An oil-in-water emulsion based on castor oil (ricinoleic acid) is currently employed as a vehicle for cyclosporin A. The formula has been slightly modified as an over-the-counter product and has been shown to reduce tear evaporation after one dose in healthy eyes as well as increasing the lipid layer in healthy and dry eyes for 8 hours after one dose.

Cationic emulsions have been also developed. Once administered, the droplets of the positively charged emulsion establish an electrostatic attraction with the eye mucus of the cornea and conjunctiva. The oily components of this heterogeneous dispersion are mineral oils.

Microemulsions are clear and form spontaneously upon mixing of components. The droplet size of microemulsions is lower than that of emulsions (20–200 nm compared with 0.1–100.0 μm for emulsions). Notwithstanding the advantages of microemulsions over emulsions, the use of microemulsions for DED is limited because they need a surfactant and cosurfactant in a high concentration to be formulated. In cases of ophthalmic formulations, PG and PEG are commonly employed as cosurfactants. New components are under development to solve the use of a cosurfactant. This is the case of a cross-linked copolymer of acrylic acid and alkyl acrylate that contains both hydrophobic and hydrophilic components within the molecule, which is being used to form stable oil-in-water emulsions with no levels of cosurfactants. The hydrophobic part of the polymer adsorbs at the oil phase and the hydrophilic portion swells in the water forming a gel network around the oil droplets, providing a high stability of the heterogeneous system.

Liposomes are vesicles that contain an aqueous core surrounded by lipophilic bilayers composed mainly of phospholipids. They can incorporate aqueous-soluble and lipophilic active substances. Depending on the number of layers, they are known as SUV (small unilamellar vesicles: 10–100 nm), LUV (large unilamellar vesicles: 100–300 nm), or MUV (multilaminar vesicles: 0.5–10.0 μm). Depending on the charge of the phospholipids, vesicles can be positive, negative, or neutral. For ophthalmic purposes, liposomes have been prepared from positively-charged phospholipids, slightly negative, or neutral liposomes. They can be prepared from phosphatidylcholine or other phospholipids. Addition of antioxidants (e.g. vitamin C or vitamin E) to liposomes is a technological tool to circumvent the oxidative degradation of phospholipids. A formulation based on liposomes has been developed to resemble the preocular tear film. Liposomes are dispersed in a solution of a bioadhesive polymer (hyaluronic acid or CMC) and trehalose (Molina-Martínez et al. 2007). These systems allow the incorporation of lipophilic and aqueous-soluble drugs. A liposome lid spray containing liposomes that are sprayed onto the closed eyelid surfaces instead of directly into the open eye is currently in the market.

Sometimes lipids can be dispersed directly in viscous polymeric solutions. This is the case of medium-chain triglycerides contained in a gel of polyacrylic acid (carbomer 980) that are presented in drops and gels. New formulations (Niosomes) are being developed with polymers other than phospholipids. As they are chemically more stable than phospholipids, they could be useful in the near future.

CALCINEURIN INHIBITORS

The efficacy of cyclosporin as an anti-inflammatory agent for DED is proven and the absence in Europe of a commercial formulation, Novagali (NOVA22007), Alcon (AL38583), Sirion/Alcon (ST603-007 (Zyclorin), Zymedis, has led several teams to try to develop new products for global commercialization, improving its tolerance and pharmacokinetic (Di Tommaso et al. 2012).

Moreover, Allergan is developing new formulations with its cyclosporine 0.005%.

Another calcineurin inhibitor, tacrolimus, has also been used for treating DED. In a recent study, topical 0.03% tacrolimus eye drops successfully improved tear stability and ocular surface status in patients with DED (Moscovici et al. 2012).

A study evaluating the efficacy and safety of two doses of pimecrolimus (0.3% and 1.0%) ophthalmic suspension in a moderate-to-severe population of patients with DED is ongoing (clinicaltrials.gov).

The safety and tolerability of LX214 ophthalmic solution (voclosporin) are being determined in healthy volunteers and in patients with DED in a phase 1 study (clinicaltrials.gov).

STEROIDS AND NON-STEROIDAL ANTI-INFLAMMATORY DRUGS

Ocular iontophoresis of EGP-437 (dexamethasone phosphate 40 mg/mL) (Eyegate Pharmaceuticals) has demonstrated statistically and clinically significant improvements in signs and symptoms of DED within a controlled adverse environment model (Patane et al. 2011).

Rimexolone (AL-2178) and loteprednol etabonate 0.5%, two soft steroids, are being studied in DED (clinicaltrials.gov).

Mapracorat (BOL-303242-X), a novel selective glucocorticoid receptor agonist (SEGRA), is being evaluated in a phase 2 study to identify the concentration and daily dosing frequency of mapracorat ophthalmic suspension in treating DED (clinicaltrials.gov).

Non-steroidal anti-inflammatory drugs are also being tested, and ISV-101 (Bromfenac In DuraSite Ophthalmic Solution) is being evaluated in volunteers with DED (clinicaltrials.gov).

OTHER ANTI-INFLAMMATORY DRUGS

In patients with Sjögren's syndrome, different monoclonal antibodies are being tested (e.g. rituximab and belimumab) in an attempt to improve dry mouth and DED.

Topical ophthalmic tofacitinib (CP-690, 550), a novel Janus kinase inhibitor from Pfizer, has demonstrated a trend for improving both signs and symptoms of DED. In a recent study, 0.001% bid, 0.003% bid, and 0.005% bid and qid doses exhibited a reasonable safety profile and were well tolerated by patients with DED in a phase 1–2 study (Liew et al. 2012).

The binding of lymphocyte function-associated antigen-1 (LFA-1) and intercellular adhesion molecule-1 (ICAM-1) is a critical step in T-cell activation in both normal immune response and inflammation. Thus, LFA-1/ICAM-1 inhibition is a therapeutic target in chronic ocular T-cell-mediated inflammation and has been validated in preclinical models of DED. An LFA-1 antagonist (SAR 1118) ophthalmic solution from SARcode Bioscience has demonstrated improvements in signs and symptoms of DED compared to placebo and appears safe when administered over 3 months in a phase 2 study (Semba et al. 2012).

Cilomilast (AL43546), a second-generation PDE4 inhibitor with anti-inflammatory effects used in chronic obstructive pulmonary disease, is being studied in animal models and patients with DED (Sadrai et al. 2012).

Topical treatment with 5% interleukin-1 receptor antagonist (IL-1Ra) has recently been shown to be effective in ameliorating the clinical signs of DED, as well as in reducing the underlying inflammation in mice. These effects were comparable with those resulting from treatment with topical methylprednisolone (Okanobo et al. 2012).

Tumor necrosis factor (TNF)-α inhibitory single-chain antibody fragment (scFv) ESBA105 is being evaluated as a future treatment in patients with severe DED, experiencing persistent ocular discomfort in a phase 2 study (clinicaltrials.gov).

The A(3) adenosine receptor—A(3)AR—is overexpressed in inflammatory cells, making A(3)AR a potential therapeutic target. Clinical studies in humans demonstrate that A(3)AR agonists induce specific anti-inflammatory activity through a molecular mechanism that entails modulation of the Wnt and the NF-κB signal transduction pathways. At present, A(3)AR agonists are being developed for the treatment of ophthalmic diseases such as DED. A dosage of 1 mg CF101—an A(3) adenosine receptor agonist—orally given bid for 12 weeks has been shown to be effective in improving corneal staining and BUT in patients with moderate-to-severe DED. The drug was well tolerated and safe in a phase 2 trial (Avni et al. 2010, Fishman et al. 2012).

Topical epigallocatechin gallate treatment has been able to reduce the clinical signs and inflammatory changes in a murine DED model by suppressing the inflammatory cytokine expression and infiltration of CD11b+ cells in the cornea (Lee et al. 2011).

The pathogenesis of DED involves the overexpression and overactivity of corneal MMP-9. PES103, a new highly soluble molecule, has been shown to inhibit MMP-9 both in vitro and in vivo. PES103 restored tear production in an animal model of reduced lacrimation, showing no significant corneal toxicity (Mori et al. 2012).

AIN457 (secukinumab), a fully human antibody to IL-17, and ACZ885 (canakinumab), a human monoclonal antibody targeted at interleukin-1β, are both undergoing a phase 2 study. This study is assessing the effects of a single intravenous dose of 10 mg/kg on the signs and symptoms of DED (clinicaltrials.gov).

Resolvin E1 belongs to a new class of endogenous immunoregulating mediators, originally identified as a metabolite of the omega-3 polyunsaturated fatty acid, eicosapentaenoic acid. Based on its proven efficacy in models of chronic inflammation, its methyl ester prodrug, RX-10005, has been investigated in a murine model of DED. Resolvin E1 improved corneal staining and goblet cell density, indicating the potential utility of resolvin analogues in the treatment of DED (de Paiva et al. 2012).

Decrease in lacrimal gland secretary function is related to age-induced DED. Lactoferrin, the main glycoprotein component of tears, has multiple functions, including anti-inflammatory effects and the promotion of cell growth. Oral lactoferrin administration preserves lacrimal gland function by attenuating oxidative damage and suppressing subsequent gland inflammation in aged mice (Kawashima et al. 2012).

SECRETAGOGUES

Cells, when functioning correctly with proper sodium chloride movement, typically serve to moisten the ocular surface. Lacovutide (Moli 1901) is designed to improve the transfer of sodium chloride in and out of cells by stimulating activity in alternative chloride channels. This compensates for the transport deficiency created by DED and moisturizes ocular surface cells.

The eicosanoid 15-(S)-HETE (hydroxyeicosatetraenoic acid) increases secretion of MUC1. Topical 15-(S)-HETE may be effective in treating ocular surface mucin deficiency in DED. Ecabet ophthalmic solution, a widely employed mucoprotective agent, and rebamipide (OPC12759) 2% ophthalmic suspension, an amino acid derivative of 2(1H)-quinolinone, used for mucosal protection, are being studied in subjects with DED (clinicaltrials.gov).

OPC-12759 (Otsuka Pharmaceuticals) stimulates secretion from cultured conjunctival goblet cells by activating the EGF receptor (EGFR) and p44/p42 mitogen-activated protein kinase (MAPK) to cause mucin secretion (Ríos et al. 2008).

DA-6034 (7-carboxymethyloxy-3¢,4¢,5-trimethoxy flavone monohydrate), a new synthetic derivative of eupatilin, increases secretion of mucin-like glycoprotein and some mucin species in the conjunctiva and cornea, and contributes to the preservation of ocular surface integrity (Choi et al. 2009).

HORMONES

The efficacy of topical androgens for the treatment of DED is being tested in clinical trials in the United States and Europe. Androgen deficiency may be a critical etiological factor in the pathogenesis of aqueous-deficient and evaporative DED during menopause, aging, and certain autoimmune diseases. The use of androgen eye drops may correct the hormonal deficiency and thus treat DED. Meibomian glands are an androgen target organ. Androgens appear to regulate meibomian gland function, improve the quality and/or quantity of lipids produced by this tissue, and promote the formation of the tear film's lipid layer. Nevertheless, Allergan and Argentis—ARG101, 102, and 103 (testosterone/progesterone)—results have not reached the expected levels. One study is assessing the safety and efficacy of testosterone 0.03% ophthalmic solution for the treatment of meibomian gland dysfunction (MGD) (clinicaltrials.gov).

OCULAR SURFACE HEALING PROMOTERS

Thymosin beta 4 (Tβ4) is a synthetic copy of the naturally occurring 43-amino acid peptide found in a variety of tissues. Tβ4 promotes and accelerates wound repair. Two recent preclinical evaluations have demonstrated that Tβ4 promotes corneal ocular surface defect healing in animal models of DED. RGN-259 (Tβ4 ophthalmic solution) mechanism of action offers potential to be a product in patients with DED. A phase 2 trial evaluating the safety and efficacy of 0.1% Tβ4 ophthalmic solution compared to vehicle on the signs and symptoms of DED in the controlled adverse environment model is ongoing (clinicaltrials.gov).

A phase 2 study of KCT-0809 (Ozagrel, an antiplatelet agent working as a thromboxane A2 synthesis inhibitor) (Kissei Pharmaceutical) is ongoing in patients with DED (clinicaltrials.gov).

NGF plays a key role in the modulation of immune reaction, trophic support, healing of ocular surface, corneal sensitivity, and tear film function. These properties of NGF make the neurotrophin a potential therapeutic agent for several corneal diseases (e.g. neurotrophic keratitis, peripheral ulcerative keratopathy, herpes infection, DED, and corneal surgery) (Lambiase et al. 2012).

MIM-D3, a small-molecule NGF peptidomimetic, from Mimetogen Pharmaceuticals, has been studied as a therapeutic agent in rats with scopolamine-induced dry eye model. MIM-D3 (1%) improved the quality and stability of the tear film, and thereby improved healing on the ocular surface in DED (Jain et al. 2011).

ALTERNATIVE THERAPIES

Increased life span is considered to be at least part of the reason for rapid growth in the number of patients with DED because there is a close association between aging and decreased secretary function in the lacrimal gland. Recent advances have led to a new way of thinking about intervention in the aging process. Calorie restriction, antioxidant use, and happiness are believed to retard functional decline in various organs, preventing age-related DED (Tsubota et al. 2010).

Acupuncture, Chinese herbal medicine, and Ayurveda have been proposed to relieve the symptoms of DED and increase watery secretion (Dhiman 2011, Jeon et al. 2010, Luo et al. 2011).

■ MGD treatment

LipiFlow (a new Food and Drug Administration-approved thermodynamic pulsatile treatment) has been demonstrated to be effective in restoring MG function and improving ocular comfort even in patients with obstructive MGD for at least 9 months (Greiner 2012). A new treatment option for obstructive MGD using invasive orifice penetration and intraductal probing has been recently developed (Maskin 2010). High price and pain are obstacles in their wide use.

New studies are investigating the genetics of MGD. Recent work has demonstrated that MGD is accompanied by multiple changes in gene expression in the meibomian gland. The nature of these alterations, including the upregulation of genes encoding small proline-rich proteins and S100 calcium binding proteins, suggests that keratinization plays an important role in the pathogenesis of MGD. In the near future, we will have genetic tests for detecting the risk of developing MGD and DED (Liu et al. 2011).

■ Pain treatment

While many patients with clear evidence of DED are asymptomatic, complaints of ocular irritation are the characteristic clinical presentation. These discomfort symptoms and pain make their life miserable. Pain elimination (analgesia) without producing anesthesia is a new research direction for DED.

Civamide, a TRPV-1 (transient receptor potential vanilloid-1), produces analgesia by decreasing the activity of sensory neurons. It appears to preferentially affect type C neurons by specific binding to a membrane receptor, the TRPV-1 receptor, which is coupled to a cation channel. Unlike local anesthetics that act to block the activity of all sensory neurons, the specificity of Civamide for type C neurons seems to limit its sensory effects to the inhibition of pain transmission, thereby not impairing the sensation of touch, pressure, heat, and vibration. Its use is being studied for postherpetic neuralgia treatment.

SYL1001 (Sylentis, Spain), a form of interference RNA that inhibits the capsaicin receptor TRPV-1, which is expressed on the surface of the eye, is being tested in the form of eye drops for treating and preventing eye discomfort associated with DED, Sjögren's, and other syndromes, and with corneal injuries, with a view to minimizing pain and improving patients' quality of life.

■ CONCLUSIONS

In the very near future, we will see amazing diagnostic and therapeutic innovations for the most frequent ophthalmic disease, DED.

■ REFERENCES

Andrés-Guerrero V, Vicario-de-la-Torre M, Molina-Martínez IT, et al. Comparison of the in vitro tolerance and in vivo efficacy of traditional timolol maleate eye drops versus new formulations with bioadhesive polymers. *Invest Ophthalmol Vis Sci* 2011; **52**:3548–3556.

Argüeso P, Gipson IK. Epithelial mucins of the ocular surface: structure, biosynthesis and function. *Exp Eye Res* 2001; **73**:281–289.

Avni I, Garzozi JJ, Barequet IS, et al. treatment of dry eye syndrome with orally administered cf101: data from a phase 2 clinical trial. *Ophthalmology* 2010; **117**:1287–1293.

Baudouin C, Labbé A, Liang H, et al. Preservatives in eyedrops: the good, the bad and the ugly. *Prog Retin Eye Res* 2010; **29**:312–334.

Choi SM, Seo MJ, Lee YG, et al. Effects of DA-6034, a flavonoid derivative, on mucin-like glycoprotein and ocular surface integrity in a rabbit model. Arzneimittelforschung 2009; **59**:498–503.

Corrales RM, Narayanan S, Fernández I, et al. Ocular mucin gene expression levels as biomarkers for the diagnosis of dry eye syndrome. *Invest Ophthalmol Vis Sci* 2011; **52**:8363–8369.

de Paiva CS, Schwartz CE, Gjörstrup P, Pflugfelder SC. Resolvin E1 (RX-10001) reduces corneal epithelial barrier disruption and protects against goblet cell loss in a murine model of dry eye. *Cornea* 2012. [Epub ahead of print]

Dhiman KS. Shushkakshipaka (dry eye syndrome): a case study. *Int J Ayurveda Res* 2011; **2**:53–55.

Di Tommaso C, Valamanesh F, Miller F, et al. A novel cyclosporin a aqueous formulation for dry eye treatment: in vitro and in vivo evaluation. *Invest Ophthalmol Vis Sci* 2012; **30**:2292–2299.

Fishman P, Bar-Yehuda S, Liang BT, Jacobson KA. Pharmacological and therapeutic effects of A(3) adenosine receptor agonists. *Drug Discov Today* 2012; **17**:359–366.

Greiner JV. A single LipiFlow thermal pulsation system treatment improves meibomian gland function and reduces dry eye symptoms for 9 months. *Curr Eye Res* 2012; **37**:272–278.

Jain P, Li R, Lama T, et al. An NGF mimetic, MIM-D3, stimulates conjunctival cell glycoconjugate secretion and demonstrates therapeutic efficacy in a rat model of dry eye. *Exp Eye Res* 2011; **93**:503–512.

Jeon JH, Shin MS, Lee MS, et al. Acupuncture reduces symptoms of dry eye syndrome: a preliminary observational study. *J Altern Complement Med* 2010; **16**:1291–1294.

Kawashima M, Kawakita T, Inaba T, et al. Dietary lactoferrin alleviates age-related lacrimal gland dysfunction in mice. *PLoS One* 2012; **7**:e33148.

Lambiase A, Micera A, Sacchetti M, et al. Alterations of tear neuromediators in dry eye disease. *Arch Ophthalmol* 2011; **129**:981–986.

Lambiase A, Sacchetti M, Bonini S. Nerve growth factor therapy for corneal disease. *Curr Opin Ophthalmol* 2012. [Epub ahead of print]

Lee HS, Chauhan SK, Okanobo A, Nallasamy N, Dana R. Therapeutic efficacy of topical epigallocatechin gallate in murine dry eye. Cornea 2011; **30**:1465–1472.

Leiske DL, Raju SR, Ketelson HA, et al. The interfacial viscoelastic properties and structures of human and animal meibomian lipids. *Exp Eye Res* 2010; **90**:598–604.

Lemp MA, Bron AJ, Baudouin C, et al. Tear osmolarity in the diagnosis and management of dry eye disease. *Am J Ophthalmol* 2011; **151**:792–798.

Liew SH, Nichols KK, Klamerus KJ, et al. Tofacitinib (CP-690,550), a Janus kinase inhibitor for dry eye disease: results from a phase 1/2 trial. *Ophthalmology* 2012. [Epub ahead of print]

Liu S, Richards SM, Lo K, et al. Changes in gene expression in human meibomian gland dysfunction. *Invest Ophthalmol Vis Sci.* 2011. [Epub ahead of print]

Luo H, Han M, Liu JP. Systematic review and meta-analysis of randomized controlled trials of Chinese herbal medicine in the treatment of Sjogren's syndrome. *Zhong Xi Yi Jie He Xue Bao* 2011; **9**:257–274.

Maskin SL. Intraductal meibomian gland probing relieves symptoms of obstructive meibomian gland dysfunction. *Cornea* 2010; **29**:1145–1152.

Molina-Martínez IT, De la Torre V, Benitez del Castillo JM, et al. Formulation of liposomal vesicles in aqueous solution with tear film characteristics. ES2006/000208 (patent), 2007.

Mori M, De Lorenzo E, Torre E, et al. A highly soluble mmp-9 inhibitor for potential treatment of dry eye syndrome. *Basic Clin Pharmacol Toxicol* 2012. doi: 10.1111/j.1742-7843.2012.00896.x. [Epub ahead of print]

Moscovici BK, Holzchuh R, Chiacchio BB, et al. Clinical treatment of dry eye using 0.03% tacrolimus eye drops. *Cornea* 2012. [Epub ahead of print]

Okanobo A, Chauhan SK, Dastjerdi MH, Kodati S, Dana R. Efficacy of topical blockade of interleukin-1 in experimental dry eye disease. *Am J Ophthalmol* 2012. [Epub ahead of print]

Patane MA, Cohen A, From S, et al. Ocular iontophoresis of EGP-437 (dexamethasone phosphate) in dry eye patients: results of a randomized clinical trial. *Clin Ophthalmol* 2011; **5**:633–643.

Ríos JD, Shatos MA, Urashima H, Dartt DA. Effect of OPC-12759 on EGF receptor activation, p44/p42 MAPK activity, and secretion in conjunctival goblet cells. *Exp Eye Res* 2008; **86**:629–636.

Sadrai Z, Stevenson W, Okanobo A, et al. PDE4 inhibition suppresses IL17-associated immunity in dry eye disease. *Invest Ophthalmol Vis Sci* 2012. [Epub ahead of print]

Semba CP, Torkildsen GL, Lonsdale JD, et al. A phase 2 randomized, double-masked, placebo-controlled study of a novel integrin antagonist (SAR 1118) for the treatment of dry eye. *Am J Ophthalmol* 2012. [Epub ahead of print]

Soria J, Duran JA, Etxebarria J, et al. Tear proteome and protein network analyses reveal a novel pentamarker panel for tear film characterization in dry eye and meibomian gland dysfunction. *J Proteomics* 2013; **78**: 94–112.

Sullivan BD, Whitmer D, Nichols KK, et al. An objective approach to dry eye severity. *Invest Ophthalmol Vis Sci* 2010; **51**:6125–6130.

Sullivan DA, Hammitt KM, Schaumberg DA, et al. Report of the TFOS/ARVO symposium on global treatments for dry eye disease: an unmet need. *Ocul Surf* 2012a; **10**:108–116.

Sullivan BD, Crews LA, Sönmez B, et al. Clinical utility of objective tests for dry eye disease: variability over time and implications for clinical trials and disease management. *Cornea* 2012b. [Epub ahead of print]

Suzuki M, Massingale ML, Ye F, et al. Tear osmolarity as a biomarker for dry eye disease severity. *Invest Ophthalmol Vis Sci* 2010; **51**:4557–4561.

Tiffany JM. The normal tear film. *Dev Ophthalmol* 2008; **41**:1–20.

Tsubota K, Kawashima M, Inaba T, et al. The era of antiaging ophthalmology comes of age: antiaging approach for dry eye treatment. *Ophthalmic Res* 2010; **44**:146–154.

Zhou L, Zhao SZ, Koh SK, et al. In-depth analysis of the human tear proteome. *J Proteomics* 2012. [Epub ahead of print]

Appendix: Diagnostic algorithms for ocular surface disease

1 OCULAR SURFACE DISORDERS (OSD)

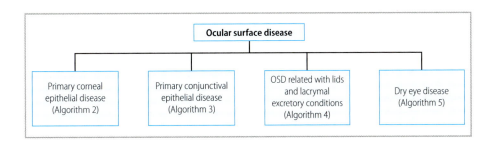

2 DIAGNOSTIC ALGORITHM FOR PRIMARY CORNEAL EPITHELIAL DISEASE

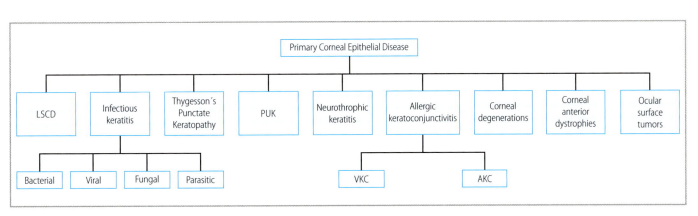

AKC, atopic keratoconjunctivitis; LSCD, limbal stem cell deficiency; PUK, peripheral ulcerative keratitis; VKC, vernal keratoconjunctivitis.

3   DIAGNOSTIC ALGORITHM PRIMARY CONJUNCTIVAL EPITHELIAL DISEASE

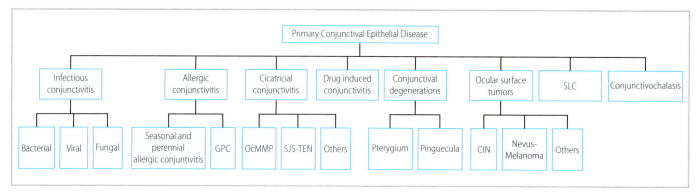

CIN, conjunctival intraepithelial neoplasia; OcMMP, ocular mucous membrane pemphigoid; SJS-TEN, Stevens–Johnson syndrome - toxic epidermal necrolysis; SLC, superior limbal conjunctivitis.

4   DIAGNOSTIC ALGORITHM FOR OSD RELATED WITH LIDS AND LACRYMAL EXCRETORY CONDITIONS

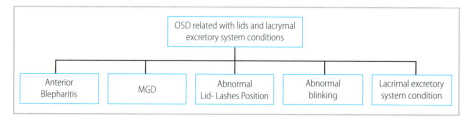

MGD, meibomian gland dysfunction.

5   DIAGNOSTIC ALGORITHM FOR DRY EYE DISEASE

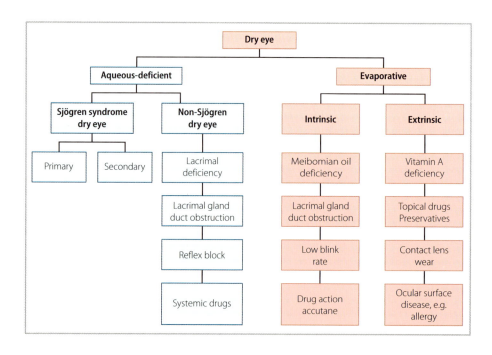

Index

Note: Page numbers in **bold** or *italic* refer to tables or figures respectively.